New Frontiers in Drug Design and Discovery

New Frontiers in Drug Design and Discovery

Editor: Sam Lehmann

FOSTER ACADEMICS
www.fosteracademics.com

www.fosteracademics.com

FOSTER ACADEMICS

Cataloging-in-Publication Data

New frontiers in drug design and discovery / edited by Sam Lehmann.
p. cm.
Includes bibliographical references and index.
ISBN 978-1-64646-636-8
1. Drugs--Design. 2. Drug development. 3. Pharmaceutical chemistry. 4. Pharmacology. I. Lehmann, Sam.
RS420 .N49 2023
615.19--dc23

Foster Academics,
118-35 Queens Blvd., Suite 400,
Forest Hills, NY 11375, USA

ISBN 978-1-64646-636-8 (Hardback)

Contents

Preface

Drug discovery refers to the process of finding potential new therapeutic entities by using a combination of translational, computational, experimental and clinical models. The process of developing new drugs based on an understanding of a biological target is known as drug design. It entails designing molecules with shapes and charge which is complementary to the molecular target with which they bind and interact. Preclinical research using animal and cell-based models, clinical trials on humans, and obtaining regulatory approval to market the drugs are the key steps involved in the development and discovery of new drugs. Modern drug discovery encompasses the identification of screening hits, medicinal chemistry and optimization of those screening hits to improve their selectivity, metabolic stability, affinity, oral bioavailability and efficacy. This book explores all the new frontiers in drug design and discovery. It covers in detail some existent theories and innovative concepts revolving around this domain. The extensive content of this book provides the readers with a thorough understanding of the subject.

The researches compiled throughout the book are authentic and of high quality, combining several disciplines and from very diverse regions from around the world. Drawing on the contributions of many researchers from diverse countries, the book's objective is to provide the readers with the latest achievements in the area of research. This book will surely be a source of knowledge to all interested and researching the field.

In the end, I would like to express my deep sense of gratitude to all the authors for meeting the set deadlines in completing and submitting their research chapters. I would also like to thank the publisher for the support offered to us throughout the course of the book. Finally, I extend my sincere thanks to my family for being a constant source of inspiration and encouragement.

Editor

1

Multi-Target Approach for Drug Discovery against Schizophrenia

Magda Kondej [1], Piotr Stępnicki [1] and Agnieszka A. Kaczor [1,2,*]

1 Department of Synthesis and Chemical Technology of Pharmaceutical Substances, Faculty of Pharmacy with Division of Medical Analytics, Medical University of Lublin, 4A Chodźki St., Lublin PL-20093, Poland; magda.kondej@onet.pl (M.K.); piotr.stepnicki93@gmail.com (P.S.)

2 School of Pharmacy, University of Eastern Finland, Yliopistonranta 1, P.O. Box 1627, Kuopio FI-70211, Finland

* Correspondence: agnieszka.kaczor@umlub.pl

Abstract: Polypharmacology is nowadays considered an increasingly crucial aspect in discovering new drugs as a number of original single-target drugs have been performing far behind expectations during the last ten years. In this scenario, multi-target drugs are a promising approach against polygenic diseases with complex pathomechanisms such as schizophrenia. Indeed, second generation or atypical antipsychotics target a number of aminergic G protein-coupled receptors (GPCRs) simultaneously. Novel strategies in drug design and discovery against schizophrenia focus on targets beyond the dopaminergic hypothesis of the disease and even beyond the monoamine GPCRs. In particular these approaches concern proteins involved in glutamatergic and cholinergic neurotransmission, challenging the concept of antipsychotic activity without dopamine D_2 receptor involvement. Potentially interesting compounds include ligands interacting with glycine modulatory binding pocket on *N*-methyl-D-aspartate (NMDA) receptors, positive allosteric modulators of α-Amino-3-hydroxy-5-methyl-4-isoxazolepropionic acid (AMPA) receptors, positive allosteric modulators of metabotropic glutamatergic receptors, agonists and positive allosteric modulators of α7 nicotinic receptors, as well as muscarinic receptor agonists. In this review we discuss classical and novel drug targets for schizophrenia, cover benefits and limitations of current strategies to design multi-target drugs and show examples of multi-target ligands as antipsychotics, including marketed drugs, substances in clinical trials, and other investigational compounds.

Keywords: antipsychotics; drug design; multi-target drugs; polypharmacology; schizophrenia

---

1. Introduction

Schizophrenia is a severe mental illness, affecting up to 1% of the population, with major public health implications. The causes of schizophrenia might be genetic or environmental or both but the complex pathomechanism of this disease is not sufficiently understood. The clinical picture of schizophrenia involves three groups of symptoms, i.e., positive, such as hallucinations, delusions and other thought disorders, negative, including social withdrawal, apathy and anhedonia, and cognitive deficits like memory and learning impairments or attention deficiencies [1]. It is generally agreed that the symptoms of schizophrenia result from disturbances in neurotransmission involving a significant number of receptors and enzymes, mainly within the dopaminergic, glutamatergic, serotoninergic, and adrenergic systems. In this regard, the dopaminergic hypothesis is still the main concept of the disease and all marketed antipsychotics target dopamine D_2 receptor. The dopaminergic hypothesis of schizophrenia evolved from the simple idea of excessive dopamine through the hypothesis combining prefrontal hypodopaminergia and striatal hyperdopaminergia and then to the current aberrant salience hypothesis [2]. However, novel findings in the field of neuroscience link schizophrenia with factors beyond the dopaminergic hypothesis and emphasize in particular the role of glutamatergic system in the development of the disease [3].

In order to treat efficiently complex neuropsychiatric diseases such as schizophrenia it is necessary to go beyond the "magic bullet" concept. This approach in drug discovery was based on the assumption that single-target drugs are safer as they have fewer side effects due to their selectivity. It turned out, however, that this is only true for single-gene diseases and the number of original single-target drugs were performing far behind expectations in the last ten years. Thus, "one-drug-one-target" paradigm has been gradually replaced by the concept of multi-target drugs (MTDs), sometimes termed "magic shotgun". From the historical perspective, MTDs, in contrast to clean single-target drugs, were sometimes referred to as dirty or promiscuous drugs. In the case of diseases with complex pathomechanisms, such as neuropsychiatric diseases or cancer, single-targets medications have been demonstrated to a great extent a failure. Most potent antipsychotics, in particular second generation or atypical antipsychotics, target simultaneously a number of aminergic G protein-coupled receptors (GPCRs). Clozapine, which is used to treat drug-resistant schizophrenia, has nanomolar affinity to several aminergic GPCRs.

In this scenario drug design and discovery today has moved from the molecular and cellular level to the systems-biology-oriented level [4] to reflect subtle events occurring on the biological networks which lead to the disease [5]. Network pharmacology involves important aspects such as connectivity, redundancy and pleiotropy of biological networks [6] which clearly shows that most drug interact with more than one target. MTDs have a number of advantages over single-target drugs, including improved efficacy due to synergistic or additive effects, better distribution in the target tissue, accelerated therapeutic efficacy in terms of clinical onset and achievement of full effect, predictable pharmacokinetic profile and fewer drug-drug interactions, lower risk of toxicity, improved patient compliance and tolerance and lower risk of target-based drug resistance due to modulation of a few targets [7]. However, it is not easy to design potent MTDs and problems arise starting from a proper target selection through affinity balancing to avoiding affinity to related off-targets.

In this review we present classical and novel drug targets for the treatment of schizophrenia, discuss benefits and limitations of MTDs and their design, as well as present multi-target antipsychotics including marketed compounds, compounds in clinical studies, and other investigational compounds. The literature search for this review was mainly based on searching PubMed database with the search terms: schizophrenia, schizophrenia drug targets, antipsychotics, multi-target antipsychotics, multi-target ligands, multi-target drugs with the focus on the references from the last five years, in particular regarding novel investigational compounds.

2. Drug Targets for the Treatment of Schizophrenia

2.1. Dopamine and Serotonin Receptors

Most of currently available antipsychotic drugs (excluding third generation drugs) act by blocking dopamine receptors in central nervous system, as seen in Table 1. This is the classical way to treat schizophrenia. The original dopamine hypothesis of schizophrenia was proposed by Carlsson (awarded a Nobel Prize in 2000) on the basis of indirect pharmacological evidence in humans and experimental animals. In humans, amphetamine causes the release of dopamine in the brain and can produce a behavioral syndrome that resembles an acute schizophrenic episode. Hallucinations are also a side effect of levodopa and dopamine agonists used in Parkinson's disease. In animals, dopamine release causes a specific pattern of stereotyped behavior that is reminiscent of the repetitive behaviors sometimes observed in patients suffering from schizophrenia. Potent D_2 receptor agonists, such as bromocriptine, lead to similar effects in animals, and these drugs, like amphetamine, aggravate the symptoms of schizophrenic patients. Moreover, dopamine antagonists and drugs blocking neuronal dopamine storage (e.g., reserpine) are effective in controlling the positive symptoms of schizophrenia and in preventing amphetamine-induced behavioral changes [8].

It is now thought that positive symptoms are the result of overactivity in the mesolimbic dopaminergic pathway (the neuronal projection from the ventral tegmental area (VTA) to the nucleus accumbens, amygdala and hippocampus) activating D_2 receptors, whereas negative symptoms may result from a lowered activity in the mesocortical dopaminergic pathway (the projection from the VTA to areas of the prefrontal cortex) where D_1 receptors predominate. Other dopaminergic pathways in the central nervous system (i.e., nigrostriatal and tuberoinfundibular) seem to function normally in schizophrenia. Thus, in terms of treatment it would be desirable to inhibit dopaminergic transmission in the limbic system but enhance this transmission in the area of prefrontal cortex [9].

Table 1. Potential clinical benefits and side effects related to the mechanisms of action of antipsychotics [10–12].

Mechanism of Action	Clinical Efficacy	Possible Side Effects
D_2 antagonism	↓Positive symptoms	Extrapyramidal symptoms (EPS) ↓Negative symptoms ↑Cognitive symptoms ↑Drowsiness
D_2 partial agonism	↓Positive symptoms ↓Negative symptoms ↓Cognitive symptoms	Little or no EPS Behavioral activation
D_3 antagonism		↑Endocrine dysfunction ↑Weight gain ↑Sexual dysfunction
5-HT_{2A} antagonism	↓Negative symptoms	↓EPS ↓Hyperprolactinemia
5-HT_{1A} partial agonism	↓Negative symptoms ↓Cognitive symptoms ↓Anxiety symptoms ↓Depressive symptoms	↓EPS ↓Hyperprolactinemia
5-HT_{2C} antagonism		↑Weight gain ↑Appetite
M_1 antagonism	↓EPS	↑Anticholinergic symptoms, e.g., dry mouth, constipation, tachycardia ↑Drowsiness ↑Cognitive impairment
M_1 agonism	↓Psychotic symptoms ↓Cognitive symptoms	
M_3 antagonism		↑Type 2 diabetes mellitus ↑Hyperglycemic hyperosmolar syndrome ↑Diabetic ketoacidosis
H_1 antagonism		↑Weight gain ↑Drowsiness ↑Hypotension
α_1-antagonism		↑Dizziness ↑Drowsiness ↑Tachycardia ↓Blood pressure ↑Orthostatic hypotension
α_2-antagonism	↓Depressive symptoms	↑Anxiety ↑Tachycardia ↑Tremor ↑Dilated pupils ↑Sweating
β-antagonism		↑Orthostatic hypotension ↑Sedation ↑Sexual dysfunction
Glutamate modulation	↓Positive symptoms ↓Negative symptoms ↓Cognitive symptoms ↓Illness progression	

Legend: ↓ Decreasing ↑ Increasing.

Besides antagonism to the dopamine D_2 receptor, majority of antipsychotic drugs, especially those classified as second generation antipsychotics also block a wide range of other receptors, such as other dopamine receptors (D_1, D_3 or D_4), serotonin (especially 5-HT_{2A} and 5-HT_{2C}), histamine (especially H_1) and α_1-adrenergic. Interaction of antipsychotics with those receptors is associated mainly with occurrence of side effects, such as sedation and drowsiness (H_1 receptors), weight gain (H_1 and 5-HT_{2C}), sexual dysfunction (5-HT_2), or orthostatic hypotension (α_1-adrenergic receptors). On the other hand, there are also hypotheses that antagonism to serotonin 5-HT_{2A} receptor may have beneficial effects when it comes to occurrence of extrapyramidal side effects, as well as to reducing negative and cognitive symptoms of schizophrenia. Basis of schizophrenia is still poorly understood and there are several hypotheses, which involve different neurotransmitters and receptors and try to explain their role in the pathogenesis of the disorder [12].

The serotonin hypothesis of schizophrenia is based on the studies of interactions between the hallucinogenic drug, LSD, and serotonin. Observations of the antipsychotic effects of drugs which are serotonin and dopamine antagonists (e.g., risperidone, clozapine) have resulted in the increased interest in serotonin receptors as a possible target for drugs used in the treatment of schizophrenia.

There are evidences that the efficacy and tolerability of the atypical antipsychotic drugs, such as clozapine, olanzapine, quetiapine, risperidone, and ziprasidone in the treatment of schizophrenia may result, in part, from their interaction with various serotonin receptors, in particular 5-HT_{2A} and 5-HT_{1A} receptors, what is the reason of growing interest in the role, which serotonin plays in the mechanism of action of antipsychotics. The antagonism to 5-HT_{2A} receptors, which is relatively potent, is connected with weaker antagonistic properties to dopamine D_2 receptors and is the only common pharmacologic feature of atypical antipsychotic drugs. The subtypes of serotonin 5-HT receptors, that are involved in the pharmacological action of second generation antipsychotics, such as clozapine, or that may potentially serve as targets for better tolerated and more effective new antipsychotic agents, include: 5-HT_{1A}, 5-HT_{2A}, 5-HT_{2C}, 5-HT_3, 5-HT_6, and 5-HT_7 receptors [13].

The distribution of serotonin 5-HT_{2A} receptor in the central nervous system is wide, but the highest concentrations occur in the cortex. 5-HT_{2A} as well as 5-HT_{1A} receptors are located on the neurons that play significant role in schizophrenia. Those are cortical and hippocampal pyramidal glutamatergic neurons and γ-aminobutyric acid (GABA) interneurons. Serotonin 5-HT_{2A} receptors localized on GABAergic interneurons stimulate the release of γ-aminobutyric acid and in that way play an important role in the regulation of the neuronal inhibition. 5-HT_{2A} receptors are distributed also in the substantia nigra and ventral tegmentum from which arise the nigrostriatal and mesocorticolimbic dopaminergic neurons. 5-HT_{2A} receptors modulate the activity of dopaminergic neurons. Antipsychotics that act by blocking serotonin 5-HT_{2A} receptor (e.g., clozapine, risperidone) lead to the increased release of dopamine in the striatum by decreasing the inhibitory effect of serotonin, what manifests clinically in reducing extrapyramidal effects. It is also suggested that combined effects of antagonism at dopamine D_2 and serotonin 5-HT_{2A} receptors in the mesolimbic circuit counteract the excessive dopamine transmission, which leads to occurrence of positive symptoms of schizophrenia. Moreover, improvement of the negative symptoms is associated with antagonism at 5-HT_{2A} receptor, due to enhanced release of both dopamine and glutamate in the mesocortical pathway [9,13].

The behavioral evidence of interactions between serotonin 5-HT_{2A} receptor and dopamine rests on the effect of 5-HT_{2A} receptor antagonists on locomotor activity stimulated by amphetamine. Namely, giving low doses of amphetamine to rodents results in producing in them locomotor hyperactivity, which is mediated by the release of dopamine from the dopaminergic neurons in the mesolimbic circuit. This amphetamine stimulated hyperactivity is observed to be inhibited by first and second generation antipsychotic drugs and is thought to be an effect of antagonism to dopamine D_2 receptor, which all of those drugs share as a mechanism of action. However, some observations proved that compounds, such as amperozide, which are antagonists selective to serotonin 5-HT_{2A} receptor and do not exhibit any affinity for dopamine D_2 receptor, also lead to lowering of hyperactivity in mice stimulated by administration of amphetamine [14]. These results support the concept that compounds that are antagonists to 5-HT_{2A} receptor may improve behavioral states associated with excessive activity of dopaminergic neurons and may serve as effective antipsychotic medications.

Typical antipsychotic drugs, beside blocking dopamine D_2 receptors in the mesolimbic circuit, act also antagonistic to D_2 receptors localized in the nigrostriatal pathway, what is thought to result in occurrence of extrapyramidal side effects. Low doses of amphetamine administered to rodents lead to producing exploratory locomotor activity, whereas high doses of amphetamine causes the occurrence of repetitive, stereotyped behaviors, which are similar to those produced by the direct agonist of dopamine D_2 receptor, apomorphine. Those stereotyped behaviors are inhibited by first generation antipsychotics, what suggests that their antagonist properties are the cause of producing extrapyramidal side effects. Contrarily, amperozide and other antagonists of the serotonin 5-HT_{2A} receptor do not reduce repetitive behaviors induced by apomorphine or high doses of amphetamine. These findings suggest that antipsychotic drugs which are antagonists to 5-HT_{2A} receptor do not cause extrapyramidal side effects, in contrast to first generation drugs, which are devoid of activity to serotonin receptors.

The majority of clinical studies of serotonin 5-HT_{2A} receptor antagonists have been carried out using ritanserin, the compound that exhibits antagonist properties to both 5-HT_{2A} and 5-HT_{2C} receptors. Its effectiveness has been studied in monotherapy, as well as an adjunct to existing treatment with antipsychotics. The studies have led to conclusions that ritanserin improves in particular negative symptoms of schizophrenia, which were poorly ameliorated in case of treatment with typical antipsychotic drugs [15].

To sum up, due to ability of antagonists of serotonin 5-HT_{2A} receptor to interfere with elevated activity of dopamine, the antagonism of this receptor is believed to contribute to improvement of both positive and negative symptoms of schizophrenia and to causing less extrapyramidal side effects than older antipsychotics [16].

The 5-HT_{1A} receptor is the subtype of serotonin receptors that is probably the best characterized in terms of functioning. It plays a significant role in modulating the activity of monoaminergic, inter alia dopaminergic, neurons. The functioning of 5-HT_{1A} receptor may be described as antagonistic to the serotonin 5-HT_{2A} receptor, when it comes to both presynaptic and postsynaptic its localization. Activation of serotonin 5-HT_{1A} inhibitory autoreceptors located in the cells of raphe nucleus leads to inhibition of those neurons. In contrast, 5-HT_{2A} receptors while activated in general cause the activation of serotonergic neurons by several mechanisms, which include a direct or indirect inhibition of GABAergic inhibitory interneurons, and a direct mechanism of excitation of other neurons, inter alia glutamatergic neurons. Both postsynaptical 5-HT_{1A} and 5-HT_{2A} receptors are located in the cortex on the pyramidal neurons. Activation of this 5-HT_{1A} receptor results in neuronal inhibition through activation of potassium current, what leads to hyperpolarization. Contrary, 5-HT_{2A} receptor while activated, facilitates neuronal output in the mechanism of activation of phospholipase C. Serotonin 5-HT_{1A} receptors are suggested to be localized also presynaptically on GABA neurons terminals and pre- or postsynaptically on the GABAergic interneurons in the dentate gyrus in the hippocampus. Basing on the opposition between those two serotonin receptors, it is thought that agents acting as 5-HT_{1A} receptor agonists are able to modulate dopaminergic transmission in the central nervous system in a similar way to antagonists to serotonin 5-HT_{2A} receptor. Agonists to 5-HT_{1A} receptor may both induce the dopamine release in the prefrontal cortex and potentiate the inhibiting effect on dopamine release of dopamine D_2 receptor antagonists [17].

In the brains of patients suffering from chronic schizophrenia, the density of serotonin 5-HT_{1A} receptors is increased, what suggests a close correlation between pathogenesis of the disease and serotonin 5-HT_{1A} receptors. These receptors are now considered as preferable target to treat schizophrenia, since there are evidences that stimulation of serotonin 5-HT_{1A} receptors may contribute to decreasing of extrapyramidal side effects induced by antipsychotics [18] and ameliorating affective disorders such as depression or anxiety [19]. Moreover, blockade of 5-HT_{1A} receptors may result in improvement of cognitive symptoms of schizophrenia [20].

It has been proved in different studies that agents which are selective agonists of serotonin 5-HT$_{1A}$ receptor, such as tandospirone or buspirone, reduced extrapyramidal side effects (e.g., bradykinesia, catalepsy) induced by antipsychotics from first generation [21]. Agonists of 5-HT$_{1A}$ receptor are thought to reduce extrapyramidal side effects induced by neuroleptics in the way of stimulating serotonin 5-HT$_{1A}$ receptors localized postsynaptically, since the inactivation of serotonergic neurons by p-chlorophenylalanine had no impact on the actions of 5-HT$_{1A}$ receptor agonists, when it comes to alleviating extrapyramidal side effects [22].

Reducing cognitive symptoms of schizophrenia is another significant role of serotonin 5-HT$_{1A}$ receptors. Cognitive dysfunction belongs to those symptoms of schizophrenia, whose treating with currently available drugs is still not very effective. Some of recently carried clinical studies have proved that the partial agonist properties of tandospirone regarding 5-HT$_{1A}$ receptor relevantly improved the deficits in cognition in schizophrenic patients. Studies carried on animals also showed that 5-HT$_{1A}$ receptor antagonists improved the cognitive deficits induced by antagonists to mACh receptor, such as scopolamine, or antagonists of *N*-methyl-D-aspartate (NMDA) receptor [23]. Although further studies are required, there are findings which suggest that serotonin 5-HT$_{1A}$ receptor antagonists may contribute to managing schizophrenia on account of ameliorating cognitive impairments [24].

Many compounds that bind to serotonin 5-HT$_{2A}$ receptors also exhibit an affinity to the structurally related serotonin 5-HT$_{2C}$ receptor. There are evidences that support the idea of an antipsychotic potential for antagonists of 5-HT$_{2C}$ receptor. One of them concerns meta-chlorophenylpiperazine (mCPP), which act as an agonist of serotonin 5-HT$_{2C}$ receptor [25]. The main action of mCPP in humans may be described as a selective activation of serotonin 5-HT$_{2C}$ receptors [26]. mCPP causes the worsening of positive symptoms in schizophrenic patients but pretreatment with mesulergine, which is an antagonist to 5-HT$_2$ receptor, results in decreased level of psychotic episodes, induced by the drug [27]. It is suspected that 5-HT$_{2C}$ receptor antagonists inhibit dopaminergic activity in mesolimbic and nigrostriatal pathways and thus contribute to reducing symptoms of schizophrenia and alleviating extrapyramidal side effects. Nonetheless, the role of this subtype of serotonin receptor in the pathogenesis of schizophrenia is still poorly understood and requires further studies [28].

Although dopamine and serotonin receptors are classical drug targets for the treatment of schizophrenia, novel drugs acting through these receptors can be developed based on novel signaling mechanisms typical for the family of GPCRs. These include allosteric modulators [29], biased ligands [30], compounds acting on receptor dimers, oligomers and mosaics [31–34] and last but not least intentionally promiscuous multi-target ligands [35].

2.2. *Adrenergic and Histaminergic Receptors*

Noradrenaline has a key role in the pathomechanism of schizophrenia although the specific role of α adrenergic receptors has been not well elucidated yet [36]. It has been hypothesized that interactions of atypical antipsychotics with α-adrenergic receptors contributes to their atypicality [37]. It was shown that antagonism at α_1 adrenergic receptors is beneficial to treat positive symptoms, in particular in acute schizophrenia while antagonism at α_2 adrenergic receptor, characteristic for clozapine and to some extent risperidone might be important to relieve negative symptoms and cognitive impairments [37]. Blockade of α adrenergic receptors may have a stabilizing effect on the dopaminergic neurotransmission in schizophrenia. In contrast, it was also reported that activation of α_{2A} adrenergic receptors in prefrontal cortex may improve cognitive functions [38]. Moreover, adjunctive α_2 adrenergic receptors antagonism increases the antipsychotic activity of risperidone and promotes cortical dopaminergic and glutamatergic, NMDA receptor-mediated neurotransmission [39]. It was also shown that blockade of α_{2C} adrenergic receptors alone or in combination with dopamine D$_2$ receptor blockade could be also beneficial in schizophrenia [38].

The histamine H$_1$ receptor is a classical off-target for antipsychotics as its blockade causes sedation and may be involved in weight gain. Although weight gain and metabolic disorders can also be attributed to blockade of adrenergic or cholinergic receptors, antagonism of histamine H_1 receptors is described as a key reason for second generation antipsychotics-induced obesity [40]. In contrast, the histamine H_3 receptor is an emerging target for novel antipsychotics [41] as selective antagonists or inverse agonists of this histamine receptor subtype are efficient in treatment cognitive deficiencies in schizophrenia [42].

2.3. Muscarinic and Nicotinic Receptors

Muscarinic receptors have a pivotal role in modulating synaptic plasticity in the prefrontal cortex and stimulation of these receptors results in long-term depression at the hippocampo-prefrontal cortex synapse [43]. A growing body of evidence indicates central role of disturbances in cholinergic neurotransmission in schizophrenia [44]. Postmortem studies indicate a reduced number of cholinergic interneurons in the ventral striatum in schizophrenia patients [45]. Furthermore, neuroimaging studies indicated that muscarinic receptors availability was significantly less in schizophrenia patients and positive symptoms of schizophrenia are negatively correlated with muscarinic receptors availability [46]. It should be emphasized that muscarinic receptor antagonists worsen cognitive and negative symptoms in schizophrenia patients and xanomeline, a muscarinic receptor agonist, ameliorates all symptoms in schizophrenia patients and corresponding animal models [43]. Based on these and other findings muscarinic hypothesis of schizophrenia has been suggested [47].

Involvement of nicotinic cholinergic receptors in the pathomechanism of schizophrenia can explain why schizophrenia patients are often heavy smokers [48,49]. It is assumed that smoking relieves particularly negative symptoms of schizophrenia. More and more evidence indicates that activation of α_7 nicotinic receptors [50] by agonists or positive allosteric modulators can be a promising strategy for the treatment of schizophrenia [51,52].

2.4. Metabotropic and Ionotropic Glutamatergic Receptors

Glutamate is one of the main excitatory neurotransmitters in the mammalian central nervous system [53]. Glutamatergic pathways linking to the cortex, the limbic system, and the thalamus regions are crucial in schizophrenia [54,55]. Abnormalities in the glutamatergic neurotransmission may influence synaptic plasticity and cortical microcircuitry, particularly NMDA receptor functioning [56]. NMDA receptors are ligand-gated ion channels, and are pivotal for excitatory neurotransmission, excitotoxicity and plasticity [57,58].

Glutamatergic hypothesis of schizophrenia is based on the observation that antagonists of *N*-methyl-D-aspartate (NMDA) receptors, such as phencyclidine or ketamine produce schizophrenia-like positive, negative, and cognitive symptoms in animal models and healthy individuals [59,60]. Glutamatergic hypothesis of schizophrenia is mainly a concept of hypofunction of NMDA receptors in this disease, however other ionotropic glutamate receptors (α-amino-3-hydroxy-5-methyl-4-isoazolepropionic acid, AMPA and kainate receptors) as well as metabotropic glutamate receptors are also involved.

In therapeutic trials compounds which promote NMDA receptor signaling were found relieve certain symptoms in patients with schizophrenia [61]. Moreover, in postmortem studies abnormalities in glutamatergic receptor density and subunit composition in the prefrontal cortex, thalamus, and temporal lobe were reported [62–64], and these are brain parts with altered stimulation during cognitive actions performed by schizophrenia patients [65]. NMDA receptor hypofunction may result in morphological and structural brain changes leading to the onset of psychosis [66,67]. It was suggested that levels of glutamate decrease with age in healthy people, but it was not found if they are influenced in case of chronic schizophrenia [68].

Antipsychotics may interfere with glutamatergic neurotransmission by influencing the release of glutamate, by modulation glutamatergic receptors, or by changing the density or subunit composition of glutamatergic receptors [55]. It was shown that antipsychotics blocking dopamine D_2 receptor increase the phosphorylation of the NR1 subunit of the NMDA receptor, thus promote its activation and consequent gene expression [69]. In this regard dopamine–glutamate interactions occur intraneuronally and intrasynaptically. There are also findings that certain second generation antipsychotics act on NMDA receptors in a distinct way than the first generation antipsychotics [70].

Abnormalities in glutamatergic neurotransmission constitute a possible drug target for schizophrenia, in particular for the treatment of cognitive impairment and negative symptoms [54,55]. Reports about hypoactivity of NMDA receptors in schizophrenia led to clinical trials with ligands stimulating this receptor [55]. Classical NMDA receptor agonists are not considered here due to excitotoxicity and neuron damage resulting from excessive NMDA receptor stimulation. In this regard, the glycine modulatory binding pocket on the NMDA receptor might be an attractive drug target [71]. Next, positive allosteric modulators of AMPA receptors [72,73] as well as orthosteric ligands and modulators of metabotropic glutamatergic receptors [74], in particular ligands acting on mGluR2/3 receptors [75] might be considered promising potential medications against schizophrenia in agreement with the glutamatergic hypothesis of this disease.

2.5. Other Drug Targets in Schizophrenia

There are also potential drug targets for the treatment of schizophrenia beyond transmembrane receptors. Most important enzymes with implications in schizophrenia include the serine/threonine kinase glycogen synthase kinase-3 (GSK-3) involved in cognitive-related processes such as neurogenesis, synaptic plasticity and neural cell survival [76], cyclic nucleotide (cNT) phosphodiestereases (PDEs)-intracellular enzymes which governs the activity of key second messenger signaling pathways in the brain [77] and acetylcholinesterase for treatment of cognitive impairments [78].

3. Multi-Target Compounds: Strategies of Design, Benefits, and Limitations

As has already been mentioned, during last twenty years most efforts in drug design and discovery followed the paradigm "one disease, one gene, one molecular target, one drug". However, novel findings in the field of systems biology and discoveries of molecular complexity of illnesses considerably moved current drug discovery efforts towards multi-target drugs [79,80]. Such compounds are able to exert numerous pharmacological actions and have emerged as magic shotguns in the treatment of multifactorial diseases in contrast to classical magic bullet approach [81].

3.1. Design of Multi-Target Compounds

Classical approaches to design multi-target ligands involve three different ways of combination of two pharmacophores, leading to a cleavable conjugate where two pharmacophores are connected by a linker (a modern form of combination therapy), a compound with overlapping pharmacophores or a highly integrated multi-target drug, as seen in Figure 1 [5]. Multi-target drugs, in particular those obtained by pharmacophore integration strategy are referred to as "master key compounds" [82,83]. Thus, MTDs are designed broadly as hybrid or conjugated drugs or as chimeric drugs from two or more pharmacophores/drugs having specific pharmacological activities [84].

Morphy and Rankovic [85] described two approaches for designing multi-target drugs: knowledge-based strategies and screening strategies. Knowledge-based techniques are based on available biological data from old drugs or other bioactive compounds, from either literature or proprietary company sources. Other methods include the screening of either diverse or focused compound libraries. Classical diversity based screening is the high-throughput screening (HTS) of large and differentiated compound collections versus one protein, and hits found are then triaged on the basis of activity at the other protein. In focused screening, compounds known to have robust activity at one protein are screened for activity at the other one. Even if only moderate activity is found for the second protein, it can supply a useful baseline for increasing that activity by incorporating structural elements from more potent selective ligands for this target [85].

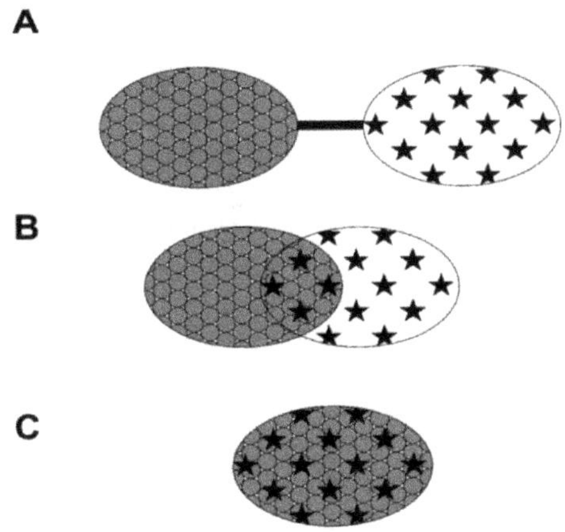

Figure 1. Strategies to design multi-target ligands. (**A**) linking of pharmacophores; (**B**) overlapping of pharmacophores; (**C**) integration of pharmacophores.

Modern in silico approaches can be also used to design multi-target ligands and can be classified into ligand-based and structure-based strategies [4]. Ligand-based target fishing strategies rely either on similarity-based screening or machine learning methods [4]. Moreover, ligand-based pharmacophores can be used. The advantage of this approach is independence from available structural information on the protein. These methods involve 2D or 3D similarity searches. Polyphramacological profiling of the compounds may also be based on three-dimensional structure-activity relationship (3D-QSAR) techniques [7]. Structure-based methods involve molecular docking (e.g., docking-based virtual screening [86] and inverse docking) or structure-based pharmacophores. The advantage of structure-based approaches in comparison to ligand-based approaches is that they do not rely on available activity data [4].

The main principle in designing multi-target compounds is the achievement of superior therapeutic efficacy and safety by targeting multiple players in pathogenic cascade simultaneously [4].

3.2. Advantages and Disadvantages of Multi-Target Ligands

Multifunctional ligands are particularly interesting as their molecules have common parts responsible for activity, and their structure is formed as a result use of pharmacophore fragments. Receiving such hybrid compounds allows not only to improve their activity, but also to positively affect pharmacokinetic parameters, similar to those shown by drugs used in therapy [81].

The main advantages of multi-target-drugs compared to single-target drugs and combination therapy include: (i) reflecting the complex pathomechanism of the disease and better therapeutic efficacy and (ii) better therapeutic safety avoidance of different bioavailabilities, pharmacokinetics, and metabolism of a combination regimen and avoidance of drug–drug interactions [87]. Multi-target mode of action is beneficial to combat drug resistance and development of tolerance and can be also a base of drug repurposing. The disadvantage of MTDs is the difficulty in designing compounds with balanced activity to multiple targets, sometimes resulting in a need to compromise activity at some targets. Moreover, compounds obtained in particular by pharmacophore linkage are often not drug-like due to high molecular mass.

4. Multi-Target Compounds to Treat Schizophrenia

4.1. Marketed Drugs—Second and Third Generation Antipsychotics

The second generation antipsychotics, which are nowadays the treatment of choice in cases of schizophrenia and also bipolar disorder, are essentially multi-target compounds. It should be emphasized, however, that many first generation antipsychotics have a complex pharmacological profile, including haloperidol, fluphenazine and even chlorpromazine, as seen in Table 2 [88].

Table 2. Relative neurotransmitter receptor affinities for first, second and third generation antipsychotics and involved side effects.

Drugs Generation	Examples	Receptors								Potential Side Effect
		D_1	D_2	D_3	D_4	$5\text{-}HT_{2A}$	α_1	H_1	M_1	
First	Chloropromazine	+	++	+++	+	+++	++	++	++	extrapyramidal symptoms such as dyskinesia, dystonias, akathisia, unwanted movements, muscle breakdown, tremors, rigidity and elevated prolactin
	Haloperidol	+	+++	+	+	0	+	0	0	
	Benperidol	0	+++	++		++	+	0	0	
	Fluspirilene	+	+++	+++		+	0	0	0	
	Thioridazine	+	++	++	+	++	++	+	+	
Second	Clozapine	++	+	++	+++	++	+		+++	hypotension, tachycardia, agranulocytosis
	Olanzapine	++	+++	+	++	+++	++	++	++	sedation, weight gain
	Risperidone	+	++	+	+	+++	++	+++	0	orthostatic hypotension, insomnia, restlessness, anxiety, headaches, agitation, extrapyramidal symptoms (EPS), rhinitis, sedation, fatigue, ocular disturbances, dizziness, palpitations, weight gain, diminished sexual desire, erectile and ejaculatory dysfunction, orthostatic dysregulation, reflex tachycardia, gastrointestinal complaints, nausea, rash, galactorrhea and amenorrhea
	Quetiapine	+	++	+++	++	+++	+++	+++	0	drowsiness, dizziness, headache, withdrawal symptoms, increased triglycerides, increased total cholesterol
	Ziprasidone	++	+++	+++	+++	+++	++	+	0	parkinsonism, headaches, rhinitis, orthostatic hypotension, tachykardia
Third	Aripiprazole	0	+++	++	+	+++	+	+	0	hyperglycaemia, headache, extrapyramidal symptoms

+++ = high, ++ = moderate, + = low, 0 = minimal to none.

Clozapine (**1**), Figure 2, is a classic example of a "dirty" drug which can be still considered a "gold standard" atypical antipsychotic due to absence of extrapyramidal syndrome (EPS), superiority in treatment of drug resistant schizophrenia and reducing suicidality [88]. Clozapine exerts severe side effects, in particular potentially life-threatening agranulocytosis, but also weight gain, diabetes, and seizures [89]. Both the effectiveness and side effects of clozapine result from its complex pharmacological profile, involving high affinity to many serotonin, dopamine, muscarinic, adrenergic, and other aminergic receptors, as seen in Figure 3 [90].

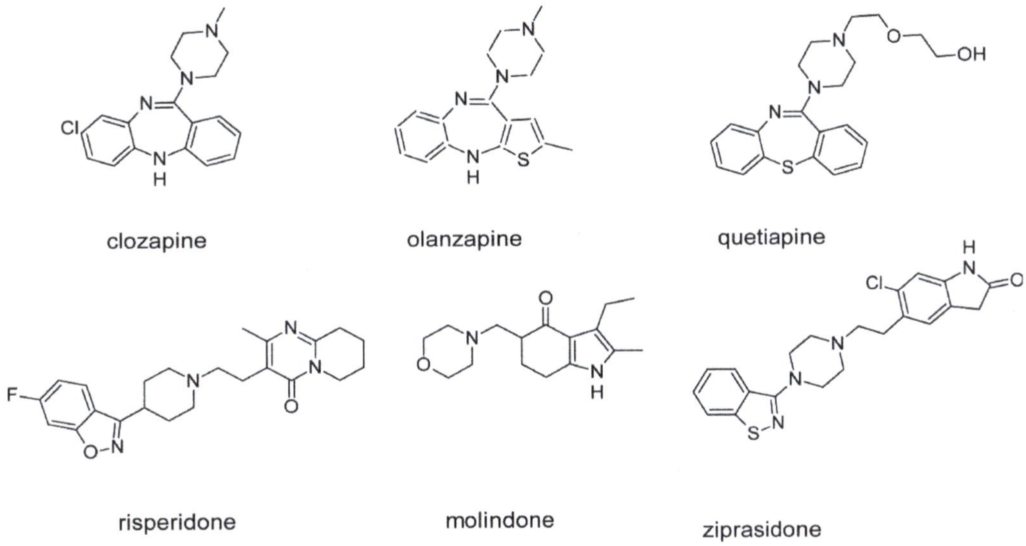

Figure 2. Examples of marketed multi-target second generation antipsychotics [1].

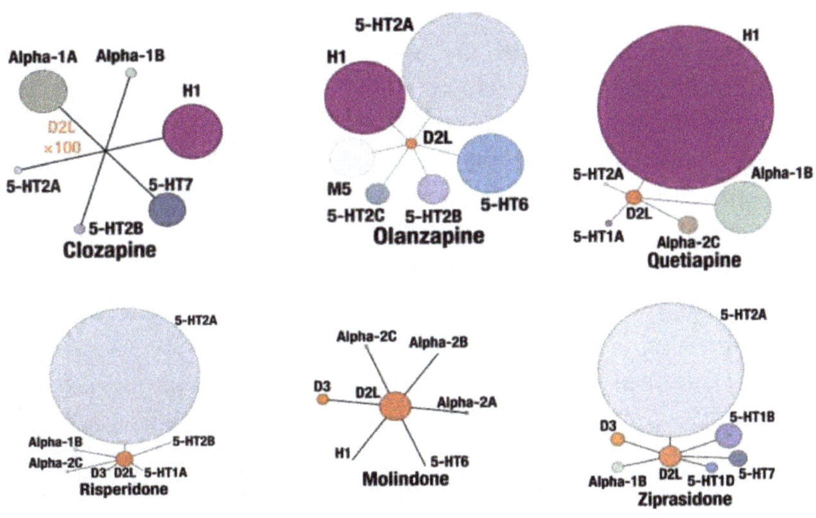

Figure 3. Pharmacological profiles of commonly used second generation antipsychotics, elaborated on the basis of [90] with modifications.

Some problems with side-effects of clozapine were solved with the introduction of another second generation antipsychotic, olanzapine (**2**), Figure 2. Olanzapine does not cause agranulocytosis but still has metabolic side effects leading to possible weight gain [91] which can be associated with histamine H_1 receptor signaling [92] and/or the −759C/T and −697G/C polymorphisms of the 5-HT_{2C} receptor gene [93]. Importantly, the side-effect profile of olanzapine can be considered beneficial, with a low incidence of EPS and little increase in prolactin during acute-phase trials [94]. Multi-receptor binding profile of olanzapine [95] involves a nanomolar affinity for dopaminergic, serotonergic, α_1 adrenergic, and muscarinic receptors, as seen in Figure 3. Olanzapine is also used to treat bipolar disorder.

Similarly, quetiapine (**3**), Figure 2, belongs to atypical antipsychotics, which, besides schizophrenia, are applied to treat bipolar disorder and major depressive disorder. Quetiapine is dopamine D_1, dopamine D_2 and serotonin 5-HT_2 receptor ligand, as seen in Figure 3. Antagonism to α_1 adrenergic and histamine H_1 receptor results in side effects like sedation and orthostatic hypotension. Moreover, there are reports about quetiapine misuse and abuse which can be linked with its high affinity for the H_1 receptor, as antihistamines agents cause rewarding action, compare Figure 3 [96].

Risperidone (**4**), Figure 2 was marketed as the first "non-clozapine" atypical antipsychotic and it is also used to treat the acute manic phase of bipolar disorder. Risperidone is a benzisoxazole derivative with nanomolar affinity for serotonin (5-HT_{2A} and 5-HT_7) and dopamine D_2 receptors (its affinity for D_3 and D_4 receptors is three times lower), Figure 3 with a 5-HT_{2A}/D_2 affinity ratio of about 20 [11]. It also has a strong affinity for adrenergic (α_1 and α_2) receptors, and some affinity for histamine (H_1) receptors [11]. Pharmacological effect of risperidone is mainly a consequence of antagonism at D_2 and 5-HT_{2A} receptors, as seen in Figure 3. Its multi-receptor profile resembles this of olanzapine, however risperidone causes sedation less frequent and orthostatic hypotension more often than olanzapine. There are also reports that this drug can increase the level of prolactin and cause arrhythmia.

Molindone (**5**), seen in Figure 2 is a dihydroindolone neuroleptic with dopamine D_2, D_3 and D_5 receptor antagonist activity and affects mainly dopaminergic neurotransmission in the CNS as seen in Figure 3. It is the second generation antipsychotic with atypical pharmacological profile. Its side effects rarely involve sedation and autonomic side effects but more often extrapyramidal side effects (more frequently than other new antipsychotics, although still less frequently than classical drugs). The application of molindone, in contrast to other atypical antipsychotics, does not usually lead to weight gain. Some patients with poor tolerance or response to other drugs can benefit from the treatment with molindone [97].

An example of modern second generation multi-target drug is ziprasidone (**6**), as shown in Figure 2. This antipsychotic is an optimized hybrid of dopamine receptor ligand (D_2 receptor agonist) and a lipophilic serotonin receptor ligand in which the D_2 agonist activity is transformed to D_2 receptor antagonist activity. It also exhibits desirable D_2/5-HT_2 ratio of 11 comparable to clozapine, as seen in Figure 3, and has lesser propensity of orthostatic hypotension. Moreover, ziprasidone has been reported not to cause significant weight gain and even to enable some weight loss in obese patients [98].

Some new second generation antipsychotics involve iloperidone (**7**), asenapine (**8**) and lurasidone (**9**), shown in Figure 4, however they have not gained popularity in clinical practice yet. Their pharmacological profiles are presented in Figure 5 [90]. From those three drugs lurasidone seems to be most important. Lurasidone has high antagonist activity at serotonin 5-HT_{2A} and 5-HT_7 receptors and weaker antagonism at dopamine D_2 receptor [99]. It has also partial agonist activity at serotonin 5-HT_{1A} receptor, considerable affinity to adrenergic α_{2A} and weaker affinity to muscarinic receptors [99]. Lurasidone is used for treatment of schizophrenia acute bipolar depression. It has low probability of side effects typical for second generation antipsychotics, but higher risk of akathisia in comparison to other atypicals [99].

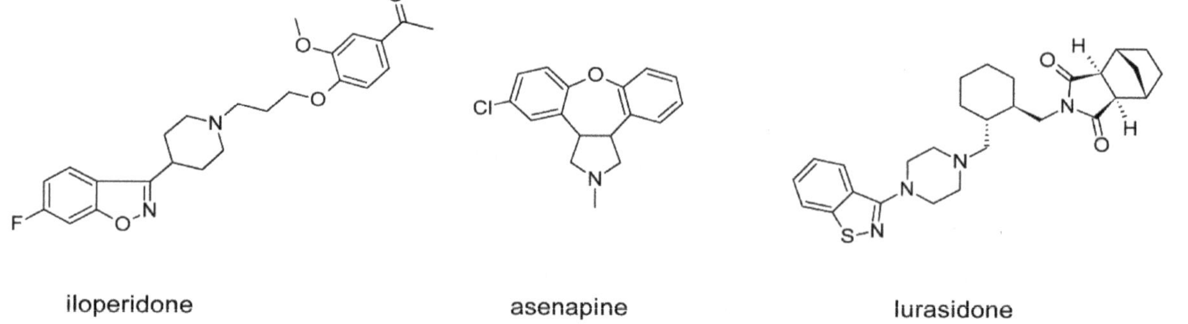

Figure 4. New second generation antipsychotics.

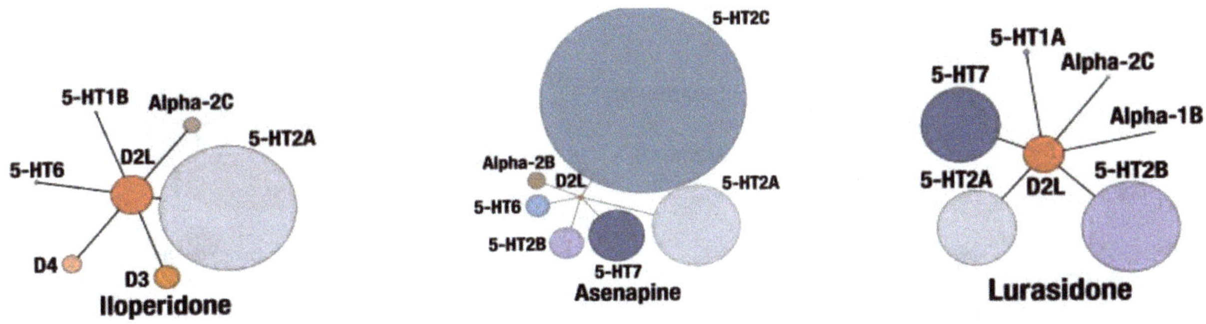

Figure 5. Pharmacological profiles of some new second generation antipsychotics, elaborated on the basis of [90] with modifications.

Third generation antipsychotics include aripiprazole (**10**), brexpiprazole (**11**) and cariprazine (**12**), as seen in Figure 6. The mechanism of action of these drugs is still mainly linked to the dopaminergic neurotransmission, shown in Figure 7, however, not to dopamine receptor antagonism but to partial or biased agonism (functional selectivity) [100,101]. Due to partial agonism properties aripiprazole is termed as "dopamine stabilizer" [102–104]. Aripiprazole was one of the first functionally selective D_2 receptor ligands identified that may stabilize the dopaminergic signaling through D_2 receptor. Although aripiprazole was first described as a partial D_2 receptor agonist, it was later demonstrated that aripiprazole could behave as a full agonist, a partial agonist, or an antagonist at D_2 receptor depending upon the signaling readout and cell type interrogated [105]. Aripiprazole is a partial agonist for inhibition of cyclic adenosine monophosphate (cAMP) accumulation through the D_2 receptor (i.e., $G\alpha$ signaling) [106–108]. In contrast, it has also been reported that aripiprazole is an antagonist in $GTP\gamma S$ binding assays with the D_2 receptor [107,109]. It was also revealed that aripiprazole failed to activate outward potassium currents following activation of the D_2 receptor in MES-23.5 cells, indirectly suggesting that it was inactive or possibly an antagonist for $G\beta\gamma$ signaling through the D_2 receptor [107]. Aripiprazole was also reported to be either an antagonist [110] or a partial agonist [111] for β-arrestin-2 recruitment.

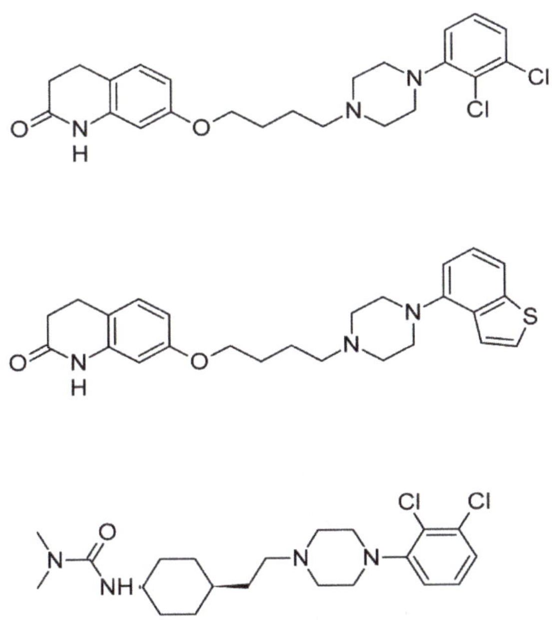

aripiprazole

brexpiprazole

cariprazine

Figure 6. The third generation antipsychotics [1].

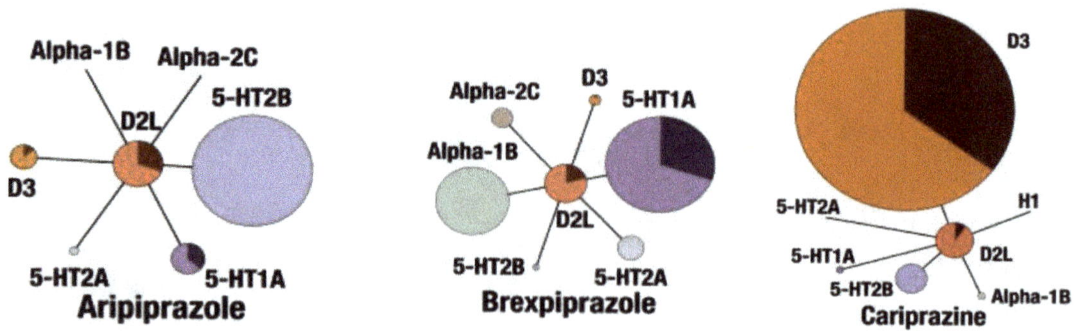

Figure 7. Pharmacological profiles of the third generation antipsychotics, elaborated on the basis of [90] with modifications.

Aripiprazole is also a partial agonist of 5-HT_{1A} and 5-HT_{2A} receptors (much weaker in the latter case) which results in functional antagonism at these receptors, as seen in Figure 7 [90]. In contrast to classical atypical drugs, aripiprazole has higher affinity for dopamine D_2 receptor than for serotonin 5-HT_{2A} receptor. Clinical application of aripiprazole includes also bipolar disorder, major depression, obsessive-compulsive disorder, and autism. Aripiprazole is characterized by efficacy similar to that of both typical and atypical antipsychotic drugs (except olanzapine and amisulpride) [112]. Aripiprazole resulted in considerably lower weight gain and lower changes in glucose and cholesterol levels in comparison to clozapine, risperidone, and olanzapine [112]. Moreover, aripiprazole led to weaker EPS, less use of antiparkinsonian drugs, and akathisia, in comparison to typical antipsychotic drugs and risperidone [112]. Furthermore, aripiprazole is characterized by better tolerability compared to other antipsychotics [113]. Adverse effects of aripiprazole may include agitation, insomnia, anxiety, headache, constipation or nausea [103].

Brexpiprazole was approved by FDA in 2015 and is a partial agonist of dopamine D_2, D_3 and serotonin 5-HT_{1A} receptors, as well as antagonist of 5-HT_{2A}, 5-HT_{2B} and 5-HT_7 receptors, as seen in Figure 7 [114]. Its pharmacological properties are close to those of aripiprazole. In comparison to aripiprazole, brexpiprazole is more potent at 5-HT_{1A} receptors and has less intrinsic activity at D_2 receptors [115]. Brexpiprazole is applied for treatment of schizophrenia and as an adjunct in major depressive disorder. The adverse effects of this drug invole akathisisa, weight gain, infections of upper respiratory tract, somnolence, headache, and nasopharyngitis.

Approval of both cariprazine and brexpiprazole was in 2015. Cariprazine is a new antipsychotic displaying unique pharmacodynamic and pharmacokinetic properties [116]. As aripiprazole and brexpiprazole, cariprazine is the dopamine D_2, D_3 and serotonin 5-HT_{1A} receptors partial agonist, as seen in Figure 7. However, its affinity for dopamine D_3 receptor is approximately ten times higher than for D_2 receptors. It is metabolized to two equipotent metabolites, desmethyl cariprazine and didesmethyl cariprazine, of which didesmethyl cariprazine has a half-life of 1 to 3 weeks [116]. Available reports indicate that cariprazine is efficient in management of cognitive and negative symptoms of schizophrenia. It also seems to have antimanic properties and it has a potential to treat bipolar depression [117]. However, currently it is not possible to evaluate antipsychotic potential of cariprazine in comparison to other antipsychotics. Cariprazine may be associated with adverse effects such as sedation, akathisia, weight gain, nausea, constipation, anxiety, dizziness [117].

The problem with the third generation antipsychotics is that they deteriorate the patient's condition in some patients suffering from schizophrenia. Thus, multi-target second generation antipsychotics are nowadays a gold standard in the schizophrenia treatment, although some patients respond better to the first generation treatment.

4.2. *Other Multi-Target Compounds for the Treatment of Schizophrenia*

Although recently implemented antipsychotics (e.g., cariprazine and brexpiprazole) are the third generation drugs, attempts are still made to design new multi-target ligands, which can be developed into second generation antipsychotics or better third generation drugs. These efforts will be presented in this chapter.

4.2.1. Modifications of Marketed Drugs

In recent years, a number of research groups studied halogenated arylpiperazines as a privileged scaffold active in CNS resulting in antipsychotics such as aripiprazole, trazodone and cariprazine [118]. The multimodal receptor profile of aripiprazole (5-HT_{1A}, 5-HT_{2A}, 5-HT_7, D_2 and D_3 receptors), as well as its functional profile as a partial agonist of D_2 and 5-HT_{1A} receptors and antagonist of 5-HT_{2A} and 5-HT_7 sites, makes it a good starting point to design compounds with antipsychotic, antidepressant, and anxiolytic activity [119]. Expanding the concept of mixed serotonin/dopamine receptor agonists as novel antipsychotics, Butini et al. designed a series of aripiprazole analogs that combined high affinity for 5-HT_{1A} and 5-HT_{2A} receptors, low affinity for D_2 receptors and high affinity for D_3 receptors. The structures of the compounds were based mainly on the 2,3-dichlorophenylpiperazine core structure, which was functionalized with isoquinoline-amide and quinolone- and isoquinoline-ether moieties, e.g., compound (**13**), compared in Figure 8. The study revealed that the optimal serotonin/dopamine receptor affinity balance was characterized by compounds with isoquinoline or benzofurane rings as heteroatomic systems [120]. As a continuation of their studies they developed a series bishetero(homo)arylpiperazines as novel and potent multifunctional ligands characterized by high affinity to D_3, 5-HT_{1A} and low occupancy at D_2 and 5-HT_{2C} receptors [121].

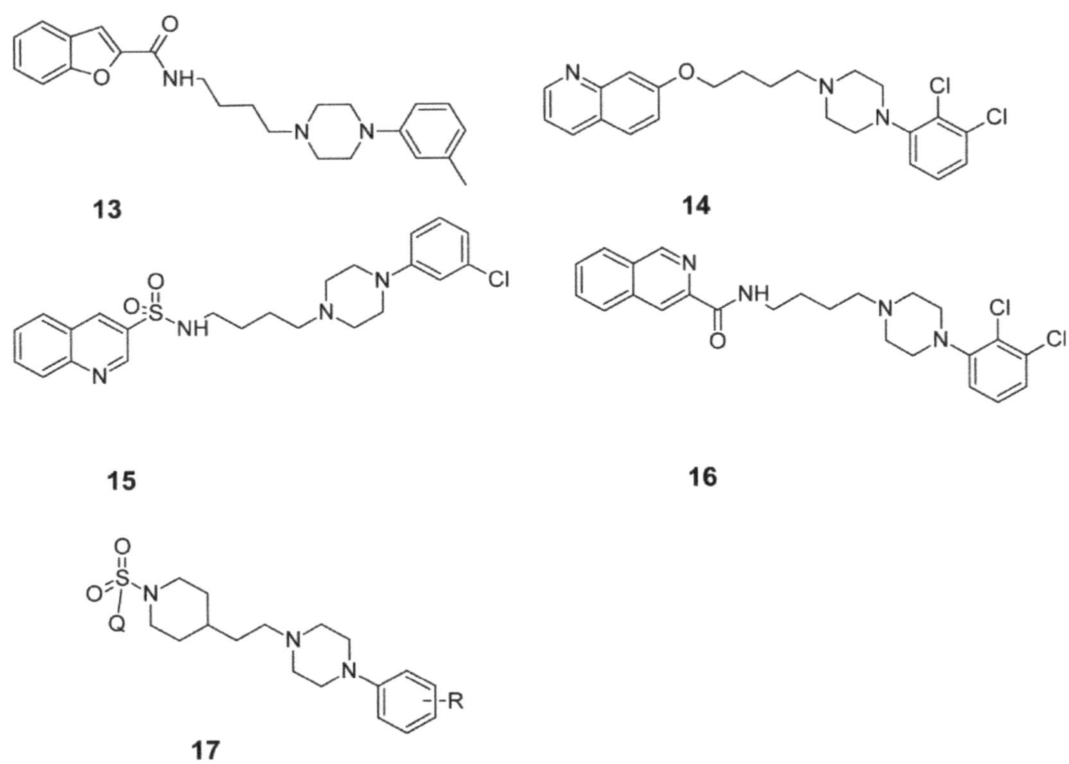

Figure 8. Novel potential multi-target antipsychotics derived from aripiprazole structure. Q: quinolone or isoquinoline.

In 2013 Zajdel et al. developed a series of new quinoline- and isoquinoline-sulfonamide analogs of aripiprazole to explore the effect of the replacement of the ether/amide moiety with sulfonamide, as well as the localization of a sulfonamide group in the azine moiety,

(**14–16**), see in Figure 8. In this study, two specific compounds displayed 5-HT_{1A} agonistic, D_2 partial agonistic and 5-HT_{2A}/5-HT_7 antagonistic activity, thus resulting in significant antidepressant activity in mice models of depression [119]. Furthermore, the 4-isoquinolinyl analog (*N*-(4-(4-(2,3-dichlorophenyl)piperazin-1-yl)butyl)isoquinoline-4-sulfonamide) not only exhibited a similar receptor binding and functional profile but also displayed significant antipsychotic activity in MK-801-induced hyperlocomotor activity in mice [119]. These results supported the study previously conducted by Zajdel and coworkers in 2012, which reported on quinoline- and isoquinoline-sulfonamide derivatives of long-chain arylpiperazines with 3- or 4-chloro-phenylpiperazine moieties as potential antidepressant, anxiolytic and antipsychotic agents [122].

Partyka et al. inspired by previous findings on a group of *N*-alkylated azinesulfonamides, synthesized a series of 15 azinesulfonamides of phenylpiperazine derivatives, based on 4-(4-{2-[4-(4-chlorophenyl)-piperazin-1-yl]-ethyl}-piperidine-1-sulfonyl)-isoquinoline with semi-rigid alkylene spacer (**17**), as seen in Figure 8, and evaluated them as multimodal dopamine/serotonin receptor ligands. The study allowed to identify compound 5-({4-(2-[4-(2,3-dichlorophenyl) piperazin-1-yl]ethyl)piperidin-1-yl}sulfonyl)quinolone which behaved as mixed D_2/5-HT_{1A}/5-HT_7 receptor antagonist. Preliminary pharmacological in vivo evaluation showed that compound was active in MK-801-evoked hyperactivity test in mice, and produced antidepressant-like activity in a mouse model of depression. Further studies in the area of CNS agents with multiple mode of action might confirmed its broad-based efficacy in the treatment of comorbid symptoms of schizophrenia/depression/anxiety [123].

In 2007 the atypical antipsychotic bifeprunox [1-(2-oxo-benzoxazolin-7-yl)-4-(3-biphenyl) methylpiperazine], with dual D_2 and 5-HT_{1A} partial agonist activity, was filed for regulatory approval with the Food and Drug Administration (FDA), however the application was rejected owing to the weakness of evidence submitted and the death of a patient involved in the clinical trials. Nevertheless, through various molecular modification studies, it was established that the phenylpiperazine moiety is responsible for its antiserotonergic and antidopaminergic activity of this compound [120]. Based on these findings and the anti-inflammatory, nitric oxide synthase inhibitory activity, antidiabetic and antifungicidal activity of biphenyl compounds, a hybrid structure comprising a biphenyl and arylpiperazine moiety with an acetyl linker was designed [124]. In this study Bhosale et al. focused on combining the beneficial effects of the biphenyl moiety of bifeprunox with the methylpiperazine moiety of the aripiprazole. The newly designed hybrid antipsychotic scaffold (**18**) is presented in Figure 9.

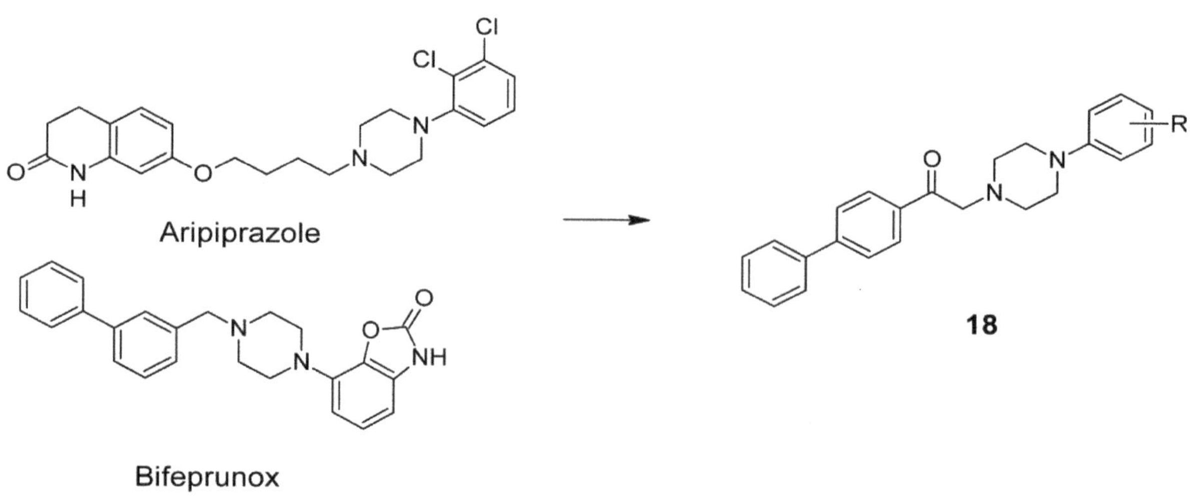

Figure 9. Design of multi-target hybrid compound based on aripiprazole and bifeprunox scaffold.

4.2.2. Other Multi-Target Compounds with Potential Application for the Treatment of Schizophrenia

It has been reported that the adjunctive usage of a neuroleptic together with selective serotonin reuptake inhibitor (SSRI), e.g., fluvoxamine, fluoxetine or citalopram is beneficial for the treatment of negative symptoms of schizophrenia without increasing EPS [125]. In this regard van Hes et al. elaborated SLV310, seen in Figure 10, (**19**), as a novel, potential antipsychotic displaying the interesting combination of potent dopamine D_2 receptor antagonism and serotonin reuptake receptor inhibition in one molecule which can be useful in treatment a broad range of symptoms in schizophrenia [126]. Subsequently the same research group obtained a series of compounds displaying D_2 receptor antagonism as well as SSRI properties by connecting the aryl piperazine of a neuroleptic with the indole moiety of a SSRI through alkyl chain in order to obtain promising antipsychotic agents, seen in Figure 10, (**20**). Optimization of length of the alkyl linker chain, substitution pattern of the indole moiety and bicyclic heteroaryl part has led to the maximally potent compound. Further, the molecular modelling studies have shown that the bifunctional activity of compound can be explained by its ability to adopt two different conformations fitting either D_2 receptor or SR pharmacophore without the disadvantages of potential pharmacokinetic interactions [127].

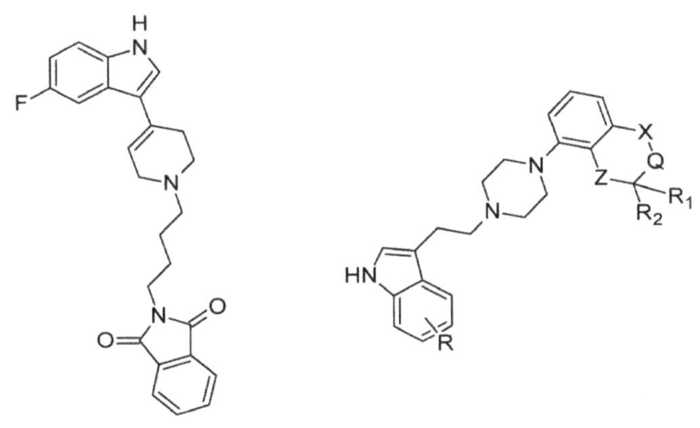

SLV310 **19** **20**

Figure 10. Dopamine D_2 receptor antagonists with selective serotonin reuptake inhibitor (SSRI) activity.

Li et al. reported synthesis and structure-activity relationships of a series of tetracyclic butyrophenones that display high affinities to serotonin 5-HT_{2A} and dopamine D_2 receptors [128]. In particular, ITI-007 (4-((6bR,10aS)-3-methyl-2,3,6b,9,10,10a-hexahydro-1H,7H-pyrido[3′,4′:4,5]pyrrolo quinoxalin-8-yl)-1-(4-fluorophenyl)-butan-1-one 4-methylbenzenesulfonate), seen in Figure 11, (**21**), was found to be a potent 5-HT_{2A} receptor antagonist, postsynaptic D_2 receptor antagonist and inhibitor of serotonin transporter [128].

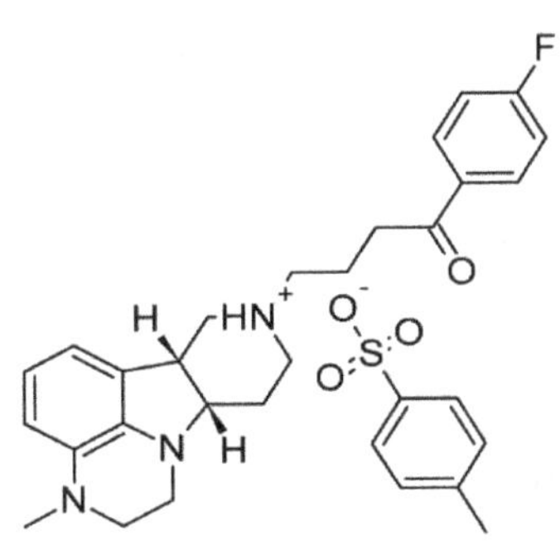

ITI-007 **21**

Figure 11. ITI-007, a potent 5-HT_{2A} receptor antagonist, postsynaptic D_2 receptor antagonist and inhibitor of serotonin transporter.

In the latest study, Zajdel et al. [129] designed, synthesized and characterized a new series of azinesulfonamides of alicyclic amine derivatives with arylpiperazine/piperidine scaffold. Structure-activity studies of this compound series disclosed that the (isoquinolin-4-ylsulfonyl)-(*S*)-pyrrolidinyl fragment and the 1,2-benzothiazol-3-yl- and benzothiophen-4-yl-piperazine fragments were beneficial for affinity to 5-HT_{1A}, 5-HT_{2A}, 5-HT_6, 5-HT_7, D_2 and D_3 receptors. Furthermore, binding of these compounds with 5-HT_6 receptor depended on the stereochemistry of the alicyclic amine. Within this compound series, (*S*)-4-((2-(2-(4-(benzo[b]thiophen-4-yl)piperazin-1-yl)ethyl) pyrrolidin-1-yl) sulfonyl) isoquinoline, seen in Figure 12, (**22**), was identified as a potential novel antipsychotic. This compound is also characterized by blockade to SERT. Because it reverses PCP-induced hyperactivity and avoidance behavior in the CAR test, (**22**) it can be used to treat positive symptoms of schizophrenia. Next, its ability to reverse the social interaction deficit in a ketamine model and memory impairment in phencyclidine (PCP)- and ketamine-disrupted conditions reveals that that drug can improve the negative symptoms and has procognitive activity. Importantly, this compound did not have cardiac toxicity and tendency of inducing catalepsy [129].

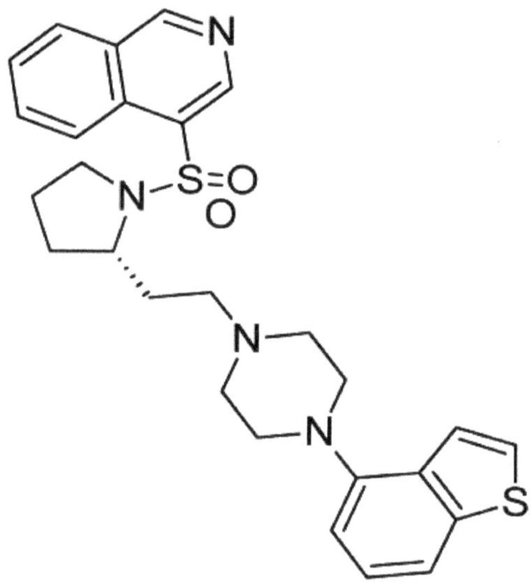

22

Figure 12. Multi-target ligand of aminergic G protein-coupled receptors (GPCRs) with SERT inhibitory properties.

In order to obtain novel antipsychotics Menegatti et al. designed and synthesized a series of N-phenylpiperazine derivatives [130]. A few compounds, i.e., 1-[1-(4-chlorophenyl)-1H-pyrazol-4-ylmethyl]-4-phenyl-piperazine (LASSBio-579, **23**, Figure 13), 1-phenyl-4-(1-phenyl-1H-[1,2,3]triazol-4-ylmethyl)-piperazine (LASSBio-580) and 1-[1-(4-chlorophenyl)-1H-[1,2,3]triazol-4-ylmethyl]-4-phenyl-piperazine (LASSBio-581) were selected based on potential antipsychotic activity. It was found that LASSBio-579 is the most promising of the three compounds, thanks to its affinity to both dopamine and serotonin receptors, in particular agonist activity at 5-HT_{1A} receptor [131]. Thus, this multi-target compound was active in animal models of psychosis and reversed the catalepsy induced by WAY 100,635, Furthermore, co-administration of sub-effective doses of LASSBio-579 with sub-effective doses of clozapine or haloperidol prevented apomorphine-induced climbing without induction of catalepsy [131].

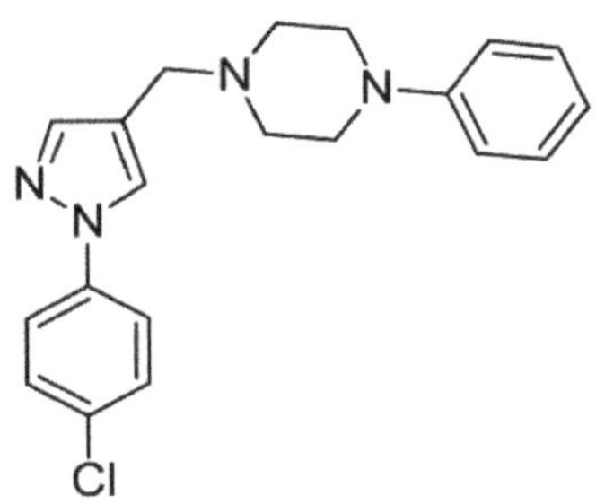

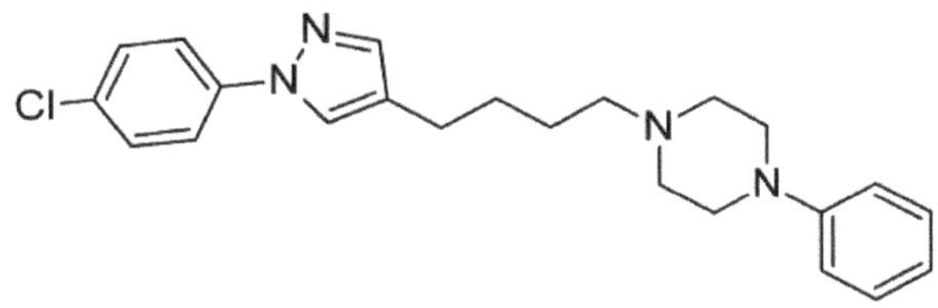

LASSBio-579 **23** LASSBio-1635 **24**

Figure 13. Potential multi-target (dopamine and serotonin receptor ligands) antipsychotics.

In 2013, another team synthesized and made a pharmacological evaluation of the antipsychotic homologues of the lead compound LASSBio-579. The applied homologation approach turned out to be appropriate for increasing the affinity of these compounds to the 5-HT_{2A} receptors, with no significant changes in the affinity for the D_2, D_4 and 5-HT_{1A} receptors. In this context, (1-(4-(1-(4-chlorophenyl)-1*H*-pyrazol-4-yl) butyl)-4-phenylpiperazine) (LASSBio-1635, **24**), Figure 13 was the most promising derivative with a ten-fold higher affinity for the 5-HT_{2A} receptor than its parent compound. Moreover, LASSBio-1635 displayed beneficial antagonistic efficacy at the 5-HT_{2A} receptors. Next, LASSBio-1635 has also a 4-fold higher affinity for α_2 adrenergic receptors in comparison to LASSBio-579 and the favorable antagonistic efficacy. This multi-target ligand fully prevented the apomorphine-induced climbing in mice and prevented the ketamine-induced hyperlocomotion at doses with no effect on the mice locomotor activity [132].

In order to search for potential multi-target antipsychotics, Kaczor et al. [86] performed structure-based virtual screening using a D_2 receptor homology model in complex with olanzapine or chlorprothixene. As a result of a screen they selected 21 compounds, which were subjected to experimental validation. From 21 compounds tested, they found ten D_2 ligands (47.6% success rate, among them D_2 receptor antagonists as expected) possessing additional affinity to other receptors tested, in particular to 5-HT_{1A} (partial agonists) and 5-HT_{2A} receptors (antagonists). The affinity of the compounds ranged from 58 nM to about 24 μM. Similarity and fragmental analysis indicated a significant structural novelty of the identified compounds. The best compound (D2AAK1, **25**) has affinity of 58 nM to D_2 receptor and nanomolar or low micromolar affinity to D_1, D_3, 5-HT_{1A} and 5-HT_{2A} receptors. D2AAK1 is an antagonist at D_2 receptor and 5-HT_{2A} receptor and a partial agonist at 5-HT_{1A} receptor which is favorable for antipsychotic activity [131]. They found one D_2 receptor antagonist (D2AAK2, **26**) that did not have a protonatable nitrogen atom which is a key structural element of the classical D_2 pharmacophore model necessary to interact with the conserved Asp(3.32). This compound exhibited over 20-fold binding selectivity for the D_2 receptor compared to the D_3 receptor. The four best compounds (D2AAK1–D2AAK4, **25–28**, Figure 14) were subjected to in vivo evaluation. In particular compound D2AAK1 decreased amphetamine-induced hyperactivity (when compared to the amphetamine-treated group), measured as spontaneous locomotor activity in mice. In addition, in a passive avoidance test this compound improved memory consolidation after acute treatment in mice. Elevated plus maze tests indicated that D2AAK1 compound induced anxiogenic activity 30 min after acute treatment and anxiolytic activity 60 min after administration [133].

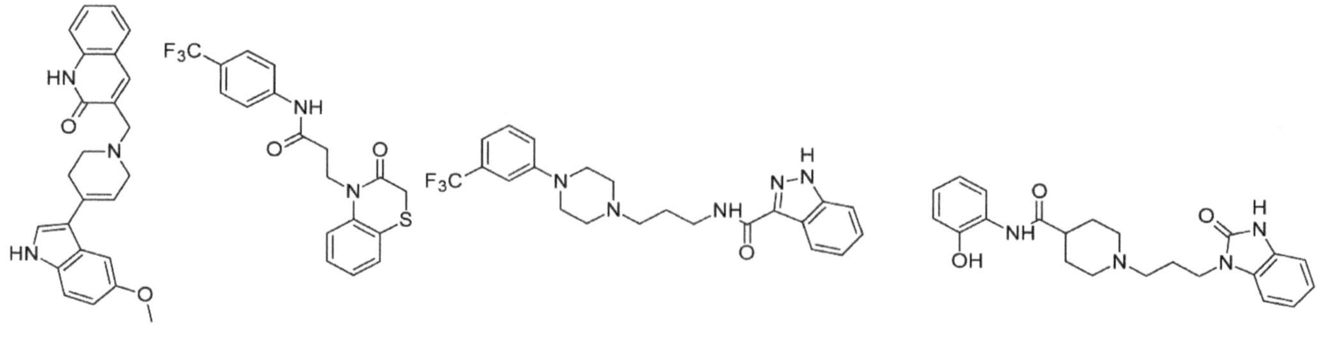

D2AAK1 **25** D2AAK2 **26** D2AAK3 **27** D2AAK4 **28**

Figure 14. Multi-target compounds obtained in structure-based virtual screening.

AVN-101 (**29**, Figure 12) is another multi-target drug candidate that has an advantageous target fingerprint of activities with prevalent affinity to serotonin receptors, mainly 5-HT_7, 5-HT_6, 5-HT_{2A}, and 5-HT_{2C}, as well as to adrenergic α_{2B}, α_{2A}, and α_{2C} and histamine H_1 and H_2 receptors. The AVN-101 exhibits positive effects in the animal models of both impaired and innate cognition. It also exhibited significant anxiolytic and anti-depressant capabilities [134].

2-[4-(6-fluorobenzisoxazol-3-yl)piperidinyl]methyl-1,2,3,4-tetrahydro-carbazol-4-one (QF2004B), a conformationally constrained butyrophenone analog (**30**, Figure 15) has a multi-receptor profile with affinities similar to those of clozapine for serotonin (5-HT_{2A}, 5-HT_{1A}, and 5-HT_{2C}), dopamine (D_1, D_2, D_3 and D_4), alpha-adrenergic (α_1, α_2), muscarinic (M_1, M_2) and histamine H_1 receptors. In addition, QF2004B mirrored the antipsychotic activity and atypical profile of clozapine in a broad battery of in vivo tests including locomotor activity, apomorphine-induced stereotypies, catalepsy, apomorphine- and DOI (2,5-dimethoxy-4-iodoamphetamine)-induced prepulse inhibition (PPI) tests. These results point to QF2004B as a new lead compound with a relevant multi-receptor interaction profile for the discovery and development of new antipsychotics [135].

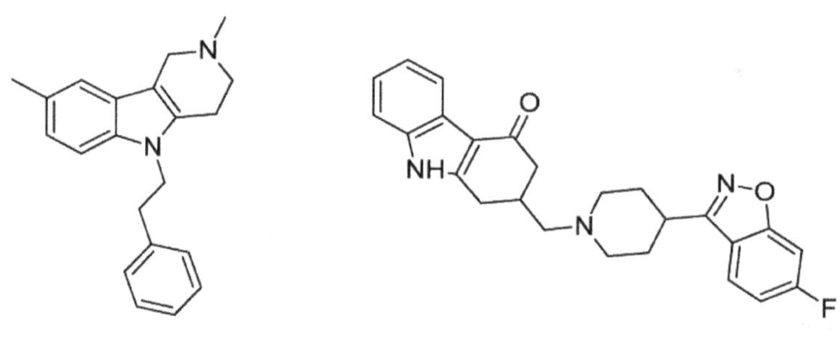

AVN-101 **29** QF2004B **30**

Figure 15. Multi-target ligands of aminergic GPCRs as potential antipsychotics.

Searching for potential multi-target antipsychotics, Huang et al. [136] obtained a series of compounds bearing benzoxazole-piperidine (piperazine) scaffold with considerable dopamine D_2 and serotonin 5-HT_{1A} and 5-HT_{2A} receptor binding affinities. The best compound (**31**, Figure 16) had high affinity to D_2, 5-HT_{1A} and 5-HT_{2A} receptors, but low affinities foroff-targets (the 5-HT_{2C} and histamine H_1 receptors and human ether-a-go-go-related gene (hERG) channels). This compound diminished apomorphine-induced climbing and DOI-induced head twitching without observable catalepsy, even at the highest dose tested making it a promising candidate for multi-target antipsychotic treatment.

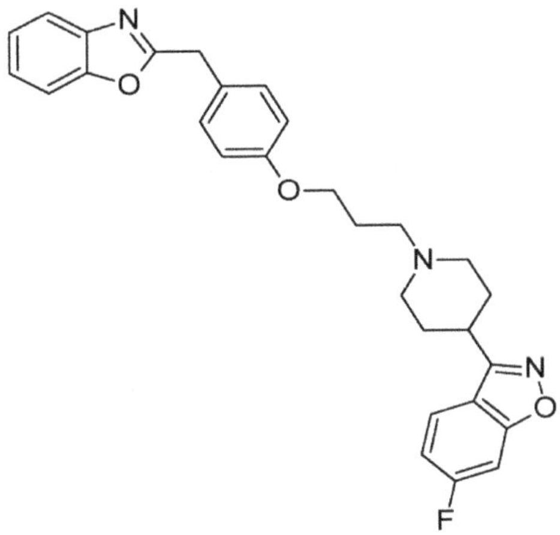

31

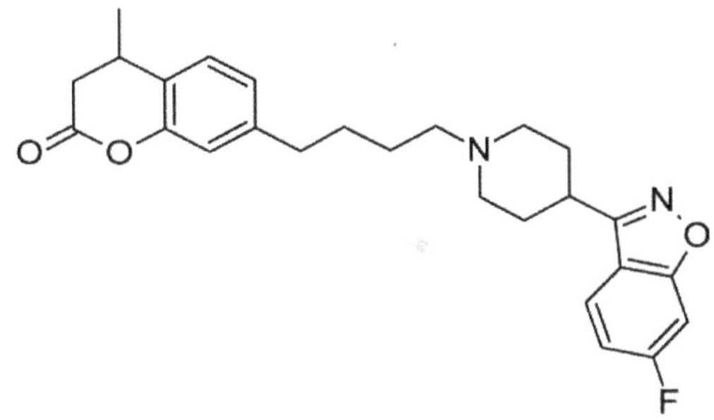

32

Figure 16. Multi-target ligands of aminergic GPCRs as potential antipsychotics with low affinity to off-targets.

Chen et al. [137] obtained potential antipsychotic coumarin derivatives, having potent dopamine D_2, D_3, and serotonin 5-HT_{1A} and 5-HT_{2A} receptor affinities. The best compound, seen in 32, Figure 16, also possesses low affinity for 5-HT_{2C} and H_1 receptors and hERG channels. In behavioral studies this compound inhibited apomorphine-induced climbing behavior, MK-801-induced hyperactivity, and the conditioned avoidance response without observable catalepsy. Further, fewer preclinical side effects were observed for (**32**) in comparison to risperidone in assays that measured prolactin secretion and weight gain.

Another group synthesized a series of benzisothiazolylpiperazine derivatives combining potent dopamine D_2 and D_3, and serotonin 5-HT_{1A} and 5-HT_{2A} receptor affinities [138]. The best compound, as seen in (**33**), Figure 17, had significant affinity for D_2, D_3, 5-HT_{1A}, and 5-HT_{2A} receptors, accompanied by a 20-fold selectivity for the D_3 versus D_2 subtype, and a low affinity for muscarinic M_1 and for hERG channels. In animal studies this compound blocked the locomotor-stimulating effects of phencyclidine, inhibited conditioned avoidance response, and improved the cognitive impairment in the novel object recognition tests in rats [138].

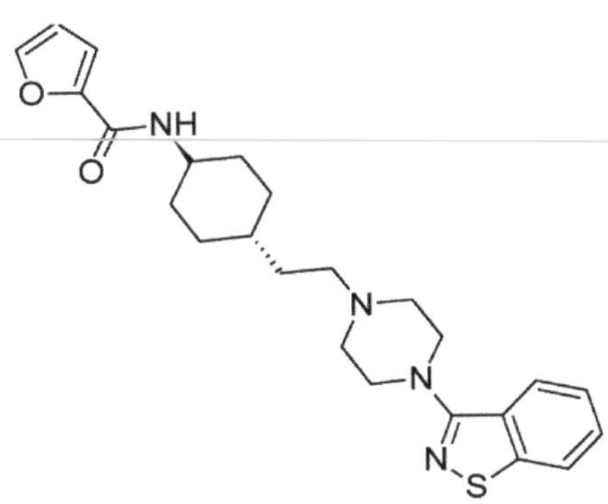

33

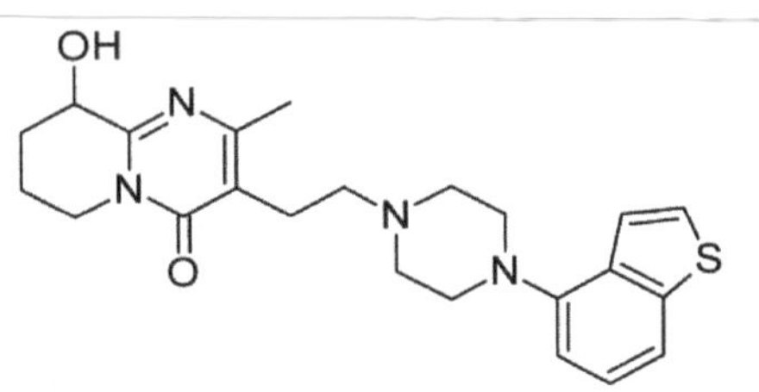

34

Figure 17. Potential multi-target antipsychotics with low probability of adverse effects.

In a recent study Xiamuxi et al. [139] reported a series of tetrahydropyridopyrimidinone derivatives, possessing potent dopamine D_2, serotonin 5-HT_{1A} and 5-HT_{2A} receptors affinities. The most promising compound, seen in (**34**), Figure 17, displayed high affinity to D_2, 5-HT_{1A}, and

$5\text{-}HT_{2A}$ receptors, with low affinity to α_{1A}, $5\text{-}HT_{2C}$, H_1 receptors and hERG channels. In animal models, this compound diminished phencyclidine-induced hyperactivity with a high threshold for catalepsy induction.

In another new study Yang et al. [140] designed a series of benzamides, with potent dopamine D_2, serotonin $5\text{-}HT_{1A}$ and $5\text{-}HT_{2A}$ receptor affinity. Two best compounds, seen in (**35**) and (**36**), Figure 18, were not only potent D_2, $5\text{-}HT_{1A}$, and $5\text{-}HT_{2A}$ receptor ligands, but they were weak binders of $5\text{-}HT_{2C}$, H_1 receptors and hERG channels. In behavioral studies these compounds decreased phencyclidine-induced hyperactivity with a high threshold for catalepsy induction.

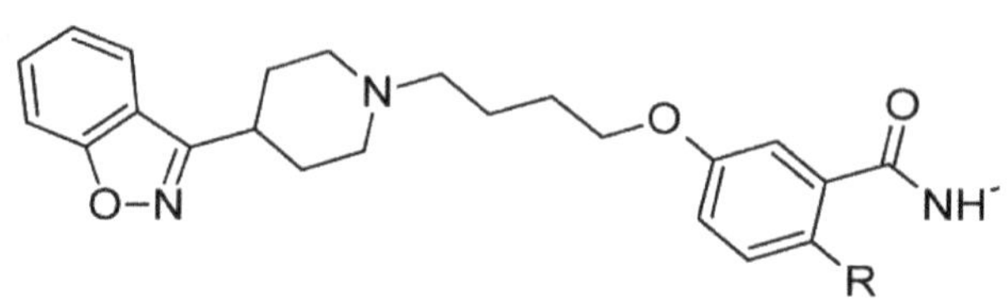

35: R=H
36: R=F

Figure 18. Benzamides as potential multi-target antipsychotics with low probability of side effects.

5. Conclusions and Perspectives

The growing pace of life promotes mental disorders. Pharmacotherapy for schizophrenia is nowadays very effective, in particular regarding treating positive symptoms of the disease, but at the same time there is a tremendous, unmet clinical need for the therapy of negative and cognitive symptoms, as well as for the management of drug resistant schizophrenia. Over the last half century, there has been only limited progress in the innovating mechanisms of action and the developing novel therapeutic agents for the treatment of schizophrenia. However, the breadth of potential goals and tested compounds clearly shows interest and importance in the pursuit of innovative drug development. A multi-target approach to drug design and discovery is now a hot topic in medicinal chemistry, in particular for the treatment of complex diseases such as schizophrenia. It should be emphasized that regarding management of schizophrenia, nothing more effective than multi-target treatment has been proposed. Involvement of nicotinic and glutamatergic targets in modern multi-target drugs can be beneficial for the treatment of negative symptoms and cognitive impairment. Another potential strategy is exploration novel signaling mechanisms concerning in particular GPCRs, such as allosteric modulation, biased signaling (functional selectivity), and receptor oligomerization. However, this approach will also be more promising when it involves multiple targets. In summary, as current multi-target antipsychotics are mainly orthosteric ligands of aminergic GPCRs with SSRI or SERT inhibitory activity in some cases, there is a huge unexplored area to include other receptors and enzymes as drug targets and to explore the wealth of signaling mechanism beyond the ternary complex model of GPCRs.

Author Contributions: M.K. wrote Section 4; P.S. wrote Section 2; A.A.K. wrote Sections 1, 3 and 5.

Abbreviations

3D QSAR	Three-dimensional structure-activity relationship
AMPA	α-Amino-3-hydroxy-5-methyl-4-isoxazolepropionic acid
cAMP	Cyclic adenosine monophosphate
CAR	Conditioned avoidance response
CNS	Central nervous system
cNT PDEs	Cyclic nucleotide phosphodiestereases
EPS	Extrapyramidal symptoms
FDA	Food and Drug Administration
GABA	γ-Aminobutyric acid
GPCRs	G protein-coupled receptors
GSK-3	Glycogen synthase kinase-3
GTP	Guanosine-5′-triphosphate
LSD	Lysergic acid diethylamide
MTDs	Multi-target drugs
NMDA	*N*-methyl-D-aspartate
PCP	Phencyclidine
SSRI	Selective serotonin reuptake inhibitor
VTA	Ventral tegmental area

References

1. Stępnicki, P.; Kondej, M.; Kaczor, A.A. Current Concepts and Treatments of Schizophrenia. *Molecules* **2018**, *23*. [CrossRef] [PubMed]
2. Lau, C.-I.; Wang, H.-C.; Hsu, J.-L.; Liu, M.-E. Does the dopamine hypothesis explain schizophrenia? *Rev. Neurosci.* **2013**, *24*, 389–400. [CrossRef] [PubMed]
3. Hu, W.; MacDonald, M.L.; Elswick, D.E.; Sweet, R.A. The glutamate hypothesis of schizophrenia: Evidence from human brain tissue studies. *Ann. N. Y. Acad. Sci.* **2015**, *1338*, 38–57. [CrossRef] [PubMed]
4. Lavecchia, A.; Cerchia, C. In silico methods to address polypharmacology: Current status, applications and future perspectives. *Drug Discov. Today* **2016**, *21*, 288–298. [CrossRef] [PubMed]
5. Korcsmáros, T.; Szalay, M.S.; Böde, C.; Kovács, I.A.; Csermely, P. How to design multi-target drugs. *Expert Opin. Drug Discov.* **2007**, *2*, 799–808. [CrossRef] [PubMed]
6. Hopkins, A.L. Network pharmacology: The next paradigm in drug discovery. *Nat. Chem. Biol.* **2008**, *4*, 682–690. [CrossRef] [PubMed]
7. Nikolic, K.; Mavridis, L.; Djikic, T.; Vucicevic, J.; Agbaba, D.; Yelekci, K.; Mitchell, J.B.O. Drug Design for CNS Diseases: Polypharmacological Profiling of Compounds Using Cheminformatic, 3D-QSAR and Virtual Screening Methodologies. *Front. Neurosci.* **2016**, *10*, 265. [CrossRef] [PubMed]
8. Bakhshi, K.; Chance, S.A. The neuropathology of schizophrenia: A selective review of past studies and emerging themes in brain structure and cytoarchitecture. *Neuroscience* **2015**, *303*, 82–102. [CrossRef] [PubMed]
9. Rang, H.P.; Ritter, J.M.; Flower, R.J.; Henderson, G. *Rang and Dale's Pharmacology*, 8th ed.; Elsevier: Amsterdam, The Netherlands, 2016.
10. Miyamoto, S.; Duncan, G.E.; Marx, C.E.; Lieberman, J.A. Treatments for schizophrenia: A critical review of pharmacology and mechanisms of action of antipsychotic drugs. *Mol. Psychiatry* **2005**, *10*, 79–104. [CrossRef] [PubMed]
11. Mauri, M.C.; Paletta, S.; Maffini, M.; Colasanti, A.; Dragogna, F.; di Pace, C.; Altamura, A.C. Clinical pharmacology of atypical antipsychotics: An update. *EXCLI J.* **2014**, *13*, 1163–1191. [PubMed]
12. Orsolini, L.; Tomasetti, C.; Valchera, A.; Vecchiotti, R.; Matarazzo, I.; Vellante, F.; Iasevoli, F.; Buonaguro, E.F.; Fornaro, M.; Fiengo, A.L.C.; et al. An update of safety of clinically used atypical antipsychotics. *Expert Opin. Drug Saf.* **2016**, *15*, 1329–1347. [CrossRef] [PubMed]
13. Meltzer, H.Y.; Nash, J.F. Effects of antipsychotic drugs on serotonin receptors. *Pharmacol. Rev.* **1991**, *43*, 587–604. [PubMed]

14. Sorensen, S.M.; Kehne, J.H.; Fadayel, G.M.; Humphreys, T.M.; Ketteler, H.J.; Sullivan, C.K.; Taylor, V.L.; Schmidt, C.J. Characterization of the 5-HT_2 receptor antagonist MDL 100907 as a putative atypical antipsychotic: Behavioral, electrophysiological and neurochemical studies. *J. Pharmacol. Exp. Ther.* **1993**, *266*, 684–691. [PubMed]
15. Miller, C.H.; Fleischhacker, W.W.; Ehrmann, H.; Kane, J.M. Treatment of neuroleptic induced akathisia with the 5-HT_2 antagonist ritanserin. *Psychopharmacol. Bull.* **1990**, *26*, 373–376. [PubMed]
16. Schmidt, C.J.; Sorensen, S.M.; Kehne, J.H.; Carr, A.A.; Palfreyman, M.G. The role of 5-HT_{2A} receptors in antipsychotic activity. *Life Sci.* **1995**, *56*, 2209–2222. [CrossRef]
17. Meltzer, H.Y.; Li, Z.; Kaneda, Y.; Ichikawa, J. Serotonin receptors: Their key role in drugs to treat schizophrenia. *Prog. Neuropsychopharmacol. Biol. Psychiatry* **2003**, *27*, 1159–1172. [CrossRef] [PubMed]
18. Millan, M.J. Improving the treatment of schizophrenia: Focus on serotonin 5-HT_{1A} receptors. *J. Pharmacol. Exp. Ther.* **2000**, *295*, 853–861. [PubMed]
19. Akimova, E.; Lanzenberger, R.; Kasper, S. The serotonin-1A receptor in anxiety disorders. *Biol. Psychiatry* **2009**, *66*, 627–635. [CrossRef] [PubMed]
20. Ogren, S.O.; Eriksson, T.M.; Elvander-Tottie, E.; D'Addario, C.; Ekström, J.C.; Svenningsson, P.; Meister, B.; Kehr, J.; Stiedl, O. The role of 5-HT_{1A} receptors in learning and memory. *Behav. Brain Res.* **2008**, *195*, 54–77. [CrossRef] [PubMed]
21. Prinssen, E.P.; Colpaert, F.C.; Koek, W. 5-HT_{1A} receptor activation and anti-cataleptic effects: High-efficacy agonists maximally inhibit haloperidol-induced catalepsy. *Eur. J. Pharmacol.* **2002**, *453*, 217–221. [CrossRef]
22. Mignon, L.; Wolf, W.A. Postsynaptic 5-HT_{1A} receptors mediate an increase in locomotor activity in the monoamine-depleted rat. *Psychopharmacology* **2002**, *163*, 85–94. [CrossRef] [PubMed]
23. Madjid, N.; Tottie, E.E.; Lüttgen, M.; Meister, B.; Sandin, J.; Kuzmin, A.; Stiedl, O.; Ogren, S.O. 5-Hydroxytryptamine 1A receptor blockade facilitates aversive learning in mice: Interactions with cholinergic and glutamatergic mechanisms. *J. Pharmacol. Exp. Ther.* **2006**, *316*, 581–591. [CrossRef] [PubMed]
24. Ohno, Y. Therapeutic role of 5-HT_{1A} receptors in the treatment of schizophrenia and Parkinson's disease. *CNS Neurosci. Ther.* **2011**, *17*, 58–65. [CrossRef] [PubMed]
25. Kennett, G.A.; Curzon, G. Evidence that mCPP may have behavioural effects mediated by central 5-HT_{1C} receptors. *Br. J. Pharmacol.* **1988**, *94*, 137–147. [CrossRef] [PubMed]
26. Kalkman, H.O. Hypersensitivity to meta-chlorophenylpiperazine (mCPP) in migraine and drug withdrawal. *Int. J. Clin. Pharmacol. Res.* **1997**, *17*, 75–77. [PubMed]
27. Krystal, J.H.; Seibyl, J.P.; Price, L.H.; Woods, S.W.; Heninger, G.R.; Aghajanian, G.K.; Charney, D.S. m-Chlorophenylpiperazine effects in neuroleptic-free schizophrenic patients. Evidence implicating serotonergic systems in the positive symptoms of schizophrenia. *Arch. Gen. Psychiatry* **1993**, *50*, 624–635. [CrossRef] [PubMed]
28. Wood, M.D.; Heidbreder, C.; Reavill, C.; Ashby, C.R., Jr.; Middlemiss, D.N. 5-HT_{2C} receptor antagonists: Potential in schizophrenia. *Drug Dev. Res.* **2001**, *54*, 88–94.
29. Foster, D.J.; Conn, P.J. Allosteric Modulation of GPCRs: New Insights and Potential Utility for Treatment of Schizophrenia and Other CNS Disorders. *Neuron* **2017**, *94*, 431–446. [CrossRef] [PubMed]
30. Urs, N.M.; Gee, S.M.; Pack, T.F.; McCorvy, J.D.; Evron, T.; Snyder, J.C.; Yang, X.; Rodriguiz, R.M.; Borrelli, E.; Wetsel, W.C.; et al. Distinct cortical and striatal actions of a β-arrestin-biased dopamine D_2 receptor ligand reveal unique antipsychotic-like properties. *Proc. Natl. Acad. Sci. USA* **2016**, *113*, E8178–E8186. [CrossRef] [PubMed]
31. Kaczor, A.A.; Selent, J. Oligomerization of G protein-coupled receptors: Biochemical and biophysical methods. *Curr. Med. Chem.* **2011**, *18*, 4606–4634. [CrossRef] [PubMed]
32. Selent, J.; Kaczor, A.A. Oligomerization of G protein-coupled receptors: Computational methods. *Curr. Med. Chem.* **2011**, *18*, 4588–4605. [CrossRef] [PubMed]
33. Kaczor, A.A.; Jörg, M.; Capuano, B. The dopamine D_2 receptor dimer and its interaction with homobivalent antagonists: Homology modeling, docking and molecular dynamics. *J. Mol. Model.* **2016**, *22*, 203. [CrossRef] [PubMed]
34. Moreno, J.L.; Miranda-Azpiazu, P.; García-Bea, A.; Younkin, J.; Cui, M.; Kozlenkov, A.; Ben-Ezra, A.; Voloudakis, G.; Fakira, A.K.; Baki, L.; et al. Allosteric signaling through an mGlu2 and 5-HT_{2A} heteromeric receptor complex and its potential contribution to schizophrenia. *Sci. Signal.* **2016**, *9*, ra5. [CrossRef] [PubMed]

35. Wong, E.H.F.; Tarazi, F.I.; Shahid, M. The effectiveness of multi-target agents in schizophrenia and mood disorders: Relevance of receptor signature to clinical action. *Pharmacol. Ther.* **2010**, *126*, 173–185. [CrossRef] [PubMed]
36. Maletic, V.; Eramo, A.; Gwin, K.; Offord, S.J.; Duffy, R.A. The Role of Norepinephrine and Its α-Adrenergic Receptors in the Pathophysiology and Treatment of Major Depressive Disorder and Schizophrenia: A Systematic Review. *Front. Psychiatry* **2017**, *8*, 42. [CrossRef] [PubMed]
37. Svensson, T.H. α-Adrenoceptor modulation hypothesis of antipsychotic atypicality. *Prog. Neuropsychopharmacol. Biol. Psychiatry* **2003**, *27*, 1145–1158. [CrossRef] [PubMed]
38. Brosda, J.; Jantschak, F.; Pertz, H.H. α_2-Adrenoceptors are targets for antipsychotic drugs. *Psychopharmacology* **2014**, *231*, 801–812. [CrossRef] [PubMed]
39. Marcus, M.M.; Wiker, C.; Frånberg, O.; Konradsson-Geuken, A.; Langlois, X.; Jardemark, K.; Svensson, T.H. Adjunctive α_2-adrenoceptor blockade enhances the antipsychotic-like effect of risperidone and facilitates cortical dopaminergic and glutamatergic, NMDA receptor-mediated transmission. *Int. J. Neuropsychopharmacol.* **2010**, *13*, 891–903. [CrossRef] [PubMed]
40. He, M.; Deng, C.; Huang, X.-F. The role of hypothalamic H1 receptor antagonism in antipsychotic-induced weight gain. *CNS Drugs* **2013**, *27*, 423–434. [CrossRef] [PubMed]
41. Ellenbroek, B.A.; Ghiabi, B. Do Histamine receptor 3 antagonists have a place in the therapy for schizophrenia? *Curr. Pharm. Des.* **2015**, *21*, 3760–3770. [CrossRef] [PubMed]
42. Sadek, B.; Saad, A.; Sadeq, A.; Jalal, F.; Stark, H. Histamine H3 receptor as a potential target for cognitive symptoms in neuropsychiatric diseases. *Behav. Brain Res.* **2016**, *312*, 415–430. [CrossRef] [PubMed]
43. Ghoshal, A.; Rook, J.M.; Dickerson, J.W.; Roop, G.N.; Morrison, R.D.; Jalan-Sakrikar, N.; Lamsal, A.; Noetzel, M.J.; Poslusney, M.S.; Wood, M.R.; et al. Potentiation of M1 Muscarinic Receptor Reverses Plasticity Deficits and Negative and Cognitive Symptoms in a Schizophrenia Mouse Model. *Neuropsychopharmacol. Off. Publ. Am. Coll. Neuropsychopharmacol.* **2016**, *41*, 598–610. [CrossRef] [PubMed]
44. Dean, B.; Scarr, E. Possible involvement of muscarinic receptors in psychiatric disorders: A focus on schizophrenia and mood disorders. *Curr. Mol. Med.* **2015**, *15*, 253–264. [CrossRef] [PubMed]
45. Holt, D.J.; Bachus, S.E.; Hyde, T.M.; Wittie, M.; Herman, M.M.; Vangel, M.; Saper, C.B.; Kleinman, J.E. Reduced density of cholinergic interneurons in the ventral striatum in schizophrenia: An in situ hybridization study. *Biol. Psychiatry* **2005**, *58*, 408–416. [CrossRef] [PubMed]
46. Raedler, T.J.; Knable, M.B.; Jones, D.W.; Urbina, R.A.; Gorey, J.G.; Lee, K.S.; Egan, M.F.; Coppola, R.; Weinberger, D.R. In vivo determination of muscarinic acetylcholine receptor availability in schizophrenia. *Am. J. Psychiatry* **2003**, *160*, 118–127. [CrossRef] [PubMed]
47. Raedler, T.J.; Bymaster, F.P.; Tandon, R.; Copolov, D.; Dean, B. Towards a muscarinic hypothesis of schizophrenia. *Mol. Psychiatry* **2007**, *12*, 232–246. [CrossRef] [PubMed]
48. Freeman, T.P.; Stone, J.M.; Orgaz, B.; Noronha, L.A.; Minchin, S.L.; Curran, H.V. Tobacco smoking in schizophrenia: Investigating the role of incentive salience. *Psychol. Med.* **2014**, *44*, 2189–2197. [CrossRef] [PubMed]
49. Parikh, V.; Kutlu, M.G.; Gould, T.J. nAChR dysfunction as a common substrate for schizophrenia and comorbid nicotine addiction: Current trends and perspectives. *Schizophr. Res.* **2016**, *171*, 1–15. [CrossRef] [PubMed]
50. Adams, C.E.; Stevens, K.E. Evidence for a role of nicotinic acetylcholine receptors in schizophrenia. *Front. Biosci. J. Virtual Libr.* **2007**, *12*, 4755–4772. [CrossRef]
51. Li, Y.; Sun, L.; Yang, T.; Jiao, W.; Tang, J.; Huang, X.; Huang, Z.; Meng, Y.; Luo, L.; Wang, X.; et al. Design and Synthesis of Novel Positive Allosteric Modulators of α7 Nicotinic Acetylcholine Receptors with the Ability To Rescue Auditory Gating Deficit in Mice. *J. Med. Chem.* **2018**. [CrossRef] [PubMed]
52. Neves, G.A.; Grace, A.A. α7 Nicotinic receptor-modulating agents reverse the hyperdopaminergic tone in the MAM model of schizophrenia. *Neuropsychopharmacol. Off. Publ. Am. Coll. Neuropsychopharmacol.* **2018**, *43*, 1712–1720. [CrossRef] [PubMed]
53. Moghaddam, B.; Javitt, D. From Revolution to Evolution: The Glutamate Hypothesis of Schizophrenia and its Implication for Treatment. *Neuropsychopharmacology* **2012**, *37*, 4–15. [CrossRef] [PubMed]
54. Yang, A.C.; Tsai, S.-J. New Targets for Schizophrenia Treatment beyond the Dopamine Hypothesis. *Int. J. Mol. Sci.* **2017**, *18*. [CrossRef] [PubMed]

55. Goff, D.C.; Coyle, J.T. The emerging role of glutamate in the pathophysiology and treatment of schizophrenia. *Am. J. Psychiatry* **2001**, *158*, 1367–1377. [CrossRef] [PubMed]
56. Harrison, P.J.; Weinberger, D.R. Schizophrenia genes, gene expression, and neuropathology: On the matter of their convergence. *Mol. Psychiatry* **2005**, *10*, 40–68. [CrossRef] [PubMed]
57. Cull-Candy, S.; Brickley, S.; Farrant, M. NMDA receptor subunits: Diversity, development and disease. *Curr. Opin. Neurobiol.* **2001**, *11*, 327–335. [CrossRef]
58. Paoletti, P.; Neyton, J. NMDA receptor subunits: Function and pharmacology. *Curr. Opin. Pharmacol.* **2007**, *7*, 39–47. [CrossRef] [PubMed]
59. Saleem, S.; Shaukat, F.; Gul, A.; Arooj, M.; Malik, A. Potential role of amino acids in pathogenesis of schizophrenia. *Int. J. Health Sci. (Quassim)* **2017**, *11*, 63–68.
60. Farber, N.B. The NMDA receptor hypofunction model of psychosis. *Ann. N. Y. Acad. Sci.* **2003**, *1003*, 119–130. [CrossRef] [PubMed]
61. Goff, D.C. Glutamate receptors in schizophrenia and antipsychotic drugs, in Neurotransmitter Receptors. In *Actions of Antipsychotic Medications*; Lidow, M.S., Ed.; CRC Press: New York, NY, USA, 2000; pp. 121–136.
62. Meador-Woodruff, J.H.; Healy, D.J. Glutamate receptor expression in schizophrenic brain. *Brain Res. Brain Res. Rev.* **2000**, *31*, 288–294. [CrossRef]
63. Gao, X.M.; Sakai, K.; Roberts, R.C.; Conley, R.R.; Dean, B.; Tamminga, C.A. Ionotropic glutamate receptors and expression of *N*-methyl-D-aspartate receptor subunits in subregions of human hippocampus: Effects of schizophrenia. *Am. J. Psychiatry* **2000**, *157*, 1141–1149. [CrossRef] [PubMed]
64. Ibrahim, H.M.; Hogg, A.J.; Healy, D.J.; Haroutunian, V.; Davis, K.L.; Meador-Woodruff, J.H. Ionotropic glutamate receptor binding and subunit mRNA expression in thalamic nuclei in schizophrenia. *Am. J. Psychiatry* **2000**, *157*, 1811–1823. [CrossRef] [PubMed]
65. Heckers, S.; Goff, D.; Schacter, D.L.; Savage, C.R.; Fischman, A.J.; Alpert, N.M.; Rauch, S.L. Functional imaging of memory retrieval in deficit vs nondeficit schizophrenia. *Arch. Gen. Psychiatry* **1999**, *56*, 1117–1123. [CrossRef] [PubMed]
66. Kondziella, D.; Brenner, E.; Eyjolfsson, E.M.; Sonnewald, U. How do glial–neuronal interactions fit into current neurotransmitter hypotheses of schizophrenia? *Neurochem. Int.* **2007**, *50*, 291–301. [CrossRef] [PubMed]
67. Stone, J.M.; Morrison, P.D.; Pilowsky, L.S. Glutamate and dopamine dysregulation in schizophrenia—A synthesis and selective review. *J. Psychopharmacol. Oxf. Engl.* **2007**, *21*, 440–452. [CrossRef] [PubMed]
68. Kaiser, L.G.; Schuff, N.; Cashdollar, N.; Weiner, M.W. Age-related glutamate and glutamine concentration changes in normal human brain: ^{1}H MR spectroscopy study at 4 T. *Neurobiol. Aging* **2005**, *26*, 665–672. [CrossRef] [PubMed]
69. Leveque, J.C.; Macías, W.; Rajadhyaksha, A.; Carlson, R.R.; Barczak, A.; Kang, S.; Li, X.M.; Coyle, J.T.; Huganir, R.L.; Heckers, S.; et al. Intracellular modulation of NMDA receptor function by antipsychotic drugs. *J. Neurosci. Off. J. Soc. Neurosci.* **2000**, *20*, 4011–4020. [CrossRef]
70. Arvanov, V.L.; Liang, X.; Schwartz, J.; Grossman, S.; Wang, R.Y. Clozapine and haloperidol modulate *N*-methyl-D-aspartate- and non-*N*-methyl-D-aspartate receptor-mediated neurotransmission in rat prefrontal cortical neurons in vitro. *J. Pharmacol. Exp. Ther.* **1997**, *283*, 226–234. [PubMed]
71. Hashimoto, K.; Malchow, B.; Falkai, P.; Schmitt, A. Glutamate modulators as potential therapeutic drugs in schizophrenia and affective disorders. *Eur. Arch. Psychiatry Clin. Neurosci.* **2013**, *263*, 367–377. [CrossRef] [PubMed]
72. Menniti, F.S.; Lindsley, C.W.; Conn, P.J.; Pandit, J.; Zagouras, P.; Volkmann, R.A. Allosteric modulators for the treatment of schizophrenia: Targeting glutamatergic networks. *Curr. Top. Med. Chem.* **2013**, *13*, 26–54. [CrossRef] [PubMed]
73. Ward, S.E.; Pennicott, L.E.; Beswick, P. AMPA receptor-positive allosteric modulators for the treatment of schizophrenia: An overview of recent patent applications. *Future Med. Chem.* **2015**, *7*, 473–491. [CrossRef] [PubMed]
74. Herman, E.J.; Bubser, M.; Conn, P.J.; Jones, C.K. Metabotropic glutamate receptors for new treatments in schizophrenia. *Handb. Exp. Pharmacol.* **2012**, 297–365. [CrossRef]
75. Li, M.-L.; Hu, X.-Q.; Li, F.; Gao, W.-J. Perspectives on the mGluR2/3 agonists as a therapeutic target for schizophrenia: Still promising or a dead end? *Prog. Neuropsychopharmacol. Biol. Psychiatry* **2015**, *60*, 66–76. [CrossRef] [PubMed]

76. O'Leary, O.; Nolan, Y. Glycogen synthase kinase-3 as a therapeutic target for cognitive dysfunction in neuropsychiatric disorders. *CNS Drugs* **2015**, *29*, 1–15. [CrossRef] [PubMed]
77. Snyder, G.L.; Vanover, K.E. PDE Inhibitors for the Treatment of Schizophrenia. *Adv. Neurobiol.* **2017**, *17*, 385–409. [CrossRef] [PubMed]
78. Singh, J.; Kour, K.; Jayaram, M.B. Acetylcholinesterase inhibitors for schizophrenia. *Cochrane Database Syst. Rev.* **2012**, *1*, CD007967. [CrossRef] [PubMed]
79. Medina-Franco, J.L.; Giulianotti, M.A.; Welmaker, G.S.; Houghten, R.A. Shifting from the single to the multitarget paradigm in drug discovery. *Drug Discov. Today* **2013**, *18*, 495–501. [CrossRef] [PubMed]
80. Zheng, H.; Fridkin, M.; Youdim, M. From Single Target to Multitarget/Network Therapeutics in Alzheimer's Therapy. *Pharmaceuticals* **2014**, *7*, 113–135. [CrossRef] [PubMed]
81. Bansal, Y.; Silakari, O. Multifunctional compounds: Smart molecules for multifactorial diseases. *Eur. J. Med. Chem.* **2014**, *76*, 31–42. [CrossRef] [PubMed]
82. Méndez-Lucio, O.; Naveja, J.J.; Vite-Caritino, H.; Prieto-Martínez, F.D.; Medina-Franco, J.L.; Méndez-Lucio, O.; Naveja, J.J.; Vite-Caritino, H.; Prieto-Martínez, F.D.; Medina-Franco, J.L. Review. One Drug for Multiple Targets: A Computational Perspective. *J. Mex. Chem. Soc.* **2016**, *60*, 168–181.
83. Talevi, A. Multi-target pharmacology: Possibilities and limitations of the "skeleton key approach" from a medicinal chemist perspective. *Front. Pharmacol.* **2015**, *6*. [CrossRef] [PubMed]
84. Wichur, T.; Malawska, B. Multifunctional ligands—A new approach in the search for drugs against multi-factorial diseases. *Postepy Hig. Med. Doswiadczalnej Online* **2015**, *69*, 1423–1434.
85. Morphy, R.; Rankovic, Z. Designed Multiple Ligands. An Emerging Drug Discovery Paradigm. *J. Med. Chem.* **2005**, *48*, 6523–6543. [CrossRef] [PubMed]
86. Kaczor, A.A.; Silva, A.G.; Loza, M.I.; Kolb, P.; Castro, M.; Poso, A. Structure-Based Virtual Screening for Dopamine D_2 Receptor Ligands as Potential Antipsychotics. *ChemMedChem* **2016**, *11*, 718–729. [CrossRef] [PubMed]
87. Bawa, P.; Pradeep, P.; Kumar, P.; Choonara, Y.E.; Modi, G.; Pillay, V. Multi-target therapeutics for neuropsychiatric and neurodegenerative disorders. *Drug Discov. Today* **2016**, *21*, 1886–1914. [CrossRef] [PubMed]
88. Roth, B.L.; Sheffler, D.J.; Kroeze, W.K. Magic shotguns versus magic bullets: Selectively non-selective drugs for mood disorders and schizophrenia. *Nat. Rev. Drug Discov.* **2004**, *3*, 353–359. [CrossRef] [PubMed]
89. Naheed, M.; Green, B. Focus on Clozapine. *Curr. Med. Res. Opin.* **2001**, *17*, 223–229. [CrossRef] [PubMed]
90. Saklad, S.R. Graphic representation of pharmacology: Development of an alternative model. *Ment. Health Clin.* **2018**, *7*, 201–206. [CrossRef] [PubMed]
91. Boyda, H.N.; Ramos-Miguel, A.; Procyshyn, R.M.; Töpfer, E.; Lant, N.; Choy, H.H.T.; Wong, R.; Li, L.; Pang, C.C.Y.; Honer, W.G.; et al. Routine exercise ameliorates the metabolic side-effects of treatment with the atypical antipsychotic drug olanzapine in rats. *Int. J. Neuropsychopharmacol.* **2014**, *17*, 77–90. [CrossRef] [PubMed]
92. He, M.; Zhang, Q.; Deng, C.; Wang, H.; Lian, J.; Huang, X.-F. Hypothalamic histamine H1 receptor-AMPK signaling time-dependently mediates olanzapine-induced hyperphagia and weight gain in female rats. *Psychoneuroendocrinology* **2014**, *42*, 153–164. [CrossRef] [PubMed]
93. Godlewska, B.R.; Olajossy-Hilkesberger, L.; Ciwoniuk, M.; Olajossy, M.; Marmurowska-Michałowska, H.; Limon, J.; Landowski, J. Olanzapine-induced weight gain is associated with the -759C/T and -697G/C polymorphisms of the *HTR2C* gene. *Pharmacogenomics J.* **2009**, *9*, 234–241. [CrossRef] [PubMed]
94. Stephenson, C.M.; Pilowsky, L.S. Psychopharmacology of olanzapine. A. review. *Br. J. Psychiatry Suppl.* **1999**, *38*, 52–58. [CrossRef]
95. Selent, J.; López, L.; Sanz, F.; Pastor, M. Multi-receptor binding profile of clozapine and olanzapine: A structural study based on the new β2 adrenergic receptor template. *ChemMedChem* **2008**, *3*, 1194–1198. [CrossRef] [PubMed]
96. Piróg-Balcerzak, A.; Habrat, B.; Mierzejewski, P. Misuse and abuse of quetiapine. *Psychiatr. Pol.* **2015**, *49*, 81–93. [CrossRef] [PubMed]
97. George, B.; Craig, S. *Brenner and Stevens' Pharmacology*, 5th ed.; Elsevier: Amsterdam, The Netherlands, 2017.
98. Hasnain, M.; Vieweg, W.V.R. Weight considerations in psychotropic drug prescribing and switching. *Postgrad. Med.* **2013**, *125*, 117–129. [CrossRef] [PubMed]

99. Fornaro, M.; de Berardis, D.; Perna, G.; Solmi, M.; Veronese, N.; Orsolini, L.; Buonaguro, E.F.; Iasevoli, F.; Köhler, C.A.; Carvalho, A.F.; et al. Lurasidone in the Treatment of Bipolar Depression: Systematic Review of Systematic Reviews. *BioMed Res. Int.* **2017**, *2017*, 3084859. [CrossRef] [PubMed]
100. Urs, N.M.; Peterson, S.M.; Caron, M.G. New Concepts in Dopamine D_2 Receptor Biased Signaling and Implications for Schizophrenia Therapy. *Biol. Psychiatry* **2017**, *81*, 78–85. [CrossRef] [PubMed]
101. Brust, T.F.; Hayes, M.P.; Roman, D.L.; Watts, V.J. New functional activity of aripiprazole revealed. Robust antagonism of D_2 dopamine receptor stimulated by $G\beta\gamma$ antagonism. *Biochem Pharmacol.* **2015**, *93*, 85–91. [CrossRef] [PubMed]
102. Tamminga, C.A. Partial dopamine agonists in the treatment of psychosis. *J. Neural Transm. Vienna Austria 1996* **2002**, *109*, 411–420. [CrossRef] [PubMed]
103. Mailman, R.B.; Murthy, V. Third generation antipsychotic drugs: Partial agonism or receptor functional selectivity? *Curr. Pharm. Des.* **2010**, *16*, 488–501. [CrossRef] [PubMed]
104. Lieberman, J.A. Dopamine partial agonists: A new class of antipsychotic. *CNS Drugs* **2004**, *18*, 251–267. [CrossRef] [PubMed]
105. Allen, J.A.; Yost, J.M.; Setola, V.; Chen, X.; Sassano, M.F.; Chen, M.; Peterson, S.; Yadav, P.N.; Huang, X.; Feng, B.; et al. Discovery of β-arrestin-biased dopamine D_2 ligands for probing signal transduction pathways essential for antipsychotic efficacy. *Proc. Natl. Acad. Sci. USA* **2011**, *108*, 18488–18493. [CrossRef] [PubMed]
106. Burris, K.D.; Molski, T.F.; Xu, C.; Ryan, E.; Tottori, K.; Kikuchi, T.; Yocca, F.D.; Molinoff, P.B. Aripiprazole, a novel antipsychotic, is a high-affinity partial agonist at human dopamine D_2 receptors. *J. Pharmacol. Exp. Ther.* **2002**, *302*, 381–389. [CrossRef] [PubMed]
107. Shapiro, D.A.; Renock, S.; Arrington, E.; Chiodo, L.A.; Liu, L.-X.; Sibley, D.R.; Roth, B.L.; Mailman, R. Aripiprazole, a novel atypical antipsychotic drug with a unique and robust pharmacology. *Neuropsychopharmacol. Off. Publ. Am. Coll. Neuropsychopharmacol.* **2003**, *28*, 1400–1411. [CrossRef] [PubMed]
108. Lawler, C.P.; Prioleau, C.; Lewis, M.M.; Mak, C.; Jiang, D.; Schetz, J.A.; Gonzalez, A.M.; Sibley, D.R.; Mailman, R.B. Interactions of the novel antipsychotic aripiprazole (OPC-14597) with dopamine and serotonin receptor subtypes. *Neuropsychopharmacol. Off. Publ. Am. Coll. Neuropsychopharmacol.* **1999**, *20*, 612–627. [CrossRef]
109. Fell, M.J.; Perry, K.W.; Falcone, J.F.; Johnson, B.G.; Barth, V.N.; Rash, K.S.; Lucaites, V.L.; Threlkeld, P.G.; Monn, J.A.; McKinzie, D.L.; et al. In vitro and in vivo evidence for a lack of interaction with dopamine D_2 receptors by the metabotropic glutamate 2/3 receptor agonists 1*S*,2*S*,5*R*,6*S*-2-aminobicyclo[3.1.0]hexane-2,6-bicaroxylate monohydrate (LY354740) and (−)-2-oxa-4-aminobicyclo[3.1.0] Hexane-4,6-dicarboxylic acid (LY379268). *J. Pharmacol. Exp. Ther.* **2009**, *331*, 1126–1136. [CrossRef] [PubMed]
110. Masri, B.; Salahpour, A.; Didriksen, M.; Ghisi, V.; Beaulieu, J.-M.; Gainetdinov, R.R.; Caron, M.G. Antagonism of dopamine D_2 receptor/β-arrestin 2 interaction is a common property of clinically effective antipsychotics. *Proc. Natl. Acad. Sci. USA* **2008**, *105*, 13656–13661. [CrossRef] [PubMed]
111. Klewe, I.V.; Nielsen, S.M.; Tarpø, L.; Urizar, E.; Dipace, C.; Javitch, J.A.; Gether, U.; Egebjerg, J.; Christensen, K.V. Recruitment of β-arrestin2 to the dopamine D_2 receptor: Insights into anti-psychotic and anti-parkinsonian drug receptor signaling. *Neuropharmacology* **2008**, *54*, 1215–1222. [CrossRef] [PubMed]
112. Ribeiro, E.L.A.; de Mendonça Lima, T.; Vieira, M.E.B.; Storpirtis, S.; Aguiar, P.M. Efficacy and safety of aripiprazole for the treatment of schizophrenia: An overview of systematic reviews. *Eur. J. Clin. Pharmacol.* **2018**. [CrossRef] [PubMed]
113. Leucht, S.; Cipriani, A.; Spineli, L.; Mavridis, D.; Orey, D.; Richter, F.; Samara, M.; Barbui, C.; Engel, R.R.; Geddes, J.R.; et al. Comparative efficacy and tolerability of 15 antipsychotic drugs in schizophrenia: A multiple-treatments meta-analysis. *Lancet Lond. Engl.* **2013**, *382*, 951–962. [CrossRef]
114. Diefenderfer, L.A.; Iuppa, C. Brexpiprazole: A review of a new treatment option for schizophrenia and major depressive disorder. *Ment. Health Clin.* **2017**, *7*, 207–212. [CrossRef] [PubMed]
115. McEvoy, J.; Citrome, L. Brexpiprazole for the Treatment of Schizophrenia: A Review of this Novel Serotonin-Dopamine Activity Modulator. *Clin. Schizophr. Relat. Psychoses* **2016**, *9*, 177–186. [CrossRef] [PubMed]
116. Campbell, R.H.; Diduch, M.; Gardner, K.N.; Thomas, C. Review of cariprazine in management of psychiatric illness. *Ment. Health Clin.* **2017**, *7*, 221–229. [CrossRef] [PubMed]

117. De Berardis, D.; Orsolini, L.; Iasevoli, F.; Prinzivalli, E.; de Bartolomeis, A.; Serroni, N.; Mazza, M.; Valchera, A.; Fornaro, M.; Vecchiotti, R.; et al. The Novel Antipsychotic Cariprazine (RGH-188): State-of-the-Art in the Treatment of Psychiatric Disorders. *Curr. Pharm. Des.* **2016**, *22*, 5144–5162. [CrossRef] [PubMed]
118. Marciniec, K.; Kurczab, R.; Książek, M.; Bębenek, E.; Chrobak, E.; Satała, G.; Bojarski, A.J.; Kusz, J.; Zajdel, P. Structural determinants influencing halogen bonding: A case study on azinesulfonamide analogs of aripiprazole as 5-HT_{1A}, 5-HT_7, and D_2 receptor ligands. *Chem. Cent. J.* **2018**, *12*, 55. [CrossRef] [PubMed]
119. Zajdel, P.; Marciniec, K.; Maślankiewicz, A.; Grychowska, K.; Satała, G.; Duszyńska, B.; Lenda, T.; Siwek, A.; Nowak, G.; Partyka, A.; et al. Antidepressant and antipsychotic activity of new quinoline- and isoquinoline-sulfonamide analogs of aripiprazole targeting serotonin 5-HT_{1A}/5-HT_{2A}/5-HT_7 and dopamine D_2/D_3 receptors. *Eur. J. Med. Chem.* **2013**, *60*, 42–50. [CrossRef] [PubMed]
120. Butini, S.; Gemma, S.; Campiani, G.; Franceschini, S.; Trotta, F.; Borriello, M.; Ceres, N.; Ros, S.; Coccone, S.S.; Bernetti, M.; et al. Discovery of a New Class of Potential Multifunctional Atypical Antipsychotic Agents Targeting Dopamine D_3 and Serotonin 5-HT_{1A} and 5-HT_{2A} Receptors: Design, Synthesis, and Effects on Behavior. *J. Med. Chem.* **2009**, *52*, 151–169. [CrossRef] [PubMed]
121. Butini, S.; Campiani, G.; Franceschini, S.; Trotta, F.; Kumar, V.; Guarino, E.; Borrelli, G.; Fiorini, I.; Novellino, E.; Fattorusso, C.; et al. Discovery of bishomo(hetero)arylpiperazines as novel multifunctional ligands targeting dopamine D_3 and serotonin 5-HT_{1A} and 5-HT_{2A} receptors. *J. Med. Chem.* **2010**, *53*, 4803–4807. [CrossRef] [PubMed]
122. Zajdel, P.; Marciniec, K.; Maślankiewicz, A.; Satała, G.; Duszyńska, B.; Bojarski, A.J.; Partyka, A.; Jastrzbska-Wisek, M.; Wróbel, D.; Wesołowska, A.; et al. Quinoline- and isoquinoline-sulfonamide derivatives of LCAP as potent CNS multi-receptor—5-HT_{1A}/5-HT_{2A}/5-HT_7 and D_2/D_3/D_4—Agents: The synthesis and pharmacological evaluation. *Bioorg. Med. Chem.* **2012**, *20*, 1545–1556. [CrossRef] [PubMed]
123. Partyka, A.; Kurczab, R.; Canale, V.; Satała, G.; Marciniec, K.; Pasierb, A.; Jastrzębska-Więsek, M.; Pawłowski, M.; Wesołowska, A.; Bojarski, A.J.; et al. The impact of the halogen bonding on D_2 and 5-HT_{1A}/5-HT_7 receptor activity of azinesulfonamides of 4-[(2-ethyl)piperidinyl-1-yl]phenylpiperazines with antipsychotic and antidepressant properties. *Bioorg. Med. Chem.* **2017**, *25*, 3638–3648. [CrossRef] [PubMed]
124. Bhosale, S.H.; Kanhed, A.M.; Dash, R.C.; Suryawanshi, M.R.; Mahadik, K.R. Design, synthesis, pharmacological evaluation and computational studies of 1-(biphenyl-4-yl)-2-[4-(substituted phenyl)-piperazin-1-yl]ethanones as potential antipsychotics. *Eur. J. Med. Chem.* **2014**, *74*, 358–365. [CrossRef] [PubMed]
125. Van Dijk, H.G.; Dapper, E.A.; Vinkers, C.H. SSRIs and depressive symptoms in schizophrenia: A. systematic review. *Tijdschr. Voor Psychiatr.* **2017**, *59*, 40–46.
126. Van Hes, R.; Smid, P.; Stroomer, C.N.J.; Tipker, K.; Tulp, M.T.M.; van der Heyden, J.A.M.; McCreary, A.C.; Hesselink, M.B.; Kruse, C.G. SLV310, a novel, potential antipsychotic, combining potent dopamine D_2 receptor antagonism with serotonin reuptake inhibition. *Bioorg. Med. Chem. Lett.* **2003**, *13*, 405–408. [CrossRef]
127. Smid, P.; Coolen, H.K.A.C.; Keizer, H.G.; van Hes, R.; de Mos, J.-P.; den Hartog, A.P.; Stork, B.; Plekkenpol, R.H.; Niemann, L.C.; Stroomer, C.N.J.; et al. Synthesis, structure-activity relationships, and biological properties of 1-heteroaryl-4-[ω-(1H-indol-3-yl)alkyl]piperazines, novel potential antipsychotics combining potent dopamine D_2 receptor antagonism with potent serotonin reuptake inhibition. *J. Med. Chem.* **2005**, *48*, 6855–6869. [CrossRef] [PubMed]
128. Li, P.; Zhang, Q.; Robichaud, A.J.; Lee, T.; Tomesch, J.; Yao, W.; Beard, J.D.; Snyder, G.L.; Zhu, H.; Peng, Y.; et al. Discovery of a Tetracyclic Quinoxaline Derivative as a Potent and Orally Active Multifunctional Drug Candidate for the Treatment of Neuropsychiatric and Neurological Disorders. *J. Med. Chem.* **2014**, *57*, 2670–2682. [CrossRef] [PubMed]
129. Zajdel, P.; Kos, T.; Marciniec, K.; Satała, G.; Canale, V.; Kamiński, K.; Hołuj, M.; Lenda, T.; Koralewski, R.; Bednarski, M.; et al. Novel multi-target azinesulfonamides of cyclic amine derivatives as potential antipsychotics with pro-social and pro-cognitive effects. *Eur. J. Med. Chem.* **2018**, *145*, 790–804. [CrossRef] [PubMed]
130. Menegatti, R.; Cunha, A.C.; Ferreira, V.F.; Perreira, E.F.; El-Nabawi, A.; Eldefrawi, A.T.; Albuquerque, E.X.; Neves, G.; Rates, S.M.; Fraga, C.A.; et al. Design, synthesis and pharmacological profile of novel dopamine D_2 receptor ligands. *Bioorg. Med. Chem.* **2003**, *11*, 4807–4813. [CrossRef]

131. Neves, G.; Antonio, C.B.; Betti, A.H.; Pranke, M.A.; Fraga, C.A.M.; Barreiro, E.J.; Noël, F.; Rates, S.M.K. New insights into pharmacological profile of LASSBio-579, a multi-target *N*-phenylpiperazine derivative active on animal models of schizophrenia. *Behav. Brain Res.* **2013**, *237*, 86–95. [CrossRef] [PubMed]
132. Pompeu, T.E.T.; Alves, F.R.S.; Figueiredo, C.D.M.; Antonio, C.B.; Herzfeldt, V.; Moura, B.C.; Rates, S.M.K.; Barreiro, E.J.; Fraga, C.A.M.; Noël, F. Synthesis and pharmacological evaluation of new N-phenylpiperazine derivatives designed as homologues of the antipsychotic lead compound LASSBio-579. *Eur. J. Med. Chem.* **2013**, *66*, 122–134. [CrossRef] [PubMed]
133. Kaczor, A.A.; Targowska-Duda, K.M.; Budzyńska, B.; Biała, G.; Silva, A.G.; Castro, M. In vitro, molecular modeling and behavioral studies of 3-{[4-(5-methoxy-1H-indol-3-yl)-1,2,3,6-tetrahydropyridin-1-yl]methyl}-1,2-dihydroquinolin-2-one (D2AAK1) as a potential antipsychotic. *Neurochem. Int.* **2016**, *96*, 84–99. [CrossRef] [PubMed]
134. Ivachtchenko, A.V.; Lavrovsky, Y.; Okun, I. AVN-101: A Multi-Target Drug Candidate for the Treatment of CNS Disorders. *J. Alzheimers Dis.* **2016**, *53*, 583–620. [CrossRef] [PubMed]
135. Brea, J.; Castro, M.; Loza, M.I.; Masaguer, C.F.; Raviña, E.; Dezi, C.; Pastor, M.; Sanz, F.; Cabrero-Castel, A.; Galán-Rodríguez, B.; et al. QF2004B, a potential antipsychotic butyrophenone derivative with similar pharmacological properties to clozapine. *Neuropharmacology* **2006**, *51*, 251–262. [CrossRef] [PubMed]
136. Huang, L.; Zhang, W.; Zhang, X.; Yin, L.; Chen, B.; Song, J. Synthesis and pharmacological evaluation of piperidine (piperazine)-substituted benzoxazole derivatives as multi-target antipsychotics. *Bioorg. Med. Chem. Lett.* **2015**, *25*, 5299–5305. [CrossRef] [PubMed]
137. Chen, Y.; Wang, S.; Xu, X.; Liu, X.; Yu, M.; Zhao, S.; Liu, S.; Qiu, Y.; Zhang, T.; Liu, B.-F.; et al. Synthesis and biological investigation of coumarin piperazine (piperidine) derivatives as potential multireceptor atypical antipsychotics. *J. Med. Chem.* **2013**, *56*, 4671–4690. [CrossRef] [PubMed]
138. Chen, X.-W.; Sun, Y.-Y.; Fu, L.; Li, J.-Q. Synthesis and pharmacological characterization of novel *N*-(trans-4-(2-(4-(benzo[d]isothiazol-3-yl)piperazin-1-yl)ethyl)cyclohexyl)amides as potential multireceptor atypical antipsychotics. *Eur. J. Med. Chem.* **2016**, *123*, 332–353. [CrossRef] [PubMed]
139. Xiamuxi, H.; Wang, Z.; Li, J.; Wang, Y.; Wu, C.; Yang, F.; Jiang, X.; Liu, Y.; Zhao, Q.; Chen, W.; et al. Synthesis and biological investigation of tetrahydropyridopyrimidinone derivatives as potential multireceptor atypical antipsychotics. *Bioorg. Med. Chem.* **2017**, *25*, 4904–4916. [CrossRef] [PubMed]
140. Yang, F.; Jiang, X.; Li, J.; Wang, Y.; Liu, Y.; Bi, M.; Wu, C.; Zhao, Q.; Chen, W.; Yin, J.; et al. Synthesis, structure-activity relationships, and biological evaluation of a series of benzamides as potential multireceptor antipsychotics. *Bioorg. Med. Chem. Lett.* **2016**, *26*, 3141–3147. [CrossRef] [PubMed]

2

The Performance of Gene Expression Signature-Guided Drug–Disease Association in Different Categories of Drugs and Diseases

Xiguang Qi [1], Mingzhe Shen [1], Peihao Fan [1], Xiaojiang Guo [1], Tianqi Wang [2], Ning Feng [3], Manling Zhang [3], Robert A. Sweet [4,5,*], Levent Kirisci [1,*] and Lirong Wang [1,*]

1 Department of Pharmaceutical Sciences, Computational Chemical Genomics Screening Center, University of Pittsburgh School of Pharmacy, 3501 Terrace St Pittsburgh, PA 15261, USA; Xiq24@pitt.edu (X.Q.); MIS216@pitt.edu (M.S.); pef14@pitt.edu (P.F.); xig53@pitt.edu (X.G.)
2 Department of Biological Sciences, University of Pittsburgh School of Arts & Sciences, Pittsburgh, PA 15260, USA; Lu_Wang@pitt.edu
3 Division of Cardiology, Vascular Medicine Institute, University of Pittsburgh School of Medicine, Pittsburgh, PA 15213, USA; FENGN@pitt.edu (N.F.); zhangm5@upmc.edu (M.Z.)
4 Department of Neurology, University of Pittsburgh School of Medicine, Pittsburgh, PA 15213, USA
5 Department of Psychiatry, University of Pittsburgh School of Medicine, Pittsburgh, PA 15213, USA
* Correspondence: sweetra@upmc.edu (R.A.S.); levent@pitt.edu (L.K.); Liw30@pitt.edu (L.W.)

Academic Editors: Marco Tutone and Anna Maria Almerico

Abstract: A gene expression signature (GES) is a group of genes that shows a unique expression profile as a result of perturbations by drugs, genetic modification or diseases on the transcriptional machinery. The comparisons between GES profiles have been used to investigate the relationships between drugs, their targets and diseases with quite a few successful cases reported. Especially in the study of GES-guided drugs–disease associations, researchers believe that if a GES induced by a drug is opposite to a GES induced by a disease, the drug may have potential as a treatment of that disease. In this study, we data-mined the crowd extracted expression of differential signatures (CREEDS) database to evaluate the similarity between GES profiles from drugs and their indicated diseases. Our study aims to explore the application domains of GES-guided drug–disease associations through the analysis of the similarity of GES profiles on known pairs of drug–disease associations, thereby identifying subgroups of drugs/diseases that are suitable for GES-guided drug repositioning approaches. Our results supported our hypothesis that the GES-guided drug–disease association method is better suited for some subgroups or pathways such as drugs and diseases associated with the immune system, diseases of the nervous system, non-chemotherapy drugs or the mTOR signaling pathway.

Keywords: gene expression signature; drug repositioning approaches; RNA expression regulation

1. Introduction

A gene expression signature (GES) is a set of comprehensive gene expression profiles that can reveal the difference between stimulated and normal cell states [1]. Current applications of GES analysis are fruitful in cancer-related areas for disease genotype classification and outcome predictions. For example, Ramaswamy, S. et al. created a GES database for diagnosing and categorizing the tumour type with an accuracy rate of 78% [2]. Wright, G. et al. developed a Bayesian rule-based algorithm to classify diffuse large B cell lymphoma into two subgroups which have a significant difference in the five-year survival rate [3]. Although the GES method is more commonly used in diagnosing cancer [2–5] and predicting the outcome of certain medical interventions [6,7], some successful cases of application on drug development have also reported [8–10].

Generally, there are two major strategies for applying GES analysis on drug development: drug–drug-based and drug–disease-based. The drug–drug-based method determines the mechanistic actions of drugs by comparing the similarity between the GES induced by a drug of interest to those of drugs with known mechanisms. If two different drugs have similar GES profiles, then they are considered to have "functional similarity", meaning they work in a similar manner. In contrast, the drug–disease-based method compares the similarity between the GES of a drug to that of a disease in order to determine its potential as a new therapeutic agent. If the GES profile of the drug is opposite to opposite to the expression pattern of the disease, then the drug is considered to have a therapeutic effect for the disease.

However, if they have similar patterns, then this drug may exacerbate the disease. Studies aimed at drug repurposing or repositioning based on GES analysis usually use one or both of these strategies [8–10]. In addition, there are studies trying to combine the GES method with other methods, such as machine learning, to increase the accuracy of compound indication prediction [11]. However, as those kinds of GES-guided drug repurposing studies usually just reported the successful predicted cases, therefore, the true accuracy of these methods needs to be assessed.

Due to the different and complex mechanisms of disease processes, the idea of an "inverse pattern of a GES between drugs and diseases for therapeutic effect" may not hold, or at least may not be suitable for all categories of drugs and diseases. In other words, a GES may be useful for certain diseases, but not for others. To our knowledge, the application domains of GES-guided drug–disease associations have not been reported. Herein, we conducted a study to validate the power of the GES-guided drug repositioning method and to further explore which specific subgroups of drug–disease pairs are more suitable for this method. Moreover, the most significant subgroup was selected as a case report of detailingwhich genes and/or pathways were more sensitive to the GES-guided drug repositioning method.

2. Results

2.1. GES Profiles Enrollment and Drug–Disease Pairs

After removing signatures from non-human assays and signatures of non-FDA (the U.S. Food and Drug Administration)-approved drugs, we found that GSE10432, GSE7036, GSE6264, GSE38713, GSE31773, GSE11393, GSE8157, GSE13887 and GSE11223 were signatures of both drugs and diseases from the same assays. We kept their disease labels except the CREEDS (crowd extracted expression of differential signatures [12]) ID of dz:297 because this case had information mis-specified (wrong disease information with its original experiment). Two GES profiles from mouse (drug:3288 and dz:724) were mis-specified as human and were also excluded from analysis. The relationship between these Gene Expression Omnibus (GEO) series (GSE) and CREEDS IDs is shown in Table 1. The proportion of data that meets the inclusion criteria is shown in Figure 1.

Table 1. The Gene Expression Omnibus (GEO) series with crowd extracted expression of differential signatures (CREEDS) IDs excluded.

GEO Series	CREEDS IDs	Excluded CREEDS IDs
GSE10432	drug:2772, dz:297	dz:297
GSE7036	drug:3292, dz:181	drug:3292
GSE6264	drug:3064, dz:582	drug:3064
GSE38713	drug:3289, drug:3194, drug:3195, dz:810	drug:3289, drug:3194, drug:3195
GSE31773	drug:2485, dz:712, dz:713, dz:714, dz:715	drug:2485
GSE11393	drug:3401, drug:3196, dz:773, dz:267	drug:3401, drug:3196
GSE8157	drug:2796, dz:880	drug:2796
GSE13887	drug:3181, dz:450	drug:3181,
GSE11223	drug:3294, drug:3287, dz:590, dz:591, dz:593, dz:589, dz:588, dz:587, dz:586, dz:585	drug:3294, drug:3287
GSE7762	drug:3288	drug:3288
GSE3248	dz:724	dz:724

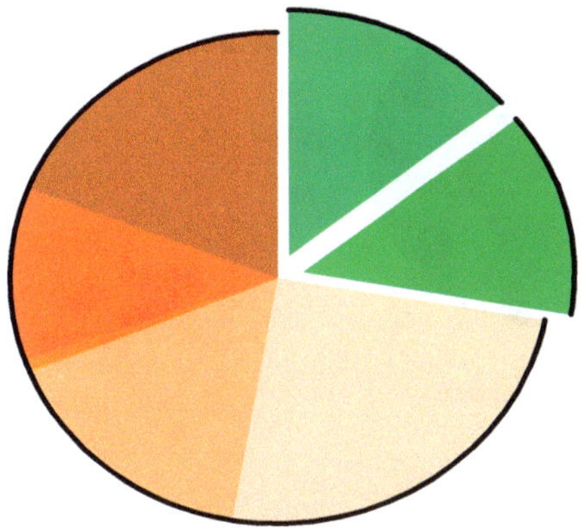

Figure 1. The proportion of data sourced from the crowd extracted expression of differential signatures (CREEDS) database. Numbers of gene signatures are shown in parentheses. "Drug and Disease Signatures Included in the Final Analysis": The proportion of drug or disease gene signatures enrolled in the final analysis. "Drug and Disease Signatures Extracted from Non-Human Assays": The proportion of drug or disease gene signatures extracted from non-human assays. "Signatures with Information Mis-Specified": The proportion of gene signatures with information errors. "Signatures from Same Assays but Labelled as Both": The proportion of gene signatures excluded because of both drug and disease sourcing from the same assay. "Drug and Disease Signatures Because of Indication Not Found": The proportion of gene signatures excluded because no FDA-labelled indication of a relationship was found for the drug or disease (including drugs not approved by FDA).

When the inclusion criteria were applied, and the signatures with no indication relationship were excluded, 230 manual disease signatures and 244 manual drug perturbation signatures from 71 unique diseases and 56 unique drugs, respectively, were enrolled in the final analysis. The average signed Jaccard indexes [12] (SJI) of 3976 unique drug–disease pairs were calculated. Among them, there were 167 pairs with a drug–disease indication from the drug labels. The remaining 3809 unique drug–disease pairs were used as the control group.

2.2. Subgroups Distribution

Among the 56 unique drugs analysed, 32 unique protein targets with 22 categories of Anatomical Therapeutic Chemical (ATC) classification were assigned. Thirteen drugs are classified as chemotherapy drugs, and 44 drugs are not (Methotrexate is both a chemotherapy and a non-chemotherapy drug due to its different main therapeutic targets when against different diseases). For transcription factor (TF) level, 12 drugs are labelled as "directly", 39 drugs are labelled as "not-directly" and 5 drugs were labelled as "non-Human" (see section *4.4. subgroup classification* for the detailed meanings of labels). Further, 71 diseases are divided into 11 ICD-11 (International Classification of Diseases 11th Revision) categories. In total, 70 subgroups belonging to five categories were assigned (Figure 2, detailed information in Table S1 and Table S2).

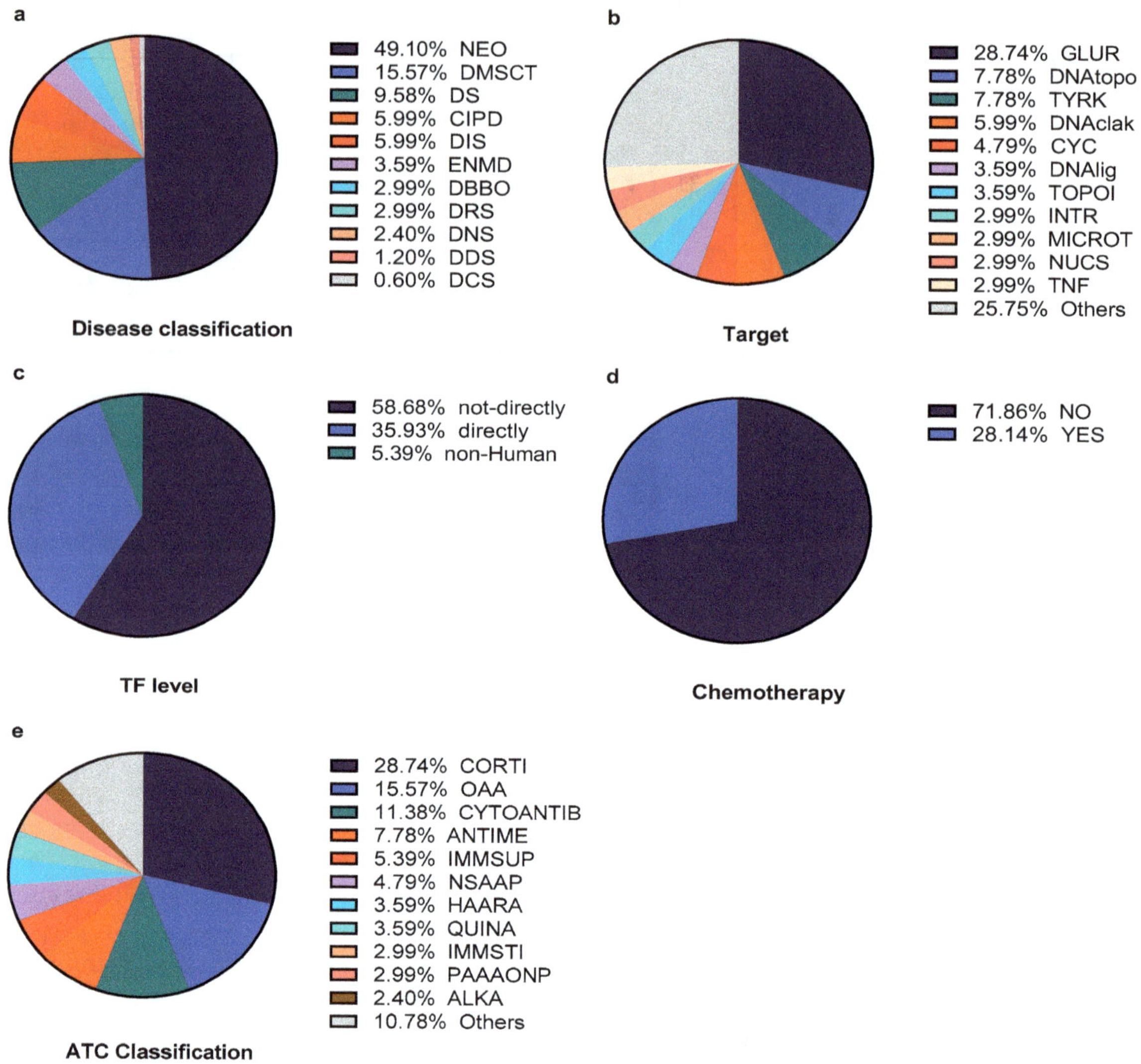

Figure 2. The subgroups proportion of unique 167 indicated drug–disease pairs of different categories. (**a**) Disease classification. NEO: neoplasms, DMSCT: diseases of the musculoskeletal system or connective tissue, DS: diseases of the skin, CIPD: certain infectious or parasitic diseases, DIS: diseases of the immune system, ENMD: endocrine, nutritional or metabolic diseases, DBBO: diseases of the blood or blood-forming organs, DRS: diseases of the respiratory system, DNS: diseases of the nervous system, DDS: diseases of the digestive system, DCS: diseases of the circulatory system. (**b**) Drug target. GLUR: glucocorticoid receptor, DNAtopo: DNA/topoisomerase-human, TYRK: tyrosine kinase, DNAclak: DNA cross-linking/alkylation, CYC: cyclooxygenase, DNAlig: DNA/ligase, TOPOI: topoisomerase-non-human, INTR: interferon receptor, MICROT: microtubules, NUCS: nucleotide synthesis, TNF: tumor necrosis factor. (**c**) TF (transcription factor) level. "Directly": drugs with TFs as its main therapeutic targets. "Not-directly" indicates drugs with main therapeutic targets which are human DNA structures or human proteins but not TFs. "Non-Human" represent drugs interacting

with protein or structures of non-human (for example, from virus or bacterial) as main therapeutic targets. (**d**) Chemotherapy. "YES" or "NO" indicates the drug is a chemotherapy drug or not. (**e**) ATC classification. CORTI: corticosteroids for systemic use, plain, OAA: other antineoplastic agents, CYTOANTIB: cytotoxic antibiotics and related substances, ANTIME: antimetabolites, IMMSUP: immunosuppressants, NSAAP: anti-inflammatory and antirheumatic products, non-steroids, HAARA: hormone antagonists and related agents, QUINA: quinolone antibacterial, IMMSTI: immunostimulants, PAAAONP: plant alkaloids and other natural products, ALKA: alkylating agents.

2.3. *Overall Score of GES Similarity of Drug-Indicted Disease Pairs Against Random Drug–Disease Pairs*

We observed significantly lower SJI similarity scores of drug–disease indication pairs than those of random drug–disease pairs (p-value of two-side t-test [13] equals to 0.02324). The average similarity score of indicated pairs is −0.00386 with a standard deviation of 0.01794 and that of random control pairs is −0.00072 with a standard deviation of 0.01750, indicating that the GES method can reflect the therapeutic effects of the drugs (The distributions of SJI in both the indication group and the control group are shown in Figure 3).

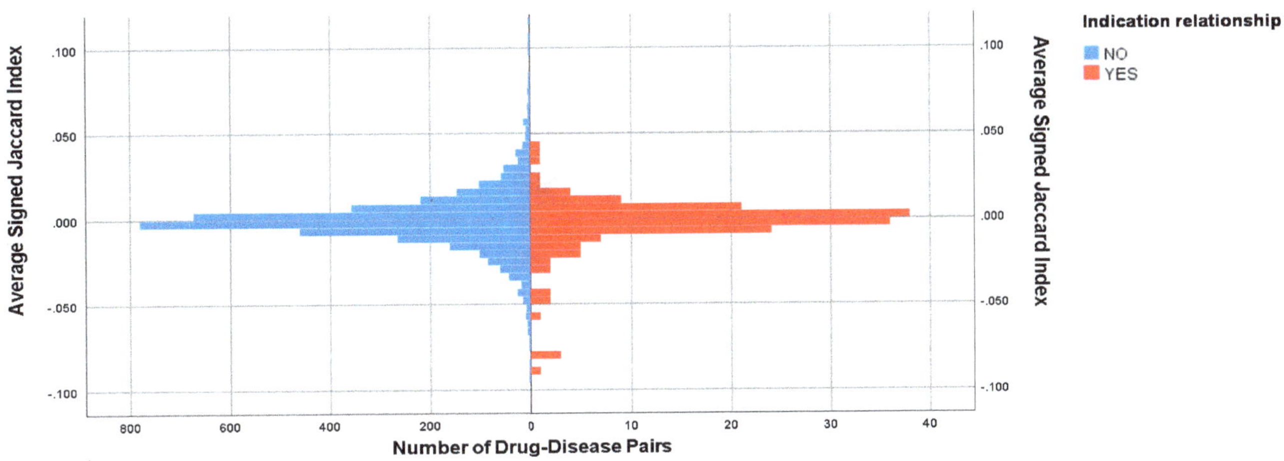

Figure 3. The distribution of signed Jaccard index in the indication group and the control group.

2.4. *Subgroup Scores of GES Similarity of Drug-Indicated Disease Pairs Against Random Drug–Disease Pairs*

We compared drugs from five different categories of subgroups: (1) disease classifications; (2) drug target; (3) TF level; (4) chemotherapy; and (5) ATC classification. The results are shown in Figure 4, detail information is listed in Table S3 and Table S4. Subgroups with important or significant (q-value according to false discover rate (FDR) lower than 0.05) results according to least squares mean partitions F tests of a generalized linear model (GLM) [14] are listed in Table 2.

Table 2. Subgroups of generalized linear model (GLM) least squares mean partitions F tests results.

Classification Category	Subgroups	Average SJI of Indicated Pairs ± SD	N	Average SJI of Control Pairs ± SD	N	Q value
Disease classification	Diseases of the blood or blood-forming organs	−0.02368 ± 0.03746	6	0.00075 ± 0.02470	138	0.01322
	Diseases of the nervous system	−0.03264 ± 0.03648	4	−0.00054 ± 0.01528	92	0.00704
Drug target classification	Interferon receptor	−0.02314 ± 0.03866	5	0.00916 ± 0.02849	115	0.00110
	Kinase mTOR	−0.05846 ± ———	1	0.00353 ± 0.01580	23	0.01755
Chemotherapy classification	Chemotherapy drugs	0.00048 ± 0.00894	47	−0.00022 ± 0.01221	1049	0.99509
	Non-chemotherapy drugs	−0.00556 ± 0.02026	120	−0.00086 ± 0.01872	2760	0.03937
ATC classification	Immunostimulants	−0.02314 ± 0.03866	5	0.00916 ± 0.02849	115	0.00110
	Other dermatological preparations	−0.05846 ± ———	1	−0.00353 ± 0.01580	23	0.01755
Transcription factor level	Directly	−0.00433 ± 0.02310	60	0.00070 ± 0.01671	1378	0.22309
	Not-directly	−0.00344 ± 0.01443	98	−0.00116 ± 0.01785	2224	0.99509
	Non-Human	−0.00533±0.01574	9	−0.00057 ± 0.01627	207	0.79080

Important subgroups or subgroups with false discover rate (FDR) q-value lower than 0.05 from GLM least squares mean partitions F tests for signed Jaccard index differences between drug-indicted disease pairs and random drug–disease pairs. "———" indicates that subgroups only have one unique drug–disease pair sample with no standard deviation.

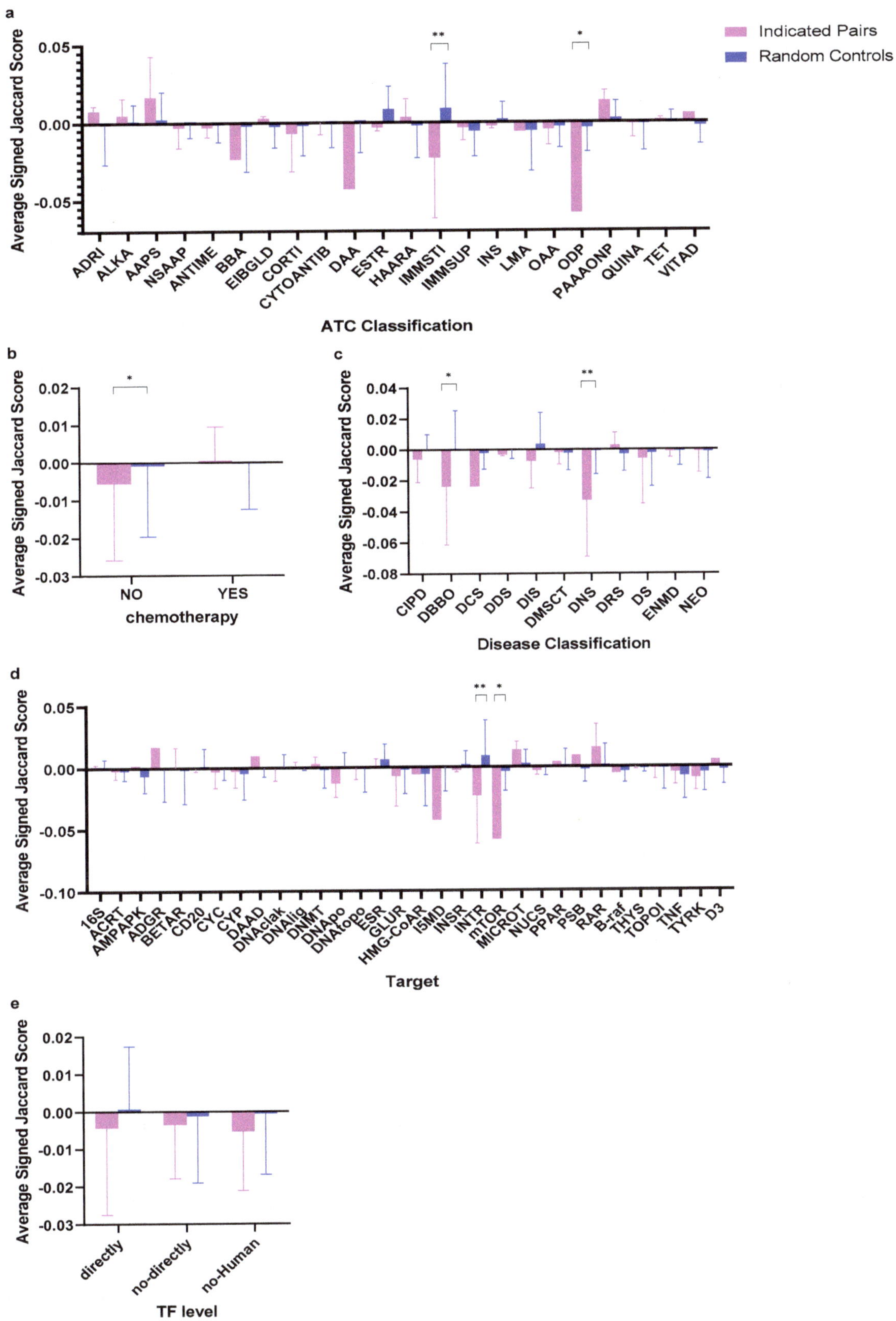

Figure 4. The average signed Jaccard index score of unique indicated drug–disease pairs split by different categories of subgroups. ** indicates FDR Q < 0.01, * indicates FDR Q < 0.05. (**a**) ATC classification. ADRI: adrenergics, inhalants, AAPS: anti-acne preparations for systemic use, EIBGLD:

blood glucose-lowering drugs, excluding insulins, DAA: direct acting antivirals, ESTR: estrogens, INS: insulins and analogues, LMA: lipid modifying agents, plain, ODP: other dermatological preparations, TET: tetracyclines, VITAD: vitamins A and D, including combinations of the two. CORTI, OAA, CYTOANTIB, ANTIME, IMMSUP, NSAAP, HAARA, QUINA, IMMSTI, PAAAONP, ALKA, see Figure 1 legend. (**b**) Chemotherapy. "YES" or "NO" indicates the drug is a chemotherapy drug or not. (**c**) Disease classification. See Figure 1 for abbreviations. (**d**) Target. 16S: 16S ribosomal RNA, ACRT: aminoimidazole caboxamide ribonucleotide transformylase, AMPAPK: AMP-activated protein kinase, ADGR: androgen receptor, BETAR: beta adrenergic receptor, CD20: CD20 antigen, CYP: cytochromes P450, DAAD: delta-aminolevulinic acid dehydratase, DNMT: DNA/methyltransferase, DNApo: DNA/polymerase, ESR: estrogen receptor, HMG-CoAR: HMG-CoA reductase, I5MD: inosine-5′-monophosphate dehydrogenase, INSR: insulin receptor, mTOR: kinase mTOR, PPAR: peroxisome proliferator-activated receptors, PSB: proteasome subunit beta, RAR: retinoic acid receptor, B-raf: serine/threonine-protein kinase B-raf, THYS: thymidylate synthase, D3: vitamin D3 receptor; GLUR, DNAtopo, TYRK, DNAclak, CYC, DNAlig, TOPOI, INTR, MICROT, NUCS, TNF see Figure 1 legend. (**e**) TF (transcription factor) level. "Directly": drugs with TFs as their main therapeutic targets. "Not-directly" indicates drugs with main therapeutic targets which are human DNA structures or human proteins but not TFs. "Non-Human" represents drugs interacting with non-human proteins or structures (for example, from viruses or bacteria) as main therapeutic targets.

2.5. Gene and Pathway Analysis on an Example Drug–Disease GES Pair

Interferon receptor (with the same drug–disease pair content as the immunostimulants subgroup), the subgroup with the lowest q-value, was chosen as a case report for the pathway analysis. The top 5% (93/1898) genes with a relatively reversed expression probability according to the relatively expression probability of a gene's ($G^{I\text{-}R\%}$, an indicator of the relative possibility difference of gene expression between the indicated group and the random control group, see below 4.5) scores are shown in Table 3. The top 10 significant biological pathways identified by the ingenuity pathway analysis are shown in Table 4.

Table 3. Top 5% genes with relatively expression probability ($G^{I\text{-}R\%}$).

Gene	$G^{I\text{-}R\%}$	Gene	$G^{I\text{-}R\%}$	Gene	$G^{I\text{-}R\%}$	Gene	$G^{I\text{-}R\%}$
MX1	−46.87%	FTL	−25.22%	USP18	−19.56%	DUSP6	−16.90%
IFIT3	−41.45%	RPL24	−25.18%	CERS2	−19.38%	TPT1	−16.66%
NME1	−40.50%	ERP29	−23.86%	RPLP0	−19.36%	RSAD2	−16.59%
RPL3	−39.19%	RSL24D1	−23.86%	KLRB1	−19.28%	ADAR	−16.48%
RPS5	−37.61%	PTMA	−23.65%	ADM	−19.23%	DDX58	−16.44%
RPL6	−36.57%	HLA-DRA	−22.88%	PLSCR1	−19.23%	APOBEC3A	−16.40%
MT1HL1	−35.52%	IFIT1	−22.22%	RPLP0P6	−19.14%	PPIB	−16.17%
MT2A	−34.80%	MX2	−22.22%	RPS3A	−19.07%	RGS2	−16.09%
RPSA	−33.55%	LDHB	−22.12%	TRIM22	−19.00%	IRF7	−16.08%
TGFBI	−33.47%	DYNLT1	−21.90%	DDX21	−18.66%	PSMA6	−16.00%
MT1X	−32.30%	ALDH1A1	−21.64%	GCH1	−18.64%	RPL9	−15.94%
HERC5	−32.15%	HSPA1A	−21.53%	GAPDH	−18.55%	OAS1	−15.91%
FAU	−31.82%	SLC25A5	−21.53%	OAS3	−18.48%	RPL31	−15.74%
PLS3	−29.66%	IFIT2	−21.38%	RPS25	−18.40%	PTTG1IP	−15.74%
HLA-A	−29.15%	RPS4X	−21.28%	NDUFB11	−18.40%	BIRC2	−15.74%
RPL22	−28.88%	EIF3E	−20.88%	SNHG6	−18.15%	MYD88	−15.67%
FBL	−28.52%	HMGN2	−20.88%	PSAT1	−18.06%	RPS14P3	−15.64%
RPS8	−27.57%	FTH1P5	−20.80%	IER2	−18.02%	FTH1	−15.62%
ISG15	−26.91%	YWHAZ	−20.72%	UXT	−17.65%	C4orf46	−15.45%
EEF1B2	−26.88%	PFDN5	−20.57%	PARP12	−17.58%	PPT1	−15.42%
PHB2	−26.48%	TMA7	−20.20%	MAFB	−17.40%	YBX1	−15.33%
MT1H	−26.29%	CCT7	−20.12%	LYZ	−17.25%		
RPL8	−26.11%	OASL	−19.89%	NARS	−17.15%		
ATF4	−25.36%	SNHG5	−19.64%	AKR1B1	−17.02%		

Table 4. Top 10 significant biological pathways according to high relatively expression probability genes.

Ingenuity Canonical Pathways	-log(p-value)	Ratio	Genes Overlapped with Datasets
EIF2 Signaling	16.50	8.02% (17/212)	ATF4, EIF3E, FAU, RPL22, RPL24, RPL3, RPL31, RPL6, RPL8, RPL9, RPLP0, RPS25, RPS3A, RPS4X, RPS5, RPS8, RPSA
Activation of IRF by Cytosolic Pattern Recognition Receptors	6.60	9.84% (6/61)	ADAR, DDX58, IFIT2, IRF7, ISG15, PPIB
Regulation of eIF4 and p70S6K Signaling	6.48	5.23% (8/153)	EIF3E, FAU, RPS25, RPS3A, RPS4X, RPS5, RPS8, RPSA
Interferon Signaling	6.34	13.90% (5/36)	IFIT1, IFIT3, ISG15, MX1, OAS1
mTOR Signaling	5.57	3.96% (8/202)	EIF3E, FAU, RPS25, RPS3A, RPS4X, RPS5, RPS8, RPSA
NRF2-mediated Oxidative Stress Response	3.80	3.23% (6/186)	ATF4, CCT7, ERP29, FTH1, FTL, PPIB
Role of Pattern Recognition Receptors in Recognition of Bacteria and Viruses	3.39	3.47% (5/144)	DDX58, IRF7, MYD88, OAS1, OAS3
Neuroinflammation Signaling Pathway	2.78	2.06% (6/291)	ATF4, BIRC2, HLA-A, HLA-DRA, IRF7, MYD88
SPINK1 General Cancer Pathway	2.63	4.92% (3/61)	MT1H, MT1X, MT2A
Systemic Lupus Erythematosus in B Cell Signaling Pathway	2.23	1.89% (5/265)	IFIT2, IFIT3, IRF7, ISG15, MYD88

These 10 pathways are reported to be involved with interferon regulation [15–27]. within inflammatory and immune responses (see Table 5).

Table 5. Top 10 pathways and their function labels.

Ingenuity Canonical Pathways	Function	Reference
EIF2 Signaling	Immune Responses	[28]
Activation of IRF by Cytosolic Pattern Recognition Receptors	Regulate Interferon	[17]
Regulation of eIF4 and p70S6K Signaling	Inflammatory	[18,29]
Interferon Signaling	Immune Responses	[30,31]
mTOR Signaling	Immune Responses	[19]
NRF2-mediated Oxidative Stress Response	Antioxidant Response	[21]
Role of Pattern Recognition Receptors in Recognition of Bacteria and Viruses	Regulate Interferon	[22]
Neuroinflammation Signaling Pathway	Inflammatory	[23]
SPINK1 General Cancer Pathway	Cancer Diagnose	[32]
Systemic Lupus Erythematosus in B Cell Signaling Pathway	Inflammatory	[33]

3. Discussion

It is well-recognized that genes with similar gene expression patterns have a similar function [34]. From the overall score, we can see that FDA-approved drugs listed in the CREEDS database and their indicated diseases generally have inverse GES patterns compared with the random controls. However, the absolute difference between the indicated group and random control group is not very obvious. For example, in a recent study [35], a significant relationship was found between drug–disease GES similarity and drug therapeutic effect using Cmap [36], with a relatively low overall area under curve (AUC) of 0.57, indicating a real, albeit weak, inverse relationship. The treatment effectors of the drugs identified in this study likely work via the interaction of the genes' protein products, with only a moderate correlation between gene expression and levels of the corresponding protein(s) [37]. Thus, an association study between drugs/diseases and gene expression/pharmaceutical effect is necessary. Also, other mechanisms, for instance, microRNA-based therapeutics, might directly orchestrate the activation/deactivation of the gene expression. However, due to the limitation of available sources, we were unable to investigate other mechanisms of action. Besides, the drugs' TF-levels were not a significant factor that reflect the indication relationship (although drugs directly interacting with TF perform slightly better with q-value of 0.22309 vs. q-value of 0.99509). In our analyses, some subgroups of drugs–diseases pairs with indication associations have positive similarity scores (which means that the drug may exacerbate the disease according to the assumption of gene expression signature similarity) or a score higher than random drug–disease pairs, but these findings were not statistically significant. On the other hand, 7 of 70 subgroups had a significantly lower similarity score when a drug–disease association is indicated.

This study may provide some hints to other future studies utilizing the GES method strategies of comparing drug–disease GES similarity for drug repositioning. That is, certain types of drugs may have a stronger ability to reverse the GES of the diseases they treat, and the disease type may also influence this ability. As such, in specific kinds of subgroups, the drug–disease pairs with higher similarities of reversed GES patterns may have greater therapeutic relationships, which means that focusing on certain kinds of diseases or drugs can increase the true positive rate of the GES-guided drug repositioning method For example, over half (4/7) of the significant subgroups (immunostimulants, interferon receptor, other dermatological preparations, and diseases of the blood or blood-forming organs) are related to diseases associated with the immune system (the disease includes in "other dermatological preparations" atopic dermatitis). This indicates that a drug with drug–disease pairs associated with the immune system tends to have lower similarity scores when compared with the diseases it indicated than random diseases. This means in a GES-guided drug repositioning analysis, an immune-associated drug is more likely to have a potential therapeutic effect on diseases that have a higher inverse similarity with it.

Chemotherapy drugs may not be as good as non-chemotherapy drugs for the GES-guided drug repositioning method (q-values: 0.99509 vs. 0.03937). Unarguably, the high diversity of chemotherapy responses to heterogenetic tumor tissues or even histologically similar tumors has been a challenging problem for a long time [37,38]. The failure of controlling the process of programmed cell death in tissue, one of the major causes of tumors, can be rectified or even overturned by activating/deactivating different pathways under various conditions [39]. This may be the reason that chemotherapy drugs are not good for the GES-guided repositioning approach. On the other hand, non-chemotherapy drugs show a significant result as they interact with cancer cells through more specific mechanisms, such as hormone regulation or mono-target therapy.

For the biological pathway analysis of the interferon receptor subgroup, we found that the genes involved in pathways directly regulated by drugs have the lowest GI-R% scores. It is reasonable that GES-guided drug repositioning methods are more sensitive to drugs directly targeting pathways related to diseases. Furthermore, the significance of mTOR signaling is in accordance with the result in which the subgroup kinase mTOR had a significant indicated-random drug–disease pairs' SJI difference. This result confirmed the high sensitivity of the GES-guided drug repositioning method to this pathway on the other side.

There are some limitations in this study. First, the tissues used for testing the drug effects may not match with the body parts/organs affected by the diseases.. Second, some bias may be caused by the limited number of the CREEDS bio-assay collection which may not have the ability to fully present the pattern of all kinds of drugs and diseases. Additionally, it is important to differentiate the types of "treatment effect". Some drugs may cure a particular disease while others may just provide symptomatic relief thereby resulting in different patterns of GES for the same disease. Also, some indicated subgroups ("kinase mTOR", and "other dermatological preparations") have too few unique drug–disease pairs (n = 1), which may weaken the analyses' power.

In this study, we systematically analyzed the similarity of gene expression profiles from known drug–disease associations, and we found that indicated pairs have a greater inverse similarity score. We found seven subgroups in which their drugs or diseases may have a greater reversed GES pattern when there is a clear therapeutic effect. These findings suggest that a GES-guided drug repositioning method should be used based on the drug or disease type differences. For example, drugs or diseases associated with the immune system, diseases of the nervous system or non-chemotherapy drugs may be a better choice for drug repositioning. Moreover, our biological pathway enrichment analysis showed that some pathways may be more sensitive to this method, such as the mTOR signaling pathway.

4. Materials and Methods

4.1. Gene Signature Data Collection and Filtering

In this study, all gene signature information was collected from a well-calibrated GES repository, the crowd extracted expression of differential signatures (CREEDS) [12] database. The CREEDS database is maintained by the Ma'ayan Lab of Icahn School of Medicine at Mount Sinai. CREEDS utilized GEO2Enrichr [40] to extract GES profiles from the National Center for Biotechnology Information (NCBI) Gene Expression Omnibus (GEO) and applied a characteristic direction (CD) model [41] to identify differentially expressed genes. This database V1.0 includes 10,797 single-gene perturbations, 2258 disease signatures and 5516 drug perturbation gene signatures. Among these signatures, 2176 manual single-gene perturbations, 828 manual disease signatures and 875 manual drug perturbation signatures were considered to be more accurate compared with the automatically generated GES by the machine learning method. The CREEDS database allows users to compare the similarity between the user-specified GES and the GESs processed and stored in the CREEDS.

We first selected the CREEDS manual GES profiles if the assays were from human tissues and/or human cell linesand if the drugs had FDA approval.

Each GES profile includes a list of up- and down-regulated genes. The SJI [12] (see below), a measurement for the similarity between two GES profiles from the paired drug–disease, was calculated. When a drug or a disease had multiple GES profiles, we calculated the SJIs of all the possible combinations, and an overall score for each unique drug–disease pair was calculated from the average of all scores from pairs sharing the same drug–disease combination. All the disease signatures and drug perturbation signatures were requested through the application program interface (API) provided by CREEDS. GES profiles were removed if they labelled for both a drug treatment and for a disease, because this may cause biased similarity. Under the criteria that (a) the GES profiles must come from assays of human cells/tissues, and (b) drugs must be approved by FDA, the remaining signatures were paired within drugs and diseases according to the indication associations. Signatures without any indicated drug–disease relationship were also excluded from further analysis. For example, cocaine was removed because its indication, local anesthesia, was not in the data of disease signatures and could not be paired. The overall data process is shown in Figure 5.

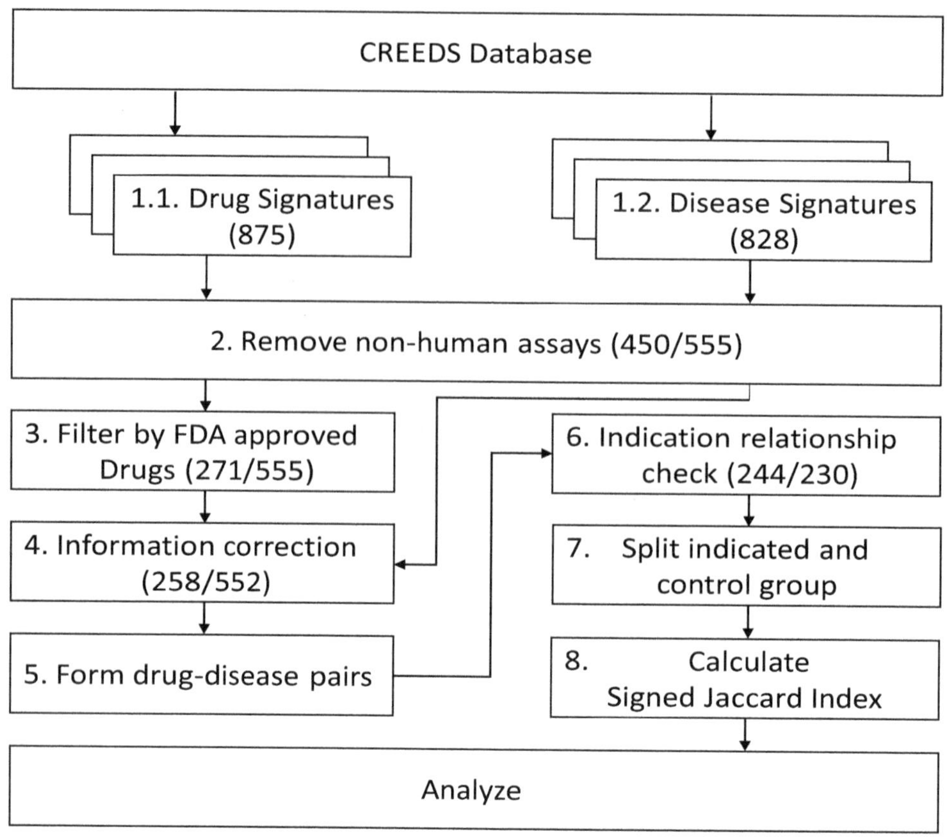

Figure 5. The flow chart of drug and disease gene signature data inclusion process. Numbers of gene signatures left in each step are shown in parentheses: (Number of drug signatures/Number of disease signatures) 1.1. and 1.2. All manual gene signatures retrieved from the CREEDS database. 2. Remove all signatures with assays not labelled as human. 3. Remove all drug signatures not from FDA-approved drugs. 4. Remove signatures with information errors or signatures labelled as both for a drug treatment and for a disease. 5. Remaining drug signatures were paired with each disease signature. 6. Remove signatures with no FDA-labelled indication relationships of drug or disease. 7. Indicated group and control group were divided according to the indication relationship from the FDA drug label. 8. Calculate the signed Jaccard index for each remaining drug–disease pair.

4.2. Similarity Calculation

In our analysis, SJI, which is based on the Jaccard similarity coefficient [42], was used to compute the similarity between GES profiles from a drug and a disease. The Jaccard similarity coefficient is a statistic used to gauge the similarity between different sample sets. It is defined as the size of the intersection divided by the size of the union of two sample sets. It is calculated as follows:

$$Jaccard\ Similarity\ Coefficient(G_1, G_2) = \frac{\text{SAME}}{\text{ALL}}$$

where G_1 and G_2 stand for two lists of differential expressed gene sets, "SAME" represents the number of same genes between two given gene sets, and "ALL" stands for all the unique genes that appeared in the two gene sets.

SJI, which combines the Jaccard similarity coefficient with the gene regulation direction is calculated as follows:

$$\textbf{Signed Jaccard index}(G_1, G_2) = \frac{J\left(G_1^{up}, G_2^{up}\right) + J\left(G_1^{down}, G_2^{down}\right) - J\left(G_1^{up}, G_2^{down}\right) - J\left(G_1^{down}, G_2^{up}\right)}{2}$$

where J means Jaccard similarity coefficient, and G^{up} and G^{down} are up- or down-regulated genes in the given gene set G, respectively. The index ranges from +1 to −1, where +1 and −1 indicate a same pattern and inverse pattern of two gene sets, respectively. Zero indicates that the two sets have no associations, or the same part is cancelled out by the inverse part. The reason to use an unranked score calculation method (SJI) is to keep in accordance with the same scoring method used in the CREEDS database. The CREEDS API (application programming interface) offers the function to calculate the SJI automatically. However, we found the API could not calculate the SJI correctly when two GES profiles are highly overlapped., therefore, all the SJIs in this study were re-calculated.

4.3. Drug-Related Information Collection

In our analysis, the source of drug-related information is listed as follows:

1. Drug target information was collected from DrugBank [43,44] Release Version 5.1.4 [45] (https://www.drugbank.ca/releases/latest#external-links). Only the targets with the main therapeutic effect in the mechanism of action section were included;
2. The human TF list was collected from the paper published by Samuel A. Lambert et al. [46];
3. ATC classifications on level 3 were collected from the WHO official website (https://www.whocc.no/atc_ddd_index/);
4. The drug indication was from section "indications and usage" of FDA label on FDA website (https://labels.fda.gov/);
5. (Drug-indicated) Disease classification was assigned to each disease based on the International Classification of Diseases 11th Revision (ICD-11), level 1.

4.4. Subgroup Classification

In our analysis, we assessed the following factors that might influence the power of the GES-guided drug repositioning method:

1. Disease classifications: A subgroup was assigned to a disease in a drug–disease pair according to the ICD-11-level 1 code of the disease;
2. Drug target subfamilies: Subgroups were divided by the main therapeutic target of each drug. To avoid group splits being too small, some same subfamilies of targets are grouped as one, such as "Beta-1 adrenergic receptor", "Beta-2 adrenergic receptor" and "Beta-3 adrenergic receptor" are grouped in the same subgroup "Beta adrenergic receptors";
3. The relationship between the drug's main therapeutic targets and human transcription factors: A TF level was assigned according to the relationship between the drugs' main therapeutic targets and human TF. Drugs with main therapeutic targets that can directly interact with at least one TF were labelled as "directly". Drugs with main therapeutic targets which are human DNA structures or human proteins but not TFs were labelled as "not-directly". Drugs interacting with non-human proteins or structures (for example, from viruses or bacteria) as main therapeutic targets were labelled as "non-Human";
4. The drug is a chemotherapy drug or not: Drugs with main therapeutic targets as "DNA cross-linking/alkylation", "DNA/ligase", "DNA/methyltransferase", "DNA/polymerase", "DNA/topoisomerase-human", "micro-tubules", "nucleotide synthesis" or "Thymidylate synthase" were defined as chemotherapy drugs
5. The drug's ATC classification: Subgroups were divided according to the Anatomical Therapeutic Chemical classification system, level 3. Drugs with multiple classifications caused by different administration routes were unified to systematic use.

4.5. Statistical Analysis and Pathway Analysis

The random control group was generated by calculating the average SJI of all possible drug–disease pairs without indicated associations to imitate a GES-guided drug repositioning screening. A t-test [13] was applied to quantify the mean differences of the SJI between drug-indicated disease pairs and random controls.

For subgroup analysis, GLM [14] least squares mean partitions F tests function was applied to estimate the mean difference between the indicated and control group since the data was unbalanced with multiple factors. A significant result of a certain subgroup indicated that the average SJI of this subgroup was significant between two indication levels (Yes/No). False discovery rate (FDR) q-value of the Benjamini–Hochberg procedure [47] was controlled to 0.05 to avoid an inflated experiment-wise type I error rate caused by multiple comparisons among all subgroups.

Data processing and statistical analysis (student t-tests, GLM, FDR calculation) were conducted using R studio 3.6.1 [48] and SAS software version 9.4. Copyright © 2019 SAS Institute Inc. Cary, NC, USA.

Differentially reversed expression genes (top 5% negative score according to the relatively reverse percentage) from the most significant subgroup will be chosen as examples to conduct biological pathway enrichment analysis.

The relatively reverse percentage is calculated as

$$Relatively\ expression\ probability\ of\ a\ gene\left(G^{I-R\%}\right) = D^{I}\% - D^{R}\%$$

where $D^I\%$ **and** $D^R\%$ stand for the percentage of the gene which is differentially expressed in all assays of indicated/random drug–diseases pairs. It is calculated as

$$D\% = \frac{NS - NR}{Total\ assays\ pairs}$$

where **NS** and **NR** represent the number of times a gene showed a same or reverse regulation direction between assays of drugs and diseases among all drug–disease assays pairs.

The $G^{I\text{-}R\%}$ ranges from 100% to -100%. A higher positive score indicates that this gene is more likely to be expressed in the same direction in indicated drug–disease assays compared with random drug–disease assays. Likewise, a lower negative score indicates that this gene has a higher probability to express reversely between indicated drug–disease assays compared with random drug–disease assays.

Biological pathway enrichment analysis was conducted by ingenuity pathway analysis (IPA, QIAGEN Inc., https://www.qiagenbioinformatics.com/products/ingenuitypathway-analysis).

Author Contributions: Conceptualization, X.Q., M.S. and L.W.; Data Curation, X.Q. and M.S.; Formal Analysis, X.Q. and P.F.; Funding Acquisition, R.A.S. and L.W.; Investigation, X.Q.; Methodology, X.Q. and L.K.; Project Administration, L.W.; Resources, L.W.; Software, X.Q.; Supervision, L.W.; Validation, X.G. and T.W.; Visualization, X.Q; Writing—original draft, X.Q.; Writing—review and editing, N.F., M.Z., R.A.S. and L.W. All authors have read and agreed to the published version of the manuscript.

Acknowledgments: The authors would like to acknowledge Zefei Li at School of Pharmacy in Sun Yat-sen University for revising the calculation process.

References

1. Alizadeh, A.A.; Eisen, M.B.; Davis, R.E.; Ma, C.; Lossos, I.S.; Rosenwald, A.; Boldrick, J.C.; Sabet, H.; Tran, T.; Yu, X.; et al. Distinct Types of Diffuse Large B-Cell Lymphoma Identified by Gene Expression Profiling. *Nature* **2000**, *403*, 503–511. [CrossRef]

2. Ramaswamy, S.P.; Tamayo, R.; Rifkin, S.; Mukherjee, C.H.; Yeang, M.; Angelo, C.; Ladd, M.; Reich, E.; Latulippe, J.P.; Mesirov, T.; et al. Multiclass Cancer Diagnosis Using Tumor Gene Expression Signatures. *Proc. Natl. Acad. Sci. USA* **2001**, *98*, 15149–15154. [CrossRef]
3. Wright, G.; Tan, B.; Rosenwald, A.; Hurt, E.H.; Wiestner, A.; Staudt, L.M. A Gene Expression-Based Method to Diagnose Clinically Distinct Subgroups of Diffuse Large B Cell Lymphoma. *Proc. Natl. Acad. Sci. USA* **2003**, *100*, 9991–9996. [CrossRef]
4. Yap, Y.L.; Zhang, X.W.; Smith, D.; Soong, R.; Hill, J. Molecular Gene Expression Signature Patterns for Gastric Cancer Diagnosis. *Comput. Biol. Chem.* **2007**, *31*, 275–287. [CrossRef]
5. Ziober, A.F.; Patel, K.R.; Alawi, F.; Gimotty, P.; Weber, R.S.; Feldman, M.M.; Chalian, A.A.; Weinstein, G.S.; Hunt, J.; Ziober, B.L. Identification of a Gene Signature for Rapid Screening of Oral Squamous Cell Carcinoma. *Clin. Cancer Res.* **2006**, *12 Pt 1*, 5960–5971. [CrossRef]
6. Chibon, F. Cancer Gene Expression Signatures—The Rise and Fall? *Eur. J. Cancer* **2000**, *49*, 2000–2009. [CrossRef] [PubMed]
7. Chen, H.Y.; Yu, S.L.; Chen, C.H.; Chang, G.C.; Chen, C.Y.; Yuan, A.; Cheng, C.L.; Wang, C.H.; Terng, H.J.; Kao, S.F.; et al. A Five-Gene Signature and Clinical Outcome in Non-Small-Cell Lung Cancer. *N. Engl. J. Med.* **2007**, *356*, 11–20. [CrossRef] [PubMed]
8. Iorio, F.; Bosotti, R.; Scacheri, E.; Belcastro, V.; Mithbaokar, P.; Ferriero, R.; Murino, L.; Tagliaferri, R.; Brunetti-Pierri, N.; Isacchi, A.; et al. Discovery of Drug Mode of Action and Drug Repositioning from Transcriptional Responses. *Proc. Natl. Acad. Sci. USA* **2010**, *107*, 14621–14626. [CrossRef] [PubMed]
9. Sirota, M.; Dudley, J.T.; Kim, J.; Chiang, A.P.; Morgan, A.A.; Sweet-Cordero, A.; Sage, J.; Butte, A.J. Discovery and Preclinical Validation of Drug Indications Using Compendia of Public Gene Expression Data. *Sci. Transl. Med.* **2011**, *3*, 96ra77. [CrossRef]
10. Hu, G.; Agarwal, P. Human Disease-Drug Network Based on Genomic Expression Profiles. *PLoS ONE* **2009**, *4*, e6536. [CrossRef]
11. Donner, Y.; Kazmierczak, S.; Fortney, K. Drug Repurposing Using Deep Embeddings of Gene Expression Profiles. *Mol. Pharm.* **2018**, *15*, 4314–4325. [CrossRef] [PubMed]
12. Wang, Z.; Monteiro, C.D.; Jagodnik, K.M.; Fernandez, N.F.; Gundersen, G.W.; Rouillard, A.D.; Jenkins, S.L.; Feldmann, A.S.; Hu, K.S.; McDermott, M.G.; et al. Extraction and Analysis of Signatures from the Gene Expression Omnibus by the Crowd. *Nat. Commun.* **2016**, *7*, 12846. [CrossRef] [PubMed]
13. Student. The Probable Error of a Mean. *Biometrika* **1908**, *6*, 1–25. [CrossRef]
14. Nelder, J.A.; Wedderburn, R.W. Generalized Linear Models. *J. R. Stat. Soc. Ser. A-Gen.* **1972**, *135*, 370. [CrossRef]
15. Bustamante, M.F.; Nurtdinov, R.N.; Río, J.; Montalban, X.; Comabella, M. Baseline Gene Expression Signatures in Monocytes from Multiple Sclerosis Patients Treated with Interferon-Beta. *PLoS ONE* **2013**, *8*, e60994. [CrossRef] [PubMed]
16. Bibeau-Poirier, A.; Servant, M.J. Roles of Ubiquitination in Pattern-Recognition Receptors and Type I Interferon Receptor Signaling. *Cytokine Servant* **2008**, *43*, 359–367. [CrossRef]
17. Honda, K.; Taniguchi, T. Irfs: Master Regulators of Signalling by Toll-Like Receptors and Cytosolic Pattern-Recognition Receptors. *Nat. Rev. Immunol. Taniguchi* **2006**, *6*, 644–658. [CrossRef]
18. Su, X.; Yu, Y.; Zhong, Y.; Giannopoulou, E.G.; Hu, X.; Liu, H.; Cross, J.R.; Rätsch, G.; Rice, C.M.; Ivashkiv, L.B. Interferon-Γ Regulates Cellular Metabolism and Mrna Translation to Potentiate Macrophage Activation. *Nat. Immunol. Ivashkiv* **2015**, *16*, 838. [CrossRef]
19. Cao, W.; Manicassamy, S.; Tang, H.; Kasturi, S.P.; Pirani, A.; Murthy, N.; Pulendran, B. Toll-Like Receptor–Mediated Induction of Type I Interferon in Plasmacytoid Dendritic Cells Requires the Rapamycin-Sensitive Pi (3) K-Mtor-P70s6k Pathway. *Nat. Immunol. Pulendran* **2008**, *9*, 1157. [CrossRef]
20. Weinstein, S.L.; Finn, A.J.; Davé, S.H.; Meng, F.; Lowell, C.A.; Sanghera, J.S.; DeFranco, A.L. Phosphatidylinositol 3-Kinase and Mtor Mediate Lipopolysaccharide-Stimulated Nitric Oxide Production in Macrophages Via Interferon-B. *J. Leukoc. Biol. DeFranco* **2000**, *67*, 405–414. [CrossRef]
21. Staitieh, B.S.; Egea, E.E.; Fan, X.; Azih, N.; Neveu, W.; Guidot, D.M. Activation of Alveolar Macrophages with Interferon-Γ Promotes Antioxidant Defenses Via the Nrf2-Are Pathway. *J. Clin. Guidot Cellular Immunol.* **2015**, *6*, 365.
22. Perry, A.K.; Gang, C.H.; Zheng, D.; Hong, T.A.; Cheng, G. Cell research Cheng. The Host Type I Interferon Response to Viral and Bacterial Infections. *Cell Res.* **2005**, *15*, 407–422. [CrossRef]

23. Vieweg, W.V.; Hasnain, M.; Howland, R.H.; Hettema, J.M.; Kogut, C.; Wood, M.A.; Pandurangi, A.K. Citalopram, Qtc Interval Prolongation, and Torsade De Pointes. How Should We Apply the Recent Fda Ruling? *Am. J. Med.* **2012**, *125*, 859–868. [CrossRef] [PubMed]
24. Honda, K.; Yanai, H.; Negishi, H.; Asagiri, M.; Sato, M.; Mizutani, T.; Shimada, N.; Ohba, Y.; Takaoka, A.; Yoshida, N.; et al. Irf-7 Is the Master Regulator of Type-I Interferon-Dependent Immune Responses. *Nature* **2005**, *434*, 772–777. [CrossRef] [PubMed]
25. Hilpert, J.; Beekman, J.M.; Schwenke, S.; Kowal, K.; Bauer, D.; Lampe, J.; Sandbrink, R.; Heubach, J.F.; Stürzebecher, S.; Reischl, J. Biological Response Genes after Single Dose Administration of Interferon B-1b to Healthy Male Volunteers. *J. Neuroimmunol.* **2008**, *199*, 115–125. [CrossRef]
26. Becker, A.M.; Dao, K.H.; Han, B.K.; Kornu, R.; Lakhanpal, S.; Mobley, A.B.; Li, Q.Z.; Lian, Y.; Wu, T.; Reimold, A.M.; et al. Sle Peripheral Blood B Cell, T Cell and Myeloid Cell Transcriptomes Display Unique Profiles and Each Subset Contributes to the Interferon Signature. *PLoS ONE* **2013**, *8*, e67003. [CrossRef]
27. Crow, M.K.; Kirou, K.A.; Wohlgemuth, J. Microarray Analysis of Interferon-Regulated Genes in Sle. *Autoimmunity* **2003**, *36*, 481–490. [CrossRef]
28. Shrestha, N.; Bahnan, W.; Wiley, D.J.; Barber, G.; Fields, K.A.; Schesser, K. Eukaryotic Initiation Factor 2 (Eif2) Signaling Regulates Proinflammatory Cytokine Expression and Bacterial Invasion. *J. Biol. Chem.* **2012**, *287*, 28738–28744. [CrossRef]
29. Flynn, A.; Proud, C.G. The Role of Eif4 in Cell Proliferation. *Cancer Surv.* **1996**, *27*, 293–310.
30. Isaacs, A. Interferon. In *Advances in Virus Research*; Elsevier: Cambridge, MA, USA, 1964; pp. 1–38.
31. Sarasin-Filipowicz, M.; Oakeley, E.J.; Duong, F.H.; Christen, V.; Terracciano, L.; Filipowicz, W.; Heim, M.H. Interferon Signaling and Treatment Outcome in Chronic Hepatitis C. *Proc. Natl. Acad. Sci. USA* **2008**, *105*, 7034–7039. [CrossRef]
32. Flavin, R.; Pettersson, A.; Hendrickson, W.K.; Fiorentino, M.; Finn, S.; Kunz, L.; Judson, G.L.; Lis, R.; Bailey, D.; Fiore, C.; et al. Fiore Spink1 Protein Expression and Prostate Cancer Progression. *Clin. Cancer Res.* **2014**, *20*, 4904–4911. [CrossRef] [PubMed]
33. Smoller, J.W. The Genetics of Stress-Related Disorders: Ptsd, Depression, and Anxiety Disorders. *Neuropsychopharmacology* **2016**, *41*, 297. [CrossRef] [PubMed]
34. Le Roch, K.G.; Zhou, Y.; Blair, P.L.; Grainger, M.; Moch, J.K.; Haynes, J.D.; De la Vega, P.; Holder, A.A.; Batalov, S.; Carucci, D.J.; et al. Carucci, and Elizabeth, A. Winzeler. Discovery of Gene Function by Expression Profiling of the Malaria Parasite Life Cycle. *Science* **2003**, *301*, 1503. [CrossRef] [PubMed]
35. Cheng, J.; Yang, L.; Kumar, V.; Agarwal, P. Systematic Evaluation of Connectivity Map for Disease Indications. *Genome Med.* **2014**, *6*, 540. [CrossRef]
36. Lamb, J.; Crawford, E.D.; Peck, D.; Modell, J.W.; Blat, I.C.; Wrobel, M.J.; Lerner, J.; Brunet, J.P.; Subramanian, A.; Ross, K.N.; et al. The Connectivity Map: Using Gene-Expression Signatures to Connect Small Molecules, Genes, and Disease. *Science* **2006**, *313*, 1929–1935. [CrossRef] [PubMed]
37. Talmadge, J.E.; Benedict, K.; Madsen, J.; Fidler, I.J. Development of Biological Diversity and Susceptibility to Chemotherapy in Murine Cancer Metastases. *Cancer Res.* **1984**, *44*, 3801–3805. [PubMed]
38. Simpson-Herren, L.; Noker, P.E.; Wagoner, S.D. Variability of Tumor Response to Chemotherapy Ii. Contribution of Tumor Heterogeneity. *Cancer Chemother. Pharmacol.* **1988**, *22*, 131–136. [CrossRef] [PubMed]
39. Zimmermann, K.C.; Bonzon, C.; Green, D.R. The Machinery of Programmed Cell Death. *Pharmacol. Ther.* **2001**, *92*, 57–70. [CrossRef]
40. Gundersen, G.W.; Jones, M.R.; Rouillard, A.D.; Kou, Y.; Monteiro, C.D.; Feldmann, A.S.; Hu, K.S.; Ma'ayan, A. Geo2enrichr: Browser Extension and Server App to Extract Gene Sets from Geo and Analyze Them for Biological Functions. *Bioinformatics* **2015**, *31*, 3060–3062. [CrossRef]
41. Clark, N.R.; Hu, K.S.; Feldmann, A.S.; Kou, Y.; Chen, E.Y.; Duan, Q.; Ma'ayan, A. The Characteristic Direction: A Geometrical Approach to Identify Differentially Expressed Genes. *BMC Bioinformatics* **2014**, *15*, 79. [CrossRef]
42. Jaccard, P. Nouvelles Recherches Sur La Distribution Florale. *Bull. Soc. Vaud. Sci. Nat.* **1908**, *44*, 223–270.
43. Wishart, D.S.; Knox, C.; Guo, A.C.; Shrivastava, S.; Hassanali, M.; Stothard, P.; Chang, Z.; Woolsey, J. Drugbank: A Comprehensive Resource for in Silico Drug Discovery and Exploration. *Nucleic Acids Res.* **2006**, *34*, D668–D672. [CrossRef] [PubMed]

44. Wishart, D.S.; Knox, C.; Guo, A.C.; Cheng, D.; Shrivastava, S.; Tzur, D.; Gautam, B.; Hassanali, M. Drugbank: A Knowledgebase for Drugs, Drug Actions and Drug Targets. *Nucleic Acids Res.* **2008**, *36*, D901–D906. [CrossRef] [PubMed]
45. Wishart, D.S.; Feunang, Y.D.; Guo, A.C.; Lo, E.J.; Marcu, A.; Grant, J.R.; Sajed, T.; Johnson, D.; Li, C.; Sayeeda, Z.; et al. Drugbank 5.0: A Major Update to the Drugbank Database for 2018. *Nucleic Acids Res.* **2017**, *46*, D1074–D1082. [CrossRef] [PubMed]
46. Lambert, S.A.; Jolma, A.; Campitelli, L.F.; Das, P.K.; Yin, Y.; Albu, M.; Chen, X.; Taipale, J.; Hughes, T.R.; Weirauch, M.T. The Human Transcription Factors. *Cell* **2018**, *172*, 650–665. [CrossRef]
47. Benjamini, Y.; Hochberg, Y. Controlling the False Discovery Rate: A Practical and Powerful Approach to Multiple Testing. *J. R. Stat. Soc.* **1995**, *57*, 289–300. [CrossRef]
48. *Team, R Core R: A Language and Environment for Statistical Computing*; R Foundation for Statistical Computing: Vienna, Austria, 2013.

3

Efficaciousness of Low Affinity Compared to High Affinity TSPO Ligands in the Inhibition of Hypoxic Mitochondrial Cellular Damage Induced by Cobalt Chloride in Human Lung H1299 Cells

Nidal Zeineh [1,†], Nunzio Denora [2,3,†], Valentino Laquintana [2], Massimo Franco [2], Abraham Weizman [4,5] and Moshe Gavish [1,*]

1 The Ruth and Bruce Rappaport Faculty of Medicine, Technion Institute of Technology, Haifa 31096, Israel; nidalz1988@gmail.com
2 Department of Pharmacy–Pharmaceutical Sciences, University of Bari "Aldo Moro", 70125 Bari, Italy; nunzio.denora@uniba.it (N.D.); valentino.laquintana@uniba.it (V.L.); massimo.franco@uniba.it (M.F.)
3 Institute for Chemical and Physical Processes (IPCF)-CNR SS Bari, Via Orabona 4, 70126 Bari, Italy
4 Research Unit at Geha Mental Health Center and Laboratory of Biological Psychiatry at Felsenstein Medical Research Center, Petah Tikva 4910002, Israel; weizmana@gmail.com
5 Sackler Faculty of Medicine, Tel Aviv University, Tel Aviv 6997801, Israel
* Correspondence: mgavish@technion.ac.il
† These authors contributed equally to this work.

Abstract: The 18 kDa translocator protein (TSPO) plays an important role in apoptotic cell death, including apoptosis induced by the hypoxia mimicking agent cobalt chloride ($CoCl_2$). In this study, the protective effects of a high (CB86; Ki = 1.6 nM) and a low (CB204; Ki = 117.7 nM) affinity TSPO ligands were investigated in H1299 lung cancer cell line exposed to $CoCl_2$. The lung cell line H1299 was chosen in the present study since they express TSPO and able to undergo programmed cell death. The examined cell death markers included: ATP synthase reversal, reactive oxygen species (ROS) generation, mitochondrial membrane potential ($\Delta\psi m$) depolarization, cellular toxicity, and cellular viability. Pretreatment of the cells with the low affinity ligand CB204 at a concentration of 100 μM suppressed significantly ($p < 0.05$ for all) $CoCl_2$-induced cellular cytotoxicity (100%), ATP synthase reversal (67%), ROS generation (82%), $\Delta\psi m$ depolarization (100%), reduction in cellular density (97%), and also increased cell viability (85%). Furthermore, the low affinity TSPO ligand CB204, was harmless when given by itself at 100 μM. In contrast, the high affinity ligand (CB86) was significantly effective only in the prevention of $CoCl_2$–induced ROS generation (39%, $p < 0.001$), and showed significant cytotoxic effects when given alone at 100 μM, as reflected in alterations in ADP/ATP ratio, oxidative stress, mitochondrial membrane potential depolarization and cell death. It appears that similar to previous studies on brain-derived cells, the relatively low affinity for the TSPO target enhances the potency of TSPO ligands in the protection from hypoxic cell death. Moreover, the high affinity TSPO ligand CB86, but not the low affinity ligand CB204, was lethal to the lung cells at high concentration (100 μM). The low affinity TSPO ligand CB204 may be a candidate for the treatment of pulmonary diseases related to hypoxia, such as pulmonary ischemia and chronic obstructive pulmonary disease COPD.

Keywords: translocator protein (TSPO); $CoCl_2$; mitochondrial membrane potential; reactive oxygen species (ROS); cell viability; cell death; lung cancer cell line

1. Introduction

In this study the hypoxic toxic agent cobalt chloride ($CoCl_2$) was used to induce hypoxic death in H1299 lung cancer cells. Hypoxia is a state in which the oxygen supply to a tissue within an organ is compromised [1]. Decreased oxygen levels or tension in a tissue results in hypoxic damage due to altered cellular signaling networks. Hypoxia may occur both in physiological conditions such as climbing to high altitudes, as well as in pathological conditions such as myocardial ischemia, chronic obstructive pulmonary disease (COPD), and obstructive sleep apnea [2]. Hypoxia affects cellular homeostasis, which may lead to reactive oxygen species (ROS) production, elevated vasoconstrictive substances, increased expression of pro-inflammatory cytokines, and increased intercellular and vascular cell adhesion molecules [3–9]. Impaired protein homeostasis in the muscle system is a well-known condition in COPD patients [10–12].

$CoCl_2$ mimics hypoxic state when applied to cell cultures [13–19]. Previous studies in neural-derived PC12 cells, demonstrated that $CoCl_2$ might induce apoptotic cell death via the P38-MAPK-caspase 3 pathway [20]. $CoCl_2$ interferes with heme production from protoporphyrin IX (PPIX) [19,21]. PPIX acts as an endogenous ligand for the mitochondrial 18 kDa translocator protein (TSPO) [22]. It was shown that decreased ROS levels due to TSPO knockdown lead to accumulation of PPIX and consequently increased heme production [23]. The hypoxia mimicking effect of $CoCl_2$ is related to its stabilizing effect on the α-subunit of HIF (hypoxia inducible transcription factor), in addition to inhibition of cytochrome-C oxidase subunit 4 (COX4) precursor processing and enhancement of its degradation [16].

Mitochondria are involved in some of the hypoxia-induced cellular injury mechanisms, and it acts as an energy source, as well as a source for metabolic signals, cellular proliferation, inflammation, and intrinsic cell death [24]. The TSPO located in the outer mitochondrial membrane plays an important role in the mitochondrial apoptotic processes [25–29], along with other cellular roles [30–32].

A previous study has indicated the role of TSPO in $CoCl_2$-induced apoptotic cell death. TSPO knockdown in U118MG glioblastoma cells, demonstrated the important role of TSPO in apoptosis induced by $CoCl_2$, including processes such as: $\Delta\psi m$ depolarization, cardiolipin peroxidation, and ROS generation. Administration of the TSPO ligand PK 11195 inhibited partially a sequence of TSPO-related processes relevant to $CoCl_2$-induced cell death reminiscent of the effects of TSPO knockdown determined in the same study [22]. In the present study, TSPO ligands characterized by a 2-phenyl-imidazo [1–a] pyridine nucleus (Scheme 1) that express various affinities were investigated (Table 1). The goal of the current study was to examine, for the first time, the protective effect of two novel TSPO ligands (CB86 and CB204), in the attenuation of the hypoxic effect of $CoCl_2$ in H1299 lung cancer cell line. The two ligands differ in their affinity to TSPO: CB204 has low affinity (Ki = 117.7 nM) and CB86 has high affinity (Ki = 1.6 nM) [33]. Among the few examples known of TSPO ligands containing hydrophilic groups, there is the 8-amino imidazopyridine CB86 ligand. In a previous study it was evaluated whether further polar substituents or ionizable functional groups could be introduced on the amino group of CB86 [33]. Data indicated that introduction of a -COOH group led to a significant decrease in affinity to TSPO, as observed for the compound CB204. Furthermore, in addition to the structure-activity relationship studies, reported by some of us, highlighting the main physicochemical factors eliciting the binding of imidazopyridines to TSPO, the pharmacological profile of these compounds by measuring their modulatory effects on the $GABA_A$ receptors was also explored [33].

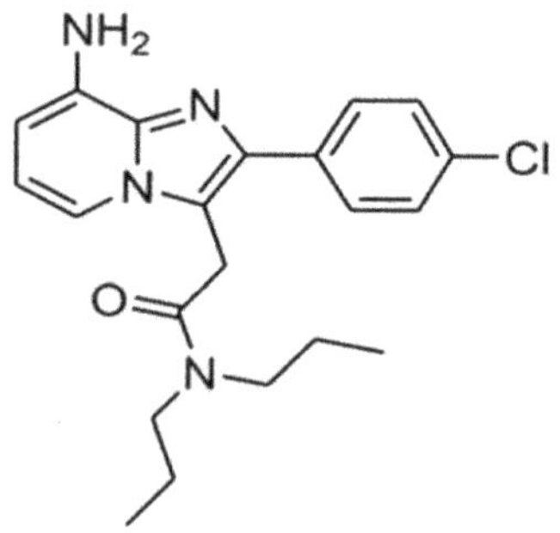

CB86

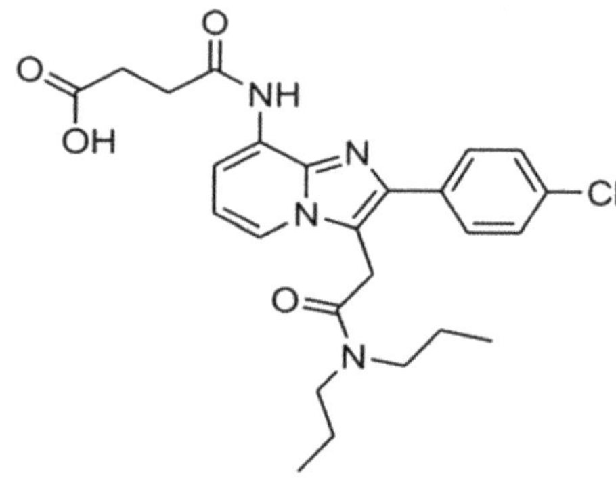

CB194

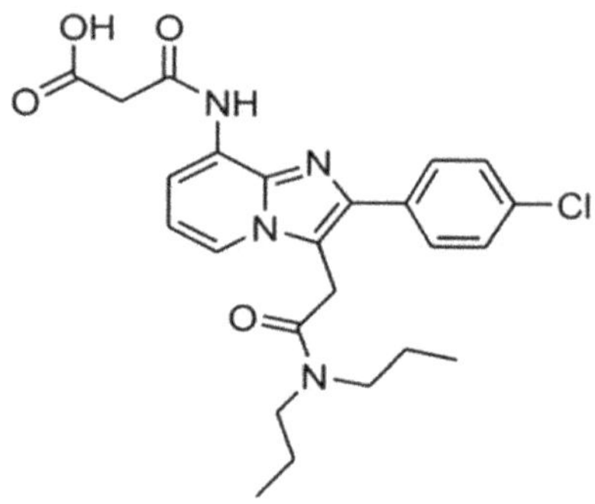

CB199

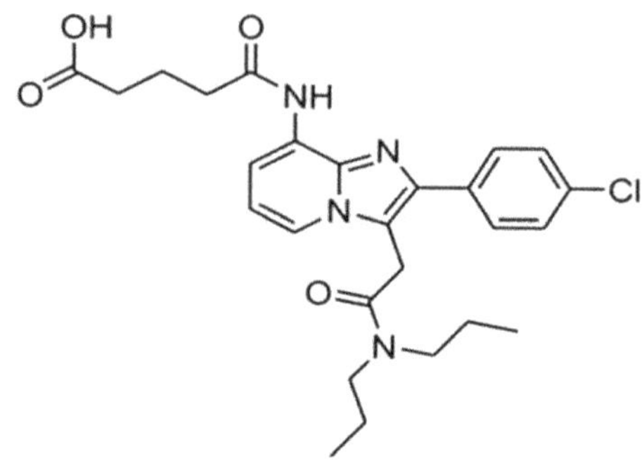

CB204

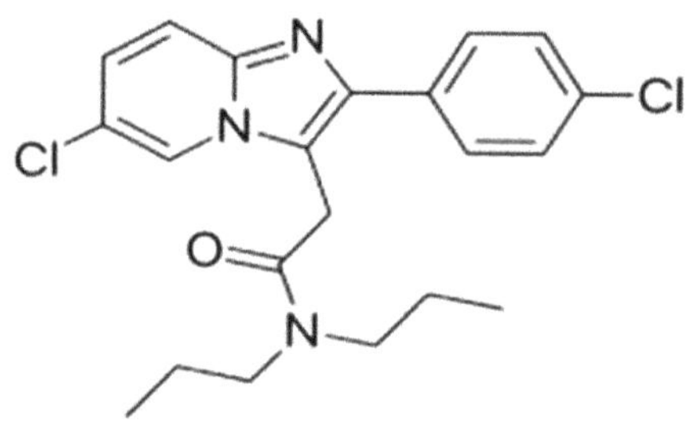

Alpidem

Scheme 1. Molecular structure of CB86, CB194, CB199, CB204, and Alpidem assayed in the present study.

Table 1. The affinity data of translocator protein (TSPO) ligands used in the current study.

Ligand Name	CB86	CB194	CB199	CB204	Alpidem
Molecular weight	384	484	470	498	404
TSPO *Ki* (nM)	1.6	285.3	193.1	117.7	0.6

CB86 and CB204 were chosen in the present study for their diverging affinities to the TSPO. This choice was prompted by previous findings with other TSPO ligands, presenting low to moderate affinity, that showed efficacy regarding cellular protective effects and without cellular toxic activity. In contrast, high affinity TSPO ligands can induce cellular toxic effects and conspicuous lethal effects at relatively high concentrations [34–36]. These previous studies were conducted on microglia, astrocytic, neuronal, and cancer cells and in animal models [35,37,38]. A previous review of numerous cell types reported that classical high affinity TSPO ligands show lethal effects at high concentrations (typically > 50 μM), but protective effects at low concentrations [39]. A subsequent experimental research reported that indeed in a paradigm of astrocytic cells challenged with ammonia, the classical high affinity TSPO ligands (PK 11195, Ro5 4864 and FGIN-1-27) induced cell death at concentrations above 50 μM, but were protective at the nM range [40]. Thus, the hypothesis of the present study was that the high affinity TSPO ligand (CB86 in Scheme 1) would show cytotoxic effects at a concentration of 100 μM, while the low affinity TSPO ligand with a comparable structure (CB204 in Scheme 1) would show cellular protective effects at the same concentration of 100 μM. We applied this to a paradigm of cells vastly different from the cells regularly used by us (lung cancer cells vs. brain cells). We attempted to confirm or disprove previous findings on the relationship between the affinity of ligands to TSPO and their cytotoxic or protective effects. Furthermore, the question was whether these cellular effects are specific for brain cells, or valid also for other types of cells as well, in our case lung cells. The present report provides new data since: (1) The TSPO ligands in the current study were not used in the previous studies; (2) low affinity and high affinity TSPO ligands based on a common structural framework are compared in one paradigm, so they can reliably represent their unique pharmacological properties; and (3) another type of cells (lung cells) are used, while in the previous similar studies brain derived cells were used. The present study was designed to provide indication whether the previous findings on the effects of TSPO ligands on brain derived cells can also be discerned with novel TSPO ligands when applied to other types of cells, and thus are not restricted to the cells of brain origin (microglia, astrocytes, and neuronal cells). Thus, the present attempted to verify and unify the image suggested by the scattered information of previous studies. We chose H1299 lung cells because they represent peripheral respiratory mitochondrial-relevant system, express TSPO and can undergo programmed cell death when exposed to cytotoxic agents [41].

Thus, the correlation between TSPO ligand affinity and their protective effects in a putative TSPO-associated hypoxic cellular model was evaluated in the present study.

2. Materials and Methods

2.1. Study Design

In this study, the H1299 lung cancer cells from human origin were used. The maintenance of the cells was performed according to the American Type Culture Collection (ATCC) instructions, as follows: Culture medium consisted of RPMI (high glucose, without L-glutamine and sodium pyruvate), supplemented with 10% Fetal Bovine Serum (FBS), 2% glutamine, and gentamycin (50 mg/mL). The serum-deprived medium contained similar components, just with 2.5 mL FCS (0.5%), instead of 50 mL (10%). According to a previous study, hypoxic damage due to exposure to toxic agent (e.g., cigarette smoke) demonstrated an association between TSPO and apoptotic cell death. Since the conditions needed were the existence of TSPO and the possibility to induce apoptosis via TSPO, H1299 fulfilled these criteria, and were chosen in the current study [41].

The cells were incubated at 37 °C in 5% CO_2 until 80–90% confluency was reached. Initially, pretreatment of the cells with the TSPO ligands: CB86, CB194, CB199, CB204, and Alpidem, at increasing concentrations was performed 24 h prior to incubation with $CoCl_2$ for another 24 h. According to the collected results, the high affinity CB86 and the low affinity CB204 TSPO ligands were chosen for the proceeding experiments.

2.2. $CoCl_2$ Exposure and Its Treatment with TSPO Ligands

According to previous studies, the $CoCl_2$ at a concentration of 0.5 mM was used in our experiments [22,42,43].

Treatment consisted of 24 h of TSPO ligand pretreatment prior to the subsequent 24 h simultaneous exposure to $CoCl_2$ and TSPO ligands/or vehicle. In more detail, pretreatment of the cells was conducted using DMSO (1%) (vehicle) in serum-deprived medium for the control groups, and ligand-containing serum-deprived medium for the experimental groups. After 24 h of pretreatment, the medium of the control groups and the ligand-containing groups was replaced by the same medium, but in the "experimental groups" it contained also 0.5 mM $CoCl_2$. Then, the groups of cells were incubated for another 24 h (the treatment), as previously described [43–45]. The pretreatment groups included: vehicle and vehicle plus ligand groups. For treatment, the groups included: Vehicle, vehicle plus ligand, vehicle plus $CoCl_2$, and vehicle plus ligand plus $CoCl_2$ groups. Following this subsequent exposure to $CoCl_2$ for 24 h, the cells were collected and processed. According to a previous study using U118MG cells [22], dose response analysis with increasing $CoCl_2$ concentrations was performed. It was shown that at concentrations of 0.3–0.5 mM cell death levels increased by 10–25%, while at concentrations above 0.6 mM cell death elevated by 40% to 90% [22]. In accord with the previous study [22], the 0.5 mM concentration of $CoCl_2$ was selected for the current experiments, in order obtain reversible and treatable cellular toxic effects. The dose response curve for H1299 cells exposed to $CoCl_2$ was very similar to the one described by us previously on U118MG cells [22].

2.3. *ADP/ATP Ratio*

White 96-well plates were used to measure the levels of ADP and ATP. After pretreatment of cells in medium with and without CB86 and CB204, followed by $CoCl_2$ exposure, the ADP/ATP ratio was measured and calculated, according to the manufacturer's protocol (MAK135; Sigma-Aldrich, St. Louis, MO, USA), as previously described [46]. Luminescence levels of the ratio between ADP and ATP were measured by ELISA using Infinite M200 Pro plate reader (Tecan, Männedorf, Switzerland), according to the instructions of the manufacturer.

2.4. *Reactive Oxygen Species (ROS) Levels*

ROS/superoxide detection assay kit (Abcam, Cambridge, UK) was used to measure ROS and superoxide levels according to the manufacturer's instructions. Following treatment of the cells as described above, they were washed using 1X wash buffer followed by application of 100 μL/well of ROS/superoxide detection solution and then incubated in dark for 60 min. ELISA with Infinite M200 Pro plate reader (Tecan, Männedorf, Switzerland) was used with standard fluorescein (excitation 488 nm and emission 520 nm) and rhodamine (excitation 550 nm and emission 610 nm) filter sets, and fluorescence levels were measured, according to the instructions of the manufacturer.

2.5. *Depolarization of the Mitochondrial Membrane Potential ($\Delta\Psi m$)*

Mitochondrial membrane potential ($\Delta\Psi$m) depolarization was assayed using the dye JC-1(5,5′,6,6′-tetrachloro-1,1′,3,3′-tetraethylbenzimidazolylcarbocyanine-chloride), as described previously [22]. JC-1 is a marker for mitochondrial function and cell health. Intact cells characterized by high $\Delta\psi_M$, the cationic lipophilic JC-1 dye selectively enters the mitochondria, forms aggregates and thus reversibly changes color from green to red inside the mitochondria (orange-red fluorescence emitting at 590 nm wavelength). In case of $\Delta\psi_M$ depolarization, monomers of JC-1 remain in the cytoplasm, and these monomers emit at 527 nm (green fluorescence). Thus, $\Delta\psi_M$ depolarization is expressed by decreased red/green ratio.

The cells were trypsinized and collected by centrifugation (660× *g*, 5 min, 4 °C). The proton ionophore carbonyl cyanide was used as a positive control, as previously described [22]. The samples were incubated in 400 μL of diluted JC-1 dye (1/500) for 30 min. Then, the cells were centrifuged (660× *g*, 5 min, 4 °C), the pellets then resuspended in 500 μL of PBS and transferred into FACS tubes. The mean fluorescence intensity (MFI) was measured using FACS device, and the results were analyzed using FlowJo (10th version, FlowJo LLC, Ashland, OR, USA). In the calculation of the mitochondrial depolarization the basal 590/527 ratio was subtracted. This is an assay demonstrating cell number-wise, namely, the percentage of the measured cell population presents mitochondrial depolarization sufficient to prevent JC-1 entry and conversion to red emitting aggregates.

2.6. Cellular Cytotoxicity Assay (LDH)

Cellular cytotoxicity levels were measured by the Cytotoxicity Detection Kit (Roche Pharmaceuticals, Basel, Switzerland), which measures the LDH enzyme levels in the medium. LDH enzyme is released from the cells when the cell membrane is disrupted in case of necrosis and late apoptosis [47].

Cytotoxicity levels were measured by an absorbance at 492 nm wavelength and a reference wavelength of 620 nm, according to the manufacturer's protocol. ELISA with spectrophotometer Zenyth 200 (Anthos, Eugendorf, Austria) was used for measurements and the results were calculated and normalized (calibrated) according to the formula given by the manufacturer.

2.7. XTT Based Colorimetric Assay

Cell viability was measured using XTT cell viability assay kit (Abcam, Cambridge, UK), according to the manufacturer's protocol. In this assay, in viable cells the 2,3-bis [2-methoxy-4-nitro-5-sulphophenyl]-2H-tetrazolium-5-carboxylanilide inner salt (XTT) is reduced by mitochondrial dehydrogenases, and this reaction leads to an orange formazan product. This assay measures cell metabolism as an indication of cell viability. The spectrophotometer Zenyth 200 (Anthos, Eugendorf, Austria) was used to assess optical density (OD) as reflected by absorbance at 492 nm wavelength and a reference wavelength of 620 nm (ELISA technology).

2.8. Cell Density

Photographs from wells of a 96-well plate with the various experimental groups were taken using a Basler scA1400–30gm camera, a CCD camera with Sony ICX285 CCD sensor (Essen Bioscience, Ann Arbor, MI, USA). The confluency of the cells was measured using the high throughput, continuous live cell imager Incucyte Zoom HD/2CLR System (Essen Bioscience, Ann Arbor, MI, USA) to assess the effects of $CoCl_2$ exposure on the density of the cells. The same number of cells were used in each assay for all wells. To ensure this, plating was done from one tube with cell suspension by collecting equal amounts from the tube for each well. In numbers, 40,000 cells per cm^2 were seeded and then the cells were cultured till they reached 80–90% confluency.

2.9. Statistical Analysis and Data Presentation

Relative changes (%) were used for comparisons among assays. GraphPad prism (GraphPad Software, San Diego, CA, USA) was used for statistical analysis. The results were expressed as mean ± SEM. One-way analysis of variance (ANOVA) was performed followed by Bonferroni's post hoc test for multiple comparisons as appropriate. $p < 0.05$ was considered as statistically significant.

3. Results

3.1. Screening of TSPO Ligand Efficacy in the Protection of Cellular Viability

Assessment of the efficacy of the TSPO ligands in the prevention of $CoCl_2$ cytotoxicity was determined using a cellular viability assay (XTT) with different TSPO ligands CB86, CB194, CB199, CB204, and alpidem, at concentrations of 1 μM, 10 μM, 25 μM, 50 μM, and 100 μM for each of them (Figure 1A–E). It was demonstrated that the high affinity CB86 ligand and the high affinity alpidem, did not protect against the cytotoxicity caused by $CoCl_2$ (0.5 mM), while the low affinity CB204 achieved significant protective capacity by 76% at a concentration of 25 μM (Figure 1C) and by 85% at 100 μM (Figure 1E). In addition, the low affinity CB194 and CB199 ligands displayed significant protection by 61% and by 59%, respectively, against $CoCl_2$ cytotoxicity only at a concentration of 100 μM (Figure 1E). According to these data (Figure 1), the high affinity ligand CB86 and the low affinity ligand CB204 at a concentration of 100 μM were chosen for further investigation of the potential effects of the affinity of the TSPO ligands in the protection from $CoCl_2$-induced cellular damage.

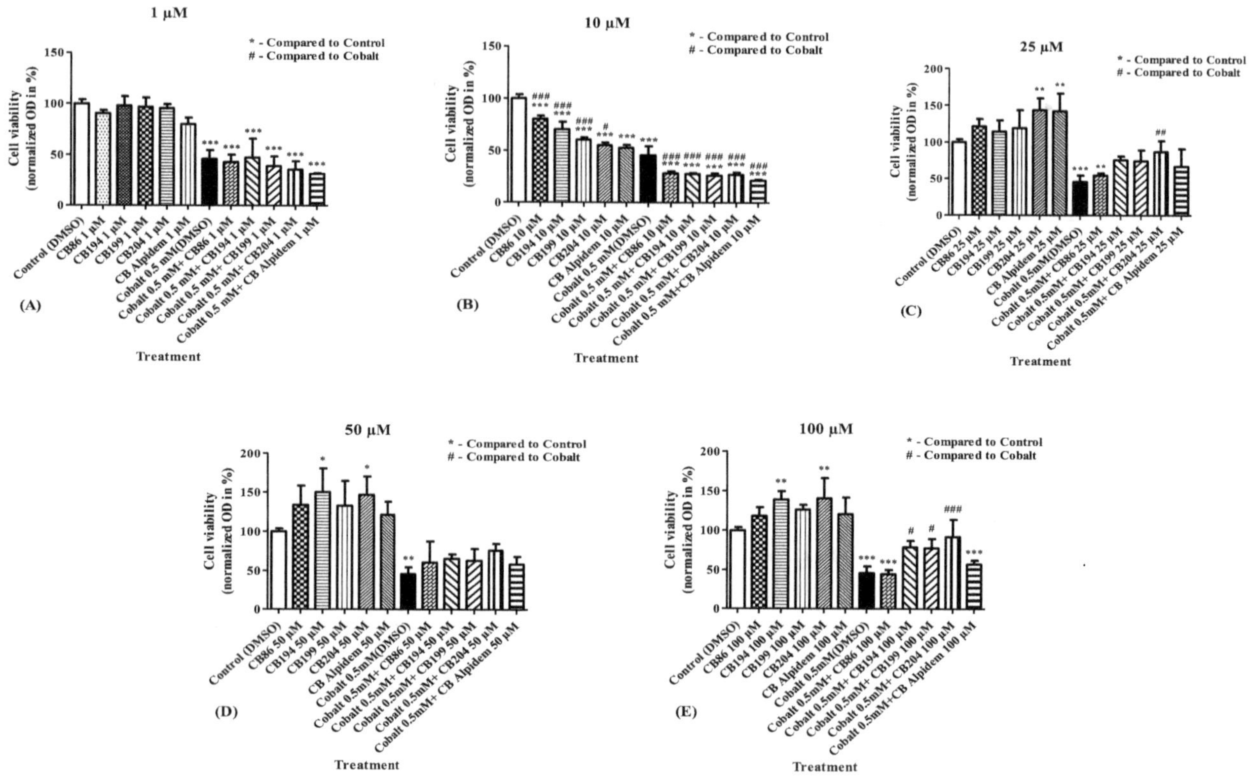

Figure 1. Determination of the ligand efficacy in inhibition of $CoCl_2$-induced decrease in cellular viability (XTT assay). Cell viability was assessed following pretreatment with TSPO ligands at various concentrations of 1 µM, 10 µM, 25 µM, 50 µM, and 100 µM (**A–E**). Results are expressed as mean ± SEM ($n = 5$ replicates in each group). # and * $p < 0.05$, ## and ** $p < 0.01$, ### and *** $p < 0.001$.

In general, going from high affinity to low affinity TSPO ligands (Table 1) was associated with larger protective effect (Figure 1).

3.2. Dose–Response Analyses for the Efficacy of CB86 and CB204 Ligands in the Prevention of $CoCl_2$-Induced Decrease in Cellular Viability

To verify the indications described in Figure 1, the modulatory effect of CB86 and CB204 on cell viability following exposure to $CoCl_2$ was assessed. The range of concentrations of these two ligands was expanded, from 1 µM to 100 µM (Figure 1), and from 5 nM to 100 µM (Figure 2), to ensure that no major concentration-dependent effects were overlooked. Dose–response assessment was performed for CB86 and CB204 using cellular viability assay (XTT). Pretreatment with increasing concentrations of CB86 did not inhibit the cytotoxic effect of 0.5 mM $CoCl_2$ at any tested concentration (Figure 2A). In contrast, the low affinity TSPO ligand CB204 at concentrations of 25 µM and 100 µM prevented 50% and 81% of the cellular damage, respectively (Figure 2B). At 100 µM, CB204 caused maintenance at control levels, i.e., cell viability was not significantly different from vehicle-exposed cells. Figures 1 and 2 show that 100 µM is the optimal concentration for CB204 capacity to provide protection from $CoCl_2$-induced cell death.

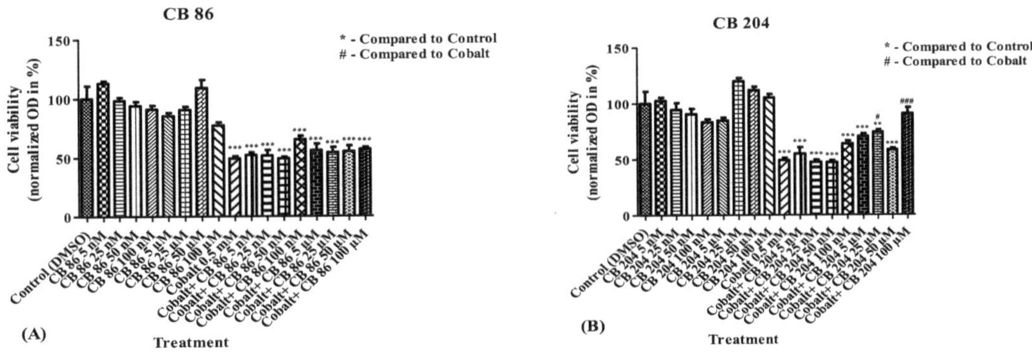

Figure 2. Dose response analysis of CB86 and CB204 ligands in inhibition of cellular viability decrease induced by $CoCl_2$. XTT assay was performed to measure the levels of cellular viability following exposure to $CoCl_2$ after pretreatment with (**A**) CB86 and (**B**) CB204 at increasing concentrations. Results are expressed as mean ± SEM ($n = 5$ replicates in each group). $^{\#}$ $p < 0.05$, $^{\#\#}$ and ** $p < 0.01$, $^{\#\#\#}$ and *** $p < 0.001$.

3.3. *ADP/ATP Ratio*

Following $CoCl_2$ exposure for 24 h, the ADP/ATP ratio significantly increased by 84% ($p < 0.001$) as compared to the control group (absolute level of ADP/ATP luminescence ratio was 0.1). This increase was not attenuated significantly by pretreatment with CB86 at a concentration of 100 μM (49%; $p > 0.05$), while pretreatment with CB204 at a concentration of 100 μM significantly attenuated (67%; $p < 0.01$) the increase in ADP/ATP ratio, as compared to the $CoCl_2$-exposed group (Figure 3).

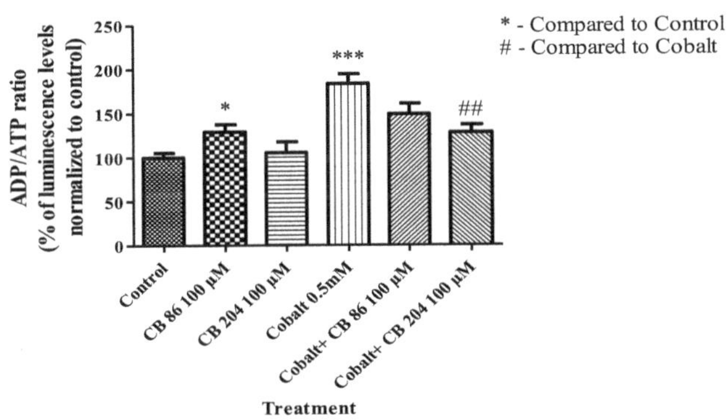

Figure 3. The ability of TSPO ligands to attenuate $CoCl_2$-induced ATP synthase reversal. ELISA was performed to measure the alterations in ADP/ATP ratio with and without pretreatment with the TSPO ligands. Results are expressed as mean ± SEM ($n = 5$ replicates in each group). * $p < 0.05$, $^{\#\#}$ $p < 0.01$, and *** $p < 0.001$.

Regarding ADP/ATP ratio, CB86 appears to have a dual effect: slightly cytotoxic by itself, but protective from the cytotoxic effects of $CoCl_2$. Reminiscent of the effects on ROS levels described in Section 3.4 (Figure 4).

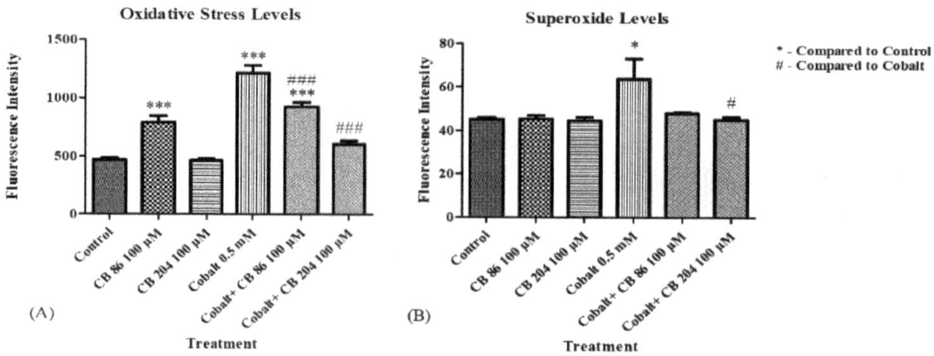

Figure 4. The protective effect of the TSPO ligands in prevention of reactive oxygen species (ROS) elevation. ELISA was performed to evaluate the levels of oxidative stress and superoxide levels. (**A**) Represents the oxidative stress levels, and (**B**) Represents the superoxide levels, with and without pretreatment with TSPO ligands. Results are expressed as mean ± SEM ($n = 6$ replicates in each group). $^{\#}$ and * $p < 0.05$, $^{\#\#\#}$ and *** $p < 0.001$.

3.4. Oxidative Stress and Superoxide Levels

ROS levels were measured following $CoCl_2$ exposure of CB86 and CB204 pretreated cells. Significant elevation in ROS levels was detected following pretreatment of the cells with CB86 ligand alone, while no elevation occurred following pretreatment with the TSPO ligand CB204 alone. $CoCl_2$ induced a significant elevation in oxidative stress levels by (158%; $p < 0.001$) as compared to the control group. Pretreatment with CB86 at a concentration of 100 μM significantly prevented (39%; $p < 0.001$) of the $CoCl_2$-induced increase in ROS generation, however remained significantly higher than the control ($p < 0.001$). In contrast, pretreatment with CB204 at a concentration of 100 μM significantly prevented 82% of the $CoCl_2$-induced elevation (at the control range; $p < 0.001$; Figure 4A). In a second assay, superoxide levels were not elevated in response to the incubation with both ligands alone. $CoCl_2$ exposure for 24 h induced a significant elevation (41%; $p < 0.05$) as compared to the control group, while pretreatment with CB86 did not prevent significantly the elevation in superoxide levels ($p > 0.05$; Figure 4B). CB204 was more effective in preventing this elevation (actually to control range; $p < 0.05$; Figure 4B).

3.5. Depolarization of the Mitochondrial Membrane Potential ($\Delta\Psi m$)

$\Delta\Psi m$ depolarization was measured by JC-1 fluorescence changes as described in the methods. Significant depolarization of the $\Delta\Psi m$ (18%; $p < 0.001$) occurred after exposure to $CoCl_2$, as compared to the control group. Pre-treatment with CB86 at a concentration of 100 μM did not show any protective effect and $\Delta\Psi m$ remained significantly different from the control group ($p < 0.001$). Pretreatment with CB204 prevented completely the depolarization of the $\Delta\Psi m$ ($p < 0.001$) induced by $CoCl_2$ (Figure 5A–G). Carbonyl cyanide chlorophenylhydrazone (CCCP) was used as a positive control and its administration resulted in a significant increase in depolarization of $\Delta\Psi m$ (by 48% vs. control raw level; $p < 0.001$) (Figure 5H).

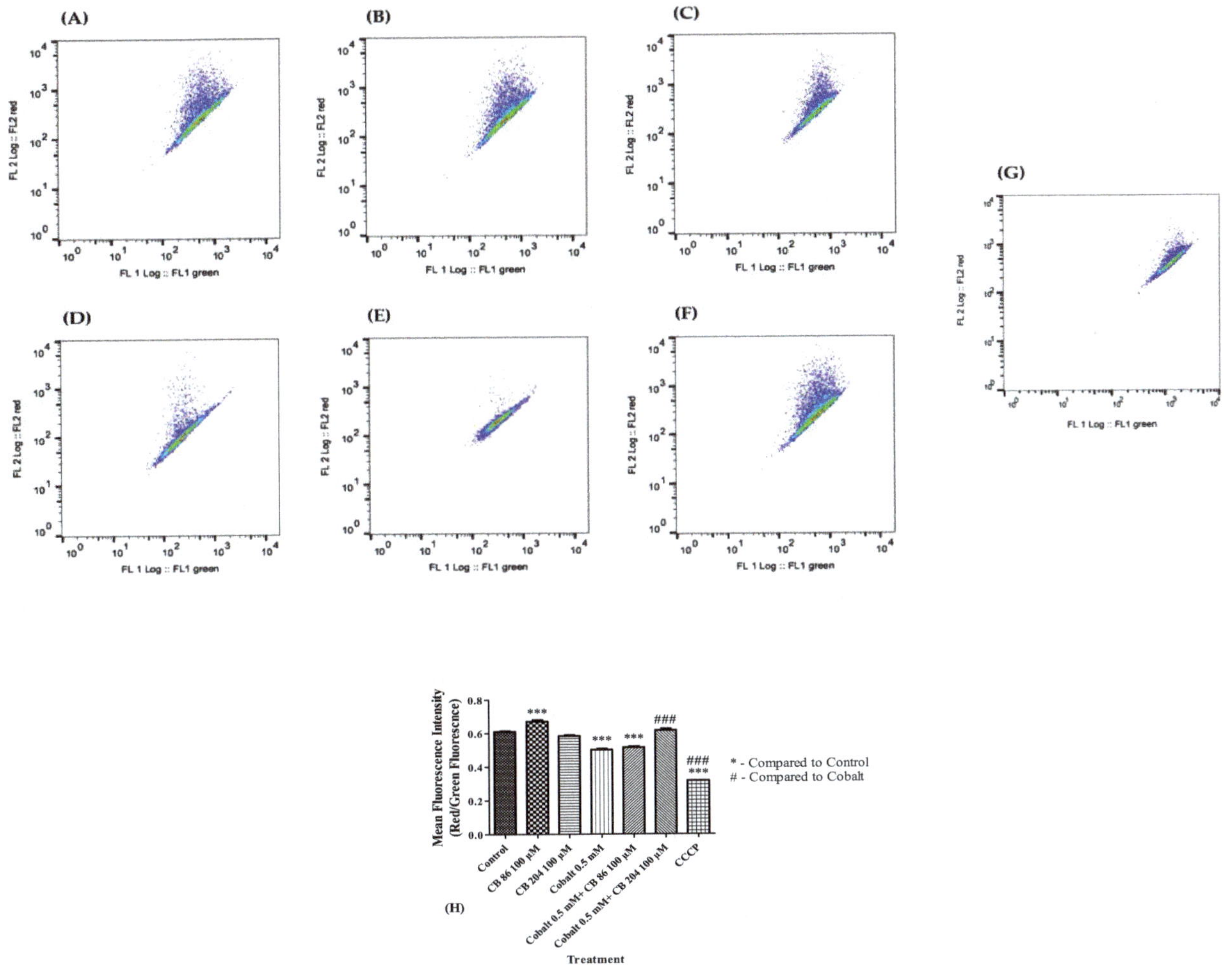

Figure 5. Comparison of the protective capacities of CB86 and CB204 in prevention of mitochondrial membrane potential depolarization. FACS was used to evaluate the $\Delta\psi m$ depolarization in (**A**) Control group, (**B**) cells pretreated with CB86 alone, (**C**) cells pretreated with CB204 alone, (**D**) cells exposed to 0.5 mM of $CoCl_2$, (**E**) cells pretreated with CB86 and exposed to $CoCl_2$, (**F**) cells pretreated with CB204 and exposed to $CoCl_2$, (**G**) positive control group exposed to CCCP, and (**H**) representative bar graph of the raw data. Results are expressed as mean ± SEM ($n = 7$ replicates in each group). ### and *** $p < 0.001$.

3.6. LDH Assay of Cell Death

Cytotoxicity levels were measured by release of LDH enzyme into the media. $CoCl_2$ exposure resulted in a significant elevation in cytotoxicity levels by 52% ($p < 0.001$) as compared to the control group (absolute LDH level measured by OD was 0.5). Pretreatment with the TSPO ligand CB86 at a concentration of 100 μM did not attenuate significantly the LDH elevation, while CB204 at a concentration of 100 μM completely prevented the LDH elevation (100%; $p < 0.001$) as compared to the $CoCl_2$-exposed group. Both CB86 and CB204 had no effect when applied alone (Figure 6).

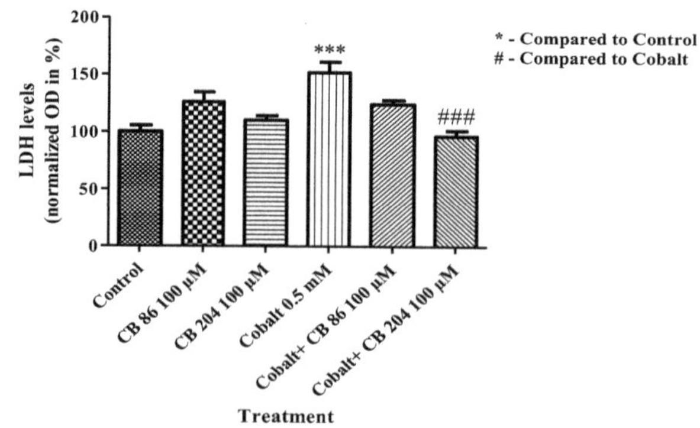

Figure 6. Prevention of $CoCl_2$-induced cellular cytotoxicity by TSPO ligands. LDH cytotoxicity assay was performed to measure cytotoxicity levels following exposure to $CoCl_2$ with or without TSPO ligands pretreatment. Results are expressed as mean ± SEM ($n = 5$ replicates in each group). ### and *** $p < 0.001$.

3.7. XTT Assay of Cell Viability

Following $CoCl_2$ exposure, cellular viability significantly decreased by 54% ($p < 0.001$) as compared to the control group. Pretreatment with CB86 at a concentration of 100 µM did not prevent the decrease in cell viability, while CB204 at a concentration of 100 µM significantly prevented the decrease in cell viability as compared to the $CoCl_2$-exposed group (85%; $p < 0.001$; Figure 7).

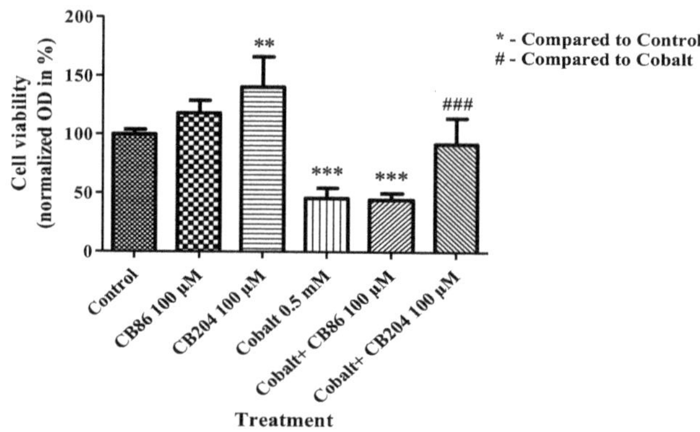

Figure 7. The protective effect of TSPO ligands in preventing the decrease in cellular viability. XTT assay was performed to measure the levels of cellular viability following $CoCl_2$ exposure with or without TSPO ligands pretreatment. Results are expressed as mean ± SEM ($n = 5$ replicates in each group). ** $p < 0.01$, ### and *** $p < 0.001$.

3.8. Cellular Density

Representative illustration of the alterations in cell density are depicted in Figure 8A–F. The density of the cells significantly decreased by 32% (Figure 8G) following exposure to 0.5 mM $CoCl_2$ for 24 h, relative to the control group (set as 100%) (Figure 8G). The application of the high affinity ligand CB86 alone at a concentration of 100 µM induced a robust reduction in cell density (by 79%; $p < 0.001$; Figure 8G). No further decrease in cell density occurred when CB86 (100 µM) was applied as a pretreatment to $CoCl_2$ exposure (by 82%; $p < 0.001$; Figure 8G). In the case of pretreatment with the low affinity ligand CB204 at a concentration of 100 µM, the density of the cells remained within the control range (Figure 8C). Also, when exposed to $CoCl_2$, the pretreatment with CB204 prevented 97% of the $CoCl_2$-induced decrease in cell density (Figure 8G). The collected data are summarized in Figure 8G.

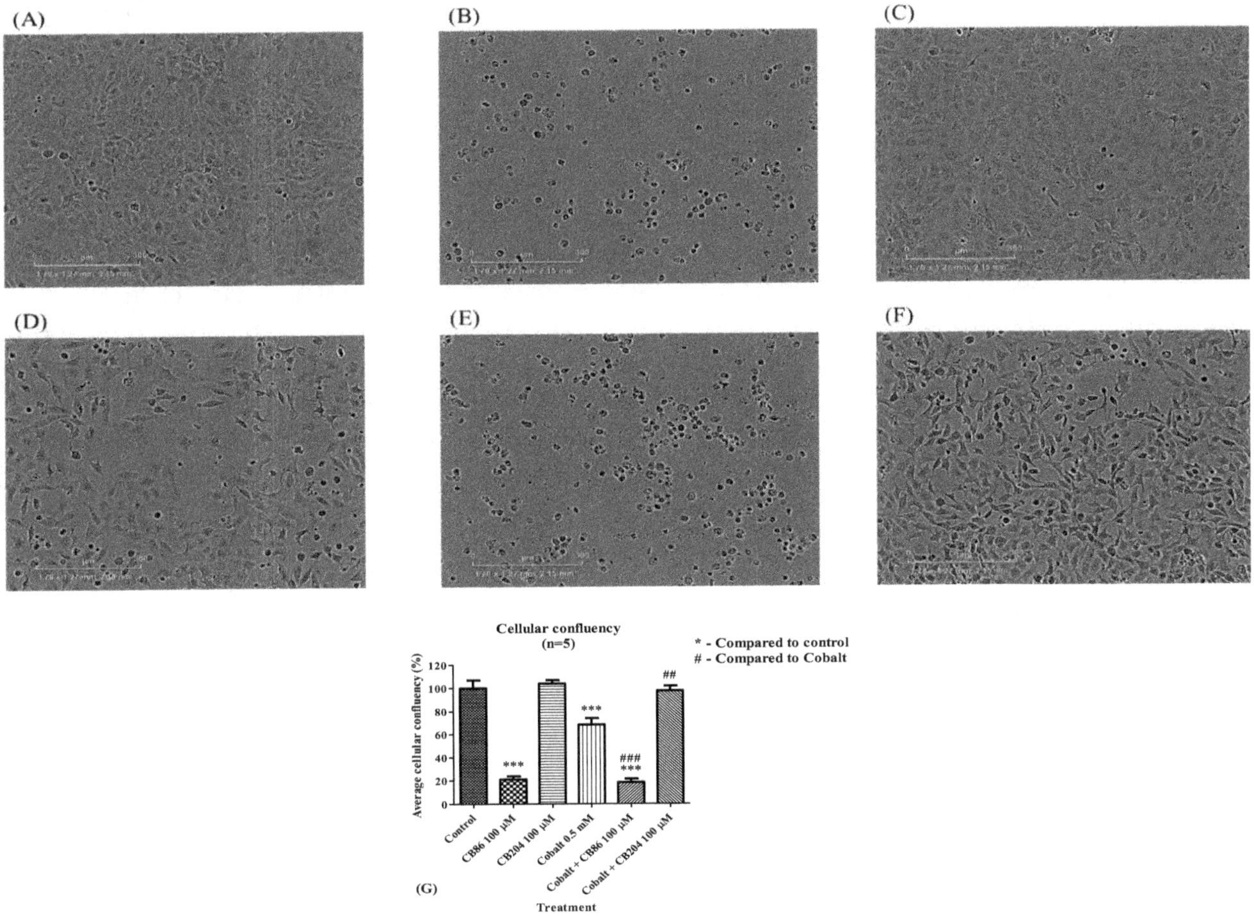

Figure 8. The effects of CB86 and CB204 on reductions of cell density caused by $CoCl_2$. Photographs showing the density of H1299 cells in (**A**) control group, (**B**) following pretreatment with the high affinity CB86 ligand alone (100 μM), (**C**) following pretreatment with the low affinity CB204 ligand alone (100 μM), (**D**) following exposure to 0.5 mM of $CoCl_2$, (**E**) following pretreatment with the high affinity CB86 at a concentration of 100 μM and exposure to 0.5 mM $CoCl_2$, (**F**) following pretreatment with the low affinity CB204 at a concentration of 100 μM and exposure to 0.5 mM $CoCl_2$, and (**G**) a bar graph summarizing the results. Results in Figure 8G are presented as mean ± SEM (n = 5 replicates in each group). $^{\#\#}$ $p < 0.01$, $^{\#\#\#}$ and *** $p < 0.001$.

In summary, CB86 (with and without $CoCl_2$) caused robust reductions in cell density, while CB204 alone has no harmful effect on cell density and prevented completely reductions in cell density induced by exposure $CoCl_2$.

3.9. Summary of the Collected Data

As the results show (Figures 3–8), application of the high affinity TSPO ligand CB86 applied alone at a concentration of 100 μM caused: (1) Increase in the ADP/ATP ratio (Figure 3); (2) increase in ROS generation, but without effect on superoxide levels (Figure 4); (3) increase in the occurrence of ΔΨm depolarization (Figure 5); (4) increase of cell membrane disruption as assessed by LDH levels in the supernatant (Figure 6). In contrast, the low affinity TSPO ligand CB204 at the same concentration (100 μM) did not induce any cytotoxic effects (Figures 3–8). The overall efficient protective effects indicate a favorable profile of the low affinity TSPO ligand CB204 (Figures 1–8) with regard to efficacy and safety in hypoxic cellular conditions.

4. Discussion

In this study, we focused on the capacity of two TSPO ligands, the high affinity CB86 and the low affinity CB204 (affinity and structure presented in Table 1 and Scheme 1) to prevent cellular damage induced by $CoCl_2$ (Figures 3–8 and Scheme 2). Based on ligand efficacy in prevention of $CoCl_2$-induced cytotoxicity (Figure 1) and dose–response analysis (Figure 2), the high affinity CB86 ligand and the low affinity CB204 ligand at a concentration of 100 μM were chosen for this study. A previous study demonstrated the protective effects of the high affinity TSPO ligand PK 11195 (25 μM), in $CoCl_2$-induced cell death, which was reminiscent to the protective effect of TSPO gene knockdown [22]. The protective effect of the TSPO ligands was established in several $CoCl_2$-induced cytotoxic assays, including ADP/ATP ratio, ROS generation, superoxide levels, LDH cytotoxicity assay, cellular viability assay (XTT), and viable cell density. The low affinity ligand CB204 significantly inhibited the cytotoxic effect of $CoCl_2$ on H1299 lung cells in all the tested assays (Figures 3–8), furthermore, it was harmless when given alone. In contrast, the high affinity ligand CB86 was ineffective in the prevention of the cytotoxicity in most of the assays, except ROS generation. Moreover, CB86 was harmful when given alone in the assay of density of viable cells (Figure 8). Our results show that the effects of TSPO ligands reported in brain cells, are not restricted to cells of the central nervous system [35,37,38], but also applicable to lung cancer cells. It would be interesting to test whether this could be true for other types of cells as well.

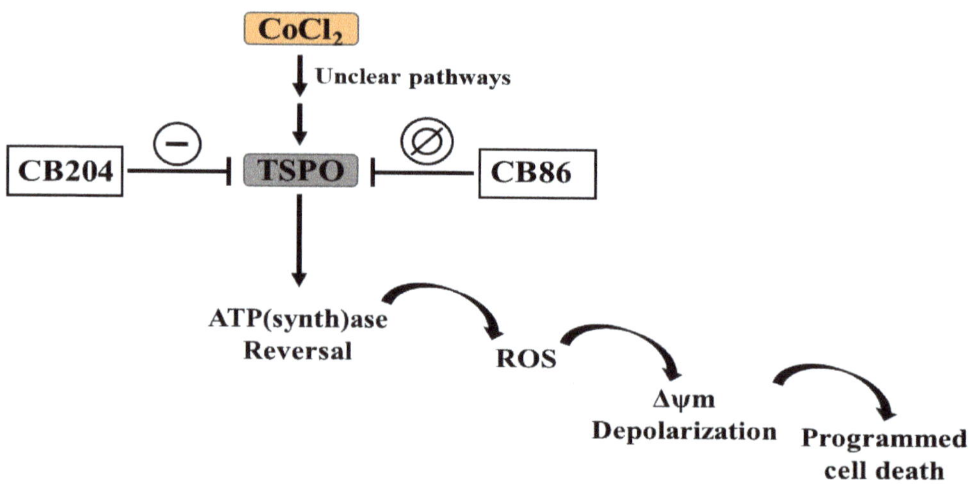

Scheme 2. The capacity of TSPO ligand to inhibit the initiation of the $CoCl_2$ cytotoxic effect and its propagation towards mitochondrial apoptosis cascade. The progression was inhibited by the low affinity CB204, but not by the high affinity CB86, TSPO ligands.

The difference in the protective capacity of the two ligands could be related to differences in their affinity to TSPO or could be related to their putative agonistic or antagonistic activities at the TSPO. Several studies attempted to identify the agonistic or antagonistic properties of TSPO ligands and to sort them as agonists and antagonists. Unfortunately, such classification of TSPO ligands was abandoned, since the same ligand may exert an agonistic activity or an antagonistic activity, depending on the investigated TSPO function [48,49]. The present study confirms the observation that high affinity TSPO ligands can exert harmful, and even lethal, cellular effects, as was described in other paradigms [34–36]. On the other hand, most importantly, the present study supports the notion that low affinity TSPO ligands, may possess protective cellular effects and are devoid of cytotoxic effects, as was demonstrated in previous studies [35,37,38].

Different ligands have varying cellular impact in nanomolar or micromolar range concentrations depending on the TSPO complex composition and the varying affinities to the TSPO complex present in a specific cell [49]. For example, the TSPO2 isoform, the main isoform at the red blood cells membrane requires micromolar concentrations for modulation of cellular functions, while the TSPO1 isoform requires nanomolar concentrations for modulation of cellular functions [49–52]. Such difference in specific ligand-interacting structural domains, within the TSPO protein or the protein complex, could explain the variability in the impact of TSPO ligands at different concentrations in different cell types. The presence of a high affinity and a low affinity binding sites can explain the dose-dependent dual effects of some TSPO ligands [39,40,53,54]. For example, the high affinity TSPO ligands PK 11195, Ro5–4864, and FGIN-1-27 at nanomolar concentrations protect U118MG human glioma cells from ammonia-induced cytotoxicity, while at micromolar concentrations the same ligands induce cytotoxic effects [36]. We suggest that this association between affinity of the ligands to TSPO and their protective potency regarding cell viability may be the rule rather than a coincidence. Yet, this notion should be investigated further in other cell types. The two ligands CB194 and CB199 with the lowest affinity (Table 1) did not show lethal cellular effect, but they may influence other TSPO functions. It is unclear whether these ligands act at the same ligand binding site, or at different ones. At present, only a restricted number of ligand binding sites were identified [36]. Previous studies showed that binding of the ligands might be influenced by the interaction between TSPO and the TSPO-associated proteins, such as mitochondrial voltage-dependent anion channels (or mitochondrial porins; VDAC) [55,56]. For example, the anticancer drugs ErPC and ErPC3, do not bind directly to TSPO, but they exert their anti-proliferative effect indirectly through TSPO [29], while TRO 19622 binds to both the TSPO and its associated protein VDAC [57].

TSPO is associated with regulation of various intracellular and mitochondrial processes. In the current study, the cytotoxic impact of CB86 on viable cellular density was accompanied by inability to protect most of the vital cellular metabolic processes. Modulation of TSPO protein expression leads to a cascade of events, including reversal of ATP synthase activity, followed by elevated ROS generation causing oxidative stress [23,29,58,59], which is associated with $\Delta\psi M$ depolarization, and eventually cell death (Scheme 2) [60]. Such a correlation between TSPO and cell death, mainly apoptotic cell death, was investigated previously. Exposure of U118MG glioblastoma cells to $CoCl_2$ resulted in increased apoptotic cell death, while TSPO knockdown prevented this cytotoxic effect of $CoCl_2$. Moreover, exposure of the cells to the proapoptotic agent $CoCl_2$ resulted in parallel increases in TSPO expression levels, as determined by Western blot and binding capacity. The same study demonstrated the role of TSPO in cellular processes leading to apoptosis [22]. Regarding another function, apart from $\Delta\Psi m$ collapse initiating the mitochondrial apoptosis cascade, TSPO via the mitochondria-to-cell-nucleus-pathway may also affect apoptosis induction due to modulation of cell nuclear gene expression for proteins that play a role in functional pathways regulating apoptosis [61]. Thus, the present observations on lung cells are similar to previous observations in brain cells, i.e., indicative of a common property, rather than a cell, tissue, or organ specific effect. However, research on different cell types, from different tissues and organs are required to further substantiate notion.

It was shown previously that 0.1–1 mM of $CoCl_2$ can mimic hypoxia in urinary bladder smooth muscle cells as well as cardiomyocytes [62,63]. In the current study in H1299 lung cancer cell line, it was shown that the $CoCl_2$-induced cascade of apoptotic events demonstrated in Scheme 2, may be prevented by TSPO ligands. The results emphasize the superiority of the low affinity TSPO ligand (CB204) in preventing cell death as well the preceding cascade of events leading to cell death as compared to the high affinity ligand (CB86). Previous studies have shown that TSPO ligands affect also cell proliferation, hence, it would also be interesting to test this for CB86 and CB204. It may be assumed that different binding domains modulate different TSPO functions.

In conclusion, our study demonstrated the robust efficacy of the low affinity TSPO ligand (CB204) in the prevention of $CoCl_2$-induced cellular damages in lung cells. The protective effect of the low affinity ligand was reflected in the inhibition of the appearance of classical makers of cytotoxicity assessed in this study. In contrast, the high affinity ligand (CB86) was effective only in the prevention of oxidative stress (ROS generation). These results may have clinical implications, namely, the potential use of the low affinity TSPO ligand CB204, but not the high affinity ligand CB86, for the treatment of lung cell pathologies related to hypoxia, such as pulmonary ischemia and COPD.

Future studies should address the following issues: the impact of TSPO knockdown and other TSPO ligands, to clarify further the role of TSPO in the $CoCl_2$-related cellular damage as well as the role of the TSPO ligands, preferably low affinity ligands, in the protection from non-$CoCl_2$-related hypoxic damage. Noteworthy, the current study, as well as a similar previous study on U118MG glioblastoma cells, were conducted on cells from human origin. Thus, it would be of interest to investigate the effects of TSPO ligands on cells of other species. The mechanism underpinning the impact of $CoCl_2$ on TSPO remains unclear (Scheme 2), further gene expression studies must be performed to identify the cellular pathways that are involved in the inhibitory effect of TSPO on in vitro and in vivo hypoxic states.

Author Contributions: Conceptualization, investigation, formal analysis, and writing—original draft preparation, N.Z.; methodology and data curation, N.Z., A.W. and M.G.; writing—review and editing, M.G., A.W., N.D., V.L. and M.F.; supervision, M.G. and A.W.; funding acquisition, M.G. and N.D. All authors have read and agreed to the published version of the manuscript.

References

1. Tuder, R.M.; Yun, J.H.; Bhunia, A.; Fijalkowska, I. Hypoxia and chronic lung disease. *J. Mol. Med.* **2007**, *85*, 1317–1324. [CrossRef]
2. Bensaid, S.; Fabre, C.; Fourneau, J.; Cieniewski-Bernard, C. Impact of different methods of induction of cellular hypoxia: Focus on protein homeostasis signaling pathways and morphology of C2C12 skeletal muscle cells differentiated into myotubes. *J. Physiol. Biochem.* **2019**, *75*, 367–377. [CrossRef] [PubMed]
3. Chen, D.; Fang, F.; Yang, Y.; Chen, J.; Xu, G.; Xu, Y.; Gao, Y. Brahma-related gene 1 (Brg1) epigenetically regulates CAM activation during hypoxic pulmonary hypertension. *Cardiovasc. Res.* **2013**, *100*, 363–373. [CrossRef] [PubMed]
4. Chen, D.; Yang, Y.; Cheng, X.; Fang, F.; Xu, G.; Yuan, Z.; Fang, M. Megakaryocytic leukemia 1 directs a histone H3 lysine 4 methyltransferase complex to regulate hypoxic pulmonary hypertension. *Hypertension* **2015**, *65*, 821–833. [CrossRef] [PubMed]
5. Janaszak-Jasiecka, A.; Siekierzycka, A.; Bartoszewska, S.; Serocki, M.; Dobrucki, L.W.; Collawn, J.F.; Bartoszewski, R. eNOS expression and NO release during hypoxia is inhibited by miR-200b in human endothelial cells. *Angiogenesis* **2018**, *21*, 711–724. [CrossRef] [PubMed]
6. Omura, J.; Satoh, K.; Kikuchi, N.; Satoh, T.; Kurosawa, R.; Nogi, M.; Sunamura, S. Protective Roles of Endothelial AMP-Activated Protein Kinase Against Hypoxia-Induced Pulmonary Hypertension in Mice. *Circ. Res.* **2016**, *119*, 197–209. [CrossRef] [PubMed]
7. Stenmark, K.R.; Fagan, K.A.; Frid, M.G. Hypoxia-induced pulmonary vascular remodeling: Cellular and molecular mechanisms. *Circ. Res.* **2006**, *99*, 675–691. [CrossRef]
8. Xu, W.; Erzurum, S.C. Endothelial cell energy metabolism, proliferation, and apoptosis in pulmonary hypertension. *Compr. Physiol.* **2011**, *1*, 357–372.
9. Ferrero, E.; Fulgenzi, A.; Belloni, D.; Foglieni, C.; Ferrero, M.E. Cellfood improves respiratory metabolism of endothelial cells and inhibits hypoxia-induced reactive oxygen species (ros) generation. *J. Physiol. Pharmacol.* **2011**, *62*, 287–293.
10. Debigaré, R.; Marquis, K.; Côté, C.H.; Tremblay, R.R.; Michaud, A.; LeBlanc, P.; Maltais, F. Catabolic/anabolic balance and muscle wasting in patients with COPD. *Chest* **2003**, *124*, 83–89. [CrossRef]
11. Egerman, M.A.; Glass, D.J. Signaling pathways controlling skeletal muscle mass. *Crit. Rev. Biochem. Mol. Biol.* **2014**, *49*, 59–68. [CrossRef] [PubMed]
12. Langen, R.C.J.; Gosker, H.R.; Remels, A.H.V.; Schols, A.M.W.J. Triggers and mechanisms of skeletal muscle wasting in chronic obstructive pulmonary disease. *Int. J. Biochem. Cell Biol.* **2013**, *45*, 2245–2256. [CrossRef] [PubMed]
13. Goldberg, M.A.; Schneider, T.J. Similarities between the Oxygen-Sensing Mechanisms Regulating the Expression of Vascular Endothelial Growth-Factor and Erythropoietin. *J. Biol. Chem.* **1994**, *269*, 4355–4359. [PubMed]

14. Griguer, C.E.; Oliva, C.R.; Kelley, E.E.; Giles, G.I.; Lancaster, J.R.; Gillespie, G.Y. Xanthine oxidase-dependent regulation of hypoxia-inducible factor in cancer cells. *Cancer Res.* **2006**, *66*, 2257–2263. [CrossRef] [PubMed]
15. Harris, G.K.; Shi, X. Signaling by carcinogenic metals and metal-induced reactive oxygen species. *Mutat. Res.* **2003**, *533*, 183–200. [CrossRef]
16. Hervouet, E.; Pecina, P.; Demont, J.; Vojtíšková, A.; Simonnet, H.; Houštěk, J.; Godinot, C. Inhibition of cytochrome c oxidase subunit 4 precursor processing by the hypoxia mimic cobalt chloride. *Biochem. Biophys. Res. Commun.* **2006**, *344*, 1086–1093. [CrossRef]
17. Leonard, S.S.; Harris, G.K.; Shi, X. Metal-induced oxidative stress and signal transduction. *Free Radic. Biol. Med.* **2004**, *37*, 1921–1942. [CrossRef]
18. Santore, M.T.; McClintock, D.S.; Lee, V.Y.; Budinger, G.S.; Chandel, N.S. Anoxia-induced apoptosis occurs through a mitochondria-dependent pathway in lung epithelial cells. *Am. J. Physiol. Lung Cell. Mol. Physiol.* **2002**, *282*, L727–L734. [CrossRef]
19. Vijayasarathy, C.; Damle, S.; Lenka, N.; Avadhani, N.G. Tissue variant effects of heme inhibitors on the mouse cytochrome c oxidase gene expression and catalytic activity of the enzyme complex. *Eur. J. Biochem.* **1999**, *266*, 191–200. [CrossRef]
20. Liu, J.; Zhu, Y.; Chen, S.; Shen, B.; Yu, F.; Zhang, Y.; Shen, R. Apocynin Attenuates Cobalt Chloride-Induced Pheochromocytoma Cell Apoptosis by Inhibiting P38-MAPK/Caspase-3 Pathway. *Cell. Physiol. Biochem.* **2018**, *48*, 208–214. [CrossRef]
21. Padmanaban, G.; Sarma, P.S. Cobalt toxicity and iron metabolism in Neurospora crassa. *Biochem. J.* **1966**, *98*, 330–334. [CrossRef] [PubMed]
22. Zeno, S.; Zaaroor, M.; Leschiner, S.; Veenman, L.; Gavish, M. CoCl(2) induces apoptosis via the 18 kDa translocator protein in U118MG human glioblastoma cells. *Biochemistry* **2009**, *48*, 4652–4661. [CrossRef] [PubMed]
23. Zeno, S.; Veenman, L.; Katz, Y.; Bode, J.; Gavish, M.; Zaaroor, M. The 18 kDa mitochondrial translocator protein (TSPO) prevents accumulation of protoporphyrin IX. Involvement of reactive oxygen species (ROS). *Curr. Mol. Med.* **2012**, *12*, 494–501. [PubMed]
24. Tang, X.; Luo, Y.X.; Chen, H.Z.; Liu, D.P. Mitochondria, endothelial cell function, and vascular diseases. *Front. Physiol.* **2014**, *5*, 175. [CrossRef] [PubMed]
25. Kugler, W.; Veenman, L.; Shandalov, Y.; Leschiner, S.; Spanier, I.; Lakomek, M.; Gavish, M. Ligands of the mitochondrial 18 kDa translocator protein attenuate apoptosis of human glioblastoma cells exposed to erucylphosphohomocholine. *Cell. Oncol.* **2008**, *30*, 435–450. [PubMed]
26. Levin, E.; Premkumar, A.; Veenman, L.; Kugler, W.; Leschiner, S.; Spanier, I.; Pasternak, G.W. The peripheral-type benzodiazepine receptor and tumorigenicity: Isoquinoline binding protein (IBP) antisense knockdown in the C6 glioma cell line. *Biochemistry* **2005**, *44*, 9924–9935. [CrossRef]
27. Shoukrun, R.; Veenman, L.; Shandalov, Y.; Leschiner, S.; Spanier, I.; Karry, R.; Gavish, M. The 18-kDa translocator protein, formerly known as the peripheral-type benzodiazepine receptor, confers proapoptotic and antineoplastic effects in a human colorectal cancer cell line. *Pharm. Genom.* **2008**, *18*, 977–988. [CrossRef]
28. Veenman, L.; Levin, E.; Weisinger, G.; Leschiner, S.; Spanier, I.; Snyder, S.H.; Gavish, M. Peripheral-type benzodiazepine receptor density and in vitro tumorigenicity of glioma cell lines. *Biochem. Pharmacol.* **2004**, *68*, 689–698. [CrossRef]
29. Veenman, L.; Shandalov, Y.; Gavish, M. VDAC activation by the 18 kDa translocator protein (TSPO), implications for apoptosis. *J. Bioenerg. Biomembr.* **2008**, *40*, 199–205. [CrossRef]
30. Gavish, M.; Bachman, I.; Shoukrun, R.; Katz, Y.; Veenman, L.; Weisinger, G.; Weizman, A. Enigma of the peripheral benzodiazepine receptor. *Pharmacol. Rev.* **1999**, *51*, 629–650.
31. Papadopoulos, V.; Baraldi, M.; Guilarte, T.R.; Knudsen, T.B.; Lacapère, J.J.; Lindemann, P.; Gavish, M. Translocator protein (18kDa): New nomenclature for the peripheral-type benzodiazepine receptor based on its structure and molecular function. *Trends Pharmacol. Sci.* **2006**, *27*, 402–409. [CrossRef] [PubMed]
32. Veenman, L.; Gavish, M. The peripheral-type benzodiazepine receptor and the cardiovascular system. Implications for drug development. *Pharmacol. Ther.* **2006**, *110*, 503–524. [CrossRef] [PubMed]
33. Denora, N.; Laquintana, V.; Pisu, M.G.; Dore, R.; Murru, L.; Latrofa, A.; Sanna, E. 2-Phenyl-imidazo[1,2-a]pyridine Compounds Containing Hydrophilic Groups as Potent and Selective Ligands for Peripheral Benzodiazepine Receptors: Synthesis, Binding Affinity and Electrophysiological Studies. *J. Med. Chem.* **2008**, *51*, 6876–6888. [CrossRef] [PubMed]

34. Azrad, M.; Zeineh, N.; Weizman, A.; Veenman, L.; Gavish, M. The TSPO Ligands 2-Cl-MGV-1, MGV-1, and PK11195 Differentially Suppress the Inflammatory Response of BV-2 Microglial Cell to LPS. *Int. J. Mol. Sci.* **2019**, *20*, 594. [CrossRef]
35. Vainshtein, A.; Veenman, L.; Shterenberg, A.; Singh, S.; Masarwa, A.; Dutta, B.; Maniv, I. Quinazoline-based tricyclic compounds that regulate programmed cell death, induce neuronal differentiation, and are curative in animal models for excitotoxicity and hereditary brain disease. *Cell Death Discov.* **2015**, *1*, 1–17. [CrossRef]
36. Veenman, L.; Vainshtein, A.; Yasin, N.; Azrad, M.; Gavish, M. Tetrapyrroles as Endogenous TSPO Ligands in Eukaryotes and Prokaryotes: Comparisons with Synthetic Ligands. *Int. J. Mol. Sci.* **2016**, *17*, 880. [CrossRef]
37. Chen, Y.; Veenman, L.; Singh, S.; Ouyang, F.; Liang, J.; Huang, W.; Gavish, M. 2-Cl-MGV-1 Ameliorates Apoptosis in the Thalamus and Hippocampus and Cognitive Deficits After Cortical Infarct in Rats. *Stroke* **2017**, *48*, 3366–3374. [CrossRef]
38. Shehadeh, M.; Palzur, E.; Apel, L.; Soustiel, J.F. Reduction of Traumatic Brain Damage by Tspo Ligand Etifoxine. *Int. J. Mol. Sci.* **2019**, *20*, 2639. [CrossRef]
39. Veenman, L.; Papadopoulos, V.; Gavish, M. Channel-like functions of the 18-kDa translocator protein (TSPO): Regulation of apoptosis and steroidogenesis as part of the host-defense response. *Curr. Pharm. Des.* **2007**, *13*, 2385–2405. [CrossRef]
40. Caballero, B.; Veenman, L.; Bode, J.; Leschiner, S.; Gavish, M. Concentration-dependent bimodal effect of specific 18 kDa translocator protein (TSPO) ligands on cell death processes induced by ammonium chloride: Potential implications for neuropathological effects due to hyperammonemia. *CNS Neurol. Disord. Drug Targets* **2014**, *13*, 574–592. [CrossRef]
41. Zeineh, N.; Nagler, R.; Gabay, M.; Weizman, A.; Gavish, M. Effects of Cigarette Smoke on TSPO-related Mitochondrial Processes. *Cells* **2019**, *8*, 694. [CrossRef] [PubMed]
42. Borcar, A.; Menze, M.A.; Toner, M.; Hand, S.C. Metabolic preconditioning of mammalian cells: Mimetic agents for hypoxia lack fidelity in promoting phosphorylation of pyruvate dehydrogenase. *Cell Tissue Res.* **2013**, *351*, 99–106. [CrossRef]
43. Kim, K.S.; Rajagopal, V.; Gonsalves, C.; Johnson, C.; Kalra, V.K. A novel role of hypoxia-inducible factor in cobalt chloride- and hypoxia-mediated expression of IL-8 chemokine in human endothelial cells. *J. Immunol.* **2006**, *177*, 7211–7224. [CrossRef] [PubMed]
44. Jones, N.M.; Kardashyan, L.; Callaway, J.K.; Lee, E.M.; Beart, P.M. Long-term functional and protective actions of preconditioning with hypoxia, cobalt chloride, and desferrioxamine against hypoxic-ischemic injury in neonatal rats. *Pediatr. Res.* **2008**, *63*, 620–624. [CrossRef] [PubMed]
45. Jung, J.Y.; Roh, K.H.; Jeong, Y.J.; Kim, S.H.; Lee, E.J.; Kim, M.S.; Kim, W.J. Estradiol protects PC12 cells against CoCl2-induced apoptosis. *Brain Res. Bull.* **2008**, *76*, 579–585. [CrossRef]
46. Wu, K.C.; Cheng, K.S.; Wang, Y.W.; Chen, Y.F.; Wong, K.L.; Su, T.H.; Leung, Y.M. Perturbation of Akt Signaling, Mitochondrial Potential, and ADP/ATP Ratio in Acidosis-Challenged Rat Cortical Astrocytes. *J. Cell Biochem.* **2017**, *118*, 1108–1117. [CrossRef]
47. Weiner, D.; Levy, Y.; Khankin, E.V.; Reznick, A.Z. Inhibition of salivary amylase activity by cigarette smoke aldehydes. *J. Physiol. Pharmacol.* **2008**, *59* (Suppl. S6), 727–737.
48. Le Fur, G.; Vaucher, N.; Perrier, M.L.; Flamier, A.; Benavides, J.; Renault, C.; Uzan, A. Differentiation between two ligands for peripheral benzodiazepine binding sites, [3H]RO5-4864 and [3H]PK 11195, by thermodynamic studies. *Life Sci.* **1983**, *33*, 449–457. [CrossRef]
49. Marginedas-Freixa, I.; Alvarez, C.L.; Moras, M.; Hattab, C.; Bouyer, G.; Chene, A.; Ostuni, M.A. Induction of ATP Release, PPIX Transport, and Cholesterol Uptake by Human Red Blood Cells Using a New Family of TSPO Ligands. *Int. J. Mol. Sci.* **2018**, *19*, 3098. [CrossRef]
50. Canat, X.; Carayon, P.; Bouaboula, M.; Cahard, D.; Shire, D.; Roque, C.; Casellas, P. Distribution profile and properties of peripheral-type benzodiazepine receptors on human hemopoietic cells. *Life Sci.* **1993**, *52*, 107–118. [CrossRef]
51. Olson, J.M.; Ciliax, B.J.; Mancini, W.R.; Young, A.B. Presence of peripheral-type benzodiazepine binding sites on human erythrocyte membranes. *Eur. J. Pharmacol.* **1988**, *152*, 47–53. [CrossRef]
52. Ostuni, M.A.; Ducroc, R.; Peranzi, G.; Tonon, M.C.; Papadopoulos, V.; Lacapere, J.J. Translocator protein (18 kDa) ligand PK 11195 induces transient mitochondrial Ca2+ release leading to transepithelial Cl- secretion in HT-29 human colon cancer cells. *Biol. Cell* **2007**, *99*, 639–647. [CrossRef] [PubMed]

53. Awad, M.; Gavish, M. Species differences and heterogeneity of solubilized peripheral-type benzodiazepine binding sites. *Biochem. Pharmacol.* **1989**, *38*, 3843–3849. [CrossRef]
54. Kanegawa, N.; Collste, K.; Forsberg, A.; Schain, M.; Arakawa, R.; Jucaite, A.; Halldin, C. In vivo evidence of a functional association between immune cells in blood and brain in healthy human subjects. *Brain Behav. Immun.* **2016**, *54*, 149–157. [CrossRef] [PubMed]
55. Garnier, M.A.R.T.I.N.E.; Dimchev, A.B.; Boujrad, N.O.U.R.E.D.D.I.N.E.; Price, J.M.; Musto, N.A.; Papadopoulos, V.A.S.S.I.L.I.O.S. In vitro reconstitution of a functional peripheral-type benzodiazepine receptor from mouse Leydig tumor cells. *Mol. Pharmacol.* **1994**, *45*, 201–211.
56. Veenman, L.; Leschiner, S.; Spanier, I.; Weisinger, G.; Weizman, A.; Gavish, M. PK 11195 attenuates kainic acid-induced seizures and alterations in peripheral-type benzodiazepine receptor (PBR) protein components in the rat brain. *J. Neurochem.* **2002**, *80*, 917–927. [CrossRef]
57. Bordet, T.; Buisson, B.; Michaud, M.; Drouot, C.; Galea, P.; Delaage, P.; Lacapere, J.J. Identification and characterization of cholest-4-en-3-one, oxime (TRO19622), a novel drug candidate for amyotrophic lateral sclerosis. *J. Pharmacol. Exp. Ther.* **2007**, *322*, 709–720. [CrossRef]
58. Caballero, B.; Veenman, L.; Gavish, M. Role of mitochondrial translocator protein (18 kDa) on mitochondrial-related cell death processes. *Recent Pat. Endocr. Metab. Immune Drug Discov.* **2013**, *7*, 86–101. [CrossRef]
59. Veenman, L.; Alten, J.; Linnemannstöns, K.; Shandalov, Y.; Zeno, S.; Lakomek, M.; Kugler, W. Potential involvement of F0F1-ATP(synth)ase and reactive oxygen species in apoptosis induction by the antineoplastic agent erucylphosphohomocholine in glioblastoma cell lines: A mechanism for induction of apoptosis via the 18 kDa mitochondrial translocator protein. *Apoptosis* **2010**, *15*, 753–768.
60. Veenman, L.; Gavish, M.; Kugler, W. Apoptosis induction by erucylphosphohomocholine via the 18 kDa mitochondrial translocator protein: Implications for cancer treatment. *Anticancer Agents Med. Chem.* **2014**, *14*, 559–577. [CrossRef]
61. Yasin, N.; Veenman, L.; Singh, S.; Azrad, M.; Bode, J.; Vainshtein, A.; Gavish, M. Classical and Novel TSPO Ligands for the Mitochondrial TSPO Can Modulate Nuclear Gene Expression: Implications for Mitochondrial Retrograde Signaling. *Int. J. Mol. Sci.* **2017**, *18*, 786. [CrossRef]
62. Sawada, N.; Yao, J.; Hiramatsu, N.; Hayakawa, K.; Araki, I.; Takeda, M.; Kitamura, M. Involvement of hypoxia-triggered endoplasmic reticulum stress in outlet obstruction-induced apoptosis in the urinary bladder. *Lab. Invest.* **2008**, *88*, 553–563. [CrossRef] [PubMed]
63. Shu, B.; Yang, W.W.; Yang, H.T. Expression pattern of E2F6 in physical and chemical hypoxia-induced apoptosis. *Sheng Li Xue Bao* **2008**, *60*, 1–10. [PubMed]

4

TRP Channels as Therapeutic Targets in Diabetes and Obesity

Andrea Zsombok [1,2,*] and Andrei V. Derbenev [1]

1 Department of Physiology, School of Medicine, Tulane University, New Orleans, LA 70112, USA; aderben@tulane.edu
2 Department of Medicine, Endocrinology Section, School of Medicine, Tulane University, New Orleans, LA 70112, USA
* Correspondence: azsombo@tulane.edu

Academic Editors: Arpad Szallasi and Susan M. Huang

Abstract: During the last three to four decades the prevalence of obesity and diabetes mellitus has greatly increased worldwide, including in the United States. Both the short- and long-term forecasts predict serious consequences for the near future, and encourage the development of solutions for the prevention and management of obesity and diabetes mellitus. Transient receptor potential (TRP) channels were identified in tissues and organs important for the control of whole body metabolism. A variety of TRP channels has been shown to play a role in the regulation of hormone release, energy expenditure, pancreatic function, and neurotransmitter release in control, obese and/or diabetic conditions. Moreover, dietary supplementation of natural ligands of TRP channels has been shown to have potential beneficial effects in obese and diabetic conditions. These findings raised the interest and likelihood for potential drug development. In this mini-review, we discuss possibilities for better management of obesity and diabetes mellitus based on TRP-dependent mechanisms.

Keywords: TRPV1; TRPM; TRPA1; obesity; diabetes mellitus; metabolism; glucose homeostasis

1. Introduction

The World Health Organization estimates that obesity doubled between 1980 and 2014, with 39% of adults being overweight and 13% being obese in 2014. In the United States the statistics are similarly alarming, more than one-third of the adults are obese and 17% of youth are also obese [1,2]. The consequences of obesity are severe including higher mortality rate, hypertension, dyslipidemia, heart disease, stroke, type 2 diabetes mellitus (T2DM), and many more.

Among the various pathophysiological conditions, T2DM is very prevalent and affects approximately 10% of the population worldwide. Lifestyle changes including weight loss can result in better glucose management; however, lifestyle changes require disciplined behavior and frequent monitoring. Unfortunately, patients often give up before reaching their goals or detectable results. In recent years, bariatric surgery has emerged as an effective treatment for improvement or remission of T2DM; however, due to the invasiveness of the procedure and potential surgical complications, bariatric surgery is not the most feasible solution. The most common treatments are still pharmacological interventions. Current pharmacological treatments mainly target the end organs by increasing insulin secretion from pancreatic beta cells (e.g., sulfonylureas), increasing tissue sensitivity to insulin (e.g., metformin), modulating the glucagon-like peptide 1 (GLP-1) system, preventing glucose reabsorption in the kidneys (SGLT2 inhibitors) or administering insulin. Despite the existing treatments, new therapeutic interventions are in great demand, therefore, every new idea, pathway, receptor, or compound (natural or synthetic) which has the potential of developing a new class of drugs for weight and/or glucose management receives attention.

Members of the transient receptor potential (TRP) family have been identified as key contributors in many physiological and pathophysiological conditions [3]. TRP channels were identified in numerous metabolically important tissues. Members of the canonical (TRPC), melastatin (TRPM), ankyrin (TRPA1), and vanilloid (TRPV) subfamilies were found to be expressed in the pancreas [3,4], liver, gastrointestinal tract [5], skeletal muscle, kidney [6–8], adipose tissue [9–12], heart [13–15], vasculature [16–18], and nervous system [19,20], including autonomic centers of the brain [21,22]. Despite that TRP channels and their natural ligands received considerable attention in the field of obesity and diabetes [4,23–28], their role in many of the metabolic processes are still debated and under investigation. This mini-review summarizes findings demonstrating functional roles of TRP channels in obese and diabetic conditions.

2. TRPV1 for the Prevention and Treatment of Obesity and Diabetes Mellitus

TRPV1 is one of the most studied TRP channels even in the context of obesity and diabetes mellitus. TRPV1, the first described member of the vanilloid subfamily, was cloned in 1997 [29]. It is a nonselective cation channel with permeability to Ca^{2+}. In the past decades TRPV1 was extensively researched and investigated as potential drug target for a variety of applications [23,30,31]. Numerous findings related to TRPV1 including its structure, species-related differences, topology, agonists, antagonists, cellular mechanisms, and pharmacological applicability can be found elsewhere including in a review by Nilius and Szallasi [23]. TRPV1 is activated by a variety of exogenous and endogenous ligands [23,32]. Among the well-known exogenous ligands, capsaicin—the pungent ingredient of hot peppers—is investigated the most for its beneficial effects on body weight and metabolism. Capsaicin-binding site of TRPV1 is intracellular [33]. Activation of TRPV1 results in influx of cations and leads to depolarization of the cell [34,35]. Capsaicin specifically binds to TRPV1; however, we have to keep in mind that capsaicin is able to cause disruption in the organization of membranes due to its localization in the lipid bilayer [36–38]. This might have important implications for delivery of drug molecules and may result in a TRPV1-independent effect.

Among the numerous physiological functions, TRPV1 has been proposed to have functional roles in a variety of metabolically important tissues including the pancreas [39,40], gastrointestinal tract [41], adipose tissue [9,12], and nervous system [21,42]. In this section, based on human and animal model studies, we provide a brief overview of TRPV1's potential for improvement of obese and diabetic conditions.

2.1. *Dietary Interventions and Possible Mechanisms in Human and Animal Model Studies*

Ingredients of spices, such as capsaicin in red peppers, are well-known for a variety of effects. Recently, Nilius and Appendino published a detailed overview about the beneficial science of spices, focusing on TRPs [28], while in this section we summarize dietary interventions and potential underlying mechanisms related to TRPV1.

Previous studies in male human subjects examined the effects of red pepper diet and demonstrated a trend for increased energy expenditure (EE), significantly higher carbohydrate oxidation, and lower lipid oxidation [43]. This increased EE immediately after a red pepper containing meal was proposed to be due to beta-adrenergic stimulation [43]. Increased carbohydrate oxidation and elevated epinephrine and norepinephrine levels following dietary red pepper ingestion were confirmed in men by another study [44].

In Japanese female subjects, diet-induced thermogenesis and lipid oxidation was higher following red pepper diet compared to the control diet [45]. On the other hand, Matsumoto and co-workers found that diet-induced thermogenesis was increased in the age- and height-matched lean control group; however, there was no thermogenic response detected in the obese group [46]. The study demonstrated that despite the identical resting sympathovagal activities, reduced sympathetic responsiveness to the capsaicin diet exists in obese females. This reduced sympathetic responsiveness likely leads to impairment of the diet-induced thermogenic response and could be an important factor in the development of obesity in female subjects [46].

A crossover study with male and female participants also aimed to determine the effect of a capsaicin-containing lunch on EE and hormone levels [47]. This study revealed increased GLP-1 levels and a decreasing trend in ghrelin levels; however, no effect on satiety, EE, and peptide YY levels were observed [47]. The negative finding on satiety was in disagreement with a previous study from the same group, in which significantly higher feelings of satiety were seen after capsaicin supplementation over two days compared to placebo [48]. The authors suggested that the satiety feeling observed after capsaicin need to be built up, and the postprandial state may mask the effects of capsaicin in general [47,48].

Many of the studies demonstrating beneficial findings of capsaicin investigated a single meal in a small group of lean subjects [45,49], while other studies focused on determining the effects of weeks long chili diet. The effect of daily ingestion of chili pepper for four weeks was investigated on the resistance of serum lipoproteins to oxidation in healthy men and women [50]. The rate of oxidation was lower following the chili pepper diet compared to the bland diet, suggesting that regular consumption of the chili diet for an extended period inhibits oxidation of serum lipoproteins; however, in addition to capsaicin, other ingredients of chili pepper can contribute to these findings [50].

On the other hand, the same group revealed no obvious beneficial or harmful effects on metabolic and vascular parameters, but suggested that four week long chili consumption may reduce resting heart rate and increase effective myocardial perfusion pressure time in men [51].

A crossover intervention study by the same group used two dietary periods of four weeks each and measured EE, serum insulin, C-peptide, and glucose levels following a bland meal after bland diet, a chili meal after bland diet, and a chili meal after chili-containing diet and suggested that regular consumption of chili may attenuate postprandial hyperinsulinemia [52].

Lejeune and co-workers revealed no difference in body weight maintenance after body weight loss following capsaicin consumption for multiple weeks compared to the placebo group [53]. However, substrate oxidation was affected by capsaicin, which was consistent with the observation of a short-term study by Yoshioka [54].

In general, as demonstrated by the abovementioned examples, in human subjects there are controversial findings regarding capsaicin containing diets, and clearly more detailed studies are necessary to make a conclusion about the dietary effects of capsaicin and TRPV1-activating supplements. We also have to note that many variables including age, metabolic status, postprandial state, sex, the diet itself (e.g., chili pepper vs. capsaicin), and many more can profoundly influence or even mask the metabolic effects in the above-discussed human studies.

Despite that the animal model studies are more mechanistic, they also revealed controversial findings about the metabolic effects of TRPV1 activation. Major dietary and topical interventions in obese and diabetic conditions were recently reviewed in more detail [4,26]. Briefly, it has been reported that TRPV1 activation with capsaicin prevented adipogenesis and obesity [9]. The study verified TRPV1 expression in 3T3-L1-preadipocytes and visceral adipose tissue from mice and humans. The findings revealed that capsaicin dose-dependently increased intracellular calcium in 3T3-L1-preadipocytes, which indicates inhibition of preadipocytes' differentiation. The capsaicin-dependent calcium increase was significantly lower in mature adipocytes compared to preadipocytes, which was consistent with the observed TRPV1 downregulation during adipogenesis [9]. This study also revealed that both db/db and ob/ob mice have lower TRPV1 expression in their visceral adipose tissue compared with the lean controls. Indeed, lower TRPV1 expression was determined in visceral and subcutaneous adipose tissue of obese men compared to lean men [9]. These observations suggest that downregulation of TRPV1 in visceral adipose tissue is a common finding both in animal models of obesity and diabetes, and in human subjects.

Dietary capsaicin (0.01%) did not affect the body weight of mice on normal chow diet; however, dietary supplementation of capsaicin to high fat diet (HFD) treated mice prevented obesity, which was not observed in TRPV1 knockout mice [9]. The prevention of obesity was associated with small adipocyte size and increased TRPV1 expression. These findings suggest that activation of TRPV1 triggers calcium influx, and leads to prevention of adipogenesis and TRPV1 downregulation that may result in attenuation of obesity in mice kept on HFD.

A more recent study evaluated the effect of dietary capsaicin (0.01%) on browning of white adipose tissue (WAT) [55]. Capsaicin diet prevented the weight gain of wild type mice on HFD, while this effect was not observed in TRPV1 knockout mice. HFD downregulated the expression of TRPV1 in epididymal and subcutaneous fat pads, and the capsaicin diet prevented this downregulation and caused browning of WAT. The prevention of obesity was associated with increased uncoupling protein 1 (UCP1) expression levels, and increased sirtuin-1 expression and activity. These findings were due to TRPV1-dependent increase of Ca^{2+} and phosphorylation of CaMKII and AMPK. TRPV1 activation elevated metabolic and ambulatory activities and induced browning of WAT likely via peroxisome proliferator-activated receptor gamma (PPAR-γ)/PRDM-16 interaction [55]. These results suggest that TRPV1 activation could be used to promote browning of WAT and thus decrease obesity (Table 1).

Table 1. Transient receptor potential (TRP) channels and their potential role in metabolism.

Title	TRPV1	TRPA1	TRPM2	TRPM3	TRPM5
Natural ligands for dietary interventions	capsaicin; red pepper; chili; capsinoids; capsiate	cinnamon; cinnamaldehyde; AITC			
Synthetic small molecule modulators	BCTC [56]; AZV1 [57]; AMG 517	methyl syringate [58]; glibenclamide [59]		CIM0216 [60]	
Pancreas	insulin + [40]	insulin + [59,61]	insulin + [62,63]	insulin + [60,64,65]	insulin + [66]
GI hormones and GI tract	GLP-1 + [47] ghrelin − [47]	GLP-1 + [67] ghrelin − [68]; peptide YY [58]; gastric and gut motility − [58,68]			GLP-1 + [69]
WAT	adipogenesis − [9]; browning + [12,55]; fat oxidation + [45,70]; leptin − [70,71]; adiponectin + [72]	fat oxidation + [68]; leptin − [73]			
BAT	thermogenesis + [12,45,46,71]	thermogenesis + [73,74]			
Nervous system	satiety + [48]; neuronal excitability + [21,22,42]; gene expression [71]	gene expression [73]	neuronal excitability [75]		neuronal excitability + [76]

AITC: allyl isothiocyanate; GLP-1: glucagon-like peptide 1; +: increase, −: decrease.

We have to mention that in addition to TRPV1, TRPV3 and TRPV4 have been shown to have functional roles in adipocytes. Recently, higher expression of TRPV3 was found in adipocytes when compared to other TRPVs. Activation of TRPV3 was shown to prevent lipid accumulation and adipogenesis by inhibiting the phosphorylation of insulin receptor substrate 1 and the expression of PPAR-γ [77]. Moreover, HFD-treated, db/db, and ob/ob mice had reduced TRPV3 expression in their visceral adipose tissue, whereas chronic treatment with TRPV3 agonists prevented adipogenesis and weight gain in HFD-treated mice [77].

In contrast, Ye and co-workers found that TRPV1, TRPV2, and TRPV4 mRNA are expressed in 3TT-F442A adipocytes, but their study showed a lack of TRPV3 mRNA. TRPV4 was expressed at the highest level [78], which confirmed previous observations revealing TRPV4 expression in adipose tissue [79]. Furthermore, Ye's paper determined that TRPV4 is a negative regulator of oxidative metabolism and it controls proinflammatory gene programming. In TRPV4 knockout mice the subcutaneous adipose tissue showed higher UCP1 mRNA and protein expression levels compared to controls. Elevated EE was found in the TRPV4 knockout mice, which was associated with the elevated thermogenic gene programming. In addition, TRPV4 knockout mice were protected from diet-induced obesity and insulin resistance [78]. Taken together, strong evidence suggests that TRPVs including TRPV1, TRPV3, and TRPV4 likely have important functional roles in adipocytes.

The effect of dietary hot pepper (1%) was determined to be beneficial to attenuate diet-induced obesity in rabbits [80]. TRPV1 mRNA was detected in various tissues of the rabbit with high similarity to human TRPV1. Rabbits fed with dietary hot pepper consumed similar amount of food; however, the hot pepper fed group gained less weight compared to the control group. This was associated with decreased adipose tissue and ratio of adipose tissue to body weight [80]. On the other hand, previous studies found that rabbits are insensitive to capsaicin and do not have resiniferatoxin binding sites [81]. It was later found that two amino acid substitutions in rabbit TRPV1 render the protein >100-fold less sensitive to vanilloids and RTX [82]. Therefore, it is debatable that the beneficial effects of dietary hot pepper observed by Yu [80] are mediated by capsaicin-dependent TRPV1 activation.

Male C57Bl/6 mice were kept on HFD for ten weeks and then received capsaicin (0.015%) supplement [70]. Dietary capsaicin resulted in lower fasting glucose, insulin, and leptin levels. In addition, it also attenuated the impairment of glucose tolerance, likely by reducing inflammatory responses and increasing fatty acid oxidation [70]. In another study by the same group, genetically obese diabetic mice (KKAy) were subjected to an HFD for two weeks then received capsaicin [72]. Dietary capsaicin reduced fasting glucose, insulin, and triglyceride levels, while adiponectin levels and its receptor expression were increased and inflammatory gene expression was decreased, resulting in reduced metabolic dysregulation.

In Swiss albino mice the effect of three month long treatment with capsaicin (2 mg/kg) plus HFD were compared with control diet and HFD [71]. The results demonstrated that capsaicin supplementation to HFD modulated hypothalamic satiety genes, altered gut microbial composition, induced browning of subcutaneous WAT, and increased thermogenesis in brown adipose tissue (BAT). Capsaicin-treated mice on HFD gained less weight than mice on HFD only. Fasting glucose levels were not different among the groups, whereas leptin and TNFα levels were decreased in the capsaicin-treated mice compared with the HFD group [71]. Hypothalamic expression of TRPV1 was downregulated in HDF mice and capsaicin treatment increased TRPV1 expression. Anorectic genes including peptide YY, brain-derived neurotrophic factor (BDNF) and CART prepropeptide were enhanced in capsaicin-treated HDF mice compared with HFD mice, while expression of orexigenic genes were reduced following capsaicin in the diet, with the exception of melanin-concentrating hormone receptor 1, hypocretin (orexin), and neuropeptide Y (NPY) [71]. The authors hypothesized that capsaicin activates vagal TRPV1 or afferent nerves in the gastrointestinal tract and thus influences hypothalamic TRPV1 and other genes' expression.

Furthermore, TRPV1 is also known to modulate insulin secretion and pancreatic function, including development of islet inflammation and type 1 diabetes mellitus. These findings were described and reviewed earlier in detail [23–26,39,83].

2.2. *Behind the Scene: Activating or Antagonizing TRPV1 for Treating Obesity and Diabetes Mellitus*

Despite that various studies investigated TRPV1 activation, it is not clear whether activation or inhibition would be a better approach for the modulation of metabolism. Capsaicin-desensitized rats were protected from obesity despite atrophied BAT [11,84,85]. The body weight of capsaicin-desensitized rats was significantly lower 14 and 32 weeks after treatment. The lower body weight was associated with reduced food intake, smaller epididymal and retroperitoneal WAT depots, smaller interscapular BAT, decreased total protein, UCP, and cytochrome oxidase in BAT; however, the resting metabolic rate and colonic temperature of the groups were not different [11].

On the other hand, adult male rats, which were neonatally treated with capsaicin, did not differ in body weight, basal plasma leptin, or fasting leptin, insulin, adiponectin, and corticosterone levels [86]. Glucose levels following intravenous glucose tolerance tests were similar in the capsaicin-treated and vehicle-treated rats [86]. However, the capsaicin-treated rats displayed reduced plasma insulin and corticosterone responses, indicating increased insulin sensitivity and lower plasma corticosterone levels [86]. The increased insulin sensitivity was also supported by euglycemic hyperinsulinemic clamp studies [87]. Koopmans and co-workers suggested that adult rats with neonatal capsaicin treatment exhibit decreased corticosterone levels, which could contribute to amplified insulin action during hyperglycemia [86].

Studies using TRPV1 knockout mice also revealed conflicting results. On one hand, TRPV1 knockout mice gained less weight following HFD compared with wild-type mice [88]. In this study wild-type and TRPV1 knockout mice had similar energy intake, but TRPV1 knockout mice had greater thermogenic capacity. In contrast, in a more recent study TRPV1 knockout mice kept on HFD became more obese than the wild-type mice kept on the same HFD [89]. TRPV1 knockout mice on HFD were significantly heavier than the wild-type mice after one month of HFD, which was mainly due to increased whole-body fat mass. Indirect calorimetry demonstrated increased food intake of TRPV1 knockout mice on day 3. Decreased physical activity was observed during the night-cycle, which was consistent with reduced night-cycle energy expenditure rates in TRPV1 knockout mice [89]. TRPV1 knockout mice also developed more severe insulin and leptin resistance and they exhibited dysfunctional hypothalamic leptin signaling.

Marshall and co-workers investigated metabolic and cardiovascular parameters and found that wild-type and TRPV1 knockout mice gain a similar amount of weight on HFD [27]. In wild-type mice, HFD was associated with increased mean arterial pressure, which was not observed in TRPV1 knockout mice. Furthermore, parameters of vascular hypertrophy showed an increase in wild-type mice on HFD compared with TRPV1 knockout mice on HFD and mice on normal chow [27]. In the HFD-treated groups, baseline glucose levels showed an increasing trend, and impaired glucose tolerance was observed. Interestingly, glucose levels normalized faster in TRPV1 knockout mice, which was indicated by the area under the curve. Interleukin 10 and 1β levels were significantly elevated in wild-type, but not in TRPV1 knockout mice [27]. Based on their findings the authors suggested that TRPV1 deletion may be protective against obesity-induced hypertension, and that TRPV1 may contribute to the development of cardiometabolic disturbances. The role of TRP channels in the cardiovascular system can be found elsewhere [90].

Promising findings have been identified with TRPV1 antagonists. Since agonists can prevent TRPV1 signaling by desensitizing the receptor [17], TRPV1 antagonists may influence TRPV1 signaling by antagonizing the receptor, and thus improve obese and/or diabetic conditions. BCTC *N*-(4-tertiarybutylphenyl)-4-(3-chloropyridin-2-yl)tetrahydropyrazine-1(2*H*)-carbox-amide, a TRPV1 antagonist has been shown to inhibit TRPV1 signaling in cultured cells and was found to decrease inflammation and neuropathic pain in vivo [91,92]. Tanaka and co-workers investigated the effect of BCTC on whole-body glucose and lipid metabolism in ob/ob mice and compared the effect of BCTC with pioglitazone, an insulin sensitizer [56]. The insulin-resistant, hyperinsulinemic ob/ob mice were treated with BCTC or pioglitazone twice a day for four weeks. Plasma glucose levels were decreased with a high dose BCTC (100 mg/kg) and the decrease was similar to pioglitazone. Plasma insulin levels showed a dose-dependent decreasing trend following BCTC treatment, but significance was observed only in the pioglitazone group [56]. Plasma triglyceride levels were significantly lower both in the BCTC and pioglitazone-treated mice, which was accompanied with a decreasing trend in calcitonin gene-related peptide. The oral glucose tolerance test indicated that BCTC increased insulin secretion, but likely in a different way than pioglitazone, even though glucose tolerance was improved by both drugs [56]. The authors also reported that BCTC did not alter insulin or glucose levels in normoglycemic control mice, indicating that inhibiting TRPV1 could be more important during the diabetic condition [56]. In summary, BCTC was shown to improve insulin resistance, which may be due to inhibiting TRPV1 in adipocytes and skeletal muscle. On the other hand, increased insulin secretion was associated with BCTC in diabetic ob/ob mice. These findings suggest that BCTC may have a dual effect by improving insulin resistance and enhancing insulin secretion in ob/ob mice. We also have to note that BCTC is an antagonist of TRPM8 and we cannot exclude a possible effect and/or interaction with TRPM8 channels [93].

More recently, at the European Association for the Study of Diabetes 2015, a novel TRPV1 antagonist, AZV1 by Astra Zeneca, was shown to improve insulin sensitivity in ob/ob mice [57]. Mice were treated daily with the TRPV1 antagonist AZV1 or vehicle for eight days. Body weight of TRPV1 antagonist-treated mice was not different compared with vehicle-treated mice; however, the glucose control of ob/ob mice was improved. Glucose levels, homeostatic model assessment and fructosamine levels of the TRPV1 antagonist-treated mice were significantly decreased compared with vehicle-treated mice. Moreover, increased liver weight was observed in the TRPV1 antagonist treated mice [57]. The data demonstrated that AZV1 was well-tolerated without effects on food intake or body weight, but it exerted an antidiabetic effect, which may be due to improved insulin sensitivity. Findings from these two studies suggest that TRPV1 antagonism could be useful for the treatment of type 2 diabetes mellitus; however, we have to note that these antagonist studies did not investigate potential temperature changes.

Taken together, the beneficial effects of TRPV1 could be valuable; however, there are numerous unanswered questions about the mechanisms underlying the findings. These include sensitization vs. desensitization, important cell types/tissues/pathways underlying the effects (e.g., pancreatic beta cells vs. sensory nerves), or the contribution of the sympathetic nervous system.

3. Role of TRPM Channels in Metabolism

Members of the TRPM family have highly variable permeability to Ca^{2+} and they lack the *N*-terminal ankyrin repeats [23,94]. TRPM channels including TRPM2, TRPM3, TRPM4, and TRPM5 were identified as candidates to play a role in the regulation of metabolism [4].

Comprehensive metabolic studies were conducted to determine insulin sensitivity of TRPM2 knockout mice [95]. TRPM2 knockout mice were more insulin-sensitive due to increased glucose metabolism in the heart. TRPM2 knockout mice exerted increased EE and elevated expression levels of metabolic genes including peroxisome proliferator-activated receptor alpha (PPARα) and PPARγ co-activator-1 alpha and 1 beta in WAT resulting in resistance to HFD. The hyperinsulinemic euglycemic clamp studies showed that TRPM2 knockout mice are more insulin-sensitive and have elevated Akt and glycogen synthase kinase 3β phosphorylation in the heart, and reduced inflammation in the liver and adipose tissue [95]. These findings demonstrated that TRPM2 likely plays an important role in whole-body metabolism.

TRPM2, in addition to TRPM3, TRPM4, and TRPM5, was described in rodent insulinoma cell lines and in mouse islets. Moreover, transcripts of TRPM2, TRPM4 and TRPM5 have been identified in human islets [96,97], suggesting that they may have an important functional role in the regulation of pancreatic function and insulin secretion. TRPM2 is activated by a variety of stimuli including reactive oxygen species (e.g., H_2O_2), glucose, and incretins [62,98,99]. In TRPM2 knockout mice plasma insulin levels were reduced and glucose clearance was impaired. This was associated with decreased insulin secretion initiated by incretins and glucose, and was supported by the observation that in the β cells of TRPM2 knockout mice the increase of intracellular Ca^{2+} was impaired following stimulation with incretins or insulin [99]. Since TRPM2 activity can be modulated by adenine dinucleotides, intracellular Ca^{2+} levels, and incretin-induced PKA phosphorylation, the regulation of TRPM2 can be more complex; however, it is undoubtedly an important mechanism for insulin secretion [62]. Involvement of TRPM2 in type 1 and type 2 diabetes mellitus has been suggested and the current hypotheses, including impairment in insulin secretion due to dysfunction of TRPM2, have been discussed in detail previously [63].

TRPM3 is important for Zn^{2+} entry in β cells and might contribute to insulin synthesis [100]. This is supported by recent studies, which demonstrated expression of TRPM3 in rat pancreatic INS-1 insulinoma cells and in mouse pancreatic islets [101]. Previously it had been revealed that pregnenolone sulfate, a canonical TRPM3 agonist, induces Ca^{2+} influx. The increase of Ca^{2+} is due to activation of TRPM3 and L-type Ca^{2+} channels, and upregulation of genes, which lead to insulin secretion [64,65]. Recently, the roles of TRPM3 and L-type Ca^{2+} channels were clarified [101]. The authors concluded that both TRPM3 and L-type Ca^{2+} channels are necessary for the pregnenolone sulfate mediated gene stimulation in INS-1 cells cultured in low-glucose medium. These data suggest that activation of TRPM3 following pregnenolone sulfate stimulation leads to an initial Ca^{2+} influx followed by activation of L-type Ca^{2+} channels [65,101].

More recently, a synthetic small-molecule TRPM3 agonist, CIM0216, has been shown to stimulate insulin release [60]. Pregnenolone sulfate, the well-known agonist of TRPM3 and CIM0216, caused Ca^{2+} increase in pancreatic islets and a dose-dependent increase of insulin release. The increase of insulin release was not observed in TRPM3-deficient islets, further confirming the findings [60].

TRPM4 has been identified in several β cell lines suggesting non-species specific TRPM4 expression [102]. TRPM4 currents were characterized with a biphasic pattern following Ca^{2+} perfusion; however, the activation and inactivation time varied among cell lines. Inhibition of TRPM4 decreased the magnitude of Ca^{2+} signals, and it has been shown that blockade of TRPM4 decreased glucose stimulated insulin secretion in INS-1 cells [103]. Marigo and co-workers suggested that in β cells, TRPM4 may have a critical role in the regulation of membrane potential oscillations during glucose stimulation [102,103]. In contrast, TRPM4 knockout mice did not show differences in glucose tolerance test and glucose-induced insulin secretion from isolated islets compared to wild-type mice [104,105]. In addition, TRPM4 was proposed to be involved in glucagon secretion [105].

TRPM5 is important for the Ca^{2+} activated cation current in pancreatic β cells since this current was reduced in TRPM5 knockout mice [66]. TRPM5 is suggested to play crucial role during glucose stimulation, and it is likely responsible for the fast glucose-induced oscillations of membrane potential and Ca^{2+} [66]. These fast oscillations are more efficient to trigger insulin release [106]. Furthermore, impaired glucose tolerance was observed in TRPM5 knockout mice, supporting an important role for TRPM5 in the regulation of metabolism [66]. Its role in the control of metabolism is further demonstrated by the existence of TRPM5 in the enteroendocrine cells in the gastrointestinal tract. Specifically, TRPM5 is expressed in the GLP-1 secreting L-cells, which are important for controlling proper glucose homeostasis [69].

In addition, TRPM5 plays a role in taste signaling, and TRPM5 knockout mice develop severe impairment in sweet, bitter, and umami taste signaling [107–109]. Interestingly, members of taste signaling pathways including TRPM5 were identified in gastrointestinal L-cells, suggesting that sweet taste signaling is directly involved in the release of GLP-1, and thus can have an important role in glucose-mediated control of metabolism [69]. Manipulation of taste is also an approach of pharmacological interventions for obesity prevention, and TRPM5 has been investigated for potential taste modifications; details can be found elsewhere [110,111]. In addition, TRPM2, TRPM4, and TRPM5 channels are identified in the brain and may play a role in neuronal excitability, cell death, or neurodegeneration; however, their functional role in autonomic centers has not been described [19,75,76] (Table 1).

4. Implications for TRPA1

TRPA1, currently the only member of the ankyrin family, was named after the high number of ankyrin repeats. TRPA1 is a voltage-dependent, Ca^{2+}-permeable cation channel. Like many of the TRP channels, TRPA1 is also modulated by herbal compounds, suggesting the potential for alternative dietary therapies. One of the natural compounds activating TRPA1 is cinnamon, a widely used spice, which originates from the bark of trees of the *Cinnamomum* genus. In one study, cinnamon treatment has been shown to improve the glucose and lipid profiles of type 2 diabetic patients [112], while other studies showed moderate improvement of glucose levels [113] or no effect [114]. We have to note that age, sex, length of the disease, and many other variables may play a role in the outcome of the human studies; therefore, it is too early to make a conclusion regarding the dietary benefits of cinnamon.

One of the main ingredients of cinnamon is cinnamaldehyde, which is a potent agonist of TRPA1. Cinnamaldehyde effect was associated with inhibition of ghrelin secretion and gastric emptying, whereas improved insulin sensitivity was observed [68]. In mice fed with high-fat high-sucrose diet, cinnamaldehyde ingestion was associated with reduced visceral adipose tissue [115] and increased fatty acid oxidation [68]. Recently it was shown that cinnamaldehyde (10 mg/kg) administration prevented the increase of weight gain caused by HFD [73]. Serum leptin levels and leptin/ghrelin ratio, a marker of weight gain, were decreased in the cinnamaldehyde-treated HFD groups. In addition, cinnamaldehyde treatment increased the expression levels of anorexigenic genes including pro-opiomelanocortin, urocortin, BDNF, and cholecystokinin [73]. The study also determined that cinnamaldehyde prevented visceral WAT accumulation, increased BAT activity and reduced inflammation, but did not affect gut microbial composition. Improved fasting blood glucose levels and glucose tolerance were observed in ob/ob mice following cinnamon extract treatment [116]. This was associated with improved insulin sensitivity, locomotor activity and improved brain activity.

Allyl isothiocyanate (AITC), an ingredient of mustard, horseradish, and wasabi, is also a potent TRPA1 agonist. It has been shown that intravenous injection of AITC induces adrenalin secretion. This response was attenuated in the presence of cholinergic blockers, suggesting activation of the adrenal sympathetic nerve through the central nervous system [117]. AITC increased thermogenesis and expression of UPC1 [74]. Recently, dietary AITC was reported to protect against free fatty acid induced insulin resistance, and it increased mitochondrial activity in skeletal muscle cells [118]. Dietary AITC reduced diet-induced obesity in C57Bl/6 mice and improved blood lipid profile compared to HFD-treated mice. AITC also reduced high fat induced hepatic steatosis and decreased hyperglycemia, hyperinsulinemia, HbA1C levels and ameliorated insulin resistance [118]. These findings suggest that activation of TRPA1 likely have beneficial effects; however, further studies are necessary to reveal the exact underlying mechanisms.

Multiple methodological approaches were used to reveal TRPA1 expression in rat pancreatic cells [61]. Expression of TRPA1 was confirmed in beta, but not in glucagon-secreting alpha cells, and activation of TRPA1 stimulated insulin release synergistically with ATP-dependent potassium channel (K_{ATP}) blockade [61]. The latter is further supported with the findings that glibenclamide, a widely used K_{ATP} channel inhibitor is an agonist of TRPA1 [59], and it has been suggested that the synergistic effect of TRPA1 and K_{ATP} channels underlies the hyperinsulinism in patients with glibenclamide treatment.

Similar to TRPM5, TRPA1 is expressed in L-cells and TRPA1 agonist administration into the duodenum or by gavage increased GLP-1 secretion [67]. On the other hand, the effect was not eliminated in TRPA1 knockout mice. GLP-1 levels did not change following activation of TRPA1 despite elevation of peptide YY, and reduced gastric emptying and food intake [58]. In dogs, following AITC, gastric and jejunum motility was increased, and this effect was prevented with ruthenium red [119]. The potential role of TRPA1 on pancreatic, adipose tissue, and the autonomic nervous system and its importance as a dietary supplement has been recently reviewed [26].

5. Conclusions

TRP channels are expressed in many tissues and organs important for the maintenance of whole body metabolism. Results from dietary supplementation of TRP ligands (e.g., capsaicin) are controversial, either showing beneficial effects on body weight, metabolism, and hormone levels, or no effects. The target tissue of the dietary supplementation is not entirely clear since many tissues including the adipose tissue, the pancreas, and even the central nervous system could be modulated by the components of the diet. TRP channels have benefits; however, currently it is not clear whether activation or inhibition, central or peripheral mechanisms, diet or topical administration, or even which tissue/organ is the most critical. In summary, further research is needed before final conclusions are available, but undoubtedly TRP channels are good potential targets for weight and diabetes management.

Acknowledgments: The authors acknowledge funding support from the National Institutes of Health (R01 DK099598 for AZs and HL122829 for AVD).

References

1. Ogden, C.L.; Carroll, M.D.; Kit, B.K.; Flegal, K.M. Prevalence of childhood and adult obesity in the United States, 2011–2012. *JAMA* **2014**, *311*, 806–814. [CrossRef] [PubMed]
2. Ogden, C.L.; Carroll, M.D.; Fryar, C.D.; Flegal, K.M. Prevalence of obesity among adults and youth: United States, 2011–2014. *NCHS Data Brief* **2015**, *219*, 1–8. [PubMed]
3. Jacobson, D.A.; Philipson, L.H. TRP channels of the pancreatic β cell. *Handb. Exp. Pharmacol.* **2007**, 409–424. [CrossRef]
4. Zhu, Z.; Luo, Z.; Ma, S.; Liu, D. TRP channels and their implications in metabolic diseases. *Pflug. Arch.* **2011**, *461*, 211–223. [CrossRef] [PubMed]
5. Yu, X.; Yu, M.; Liu, Y.; Yu, S. TRP channel functions in the gastrointestinal tract. *Semin. Immunopathol.* **2016**, *38*, 385–396. [CrossRef] [PubMed]
6. Kunert-Keil, C.; Bisping, F.; Kruger, J.; Brinkmeier, H. Tissue-specific expression of TRP channel genes in the mouse and its variation in three different mouse strains. *BMC Genom.* **2006**, *7*, 159. [CrossRef] [PubMed]
7. Feng, N.H.; Lee, H.H.; Shiang, J.C.; Ma, M.C. Transient receptor potential vanilloid type 1 channels act as mechanoreceptors and cause substance p release and sensory activation in rat kidneys. *Am. J. Physiol. Ren. Physiol.* **2008**, *294*, F316–F325. [CrossRef] [PubMed]
8. Tomilin, V.; Mamenko, M.; Zaika, O.; Pochynyuk, O. Role of renal TRP channels in physiology and pathology. *Semin. Immunopathol.* **2016**, *38*, 371–383. [CrossRef] [PubMed]
9. Zhang, L.L.; Liu, D.Y.; Ma, L.Q.; Luo, Z.D.; Cao, T.B.; Zhong, J.; Yan, Z.C.; Wang, L.J.; Zhao, Z.G.; Zhu, S.J.; et al. Activation of transient receptor potential vanilloid type-1 channel prevents adipogenesis and obesity. *Circ. Res.* **2007**, *100*, 1063–1070. [CrossRef] [PubMed]
10. Lee, G.R.; Shin, M.K.; Yoon, D.J.; Kim, A.R.; Yu, R.; Park, N.H.; Han, I.S. Topical application of capsaicin reduces visceral adipose fat by affecting adipokine levels in high-fat diet-induced obese mice. *Obesity* **2013**, *21*, 115–122. [CrossRef] [PubMed]
11. Cui, J.; Himms-Hagen, J. Long-term decrease in body fat and in brown adipose tissue in capsaicin-desensitized rats. *Am. J. Physiol.* **1992**, *262*, R568–R573. [PubMed]
12. Baboota, R.K.; Singh, D.P.; Sarma, S.M.; Kaur, J.; Sandhir, R.; Boparai, R.K.; Kondepudi, K.K.; Bishnoi, M. Capsaicin induces "brite" phenotype in differentiating 3T3-L1 preadipocytes. *PLoS ONE* **2014**, *9*, e103093.
13. Zvara, A.; Bencsik, P.; Fodor, G.; Csont, T.; Hackler, L., Jr.; Dux, M.; Furst, S.; Jancso, G.; Puskas, L.G.; Ferdinandy, P. Capsaicin-sensitive sensory neurons regulate myocardial function and gene expression pattern of rat hearts: A DNA microarray study. *FASEB J.* **2006**, *20*, 160–162. [CrossRef] [PubMed]
14. Watanabe, H.; Murakami, M.; Ohba, T.; Ono, K.; Ito, H. The pathological role of transient receptor potential channels in heart disease. *Circ. J.* **2009**, *73*, 419–427. [CrossRef] [PubMed]
15. Thilo, F.; Liu, Y.; Schulz, N.; Gergs, U.; Neumann, J.; Loddenkemper, C.; Gollasch, M.; Tepel, M. Increased transient receptor potential vanilloid type 1 (TRPV1) channel expression in hypertrophic heart. *Biochem. Biophys. Res. Commun.* **2010**, *401*, 98–103. [CrossRef] [PubMed]
16. Liu, D.; Maier, A.; Scholze, A.; Rauch, U.; Boltzen, U.; Zhao, Z.; Zhu, Z.; Tepel, M. High glucose enhances transient receptor potential channel canonical type 6-dependent calcium influx in human platelets via phosphatidylinositol 3-kinase-dependent pathway. *Arterioscler. Thromb. Vasc. Biol.* **2008**, *28*, 746–751. [CrossRef] [PubMed]
17. Lizanecz, E.; Bagi, Z.; Pasztor, E.T.; Papp, Z.; Edes, I.; Kedei, N.; Blumberg, P.M.; Toth, A. Phosphorylation-dependent desensitization by anandamide of vanilloid receptor-1 (TRPV1) function in rat skeletal muscle arterioles and in chinese hamster ovary cells expressing TRPV1. *Mol. Pharmacol.* **2006**, *69*, 1015–1023. [PubMed]

18. Toth, A.; Czikora, A.; Pasztor, E.T.; Dienes, B.; Bai, P.; Csernoch, L.; Rutkai, I.; Csato, V.; Manyine, I.S.; Porszasz, R.; et al. Vanilloid receptor-1 (TRPV1) expression and function in the vasculature of the rat. *J. Histochem. Cytochem.* **2014**, *62*, 129–144. [CrossRef] [PubMed]
19. Vennekens, R.; Menigoz, A.; Nilius, B. Trps in the brain. *Rev. Physiol. Biochem. Pharmacol.* **2012**, *163*, 27–64. [PubMed]
20. Morelli, M.B.; Amantini, C.; Liberati, S.; Santoni, M.; Nabissi, M. TRP channels: New potential therapeutic approaches in CNS neuropathies. *CNS Neurol. Disord. Drug Targets* **2013**, *12*, 274–293. [CrossRef] [PubMed]
21. Gao, H.; Miyata, K.; Bhaskaran, M.D.; Derbenev, A.V.; Zsombok, A. Transient receptor potential vanilloid type 1-dependent regulation of liver-related neurons in the paraventricular nucleus of the hypothalamus diminished in the type 1 diabetic mouse. *Diabetes* **2012**, *61*, 1381–1390. [CrossRef] [PubMed]
22. Zsombok, A.; Bhaskaran, M.D.; Gao, H.; Derbenev, A.V.; Smith, B.N. Functional plasticity of central TRPV1 receptors in brainstem dorsal vagal complex circuits of streptozotocin-treated hyperglycemic mice. *J. Neurosci.* **2011**, *31*, 14024–14031. [CrossRef] [PubMed]
23. Nilius, B.; Szallasi, A. Transient receptor potential channels as drug targets: From the science of basic research to the art of medicine. *Pharmacol. Rev.* **2014**, *66*, 676–814. [CrossRef] [PubMed]
24. Suri, A.; Szallasi, A. The emerging role of TRPV1 in diabetes and obesity. *Trends Pharmacol. Sci.* **2008**, *29*, 29–36. [CrossRef] [PubMed]
25. Zsombok, A. Vanilloid receptors—Do they have a role in whole body metabolism? Evidence from TRPV1. *J. Diabetes Its Complicat.* **2013**, *27*, 287–292. [CrossRef] [PubMed]
26. Derbenev, A.V.; Zsombok, A. Potential therapeutic value of TRPV1 and TRPA1 in diabetes mellitus and obesity. *Semin. Immunopathol.* **2016**, *38*, 397–406. [CrossRef] [PubMed]
27. Marshall, N.J.; Liang, L.; Bodkin, J.; Dessapt-Baradez, C.; Nandi, M.; Collot-Teixeira, S.; Smillie, S.J.; Lalgi, K.; Fernandes, E.S.; Gnudi, L.; et al. A role for TRPV1 in influencing the onset of cardiovascular disease in obesity. *Hypertension* **2013**, *61*, 246–252. [CrossRef] [PubMed]
28. Nilius, B.; Appendino, G. Spices: The savory and beneficial science of pungency. *Rev. Physiol. Biochem. Pharmacol.* **2013**, *164*. [CrossRef]
29. Caterina, M.J.; Schumacher, M.A.; Tominaga, M.; Rosen, T.A.; Levine, J.D.; Julius, D. The capsaicin receptor: A heat-activated ion channel in the pain pathway. *Nature* **1997**, *389*, 816–824. [PubMed]
30. Szallasi, A.; Cortright, D.N.; Blum, C.A.; Eid, S.R. The vanilloid receptor TRPV1: 10 years from channel cloning to antagonist proof-of-concept. *Nat. Rev. Drug Discov.* **2007**, *6*, 357–372. [CrossRef] [PubMed]
31. Moran, M.M.; McAlexander, M.A.; Biro, T.; Szallasi, A. Transient receptor potential channels as therapeutic targets. *Nat. Rev. Drug Discov.* **2011**, *10*, 601–620. [CrossRef] [PubMed]
32. Van Der Stelt, M.; Di Marzo, V. Endovanilloids. Putative endogenous ligands of transient receptor potential vanilloid 1 channels. *Eur. J. Biochem.* **2004**, *271*, 1827–1834. [CrossRef] [PubMed]
33. Jordt, S.E.; Julius, D. Molecular basis for species-specific sensitivity to "hot" chili peppers. *Cell* **2002**, *108*, 421–430. [CrossRef]
34. Tominaga, M.; Tominaga, T. Structure and function of TRPV1. *Pflug. Arch.* **2005**, *451*, 143–150. [CrossRef] [PubMed]
35. Rosenbaum, T.; Simon, S.A. TRPV1 receptors and signal transduction. In *TRP Ion Channel Function in Sensory Transduction and Cellular Signaling Cascades*; Liedtke, W.B., Heller, S., Eds.; CRC Press/Taylor & Francis: Boca Raton, FL, USA, 2007.
36. Aranda, F.J.; Villalain, J.; Gomez-Fernandez, J.C. Capsaicin affects the structure and phase organization of phospholipid membranes. *Biochim. Biophys. Acta* **1995**, *1234*, 225–234. [CrossRef]
37. Swain, J.; Kumar Mishra, A. Location, partitioning behavior, and interaction of capsaicin with lipid bilayer membrane: Study using its intrinsic fluorescence. *J. Phys. Chem. B* **2015**, *119*, 12086–12093. [CrossRef] [PubMed]
38. Torrecillas, A.; Schneider, M.; Fernandez-Martinez, A.M.; Ausili, A.; de Godos, A.M.; Corbalan-Garcia, S.; Gomez-Fernandez, J.C. Capsaicin fluidifies the membrane and localizes itself near the lipid-water interface. *ACS Chem. Neurosci.* **2015**, *6*, 1741–1750. [CrossRef] [PubMed]
39. Razavi, R.; Chan, Y.; Afifiyan, F.N.; Liu, X.J.; Wan, X.; Yantha, J.; Tsui, H.; Tang, L.; Tsai, S.; Santamaria, P.; et al. TRPV1^{+} sensory neurons control beta cell stress and islet inflammation in autoimmune diabetes. *Cell* **2006**, *127*, 1123–1135. [CrossRef] [PubMed]

40. Akiba, Y.; Kato, S.; Katsube, K.; Nakamura, M.; Takeuchi, K.; Ishii, H.; Hibi, T. Transient receptor potential vanilloid subfamily 1 expressed in pancreatic islet beta cells modulates insulin secretion in rats. *Biochem. Biophys. Res. Commun.* **2004**, *321*, 219–225. [CrossRef] [PubMed]
41. Wang, P.; Yan, Z.; Zhong, J.; Chen, J.; Ni, Y.; Li, L.; Ma, L.; Zhao, Z.; Liu, D.; Zhu, Z. Transient receptor potential vanilloid 1 activation enhances gut glucagon-like peptide-1 secretion and improves glucose homeostasis. *Diabetes* **2012**, *61*, 2155–2165. [CrossRef] [PubMed]
42. Zsombok, A.; Jiang, Y.; Gao, H.; Anwar, I.J.; Rezai-Zadeh, K.; Enix, C.L.; Munzberg, H.; Derbenev, A.V. Regulation of leptin receptor-expressing neurons in the brainstem by TRPV1. *Physiol. Rep.* **2014**, *2*, e12160. [CrossRef] [PubMed]
43. Yoshioka, M.; Lim, K.; Kikuzato, S.; Kiyonaga, A.; Tanaka, H.; Shindo, M.; Suzuki, M. Effects of red-pepper diet on the energy metabolism in men. *J. Nutr. Sci. Vitaminol.* **1995**, *41*, 647–656. [CrossRef] [PubMed]
44. Lim, K.; Yoshioka, M.; Kikuzato, S.; Kiyonaga, A.; Tanaka, H.; Shindo, M.; Suzuki, M. Dietary red pepper ingestion increases carbohydrate oxidation at rest and during exercise in runners. *Med. Sci. Sports Exerc.* **1997**, *29*, 355–361. [CrossRef] [PubMed]
45. Yoshioka, M.; St-Pierre, S.; Suzuki, M.; Tremblay, A. Effects of red pepper added to high-fat and high-carbohydrate meals on energy metabolism and substrate utilization in Japanese women. *Br. J. Nutr.* **1998**, *80*, 503–510. [PubMed]
46. Matsumoto, T.; Miyawaki, C.; Ue, H.; Yuasa, T.; Miyatsuji, A.; Moritani, T. Effects of capsaicin-containing yellow curry sauce on sympathetic nervous system activity and diet-induced thermogenesis in lean and obese young women. *J. Nutr. Sci. Vitaminol.* **2000**, *46*, 309–315. [CrossRef] [PubMed]
47. Smeets, A.J.; Westerterp-Plantenga, M.S. The acute effects of a lunch containing capsaicin on energy and substrate utilisation, hormones, and satiety. *Eur. J. Nutr.* **2009**, *48*, 229–234. [CrossRef] [PubMed]
48. Westerterp-Plantenga, M.S.; Smeets, A.; Lejeune, M.P. Sensory and gastrointestinal satiety effects of capsaicin on food intake. *Int. J. Obes.* **2005**, *29*, 682–688. [CrossRef] [PubMed]
49. Yoshioka, M.; Doucet, E.; Drapeau, V.; Dionne, I.; Tremblay, A. Combined effects of red pepper and caffeine consumption on 24 h energy balance in subjects given free access to foods. *Br. J. Nutr.* **2001**, *85*, 203–211. [CrossRef] [PubMed]
50. Ahuja, K.D.; Ball, M.J. Effects of daily ingestion of chilli on serum lipoprotein oxidation in adult men and women. *Br. J. Nutr.* **2006**, *96*, 239–242. [CrossRef]
51. Ahuja, K.D.; Robertson, I.K.; Geraghty, D.P.; Ball, M.J. The effect of 4-week chilli supplementation on metabolic and arterial function in humans. *Eur. J. Clin. Nutr.* **2007**, *61*, 326–333. [CrossRef] [PubMed]
52. Ahuja, K.D.; Robertson, I.K.; Geraghty, D.P.; Ball, M.J. Effects of chili consumption on postprandial glucose, insulin, and energy metabolism. *Am. J. Clin. Nutr.* **2006**, *84*, 63–69. [PubMed]
53. Lejeune, M.P.; Kovacs, E.M.; Westerterp-Plantenga, M.S. Effect of capsaicin on substrate oxidation and weight maintenance after modest body-weight loss in human subjects. *Br. J. Nutr.* **2003**, *90*, 651–659. [CrossRef] [PubMed]
54. Yoshioka, M.; St-Pierre, S.; Drapeau, V.; Dionne, I.; Doucet, E.; Suzuki, M.; Tremblay, A. Effects of red pepper on appetite and energy intake. *Br. J. Nutr.* **1999**, *82*, 115–123. [PubMed]
55. Baskaran, P.; Krishnan, V.; Ren, J.; Thyagarajan, B. Capsaicin induces browning of white adipose tissue and counters obesity by activating TRPV1 dependent mechanism. *Br. J. Pharmacol.* **2016**, *173*, 2369–2389. [CrossRef] [PubMed]
56. Tanaka, H.; Shimaya, A.; Kiso, T.; Kuramochi, T.; Shimokawa, T.; Shibasaki, M. Enhanced insulin secretion and sensitization in diabetic mice on chronic treatment with a transient receptor potential vanilloid 1 antagonist. *Life Sci.* **2011**, *88*, 559–563. [CrossRef] [PubMed]
57. Fredin, M.F.; Kjellstedt, A.; Smith, D.M.; Oakes, N. The novel TRPV1 antagonist, AZV1, improves insulin sensitivity in ob/ob mice. In Proceedings of European Association for the Study of Diabetes 2015, Stockholm, Sweden, 14–18 September 2015.
58. Kim, M.J.; Son, H.J.; Song, S.H.; Jung, M.; Kim, Y.; Rhyu, M.R. The TRPA1 agonist, methyl syringate suppresses food intake and gastric emptying. *PLoS ONE* **2013**, *8*, e71603. [CrossRef] [PubMed]
59. Babes, A.; Fischer, M.J.; Filipovic, M.; Engel, M.A.; Flonta, M.L.; Reeh, P.W. The anti-diabetic drug glibenclamide is an agonist of the transient receptor potential ankyrin 1 (TRPA1) ion channel. *Eur. J. Pharmacol.* **2013**, *704*, 15–22. [CrossRef] [PubMed]

60. Held, K.; Kichko, T.; De Clercq, K.; Klaassen, H.; Van Bree, R.; Vanherck, J.C.; Marchand, A.; Reeh, P.W.; Chaltin, P.; Voets, T.; et al. Activation of TRPM3 by a potent synthetic ligand reveals a role in peptide release. *Proc. Natl. Acad. Sci. USA* **2015**, *112*, E1363–E1372. [CrossRef] [PubMed]
61. Cao, D.S.; Zhong, L.; Hsieh, T.H.; Abooj, M.; Bishnoi, M.; Hughes, L.; Premkumar, L.S. Expression of transient receptor potential ankyrin 1 (TRPA1) and its role in insulin release from rat pancreatic beta cells. *PLoS ONE* **2012**, *7*, e38005. [CrossRef] [PubMed]
62. Uchida, K.; Tominaga, M. TRPM2 modulates insulin secretion in pancreatic beta-cells. *Islets* **2011**, *3*, 209–211. [CrossRef] [PubMed]
63. Uchida, K.; Tominaga, M. The role of TRPM2 in pancreatic beta-cells and the development of diabetes. *Cell Calcium* **2014**, *56*, 332–339. [CrossRef] [PubMed]
64. Mayer, S.I.; Muller, I.; Mannebach, S.; Endo, T.; Thiel, G. Signal transduction of pregnenolone sulfate in insulinoma cells: Activation of Egr-1 expression involving TRPM3, voltage-gated calcium channels, ERK, and ternary complex factors. *J. Biol. Chem.* **2011**, *286*, 10084–10096. [CrossRef] [PubMed]
65. Wagner, T.F.; Loch, S.; Lambert, S.; Straub, I.; Mannebach, S.; Mathar, I.; Dufer, M.; Lis, A.; Flockerzi, V.; Philipp, S.E.; et al. Transient receptor potential M3 channels are ionotropic steroid receptors in pancreatic beta cells. *Nat. Cell Biol.* **2008**, *10*, 1421–1430. [CrossRef] [PubMed]
66. Colsoul, B.; Schraenen, A.; Lemaire, K.; Quintens, R.; Van Lommel, L.; Segal, A.; Owsianik, G.; Talavera, K.; Voets, T.; Margolskee, R.F.; et al. Loss of high-frequency glucose-induced Ca^{2+} oscillations in pancreatic islets correlates with impaired glucose tolerance in *TRPM5*$^{-/-}$ mice. *Proc. Natl. Acad. Sci. USA* **2010**, *107*, 5208–5213. [CrossRef] [PubMed]
67. Emery, E.C.; Diakogiannaki, E.; Gentry, C.; Psichas, A.; Habib, A.M.; Bevan, S.; Fischer, M.J.; Reimann, F.; Gribble, F.M. Stimulation of GLP-1 secretion downstream of the ligand-gated ion channel TRPA1. *Diabetes* **2015**, *64*, 1202–1210. [CrossRef] [PubMed]
68. Camacho, S.; Michlig, S.; de Senarclens-Bezencon, C.; Meylan, J.; Meystre, J.; Pezzoli, M.; Markram, H.; le Coutre, J. Anti-obesity and anti-hyperglycemic effects of cinnamaldehyde via altered ghrelin secretion and functional impact on food intake and gastric emptying. *Sci. Rep.* **2015**, *5*, 7919. [CrossRef] [PubMed]
69. Jang, H.J.; Kokrashvili, Z.; Theodorakis, M.J.; Carlson, O.D.; Kim, B.J.; Zhou, J.; Kim, H.H.; Xu, X.; Chan, S.L.; Juhaszova, M.; et al. Gut-expressed gustducin and taste receptors regulate secretion of glucagon-like peptide-1. *Proc. Natl. Acad. Sci. USA* **2007**, *104*, 15069–15074. [CrossRef] [PubMed]
70. Kang, J.H.; Goto, T.; Han, I.S.; Kawada, T.; Kim, Y.M.; Yu, R. Dietary capsaicin reduces obesity-induced insulin resistance and hepatic steatosis in obese mice fed a high-fat diet. *Obesity* **2010**, *18*, 780–787. [CrossRef]
71. Baboota, R.K.; Murtaza, N.; Jagtap, S.; Singh, D.P.; Karmase, A.; Kaur, J.; Bhutani, K.K.; Boparai, R.K.; Premkumar, L.S.; Kondepudi, K.K.; et al. Capsaicin-induced transcriptional changes in hypothalamus and alterations in gut microbial count in high fat diet fed mice. *J. Nutr. Biochem.* **2014**, *25*, 893–902. [CrossRef] [PubMed]
72. Kang, J.H.; Tsuyoshi, G.; Le Ngoc, H.; Kim, H.M.; Tu, T.H.; Noh, H.J.; Kim, C.S.; Choe, S.Y.; Kawada, T.; Yoo, H.; et al. Dietary capsaicin attenuates metabolic dysregulation in genetically obese diabetic mice. *J. Med. Food* **2011**, *14*, 310–315. [CrossRef] [PubMed]
73. Khare, P.; Jagtap, S.; Jain, Y.; Baboota, R.K.; Mangal, P.; Boparai, R.K.; Bhutani, K.K.; Sharma, S.S.; Premkumar, L.S.; Kondepudi, K.K.; et al. Cinnamaldehyde supplementation prevents fasting-induced hyperphagia, lipid accumulation, and inflammation in high-fat diet-fed mice. *BioFactors* **2016**, *42*, 201–211. [PubMed]
74. Yoshida, T.; Yoshioka, K.; Wakabayashi, Y.; Nishioka, H.; Kondo, M. Effects of capsaicin and isothiocyanate on thermogenesis of interscapular brown adipose tissue in rats. *J. Nutr. Sci. Vitaminol.* **1988**, *34*, 587–594. [CrossRef] [PubMed]
75. Alim, I.; Teves, L.; Li, R.; Mori, Y.; Tymianski, M. Modulation of NMDAR subunit expression by TRPM2 channels regulates neuronal vulnerability to ischemic cell death. *J. Neurosci.* **2013**, *33*, 17264–17277. [CrossRef] [PubMed]
76. Lee, C.R.; Patel, J.C.; O'Neill, B.; Rice, M.E. Inhibitory and excitatory neuromodulation by hydrogen peroxide: Translating energetics to information. *J. Physiol.* **2015**, *593*, 3431–3446. [CrossRef] [PubMed]
77. Cheung, S.Y.; Huang, Y.; Kwan, H.Y.; Chung, H.Y.; Yao, X. Activation of transient receptor potential vanilloid 3 channel suppresses adipogenesis. *Endocrinology* **2015**, *156*, 2074–2086. [CrossRef] [PubMed]

78. Ye, L.; Kleiner, S.; Wu, J.; Sah, R.; Gupta, R.K.; Banks, A.S.; Cohen, P.; Khandekar, M.J.; Bostrom, P.; Mepani, R.J.; et al. TRPV4 is a regulator of adipose oxidative metabolism, inflammation, and energy homeostasis. *Cell* **2012**, *151*, 96–110. [CrossRef] [PubMed]
79. Liedtke, W.; Choe, Y.; Marti-Renom, M.A.; Bell, A.M.; Denis, C.S.; Sali, A.; Hudspeth, A.J.; Friedman, J.M.; Heller, S. Vanilloid receptor-related osmotically activated channel (VR-OAC), a candidate vertebrate osmoreceptor. *Cell* **2000**, *103*, 525–535. [CrossRef]
80. Yu, Q.; Wang, Y.; Yu, Y.; Li, Y.; Zhao, S.; Chen, Y.; Waqar, A.B.; Fan, J.; Liu, E. Expression of TRPV1 in rabbits and consuming hot pepper affects its body weight. *Mol. Biol. Rep.* **2012**, *39*, 7583–7589. [CrossRef] [PubMed]
81. Szallasi, A.; Blumberg, P.M. [^{3}H]resiniferatoxin binding by the vanilloid receptor: Species-related differences, effects of temperature and sulfhydryl reagents. *Naunyn-Schmiedeberg's Arch. Pharmacol.* **1993**, *347*, 84–91. [CrossRef]
82. Gavva, N.R.; Klionsky, L.; Qu, Y.; Shi, L.; Tamir, R.; Edenson, S.; Zhang, T.J.; Viswanadhan, V.N.; Toth, A.; Pearce, L.V.; et al. Molecular determinants of vanilloid sensitivity in TRPV1. *J. Biol. Chem.* **2004**, *279*, 20283–20295. [CrossRef] [PubMed]
83. Tsui, H.; Razavi, R.; Chan, Y.; Yantha, J.; Dosch, H.M. "Sensing" autoimmunity in type 1 diabetes. *Trends Mol. Med.* **2007**, *13*, 405–413. [CrossRef] [PubMed]
84. Cui, J.; Himms-Hagen, J. Rapid but transient atrophy of brown adipose tissue in capsaicin-desensitized rats. *Am. J. Physiol.* **1992**, *262*, R562–R567. [PubMed]
85. Cui, J.; Zaror-Behrens, G.; Himms-Hagen, J. Capsaicin desensitization induces atrophy of brown adipose tissue in rats. *Am. J. Physiol.* **1990**, *259*, R324–R332. [PubMed]
86. Van de Wall, E.H.; Wielinga, P.Y.; Strubbe, J.H.; van Dijk, G. Neonatal capsaicin causes compensatory adjustments to energy homeostasis in rats. *Physiol. Behav.* **2006**, *89*, 115–121. [CrossRef] [PubMed]
87. Koopmans, S.J.; Leighton, B.; DeFronzo, R.A. Neonatal de-afferentation of capsaicin-sensitive sensory nerves increases in vivo insulin sensitivity in conscious adult rats. *Diabetologia* **1998**, *41*, 813–820. [CrossRef] [PubMed]
88. Motter, A.L.; Ahern, G.P. TRPV1-null mice are protected from diet-induced obesity. *FEBS Lett.* **2008**, *582*, 2257–2262. [CrossRef] [PubMed]
89. Lee, E.; Jung, D.Y.; Kim, J.H.; Patel, P.R.; Hu, X.; Lee, Y.; Azuma, Y.; Wang, H.F.; Tsitsilianos, N.; Shafiq, U.; et al. Transient receptor potential vanilloid type-1 channel regulates diet-induced obesity, insulin resistance, and leptin resistance. *FASEB J.* **2015**, *29*, 3182–3192. [CrossRef] [PubMed]
90. Yue, Z.; Xie, J.; Yu, A.S.; Stock, J.; Du, J.; Yue, L. Role of trp channels in the cardiovascular system. *Am. J. Physiol. Heart Circ. Physiol.* **2015**, *308*, H157–H182. [CrossRef]
91. Pomonis, J.D.; Harrison, J.E.; Mark, L.; Bristol, D.R.; Valenzano, K.J.; Walker, K. *N*-(4-Tertiarybutylphenyl)-4-(3-cholorphyridin-2-yl)tetrahydropyrazine-1(2*H*)-carbox-amide (BCTC), a novel, orally effective vanilloid receptor 1 antagonist with analgesic properties: II. In vivo characterization in rat models of inflammatory and neuropathic pain. *J. Pharmacol. Exp. Ther.* **2003**, *306*, 387–393. [PubMed]
92. Valenzano, K.J.; Grant, E.R.; Wu, G.; Hachicha, M.; Schmid, L.; Tafesse, L.; Sun, Q.; Rotshteyn, Y.; Francis, J.; Limberis, J.; et al. *N*-(4-tertiarybutylphenyl)-4-(3-chloropyridin-2-yl)tetrahydropyrazine-1(2*H*)-carbox-amide (BCTC), a novel, orally effective vanilloid receptor 1 antagonist with analgesic properties: I. In vitro characterization and pharmacokinetic properties. *J. Pharmacol. Exp. Ther.* **2003**, *306*, 377–386. [CrossRef] [PubMed]
93. Behrendt, H.J.; Germann, T.; Gillen, C.; Hatt, H.; Jostock, R. Characterization of the mouse cold-menthol receptor TRPM8 and vanilloid receptor type-1 VR1 using a fluorometric imaging plate reader (FLIPR) assay. *Br. J. Pharmacol.* **2004**, *141*, 737–745. [CrossRef] [PubMed]
94. Nilius, B.; Owsianik, G.; Voets, T.; Peters, J.A. Transient receptor potential cation channels in disease. *Physiol. Rev.* **2007**, *87*, 165–217. [CrossRef] [PubMed]
95. Zhang, Z.; Zhang, W.; Jung, D.Y.; Ko, H.J.; Lee, Y.; Friedline, R.H.; Lee, E.; Jun, J.; Ma, Z.; Kim, F.; et al. TRPM2 Ca^{2+} channel regulates energy balance and glucose metabolism. *Am. J. Physiol. Endocrinol. Metab.* **2012**, *302*, E807–E816. [CrossRef] [PubMed]
96. Colsoul, B.; Vennekens, R.; Nilius, B. Transient receptor potential cation channels in pancreatic beta cells. *Rev. Physiol. Biochem. Pharmacol.* **2011**, *161*, 87–110. [PubMed]
97. Colsoul, B.; Nilius, B.; Vennekens, R. Transient receptor potential (TRP) cation channels in diabetes. *Curr. Top. Med. Chem.* **2013**, *13*, 258–269. [CrossRef] [PubMed]

98. Togashi, K.; Hara, Y.; Tominaga, T.; Higashi, T.; Konishi, Y.; Mori, Y.; Tominaga, M. TRPM2 activation by cyclic ADP-ribose at body temperature is involved in insulin secretion. *EMBO J.* **2006**, *25*, 1804–1815. [CrossRef] [PubMed]
99. Uchida, K.; Dezaki, K.; Damdindorj, B.; Inada, H.; Shiuchi, T.; Mori, Y.; Yada, T.; Minokoshi, Y.; Tominaga, M. Lack of TRPM2 impaired insulin secretion and glucose metabolisms in mice. *Diabetes* **2011**, *60*, 119–126. [CrossRef] [PubMed]
100. Wagner, T.F.; Drews, A.; Loch, S.; Mohr, F.; Philipp, S.E.; Lambert, S.; Oberwinkler, J. TRPM3 channels provide a regulated influx pathway for zinc in pancreatic beta cells. *Pflug. Arch.* **2010**, *460*, 755–765. [CrossRef] [PubMed]
101. Muller, I.; Rossler, O.G.; Thiel, G. Pregnenolone sulfate activates basic region leucine zipper transcription factors in insulinoma cells: Role of voltage-gated Ca^{2+} channels and transient receptor potential melastatin 3 channels. *Mol. Pharmacol.* **2011**, *80*, 1179–1189. [CrossRef] [PubMed]
102. Marigo, V.; Courville, K.; Hsu, W.H.; Feng, J.M.; Cheng, H. TRPM4 impacts on Ca^{2+} signals during agonist-induced insulin secretion in pancreatic beta-cells. *Mol. Cell. Endocrinol.* **2009**, *299*, 194–203. [CrossRef] [PubMed]
103. Cheng, H.; Beck, A.; Launay, P.; Gross, S.A.; Stokes, A.J.; Kinet, J.P.; Fleig, A.; Penner, R. TRPM4 controls insulin secretion in pancreatic beta-cells. *Cell Calcium* **2007**, *41*, 51–61. [CrossRef] [PubMed]
104. Vennekens, R.; Olausson, J.; Meissner, M.; Bloch, W.; Mathar, I.; Philipp, S.E.; Schmitz, F.; Weissgerber, P.; Nilius, B.; Flockerzi, V.; et al. Increased IgE-dependent mast cell activation and anaphylactic responses in mice lacking the calcium-activated nonselective cation channel TRPM4. *Nat. Immunol.* **2007**, *8*, 312–320. [CrossRef] [PubMed]
105. Nelson, P.L.; Zolochevska, O.; Figueiredo, M.L.; Soliman, A.; Hsu, W.H.; Feng, J.M.; Zhang, H.; Cheng, H. Regulation of Ca^{2+}-entry in pancreatic alpha-cell line by transient receptor potential melastatin 4 plays a vital role in glucagon release. *Mol. Cell. Endocrinol.* **2011**, *335*, 126–134. [CrossRef] [PubMed]
106. Berggren, P.O.; Yang, S.N.; Murakami, M.; Efanov, A.M.; Uhles, S.; Kohler, M.; Moede, T.; Fernstrom, A.; Appelskog, I.B.; Aspinwall, C.A.; et al. Removal of Ca^{2+} channel beta3 subunit enhances Ca^{2+} oscillation frequency and insulin exocytosis. *Cell* **2004**, *119*, 273–284. [CrossRef] [PubMed]
107. Perez, C.A.; Huang, L.; Rong, M.; Kozak, J.A.; Preuss, A.K.; Zhang, H.; Max, M.; Margolskee, R.F. A transient receptor potential channel expressed in taste receptor cells. *Nat. Neurosci.* **2002**, *5*, 1169–1176. [CrossRef] [PubMed]
108. Huang, Y.A.; Roper, S.D. Intracellular Ca^{2+} and TRPM5-mediated membrane depolarization produce ATP secretion from taste receptor cells. *J. Physiol.* **2010**, *588*, 2343–2350. [CrossRef] [PubMed]
109. Palmer, R.K. The pharmacology and signaling of bitter, sweet, and umami taste sensing. *Mol. Interv.* **2007**, *7*, 87–98. [CrossRef] [PubMed]
110. Sprous, D.; Palmer, K.R. The T1R2/T1R3 sweet receptor and TRPM5 ion channel taste targets with therapeutic potential. *Prog. Mol. Biol. Transl. Sci.* **2010**, *91*, 151–208. [PubMed]
111. Palmer, R.K.; Lunn, C.A. TRP channels as targets for therapeutic intervention in obesity: Focus on TRPV1 and TRPM5. *Curr. Top. Med. Chem.* **2013**, *13*, 247–257. [CrossRef] [PubMed]
112. Khan, A.; Safdar, M.; Ali Khan, M.M.; Khattak, K.N.; Anderson, R.A. Cinnamon improves glucose and lipids of people with type 2 diabetes. *Diabetes Care* **2003**, *26*, 3215–3218. [CrossRef] [PubMed]
113. Mang, B.; Wolters, M.; Schmitt, B.; Kelb, K.; Lichtinghagen, R.; Stichtenoth, D.O.; Hahn, A. Effects of a cinnamon extract on plasma glucose, HbA, and serum lipids in diabetes mellitus type 2. *Eur. J. Clin. Investig.* **2006**, *36*, 340–344. [CrossRef] [PubMed]
114. Vanschoonbeek, K.; Thomassen, B.J.; Senden, J.M.; Wodzig, W.K.; van Loon, L.J. Cinnamon supplementation does not improve glycemic control in postmenopausal type 2 diabetes patients. *J. Nutr.* **2006**, *136*, 977–980. [PubMed]
115. Tamura, Y.; Iwasaki, Y.; Narukawa, M.; Watanabe, T. Ingestion of cinnamaldehyde, a TRPA1 agonist, reduces visceral fats in mice fed a high-fat and high-sucrose diet. *J. Nutr. Sci. Vitaminol.* **2012**, *58*, 9–13. [CrossRef] [PubMed]
116. Sartorius, T.; Peter, A.; Schulz, N.; Drescher, A.; Bergheim, I.; Machann, J.; Schick, F.; Siegel-Axel, D.; Schurmann, A.; Weigert, C.; et al. Cinnamon extract improves insulin sensitivity in the brain and lowers liver fat in mouse models of obesity. *PLoS ONE* **2014**, *9*, e92358. [CrossRef] [PubMed]

117. Iwasaki, Y.; Tanabe, M.; Kobata, K.; Watanabe, T. Trpa1 agonists—Allyl isothiocyanate and cinnamaldehyde—Induce adrenaline secretion. *Biosci. Biotechnol. Biochem.* **2008**, *72*, 2608–2614. [CrossRef] [PubMed]
118. Ahn, J.; Lee, H.; Im, S.W.; Jung, C.H.; Ha, T.Y. Allyl isothiocyanate ameliorates insulin resistance through the regulation of mitochondrial function. *J. Nutr. Biochem.* **2014**, *25*, 1026–1034. [CrossRef] [PubMed]
119. Doihara, H.; Nozawa, K.; Kawabata-Shoda, E.; Kojima, R.; Yokoyama, T.; Ito, H. Molecular cloning and characterization of dog TRPA1 and AITC stimulate the gastrointestinal motility through TRPA1 in conscious dogs. *Eur. J. Pharmacol.* **2009**, *617*, 124–129. [CrossRef] [PubMed]

5

Computer-Driven Development of an in Silico Tool for Finding Selective Histone Deacetylase 1 Inhibitors

Hajar Sirous [1,*], Giuseppe Campiani [2], Simone Brogi [3,*], Vincenzo Calderone [3] and Giulia Chemi [2,†]

1 Bioinformatics Research Center, School of Pharmacy and Pharmaceutical Sciences, Isfahan University of Medical Sciences, Isfahan 81746-73461, Iran

2 Department of Biotechnology, Chemistry and Pharmacy, DoE Department of Excellence 2018–2022, University of Siena, via Aldo Moro 2, 53100 Siena, Italy; campiani@unisi.it (G.C.); GChemi001@dundee.ac.uk (G.C.)

3 Department of Pharmacy, University of Pisa, via Bonanno 6, 56126 Pisa, Italy; vincenzo.calderone@unipi.it

* Correspondence: h_sirous@pharm.mui.ac.ir (H.S.); simone.brogi@unipi.it (S.B.)

† Present address: Wellcome Centre for Anti-Infectives Research, Drug Discovery Unit, Division of Biological Chemistry and Drug Discovery, University of Dundee, Dundee DD1 5EH, UK.

Academic Editors: Marco Tutone and Anna Maria Almerico

Abstract: Histone deacetylases (HDACs) are a class of epigenetic modulators overexpressed in numerous types of cancers. Consequently, HDAC inhibitors (HDACIs) have emerged as promising antineoplastic agents. Unfortunately, the most developed HDACIs suffer from poor selectivity towards a specific isoform, limiting their clinical applicability. Among the isoforms, HDAC1 represents a crucial target for designing selective HDACIs, being aberrantly expressed in several malignancies. Accordingly, the development of a predictive in silico tool employing a large set of HDACIs (aminophenylbenzamide derivatives) is herein presented for the first time. Software Phase was used to derive a 3D-QSAR model, employing as alignment rule a common-features pharmacophore built on 20 highly active/selective HDAC1 inhibitors. The 3D-QSAR model was generated using 370 benzamide-based HDACIs, which yielded an excellent correlation coefficient value ($R^2 = 0.958$) and a satisfactory predictive power ($Q^2 = 0.822$; $Q^2_{F3} = 0.894$). The model was validated ($r^2_{ext\_ts} = 0.794$) using an external test set (113 compounds not used for generating the model), and by employing a decoys set and the receiver-operating characteristic (ROC) curve analysis, evaluating the Güner–Henry score (GH) and the enrichment factor (EF). The results confirmed a satisfactory predictive power of the 3D-QSAR model. This latter represents a useful filtering tool for screening large chemical databases, finding novel derivatives with improved HDAC1 inhibitory activity.

Keywords: 3D-QSAR; pharmacophore modeling; ligand-based model; HDACs; isoform-selective histone deacetylase inhibitors; aminophenylbenzamide

---

1. Introduction

Epigenetic defects in gene expression are well known in the onset and progression of cancer. In this context, pharmacological targeting of proteins of the cellular epigenetic machinery has provided opportunities for anti-cancer drug design [1,2]. Among epigenetic enzymes, histone deacetylases (HDACs) hold a fundamental role in regulating gene expression through histone post-translational modifications [3–5].

HDACs catalyze the removal of acetyl groups from the acetylated ε-amino termini of lysine residues located at the tails of the nucleosomal histones core. Histone deacetylation process leads to condensed chromatin structure which concomitantly restricts the accessibility of related transcriptional factors to their target genes, thereby suppressing gene expression including tumor suppressor genes [6–8]. The abnormal regulation of this process culminates with the high expression level of HDACs. This event has been observed in the development of several human cancers. Consequently, effective inhibition of HDACs has recently gained importance as a valid therapeutic strategy to reverse aberrant epigenetic changes associated with cancer [9–11]. HDAC inhibitors (HDACIs) induce histone hyperacetylation and subsequent transcriptional re-activation of suppressed genes which are correlated with a variety of effects on tumor cells including apoptosis, differentiation, cell cycle arrest, inhibition of proliferation and cytostasis [12,13].

The HDAC family comprises 18 isoforms in mammalian cells which are categorized into four main classes (class I-IV) based on their structural and functional characteristics. HDACs belonging to class I (HDAC1–3 and 8), II (HDACs 4–7, 9 and 10) and IV (HDAC11) are all zinc-dependent metalloenzymes, while class III HDACs, also known as the sirtuins (SIRT1-7), requires NAD^+ as a cofactor for their catalytic function [6,14].

Extensive efforts over recent decades have led to the identification of four chemically diverse classes of HDACIs as potent antineoplastic agents including, hydroxamates, benzamides, cyclic peptides, and short-chain fatty acids [3]. The main breakthrough in developing these inhibitors was achieved by the US FDA approval of Vorinostat [15], Belinostat [16], Panobinostat (hydroxamate-based inhibitors) [17], Romidepsin (a cyclic peptide) [18] and Chidamide (a benzamide-based inhibitor) [19] for the treatment of lymphoma and myeloma. Moreover, several HDACIs such as Mocetinostat [20], Entinostat [21], Tacedinaline [22], Givinostat [23], and Abexinostat [24] are currently in clinical trials for treating various types of cancers. The structures of several approved and clinical HDACIs are shown in Figure 1.

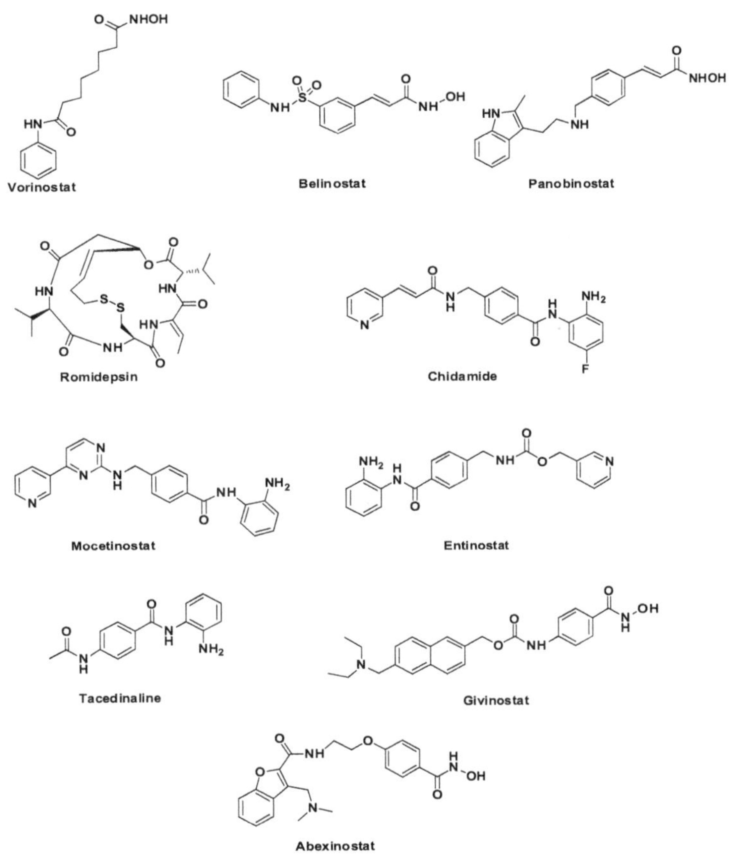

Figure 1. HDACIs approved by FDA and/or in clinical trials.

Despite these successes, the most known HDACIs target multiple HDAC isoforms and this poor selectivity represents a major drawback which limits their broad clinical utility [25,26]. Isoform-selective

HDACIs would offer superior therapeutic advantages due to limited off-target and undesirable effects, improved clinical efficacy and better tolerability [27,28]. Moreover, isoform-selective inhibitors would provide chemical tools to delineate the precise roles of individual HDAC isoforms in human diseases, including rare disorders [29]. Therefore, in recent years, identification of highly potent inhibitors with strict selectivity towards a specific isoform have caught more attention in the development of novel HDACIs for the epigenetic therapy [30–33]. In this context, due to the pivotal role of HDAC1 in the angiogenesis, proliferation, and survival of mammalian carcinoma cells, this isoform is particularly being sought as a preferred target for successful design of selective HDACIs [34–38].

A wide range of hydroxamic acid derivatives are known to be potent pan-inhibitors of several HDAC isoforms [39,40]. Accordingly, in recent years, there has been considerable interest in developing non-hydroxamate HDACIs with satisfactory selectivity towards a specific isoform. In this context, aminophenylbenzamide derivatives represent an important class of non-hydroxamate HDACIs owing to their potent HDAC inhibition along with desirable pharmacokinetic profile and excellent selectivity for HDAC class I enzyme. Furthermore, inhibitors containing an ortho-aminobenzamide typically exhibit relatively greater levels of selectivity for class I HDACs, particularly HDAC1 [35,41]. In addition, hydroxamic-derived inhibitors often suffer from some serious pharmacokinetic issues including poor metabolic stability, rapid clearance, undesirable oral absorption, and short half-life in plasma, whereas benzamides-based inhibitors show better metabolic stability and oral bioavailability [42–45]. For these solid reasons, renewed efforts are being directed towards the further exploration of innovative aminophenylbenzamide chemotypes as privileged and valuable scaffolds to develop isoform-selective HDACIs [46–48].

Recently, in silico techniques, including ligand-based methods such as pharmacophore modeling and three-dimensional quantitative structural activity relationship (3D-QSAR), have efficiently contributed to guide the discovery of novel bioactive molecules, with reduced costs in terms of money and time [49–51]. In fact, QSAR methods provide relationships between physicochemical properties of a series of compounds and their biological activities to obtain a reliable statistical model for predicting the activities of new chemical entities. The fundamental principle of the technique is that the change in structural properties determines modifications in biological activities of the compounds. In the classical QSAR approaches, affinities of ligands to their binding sites, inhibition constants, rate constants, and other biological data have been correlated with molecular properties including lipophilicity, polarizability, electronic and steric properties (Hansch analysis) or with structural features (Free-Wilson analysis). However, classical QSAR approach has only a limited utility for designing new molecules due to the lack of consideration of the 3D structure of the selected compounds. Accordingly, 3D-QSAR has emerged as a natural extension to the classical Hansch and Free-Wilson approaches, which exploits the three-dimensional properties of the ligands to predict their biological activities employing robust chemometric techniques such as partial least squares (PLS). The success of these methods can be attributed to several factors including identification of important features for the activity, rationalization of activity trends in molecules under study, prediction of the specific activity for a selected target or undesirable effects of new compounds. On the other hand, ligand-based methods have been used in virtual screening campaigns of chemical databases to find novel hits with improved potency and can be combined with other computational and experimental workflows to discover new potential drugs [52–57].

Until now, only limited number of 3D-QSAR studies for hydroxamate set of HDACIs have been reported [58–64]. However, to the best of our knowledge, no previous attempt has been made to seek the structural and chemical features of aminophenylbenzamide governing their HDAC inhibitory activities employing 3D-QSAR methodology along with a large set of compounds. Given the aforementioned therapeutic significance of this class of inhibitors, we developed and validated a 3D-QSAR model using a comprehensive set of previously reported benzamide derivatives as selective HDAC1 inhibitors. From this perspective, the software Phase, implemented in Maestro, was employed to explore a common-features pharmacophore hypothesis based on highly active ligands. This hypothesis was then used as an alignment rule to derive a predictive 3D-QSAR model [65]. Such an in silico tool could aid not only in forecasting the HDAC1 inhibitory activity of newly designed chemical entities, but also offer a robust foundation for designing new selective HDACIs with increased binding affinities to HDAC1. Accordingly, the developed model could have a relevant implication in drug discovery campaign for searching isoform-selective HDACIs.

2. Results and Discussion

The application of 3D-QSAR methodology in the design of HDACIs has received little attention to date and only a few instances of field-based QSAR models (comparative molecular field analysis (CoMFA) and comparative similarity indices analysis (CoMSIA) methods) have been reported for hydroxamate-based inhibitors [58–64]. However, this approach has not been carried out for a large set of benzamide-based derivatives behaving as HDACIs. On the other hand, we have recently developed a series of predictive 3D-QSAR models for different purposes including the identification or rational design of new chemical entities for different targets [53,55], and the prediction of undesirable effects of novel molecules such as potential *h*ERG K^+ channel related cardiotoxicity [57]. In all these cases, Phase was used to develop a computational tool using a pharmacophore-based alignment that links the information of pivotal functional groups of the ligands with their biological activity [65]. The fruitful results of the above-mentioned molecular modeling studies as well as therapeutic significance of benzamide chemotypes as valuable isoform-selective HDACIs inspired us to derive a pharmacophore-based 3D-QSAR model to be used as a screening filtering tool able to quantitatively predict the HDAC1 inhibitory activity of newly designed ligands.

2.1. Data Set Preparation

A comprehensive data set of 370 diverse HDACIs based on benzamide scaffold with functional biological activity expressed as IC_{50} (see the Supplementary Materials for further details) with a range of HDAC1 inhibitory activities spanning five orders of magnitude (from 6.0 nM of compound **17** to 50 μM of compound **132**, Table S1) were selected from literature for developing a predictive 3D-QSAR model. Subsequently, an extensive conformational search for each ligand was performed employing MacroModel software (see experimental section for further details). Conformational analysis is crucial to enhance both the quality of the alignment for the molecules used to generate the 3D-QSAR model and the reliability of the in silico tool [53–57]. After the exhaustive conformational analysis of the selected ligands (Table S1), the generation of the 3D-QSAR model was started.

2.2. Pharmacophore Modeling and 3D-QSAR Model Generation

As a first step to develop the 3D-QSAR model, 20 most active compounds with IC_{50} values $\leq$ 10 nM included in the data set (ligands **1–20**, Figure 2, Table S1) were considered to find out common pharmacophore hypotheses that were subsequently scored and ranked by the software Phase. This means that the highly active compounds possess common features that are responsible for the activity exploited by a 3D pharmacophore hypothesis. Therefore, a pharmacophore hypothesis provides a rational picture of primary chemical features of ligands responsible for HDAC1 inhibitory activity and therefore can be used as a reliable alignment rule for the 3D-QSAR model development.

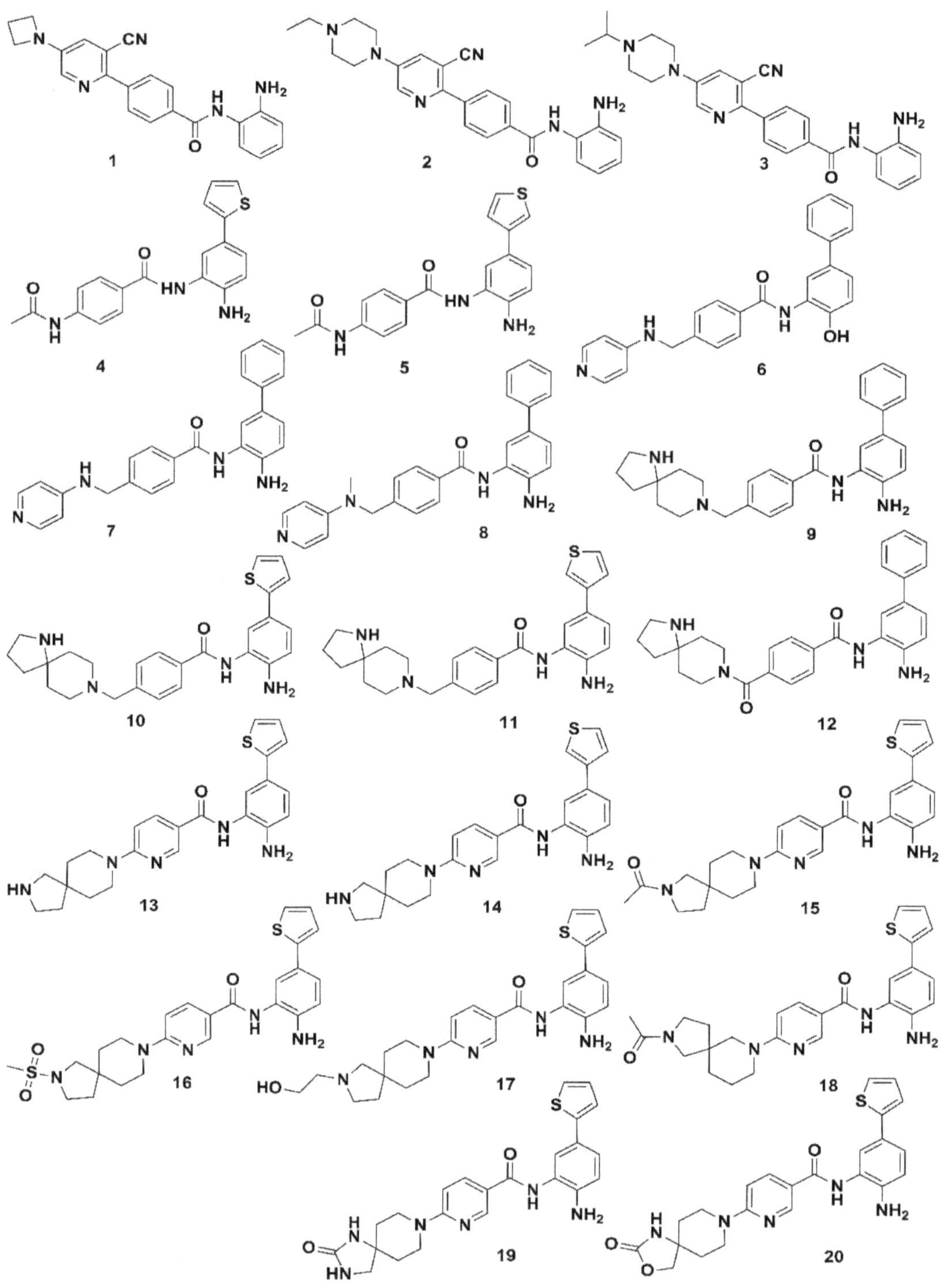

Figure 2. Chemical structure of highly active compounds against HDAC1 (IC_{50} comprised between 0.004 μM and 0.01 μM) used for generating a common-features pharmacophore.

To have optimal combination of sites or features shared by the most active ligands, the minimum and maximum number of site points were set on 5. This means that we selected 5 as maximum features to include in the pharmacophore models. Among the 26 common pharmacophore hypotheses generated by the software Phase, only those models which showed superior alignment with the active compounds were identified by calculating the survival score. The survival scoring function of Phase module identifies the best candidate hypothesis from the generated models and offers an overall ranking of all the hypotheses. The scoring algorithm includes contributions from the alignment of site points and vectors, volume overlap, selectivity, number of ligands matched, relative conformational energy, and activity. To identify pharmacophore models with more active and less inactive features, all models were mapped to inactive compounds and scored. If inactives score well, the hypothesis could be invalid because it does not discriminate between actives and inactives. Therefore, adjusted survival score was calculated by subtracting the inactive score from the survival score of these pharmacophores.

After the scoring, the model ADDRR, herein referred to ADDRR hypothesis, with the maximum adjusted survival score (3.769) and lowest relative conformational energy, was selected as the top-ranked hypothesis among the generated 3D model hypotheses. The different scoring parameters for the selected hypothesis (ADDRR) were provided in Table 1. The 3D spatial arrangement of all features with inter-feature distance constraints of ADDRR are presented in Figure 3. As shown in this figure, the hypothesis was characterized by the five main features: one hydrogen-bond acceptor (A), two hydrogen-bond donors (D), and two aromatic rings (R).

Table 1. The different scoring parameters for the best pharmacophore hypothesis, matching all 20 highly active compounds used.

HYPO ID	Survival	Survival—Inactive	Site	Vector	Volume	Selectivity	Matches	Energy	Activity	Inactive
ADDRR	3.769	1.841	0.97	0.999	0.798	1.578	20	0.006	2.097	1.928

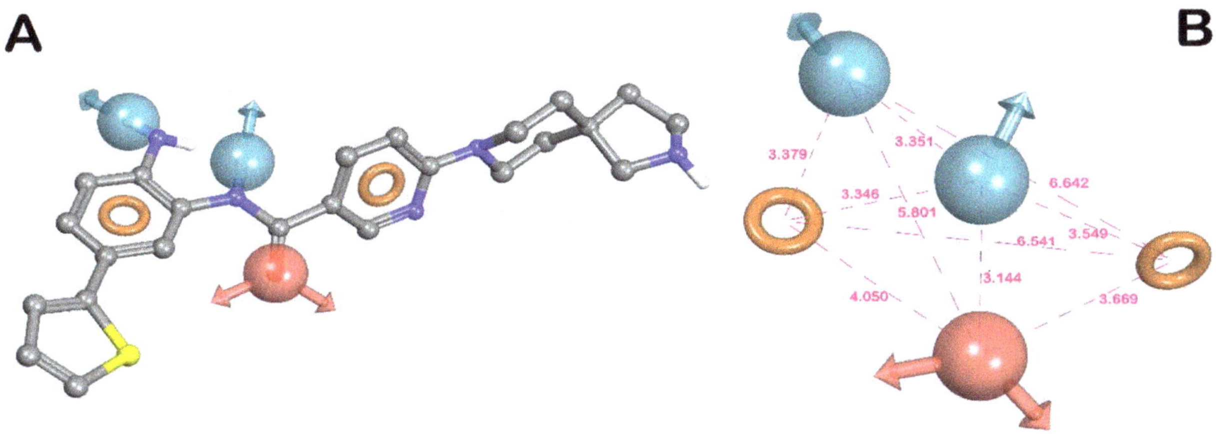

Figure 3. (**A**) Superposition of highly active compound **13** and ADDRR hypothesis. (**B**) ADDRR hypothesis and its inter-feature distances. Features are as follows: H-bond acceptor = A, red vector; H-bond donor = D, blue vectors; aromatic feature = R, orange ring (pictures were generated by means of Maestro software).

Figure 3A depicts one of the most active ligands in the set (compound **13**, Table S1), mapped onto the ADDRR pharmacophore. As depicted in the mentioned figure, compound **13** thoroughly fits all features of the pharmacophore model, underlining the previous findings on structural components required for interacting with the HDAC1 binding site [66–68]. As illustrated in Figure 3, the carbonyl oxygen of the benzamide group served as a hydrogen-bond acceptor (HBA) feature, while two hydrogen-bond donor (HBD) features were mapped to the protons of the 2-aminophenyl NH_2 and amide NH. Furthermore, out of two aromatic features, one was mapped to the phenyl ring of the 2-aminophenyl. The other aromatic feature was mapped to the pyridine ring of the nicotinamide moiety. This hypothesis was well corroborated by accepted common pharmacophore model for HDACIs comprising the zinc binding group (ZBG), a linker and a cap group as established by computational and biophysical studies reported for HDAC1 inhibitors [66–70]. Based on the current study, the aniline groups of the benzamide-based inhibitors are served as ZBG, coordinating the catalytic zinc ion in the HDAC1 active site. Moreover, it is well known that H-bonds formation with key residues of HDAC1 active site are commonly found for the ZBG of this class of HDAC1 inhibitors. In particular, in addition to the zinc ion coordination, protons of the 2-aminophenyl NH_2 group could also establish hydrogen bonds with His140 and His141, while the carbonyl oxygen of the benzamide portion could also form another hydrogen binding interaction with hydroxyl group of

Tyr303. It has been reported that NH of amide could offer the appropriate HBD vector to address the Gly149 through H-bond formation. The presence of two aromatic features capable of participating in π-π stacking interactions with hydrophobic residues Phe150, Tyr204, Phe205, and Tyr303, represents another important requisite for further stabilization of ligand binding. These residues were located in a long and narrow hydrophobic tube-like channel and thus interaction with them allow tubular access of ligand into active site [66,67,69,70]. Accordingly, the above-mentioned ADDRR hypothesis imparts the key features of ligand for providing the relevant interactions with the HDAC1 active site.

The ADDRR pharmacophore hypothesis was then employed as alignment rule to derive the 3D-QSAR model. In this step, the compounds were randomly divided into training (70%) and test sets (30%) taking into account that the response range was well-covered in both sets (Table S1). This choice was made to warrant the inclusion of the positive information originating from 70% of the compounds enclosed in the training set (corresponding to 259 compounds), for the development of the computational tool. Moreover, the compounds kept in the test set (30%, 111 compounds) ensures an appropriate assessment of the predictive power of the generated model through an exhaustive internal validation. The atom-based version of Phase's 3D-QSAR workflow was preferred to the pharmacophore-based one. Such a choice allowed us to take into account contributions associated with all the important structural features other than pharmacophore for HDAC1 inhibitory activity such as the steric clashes. To enhance the model accuracy and evade overfitting phenomenon, models containing one up to seven factors were generated for the studied data set. Statistical parameters for each model are provided in Table 2. Model featuring seven factors was preferred and selected because it better performed in comparison with other models. The reliability of the selected model is justified by the fact that all statistical parameters were in acceptable range. In this regard, the correlation and cross-validated correlation coefficients (R^2 = 0.958 and Q^2 = 0.822, respectively) of the selected model along with the Pearson R-value (R-Pearson = 0.915) were extremely satisfactory, indicating a close correspondence between estimated and experimental IC_{50} values. Moreover, the high Fisher ratio (F = 822.1) suggested a statistically significant regression model, which was further supported by the small value of the variance ratio ($P = 4.377 \times 10^{-169}$), an indication of a high degree of confidence. Finally, the small values of the standard deviation and the root-mean-square error (SD: 0.178 and RMSE: 0.281, respectively) also provided indication about the robustness of the developed computational model. Moreover, the Q^2_{F3} value clearly indicates that the 3D-QSAR model with seven factors is robust.

Table 2. 3D-QSAR statistical parameters of the seven Latent Variables (LVs) Phase-derived sets of models.

LVs	R^{2a}	SD [b]	F [c]	P [d]	RMSE [e]	Q^{2f}	Q^2_{F3} [g]	R-Pearson [h]
1	0.3408	0.6978	132.9	4.699×10^{-22}	0.5199	0.3886	0.635	0.6747
2	0.6273	0.5257	215.5	1.344×10^{-55}	0.3979	0.6420	0.791	0.8282
3	0.7620	0.4209	272.2	3.629×10^{-79}	0.3615	0.7045	0.823	0.8579
4	0.8775	0.3025	455.0	1.704×10^{-144}	0.3514	0.7207	0.833	0.8690
5	0.9159	0.2512	551.0	9.327×10^{-134}	0.2971	0.8004	0.881	0.9003
6	0.9433	0.2067	698.6	6.590×10^{-134}	0.2865	0.8143	0.890	0.9100
7	0.9582	0.1778	822.1	4.377×10^{-169}	0.2808	0.8217	0.894	0.9152

[a] R^2: value of r^2 of the regression. [b] SD: standard deviation of the regression. [c] F: variance ratio. [d] P: significance level of variance ratio. [e] RMSE: root-mean-square error in the test set predictions. [f] Q^2: value of Q^2 for the predicted activities. [g] Q^2_{F3}: value of Q^2_{F3} for the predicted activities calculated as reported in Materials and Methods section. [h] R-Pearson: correlation between the predicted and observed selectivity index values for the test set.

A scatter plot of experimental versus predicted activities was generated to assess the results (Figure 4). Based on this plot, the IC_{50} values were reliably predicted for both training and test set molecules (Table S1). This plot along with the aforementioned statistical features clearly imply the significance of the approach and indicate a QSAR model with a robust predictive power.

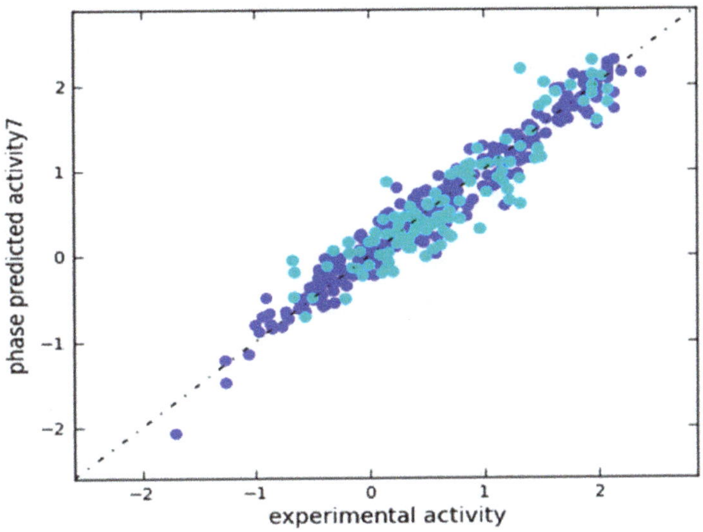

Figure 4. Scatter plot for the predicted (Phase-predicted activity) and the observed (experimental activity) pIC_{50} values (μM) as calculated by the 3D-QSAR model applied to the training set (blue) and test set (cyan) compounds.

Three-dimensional aspects obtained from the QSAR model were visualized using 3D plots of the crucial volume elements occupied by ligands. Such plots allow the visual analysis of important features of ligand structures along with their contributions to the biological activity. The 3D plot representation of the whole model, superimposed to the highly (**3**, **10**, and **13**), moderate (**22, 213,** and **239**), and less active derivatives (**218, 279**, and **299**), is depicted in Figure 5. In this illustration, the blue and red cubes indicate the positive and negative coefficients, respectively. In fact, blue cubes refer to ligand regions in which the specific feature is important for better activity, whereas the red cubes are indicative of a particular structural feature or functional group which is not essential for the activity or is likely to decrease the activity. Cubes with small positive and negative coefficients, which therefore did not greatly affect the activity, were filtered out by setting a 1.50×10^{-2} coefficient threshold. Remarkably, compounds **10** and **13** (Figure 5A,B, respectively) as well as other highly active ligands, mainly lodge in the blue regions, while the less active compounds such as **218** and **299** (Figure 5G,I, respectively) largely resides on the red regions. Moreover, regarding some compounds with moderate activity and generally all compounds with limited activity, we also observed a significant inability to match all the pharmacophore features, according to the decrease of inhibitory potencies.

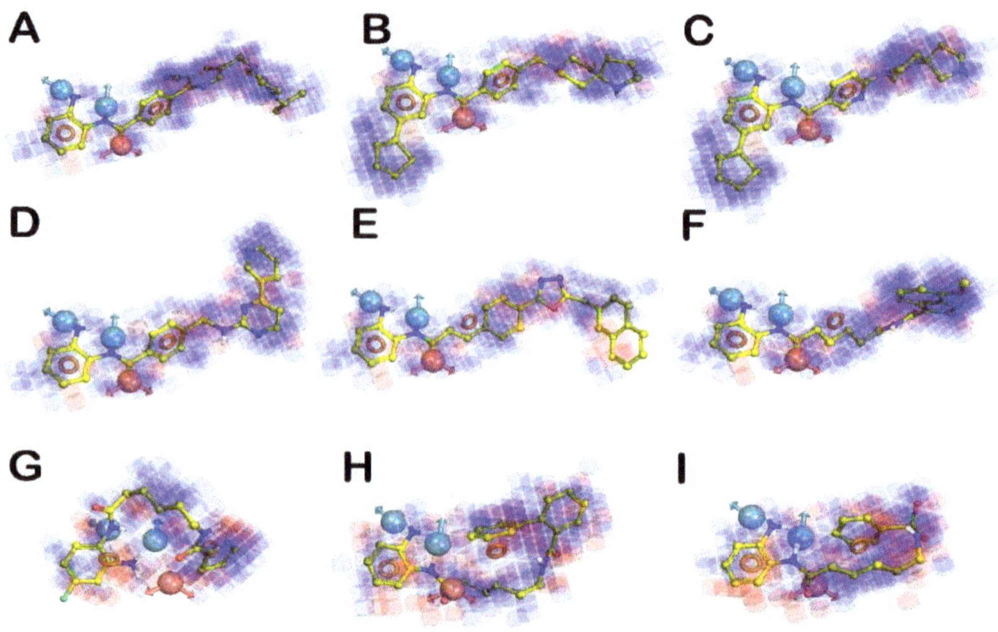

Figure 5. (**A–C**) Superposition of highly active compounds **3**, **10**, and **13**, respectively with the 3D-QSAR model. (**D–F**) Superposition of moderate active compounds **22** (Mocetinostat), **213**, and **239**, respectively with the 3D-QSAR model. (**G–I**) Superposition of less active compounds **218**, **279**, and **299**, respectively with the 3D-QSAR model. The picture was generated by means of Maestro software (Schrödinger, LLC, New York, NY, USA, 2015).

2.3. In Silico 3D-QSAR Model Validation

2.3.1. Validation Using External Test Set

After the generation of the 3D-QSAR model, a preliminary in silico validation was performed using an external test set selected from the literature that have not been used for generating the computational model. This set was composed of 113 compounds with different inhibitory activities against HDAC1 (ranging from 5.8 nM to 1140 nM; Table S2 in the Supplementary Materials). As reported in Table S2, our model was satisfactorily efficient in estimating the HDAC1 inhibitory activity of compounds included in the external test set. In the scatter plot depicted in Figure 6, the experimental and predicted pIC_{50} values of these compounds are also displayed, offering a reasonable correlation coefficient ($r^2_{ext\_ts}$ = 0.794). This result provided further confirmation that the correlation shown by the model is not accidental.

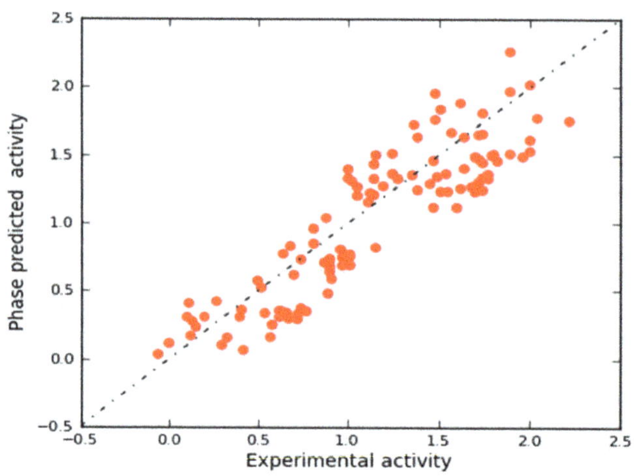

Figure 6. Scatter plot for the predicted (Phase-predicted activity) and observed (experimental activity) pIC_{50} values (μM) as calculated by the 3D-QSAR model with 7 factors applied to the external test set.

2.3.2. Validation Using Decoy Set and Receiver-Operating Characteristic (ROC) Curve Approach

For a further validation and to assess the performance of the developed 3D-QSAR model, we employed a validation method based on generation of decoys set. This procedure is usually employed to evaluate the capability of in silico tools such as 3D-QSAR models to discriminate between active or inactive molecules [71–75]. Starting from highly active compounds (ligands 1–20 in Table S1), 86 additional compounds with good activity against HDAC1 (cutoff IC_{50} < 35 nM; Tables S1 and S2) were selected from the training, test and external validation sets for a total of 106 compounds (Table S3) from which decoys were generated. For this set of active ligands, DUD-E server generated 5764 decoys. After an appropriate minimization and conformational search of decoys, we have combined them with the active molecules (referred as A in Figure 7A) for a total of 5870 compounds (referred as D in Figure 7A) that were then subjected to a virtual screening using the developed 3D-QSAR model. Interestingly, the results of this evaluation supported the validity of the proposed model. Analysis of the database screening results (Figure 7A) indicated a trend in which inactive compounds fail to completely satisfy all the pharmacophore features, thus making their predicted activity very poor or absent. In contrast, the 3D-QSAR model was reasonably efficient in the estimation of HDAC1 inhibitory activity of active compounds.

A: Parameters	Values
Total molecules in database (D)	5870
Total number of actives in database (A)	106
Total hits (Ht)	30
Active hits (Ha)	26
%Yield of actives (YA)	86.67
%Ratio of actives (RA)	24.53
Enrichment factor (EF)	48.33
Goodness hit of score (GH)	0.71

B: ROC curve

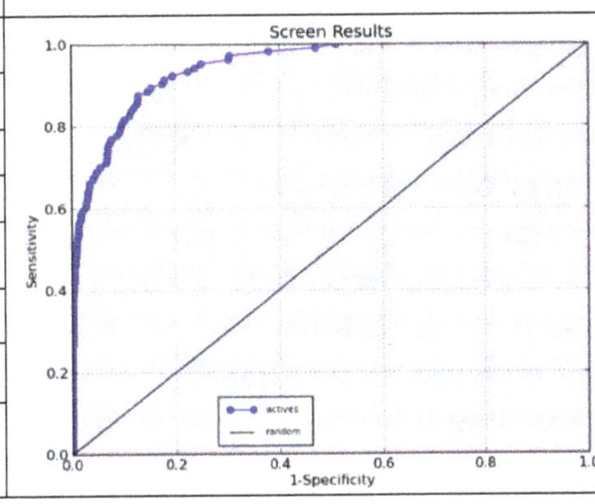

Figure 7. (**A**) EF and GH scores obtained by the application of 3D-QSAR model in a database screening; and (**B**) receiver-operating characteristic (ROC) curve generated from database screening.

According to the screening results (Figure 7A), the top 30 ranked compounds were considered to be hits (Ht). This cutoff value could represent a suitable number of molecules (about 1% of database) to be purchased after a virtual screening campaign. Remarkably, among Ht, 26 (Ha) compounds belonged to the set of 106 known HDAC1 inhibitors. Furthermore, this qualitative analysis was well supported by the calculation of some statistical parameters such as EF and GH score (see Materials and Methods section for calculation details). In this regard, the calculated EF was 48.33, which implies that it could be about 48.33 times more probable to select active compounds from the hit list compared with random selection from the complete database. The estimated GH score value of 0.71, larger than 0.5, indicates a great reliability of the model (Figure 7A). This suggests that the developed computational model can serve as efficient tool in virtual screening studies to find out novel chemical entities behaving as selective HDAC1 inhibitors.

The applicability of the proposed 3D-QSAR model was further evaluated by means of the receiver-operating characteristic (ROC) curve. The ROC curve approach is a well-recognized metric used as an objective way to assess the balance between model sensitivity (capability to discover true positives) and specificity (capability to avoid false positives) [55,57,76,77]. For this purpose, 5870 compounds employed in the previous validation step, were ranked according to their predicted activity values as estimated by the 3D-QSAR model. The output of the ROC curve provided a score for appraising the overall performance of the model. In particular, the closer the ROC score is to 1.0, the better is the model at discriminating active from inactive compounds. ROC curve analysis of our in silico model yielded a satisfactory Area Under the Curve (AUC) score of 0.94 (Figure 7B), providing additional evidence about the predictivity of the developed 3D-QSAR model.

3. Materials and Methods

3.1. Hardware and Software Specifications

All computational tasks in this study were carried out using molecular modeling package from Schrödinger suite 2015 (Schrödinger, Inc., LLC, New York, NY, USA) installed on an Intel(R) Xeon(R) CPU E5-2620 v2 @ 3.30 GHz, 64 GB RAM with 12 processors, and a 2GB graphics card of NVIDIA Quadro K2200 running Ubuntu 10.04 LTS (long-term support) as operating system. Access to the Schrödinger modules as well as the capability to organize and analyze data was provided by Maestro as a portal interface of Schrödinger [78].

3.2. Ligands and Data Set Preparation

A comprehensive set of HDAC1 inhibitors characterized by the 2-aminophenylbenzamide scaffold with known IC_{50} values that vary over a wide range was collected from the literature [66,67,79–92] and the bindingDB database [93]. The selection criterion for the compounds to be included in the set was that their HDAC1 inhibition was evaluated using the same fluorescent assay based on the fluorogenic substrate Fluor-de-Lys. This inclusion criterion allowed us to obtain a homogeneous set of compounds regarding their biological evaluation. This step is crucial to develop a predictive model since the data selection is pivotal for adding the correct information to a software for developing computational models. The 3D structures of all ligands were built using the builder panel in the Maestro. For the molecules possessing known stereochemistry, the absolute configuration was specified during the drawing of the compounds. All structures were treated by LigPrep module of Schrödinger suite 2015 [94] in order to generate the most probable ionization state at the cellular pH value (7.4 ± 0.2) as reported by us [95–97]. Moreover, the OPLS-AA_2005 force field was used for optimization, which produces the lowest energy conformer of the ligand [98]. The prepared ligands were then submitted to MacroModel software [99] in order to obtain an exhaustive conformational analysis using the OPLS-AA_2005 as force field. The solvent effects are simulated employing the analytical Generalized-Born/Surface-Area (GB/SA) model [100], and no cutoff for non-bonded interactions was selected. Molecular energy minimizations were performed using Polak–Ribiere conjugate gradient (PRCG) method with 2000 maximum iterations and 0.001 gradient convergence threshold. The conformational searches were carried out by employing MCMM (Monte Carlo Multiple Minimum) torsional sampling method. Automatic setup with 21 kJ/mol (5.02 kcal/mol) in the energy window for saving structure and a 0.5 Å cutoff distance for redundant conformers was used.

3.3. 3D-QSAR Model Generation

The software package Phase 4.2 [101], implemented in Maestro suite, was used to generate pharmacophore hypotheses and 3D-QSAR models for HDAC1 inhibitors based on 2-aminophenylbenzamide scaffold. Given a set of molecules with high affinity for a particular protein target, this software uses fine-grained conformational sampling and a range of scoring techniques to identify a common-features pharmacophore hypothesis, which conveys 3D structural characteristics that are critical for the activity. Pharmacophore feature sites for the molecules were specified by a set of features well-defined in Phase as hydrogen-bond acceptor (A), hydrogen-bond donor (D), hydrophobic group (H), negatively charged group (N), positively charged group (P) and aromatic ring (R). No user-defined feature was employed for the present study. The ligands prepared as reported in the previous step, were imported into the "develop common pharmacophore hypotheses" panel of Phase with their respective biological activity values. Twenty active compounds (Figure 2 and in Table S1 in the Supplementary Materials) possessing highly inhibitory potency against HDAC1 were selected for generating the pharmacophore hypotheses. Common-features pharmacophore hypotheses were identified, scored, and ranked by means of conformational analysis and tree-based partitioning techniques. In the score hypotheses step, common pharmacophores are examined, and a scoring procedure is applied to identify the pharmacophore from each surviving n-dimensional box that yields the best alignment of the active set ligands. This pharmacophore provides the means to explain how the active molecules bind to the receptor.

The best ranked pharmacophore model obtained by Phase (ADDRR, shown in Figure 3A superimposed to aminophenylnicotinamide analogue **13**), consisted of five features: one hydrogen-bond acceptor (A), two hydrogen-bond donors (D), and two aromatic functions (R). The inter-feature distances (Figure 3B) were measured by using the site measurements tool implemented in the software Phase. This pharmacophore was used as alignment rule for further 3D-QSAR analysis. All the molecules used for the QSAR studies (Table S1) were aligned to the selected pharmacophore hypothesis. In the present study, we set a pIC_{50} threshold for the selection of active and inactive ligands. These pIC_{50} values were also used as the dependent variable in the 3D-QSAR calculations. In particular, compounds that showed an IC_{50} comprised between 5 and 50 μM were considered to be inactive ligands. Moderate inhibitors were considered compounds with IC_{50} between 10 nM and 5 μM, while compounds possessing an $IC_{50} \leq 10$ nM were assigned as potent inhibitors of HDAC1 and consequently as actives during 3D-QSAR model generation. Remarkably, to avoid possible faults arising from the inclusion in the set of molecules with uncertain activity, only molecules with experimentally definite inhibitory activity have been selected to develop the in silico model. Atom-based QSAR models were developed for ADDRR hypothesis using 259 compounds in the training set (370 compounds were randomly divided 70% in the training and 30% in the test set) and a grid spacing of 0.5 Å. QSAR models were generated by means of PLS method. An internal validation was achieved employing leave-n-out (LnO) technique as specified in Phase user manual (Phase, version 4.2, User Manual, Schrödinger press, LLC, New York, NY, 2015). As reported by Todeschini et al. the internal validation results generally expressed in terms of Q^2 metrics should be amended introducing $Q^2{}_{F3}$ metrics for the internal validation of the QSAR models [102]. For this purpose, we calculated these metrics (Table 2) employing the formula reported below (Equation (1)).

$$Q^2_{F3} = 1 - \frac{\sum_{i=1}^{n_{OUT}} (y_i - \hat{y}_{i/i})^2 / n_{OUT}}{\sum_{i=1}^{n_{TR}} \left(y_i - \bar{y}_{TR}\right)^2 / n_{TR}} \tag{1}$$

where y_i is the experimental response of the ith object, $\hat{y}_{i/i}$ is the predicted response when the ith object is not in the training set, n_{TR} and n_{OUT} are the number of training and prediction objects, respectively, and $\bar{y}_{TR}$ is the average value of the training set experimental responses. Moreover, to avoid overfitting/underfitting phenomena, we considered 7 factors that is an appropriate for the number of selected compounds. In fact, although there is no limit on the maximum number of factors, but as a general rule, we stopped adding factors when the standard deviation of regression is approximately equal to the experimental error (calculated as median error among the selected compounds).

3.4. *In Silico 3D-QSAR Model Validation*

After the generation of the 3D-QSAR model, a preliminary in silico validation was performed using a large external test set of compounds (113 molecules) selected from the literature [83,84,89,103–106] (Table S2 in the Supplementary Materials) that have not been used for generating and cross validating the model. These compounds were prepared by using Maestro, LigPrep, and MacroModel, adopting the same procedure for preparing the molecules used to derive the model. Moreover, to further assess that the chosen model with 7 factors better performs with respect to the other Phase-derived models, we applied the validation method employing the external test set to all the generated QSAR models (Table 2). This workflow established that the model with 7 factors is the best performing model of the series in predicting the activity of the external test set with a correlation coefficient $r^2{}_{ext\_ts} = 0.794$

(Figure 6) (LVs 1, $r^2_{ext\_ts} = 0.421$; LVs 2, $r^2_{ext\_ts} = 0.698$; LVs 3, $r^2_{ext\_ts} = 0.657$; LVs 4, $r^2_{ext\_ts} = 0.712$; LVs 5, $r^2_{ext\_ts} = 0.735$; LVs 6, $r^2_{ext\_ts} = 0.787$; Figures S1–S6, respectively).

Further validation of the model was done by enrichment study using decoy test [107]. For this purpose, the Enhanced (DUD-E) web server [108] was employed to generate a set of useful decoys generated from a collection of 106 active compounds from three sources: 1) active compounds used to develop the pharmacophore model, 2) other compounds with good activity against HDAC1 used in 3D-QSAR studies and 3) the most active compounds of the external test set. This collection consisted of 106 active compounds with $IC_{50} \leq 35$ nM (Table S3). For this set of active ligands, the DUD-E server provided 5764 inactive ligands (redundant structures in the output files were deleted) from a subset of the ZINC database filtered using the Lipinski's rules for drug-likeness, for a total of 5870 compounds (5764 inactives plus 106 actives). Each of these inactive decoys was selected to bear a resemblance to the physicochemical properties of the reference ligand but differ from it in terms of 2D structure (e.g., large difference of Tanimoto coefficient between decoys and active molecules). Although largely used, the approach based on decoys sets presents some limitations (i.e., the decoy sets often span a small, synthetically feasible subset of molecular space and are restricted in physicochemical similarity compared with actives). After the generation, the decoys sets were downloaded as 126 smiles files and imported into Maestro and submitted to LigPrep application to properly convert smiles into 3D structures as well as for removing potential erroneous structures. Subsequently, to perform a minimization and a conformational search of the obtained structures MacroModel program was employed (same parameters for ligands preparation were applied). A single file containing conformers of active molecules and decoys was created and submitted to Phase software for predicting the inhibitory activity of database against HDAC1 using the developed 3D-QSAR model and employing "search for matches" option. After decoys generation and activity evaluation, the Güner–Henry score, i.e., goodness of hit list (GH) and enrichment factor (EF) values were estimated by Equations (2) and (3), respectively.

$$EF = \frac{Ha/Ht}{(A/D)} \tag{2}$$

$$GH = \left\{\frac{Ha * (3A + Ht)}{4HtA}\right\} * \left[1 - \frac{(Ht - Ha)}{(D - A)}\right] \tag{3}$$

where Ht represents the total number of compounds in the hit list found by virtual screening, Ha is the total actives found by virtual screening considering the top 30-ranked position (positions comprise within the cutoff value). The total number of compounds (Ht) might represent the number of molecules to purchase after a virtual screening protocol and almost the 1% of the considered database (D). A represents the total of the active derivatives enclosed in the database, and D stands for the total number of molecules existing in the set. The range of GH score varies from 0 to 1. The GH score 0 means a null model, while the GH score 1 denotes generation of an ideal model. Moreover, the % yield of actives (% YA) and % ratio of actives (% RA) were evaluated by Equations (4) and (5), respectively.

$$\%YA = \left[\left(\frac{Ha}{Ht}\right) * 100\right] \tag{4}$$

$$\%RA = \left[\left(\frac{Ha}{A}\right) * 100\right] \tag{5}$$

Moreover, to assess the predictive power of the 3D-QSAR model, a ROC was employed through an Enrichment Calculator (enrichment.py) script [55–57,76]. The mentioned script calculates the enrichment metrics, including area under the receiver-operating characteristic curve (AUC), from virtual screening by means of the output structure file and a list of known active molecules. The output of the screening protocol, using active molecules and decoys, consisted of a list of molecules ranked by the predicted activity from the top-predicted molecules as estimated by the 3D-QSAR model. These ranking data along with a list file of active molecules were submitted to the enrichment.py application.

4. Conclusions

The present study describes the generation of a ligand-based pharmacophore model (ADDRR) for a subset of 20 highly active aminophenylbenzamide derivatives reported as selective HDAC1 inhibitors by employing the software Phase implemented in the Schrödinger molecular modeling suite. With the aid of pharmacophore-based alignment rule, a meaningful 3D-QSAR model was derived and validated employing of the QSAR models a large set of benzamide-based HDAC1 inhibitors (training set, test set, and an external test set for a total of 483 molecules) by using PLS analysis. The main objective of this approach was to develop an in-house computational tool for the prediction of HDAC1 inhibitory activity during the design of innovative aminophenylbenzamide chemotypes as privileged therapeutic scaffold in the isoform-selective HDACIs research. The validation outcomes confirmed that the proposed 3D-QSAR model is endowed with satisfactory predictive power taking into account favorable structural requirements responsible for HDAC1 inhibitory activity. This aspect has been computationally investigated since the selectivity is implicit in the template molecules; however prospective validation is needed to exploit the performance of the model. In fact, the developed 3D-QSAR model can be used for rationally designing novel and selective HDACIs. Moreover, based on the computational investigation, the developed model possesses a rationale for virtual screening campaign, with huge potential in isoform-selective HDACIs drug discovery, and it can effectively provide a set of guidelines for the design and optimization of novel derivatives with greater activity towards HDAC1.

Author Contributions: Conceptualization, H.S. and S.B.; methodology, H.S., G.C. (Giulia Chemi) and S.B.; software, H.S., G.C. (Giulia Chemi) and S.B.; validation, H.S., G.C. (Giulia Chemi) and S.B.; formal analysis, H.S., G.C. (Giulia Chemi), G.C. (Giuseppe Campiani), V.C. and S.B.; investigation, H.S., G.C. (Giulia Chemi); data curation, H.S., G.C. (Giulia Chemi), G.C. (Giuseppe Campiani), V.C. and S.B.; writing—original draft preparation, H.S. and S.B.; writing—review and editing, H.S., G.C. (Giulia Chemi), S.B., G.C. (Giuseppe Campiani), V.C.; supervision, S.B. All authors have read and agreed to the published version of the manuscript.

Acknowledgments: The authors thank Lorenzo Chemi for the technical assistance during the calculation of Q^2_{F3}.

References

1. Conway, S.J.; Woster, P.M.; Greenlee, W.J.; Georg, G.; Wang, S. Epigenetics: Novel Therapeutics Targeting Epigenetics. *J. Med. Chem.* **2016**, *59*, 1247–1248. [CrossRef]
2. Yoo, C.B.; Jones, P.A. Epigenetic therapy of cancer: Past, present and future. *Nat. Rev. Drug Discov.* **2006**, *5*, 37–50. [CrossRef]
3. Bertrand, P. Inside HDAC with HDAC inhibitors. *Eur. J. Med. Chem.* **2010**, *45*, 2095–2116. [CrossRef]
4. Falkenberg, K.J.; Johnstone, R.W. Histone deacetylases and their inhibitors in cancer, neurological diseases and immune disorders. *Nat. Rev. Drug Discov.* **2014**, *13*, 673–691. [CrossRef]
5. Paris, M.; Porcelloni, M.; Binaschi, M.; Fattori, D. Histone deacetylase inhibitors: From bench to clinic. *J. Med. Chem* **2008**, *51*, 1505–1529. [CrossRef]
6. de Ruijter, A.J.; van Gennip, A.H.; Caron, H.N.; Kemp, S.; van Kuilenburg, A.B. Histone deacetylases (HDACs): Characterization of the classical HDAC family. *Biochem. J.* **2003**, *370*, 737–749. [CrossRef]
7. Kouzarides, T. Chromatin modifications and their function. *Cell* **2007**, *128*, 693–705. [CrossRef]
8. Rodriquez, M.; Aquino, M.; Bruno, I.; De Martino, G.; Taddei, M.; Gomez-Paloma, L. Chemistry and biology of chromatin remodeling agents: State of art and future perspectives of HDAC inhibitors. *Curr. Med. Chem.* **2006**, *13*, 1119–1139. [CrossRef]

9. Bolden, J.E.; Peart, M.J.; Johnstone, R.W. Anticancer activities of histone deacetylase inhibitors. *Nat. Rev. Drug Discov.* **2006**, *5*, 769–784. [CrossRef]
10. Marks, P.A.; Dokmanovic, M. Histone deacetylase inhibitors: Discovery and development as anticancer agents. *Expert Opin. Investig. Drugs* **2005**, *14*, 1497–1511. [CrossRef]
11. Minucci, S.; Pelicci, P.G. Histone deacetylase inhibitors and the promise of epigenetic (and more) treatments for cancer. *Nat. Rev. Cancer* **2006**, *6*, 38–51. [CrossRef]
12. Brittain, D.; Weinmann, H.; Ottow, E. Recent Advances in the Medicinal Chemistry of Histone Deacetylase Inhibitors. *Annu. Rep. Med. Chem.* **2007**, *42*, 337–348. [CrossRef]
13. Miller, T.A. Patent status of histone deacetylase inhibitors. *Expert Opin. Ther. Pat.* **2005**, *14*, 791–804. [CrossRef]
14. Gregoretti, I.; Lee, Y.-M.; Goodson, H.V. Molecular Evolution of the Histone Deacetylase Family: Functional Implications of Phylogenetic Analysis. *J. Mol. Biol.* **2004**, *338*, 17–31. [CrossRef]
15. Duvic, M.; Talpur, R.; Ni, X.; Zhang, C.; Hazarika, P.; Kelly, C.; Chiao, J.H.; Reilly, J.F.; Ricker, J.L.; Richon, V.M.; et al. Phase 2 trial of oral vorinostat (suberoylanilide hydroxamic acid, SAHA) for refractory cutaneous T-cell lymphoma (CTCL). *Blood* **2006**, *109*, 31–39. [CrossRef]
16. Lee, H.Z.; Kwitkowski, V.E.; Del Valle, P.L.; Ricci, M.S.; Saber, H.; Habtemariam, B.A.; Bullock, J.; Bloomquist, E.; Li Shen, Y.; Chen, X.H.; et al. FDA Approval: Belinostat for the Treatment of Patients with Relapsed or Refractory Peripheral T-cell Lymphoma. *Clin. Cancer Res.* **2015**, *21*, 2666–2670. [CrossRef]
17. Garnock-Jones, K.P. Panobinostat: First Global Approval. *Drugs* **2015**, *75*, 695–704. [CrossRef]
18. VanderMolen, K.M.; McCulloch, W.; Pearce, C.J.; Oberlies, N.H. Romidepsin (Istodax, NSC 630176, FR901228, FK228, depsipeptide): A natural product recently approved for cutaneous T-cell lymphoma. *J. Antibiot.* **2011**, *64*, 525–531. [CrossRef]
19. Qiao, Z.; Ren, S.; Li, W.; Wang, X.; He, M.; Guo, Y.; Sun, L.; He, Y.; Ge, Y.; Yu, Q. Chidamide, a novel histone deacetylase inhibitor, synergistically enhances gemcitabine cytotoxicity in pancreatic cancer cells. *Biochem. Biophys. Res. Commun.* **2013**, *434*, 95–101. [CrossRef]
20. Garcia-Manero, G.; Assouline, S.; Cortes, J.; Estrov, Z.; Kantarjian, H.; Yang, H.; Newsome, W.M.; Miller, W.H.; Rousseau, C.; Kalita, A.; et al. Phase 1 study of the oral isotype specific histone deacetylase inhibitor MGCD0103 in leukemia. *Blood* **2008**, *112*, 981–989. [CrossRef]
21. Knipstein, J.; Gore, L. Entinostat for treatment of solid tumors and hematologic malignancies. *Expert Opin. Investig. Drugs* **2011**, *20*, 1455–1467. [CrossRef]
22. Gediya, L.K.; Belosay, A.; Khandelwal, A.; Purushottamachar, P.; Njar, V.C.O. Improved synthesis of histone deacetylase inhibitors (HDIs) (MS-275 and CI-994) and inhibitory effects of HDIs alone or in combination with RAMBAs or retinoids on growth of human LNCaP prostate cancer cells and tumor xenografts. *Bioorg. Med. Chem.* **2008**, *16*, 3352–3360. [CrossRef] [PubMed]
23. Finazzi, G.; Vannucchi, A.M.; Martinelli, V.; Ruggeri, M.; Nobile, F.; Specchia, G.; Pogliani, E.M.; Olimpieri, O.M.; Fioritoni, G.; Musolino, C.; et al. A phase II study of Givinostat in combination with hydroxycarbamide in patients with polycythaemia vera unresponsive to hydroxycarbamide monotherapy. *Br. J. Haematol.* **2013**, *161*, 688–694. [CrossRef] [PubMed]
24. Evens, A.M.; Balasubramanian, S.; Vose, J.M.; Harb, W.; Gordon, L.I.; Langdon, R.; Sprague, J.; Sirisawad, M.; Mani, C.; Yue, J.; et al. A Phase I/II Multicenter, Open-Label Study of the Oral Histone Deacetylase Inhibitor Abexinostat in Relapsed/Refractory Lymphoma. *Clin. Cancer Res.* **2015**, *22*, 1059–1066. [CrossRef]
25. Bruserud, O.; Stapnes, C.; Ersvær, E.; Gjertsen, B.; Ryningen, A. Histone Deacetylase Inhibitors in Cancer Treatment: A Review of the Clinical Toxicity and the Modulation of Gene Expression in Cancer Cells. *Curr. Pharm. Biotechnol.* **2007**, *8*, 388–400. [CrossRef]
26. Subramanian, S.; Bates, S.E.; Wright, J.J.; Espinoza-Delgado, I.; Piekarz, R.L. Clinical Toxicities of Histone Deacetylase Inhibitors. *Pharmaceuticals* **2010**, *3*, 2751–2767. [CrossRef]
27. Karagiannis, T.C.; El-Osta, A. Will broad-spectrum histone deacetylase inhibitors be superseded by more specific compounds? *Leukemia* **2006**, *21*, 61–65. [CrossRef]
28. Roche, J.; Bertrand, P. Inside HDACs with more selective HDAC inhibitors. *Eur. J. Med. Chem.* **2016**, *121*, 451–483. [CrossRef]
29. Brindisi, M.; Saraswati, A.P.; Brogi, S.; Gemma, S.; Butini, S.; Campiani, G. Old but Gold: Tracking the New Guise of Histone Deacetylase 6 (HDAC6) Enzyme as a Biomarker and Therapeutic Target in Rare Diseases. *J. Med. Chem.* **2020**, *63*, 23–39. [CrossRef]

30. Bieliauskas, A.V.; Pflum, M.K.H. Isoform-selective histone deacetylase inhibitors. *Chem. Soc. Rev.* **2008**, *37*, 1402. [CrossRef]
31. Guha, M. HDAC inhibitors still need a home run, despite recent approval. *Nat. Rev. Drug Discov.* **2015**, *14*, 225–226. [CrossRef] [PubMed]
32. Ononye, S.N.; van Heyst, M.; Falcone, E.M.; Anderson, A.C.; Wright, D.L. Toward isozyme-selective inhibitors of histone deacetylase as therapeutic agents for the treatment of cancer. *Pharm. Pat. Anal.* **2012**, *1*, 207–221. [CrossRef] [PubMed]
33. Zhang, L.; Han, Y.; Jiang, Q.; Wang, C.; Chen, X.; Li, X.; Xu, F.; Jiang, Y.; Wang, Q.; Xu, W. Trend of Histone Deacetylase Inhibitors in Cancer Therapy: Isoform Selectivity or Multitargeted Strategy. *Med. Res. Rev.* **2015**, *35*, 63–84. [CrossRef] [PubMed]
34. Glaser, K.B.; Li, J.; Staver, M.J.; Wei, R.-Q.; Albert, D.H.; Davidsen, S.K. Role of Class I and Class II histone deacetylases in carcinoma cells using siRNA. *Biochem. Biophys. Res. Commun.* **2003**, *310*, 529–536. [CrossRef]
35. Hu, E.; Dul, E.; Sung, C.-M.; Chen, Z.; Kirkpatrick, R.; Zhang, G.-F.; Johanson, K.; Liu, R.; Lago, A.; Hofmann, G.; et al. Identification of Novel Isoform-Selective Inhibitors within Class I Histone Deacetylases. *J. Pharmacol. Exp. Ther.* **2003**, *307*, 720–728. [CrossRef]
36. Kawai, H.; Li, H.; Avraham, S.; Jiang, S.; Avraham, H.K. Overexpression of histone deacetylase HDAC1 modulates breast cancer progression by negative regulation of estrogen receptor? *Int. J. Cancer* **2003**, *107*, 353–358. [CrossRef]
37. Rikimaru, T.; Taketomi, A.; Yamashita, Y.-I.; Shirabe, K.; Hamatsu, T.; Shimada, M.; Maehara, Y. Clinical Significance of Histone Deacetylase 1 Expression in Patients with Hepatocellular Carcinoma. *Oncology* **2007**, *72*, 69–74. [CrossRef]
38. Senese, S.; Zaragoza, K.; Minardi, S.; Muradore, I.; Ronzoni, S.; Passafaro, A.; Bernard, L.; Draetta, G.F.; Alcalay, M.; Seiser, C.; et al. Role for Histone Deacetylase 1 in Human Tumor Cell Proliferation. *Mol. Cell Biol.* **2007**, *27*, 4784–4795. [CrossRef]
39. Khan, N.; Jeffers, M.; Kumar, S.; Hackett, C.; Boldog, F.; Khramtsov, N.; Qian, X.; Mills, E.; Berghs, S.C.; Carey, N.; et al. Determination of the class and isoform selectivity of small-molecule histone deacetylase inhibitors. *Biochem. J.* **2007**, *409*, 581–589. [CrossRef]
40. Shen, S.; Kozikowski, A.P. Why Hydroxamates May Not Be the Best Histone Deacetylase Inhibitors-What Some May Have Forgotten or Would Rather Forget? *ChemMedChem* **2016**, *11*, 15–21. [CrossRef]
41. Beckers, T.; Burkhardt, C.; Wieland, H.; Gimmnich, P.; Ciossek, T.; Maier, T.; Sanders, K. Distinct pharmacological properties of second generation HDAC inhibitors with the benzamide or hydroxamate head group. *Int. J. Cancer* **2007**, *121*, 1138–1148. [CrossRef] [PubMed]
42. Bonfils, C.; Kalita, A.; Dubay, M.; Siu, L.L.; Carducci, M.A.; Reid, G.; Martell, R.E.; Besterman, J.M.; Li, Z. Evaluation of the Pharmacodynamic Effects of MGCD0103 from Preclinical Models to Human Using a Novel HDAC Enzyme Assay. *Clin. Cancer Res.* **2008**, *14*, 3441–3449. [CrossRef] [PubMed]
43. Chou, C.J.; Herman, D.; Gottesfeld, J.M. Pimelic Diphenylamide 106 Is a Slow, Tight-binding Inhibitor of Class I Histone Deacetylases. *J. Biol. Chem.* **2008**, *283*, 35402–35409. [CrossRef] [PubMed]
44. Kelly, W.K.; Richon, V.M.; O'Connor, O.; Curley, T.; MacGregor-Curtelli, B.; Tong, W.; Klang, M.; Schwartz, L.; Richardson, S.; Rosa, E.; et al. Phase I clinical trial of histone deacetylase inhibitor: Suberoylanilide hydroxamic acid administered intravenously. *Clin. Cancer Res.* **2003**, *9*, 3578–3588.
45. Nagaoka, Y.; Maeda, T.; Kawai, Y.; Nakashima, D.; Oikawa, T.; Shimoke, K.; Ikeuchi, T.; Kuwajima, H.; Uesato, S. Synthesis and cancer antiproliferative activity of new histone deacetylase inhibitors: Hydrophilic hydroxamates and 2-aminobenzamide-containing derivatives. *Eur. J. Med. Chem.* **2006**, *41*, 697–708. [CrossRef]
46. Moradei, O.M.; Mallais, T.C.; Frechette, S.; Paquin, I.; Tessier, P.E.; Leit, S.M.; Fournel, M.; Bonfils, C.; Trachy-Bourget, M.-C.; Liu, J.; et al. Novel Aminophenyl Benzamide-Type Histone Deacetylase Inhibitors with Enhanced Potency and Selectivity. *J. Med. Chem.* **2007**, *50*, 5543–5546. [CrossRef]
47. Suzuki, T.; Miyata, N. Non-hydroxamate Histone Deacetylase Inhibitors. *Curr. Med. Chem.* **2005**, *12*, 2867–2880. [CrossRef]
48. Wang, D.-F.; Helquist, P.; Wiech, N.L.; Wiest, O. Toward Selective Histone Deacetylase Inhibitor Design: Homology Modeling, Docking Studies, and Molecular Dynamics Simulations of Human Class I Histone Deacetylases. *J. Med. Chem.* **2005**, *48*, 6936–6947. [CrossRef]

49. Chemi, G.; Brogi, S. Breakthroughs in Computational Approaches for Drug Discovery. *J. Drug Res. Dev.* **2017**, *3*. [CrossRef]
50. Verma, J.; Khedkar, V.; Coutinho, E. 3D-QSAR in Drug Design—A Review. *Curr. Top. Med. Chem.* **2010**, *10*, 95–115. [CrossRef]
51. Yang, S.-Y. Pharmacophore modeling and applications in drug discovery: Challenges and recent advances. *Drug Discov. Today* **2010**, *15*, 444–450. [CrossRef]
52. Cherkasov, A.; Muratov, E.N.; Fourches, D.; Varnek, A.; Baskin, I.I.; Cronin, M.; Dearden, J.; Gramatica, P.; Martin, Y.C.; Todeschini, R.; et al. QSAR Modeling: Where Have You Been? Where Are You Going To? *J. Med. Chem.* **2014**, *57*, 4977–5010. [CrossRef] [PubMed]
53. Brogi, S.; Corelli, F.; Di Marzo, V.; Ligresti, A.; Mugnaini, C.; Pasquini, S.; Tafi, A. Three-dimensional quantitative structure–selectivity relationships analysis guided rational design of a highly selective ligand for the cannabinoid receptor 2. *Eur. J. Med. Chem.* **2011**, *46*, 547–555. [CrossRef] [PubMed]
54. Brogi, S.; Papazafiri, P.; Roussis, V.; Tafi, A. 3D-QSAR using pharmacophore-based alignment and virtual screening for discovery of novel MCF-7 cell line inhibitors. *Eur. J. Med. Chem.* **2013**, *67*, 344–351. [CrossRef] [PubMed]
55. Zaccagnini, L.; Brogi, S.; Brindisi, M.; Gemma, S.; Chemi, G.; Legname, G.; Campiani, G.; Butini, S. Identification of novel fluorescent probes preventing PrP Sc replication in prion diseases. *Eur. J. Med. Chem.* **2017**, *127*, 859–873. [CrossRef] [PubMed]
56. Brogi, S.; Brindisi, M.; Joshi, B.P.; Sanna Coccone, S.; Parapini, S.; Basilico, N.; Novellino, E.; Campiani, G.; Gemma, S.; Butini, S. Exploring clotrimazole-based pharmacophore: 3D-QSAR studies and synthesis of novel antiplasmodial agents. *Bioorg. Med. Chem. Lett.* **2015**, *25*, 5412–5418. [CrossRef] [PubMed]
57. Chemi, G.; Gemma, S.; Campiani, G.; Brogi, S.; Butini, S.; Brindisi, M. Computational Tool for Fast in silico Evaluation of hERG K+ Channel Affinity. *Front. Chem.* **2017**, *5*. [CrossRef]
58. Liu, B.; Lu, A.J.; Liao, C.Z.; Liu, H.B.; Zhou, J.J. 3D-QSAR of Sulfonamide Hydroxamic Acid HDAC Inhibitors. *Acta Phys. Chim. Sin.* **2005**, *21*, 333–337. [CrossRef]
59. Guo, Y.; Xiao, J.; Guo, Z.; Chu, F.; Cheng, Y.; Wu, S. Exploration of a binding mode of indole amide analogues as potent histone deacetylase inhibitors and 3D-QSAR analyses. *Bioorg. Med. Chem.* **2005**, *13*, 5424–5434. [CrossRef]
60. Juvale, D.C.; Kulkarni, V.V.; Deokar, H.S.; Wagh, N.K.; Padhye, S.B.; Kulkarni, V.M. 3D-QSAR of histone deacetylase inhibitors: Hydroxamate analogues. *Org. Biomol. Chem.* **2006**, *4*, 2858. [CrossRef]
61. Ragno, R.; Simeoni, S.; Valente, S.; Massa, S.; Mai, A. 3-D QSAR Studies on Histone Deacetylase Inhibitors. A GOLPE/GRID Approach on Different Series of Compounds. *J. Chem. Inf. Model.* **2006**, *46*, 1420–1430. [CrossRef] [PubMed]
62. Chen, Y.; Li, H.; Tang, W.; Zhu, C.; Jiang, Y.; Zou, J.; Yu, Q.; You, Q. 3D-QSAR studies of HDACs inhibitors using pharmacophore-based alignment. *Eur. J. Med. Chem.* **2009**, *44*, 2868–2876. [CrossRef] [PubMed]
63. Wang, D.-F.; Wiest, O.; Helquist, P.; Lan-Hargest, H.-Y.; Wiech, N.L. QSAR Studies of PC-3 cell line inhibition activity of TSA and SAHA-like hydroxamic acids. *Bioorg. Med. Chem. Lett.* **2004**, *14*, 707–711. [CrossRef] [PubMed]
64. Xie, A.; Liao, C.; Li, Z.; Ning, Z.; Hu, W.; Lu, X.; Shi, L.; Zhou, J. Quantitative Structure-Activity Relationship Study of Histone Deacetylase Inhibitors. *Anti-Cancer Agents Med. Chem.* **2004**, *4*, 273–299. [CrossRef] [PubMed]
65. Dixon, S.L.; Smondyrev, A.M.; Knoll, E.H.; Rao, S.N.; Shaw, D.E.; Friesner, R.A. PHASE: A new engine for pharmacophore perception, 3D QSAR model development, and 3D database screening: 1. Methodology and preliminary results. *J. Comput. Aided Mol. Des.* **2006**, *20*, 647–671. [CrossRef] [PubMed]
66. Abdizadeh, T.; Kalani, M.R.; Abnous, K.; Tayarani-Najaran, Z.; Khashyarmanesh, B.Z.; Abdizadeh, R.; Ghodsi, R.; Hadizadeh, F. Design, synthesis and biological evaluation of novel coumarin-based benzamides as potent histone deacetylase inhibitors and anticancer agents. *Eur. J. Med. Chem.* **2017**, *132*, 42–62. [CrossRef]
67. Hamblett, C.L.; Methot, J.L.; Mampreian, D.M.; Sloman, D.L.; Stanton, M.G.; Kral, A.M.; Fleming, J.C.; Cruz, J.C.; Chenard, M.; Ozerova, N.; et al. The discovery of 6-amino nicotinamides as potent and selective histone deacetylase inhibitors. *Bioorg. Med. Chem. Lett.* **2007**, *17*, 5300–5309. [CrossRef]
68. Sixto-López, Y.; Bello, M.; Correa-Basurto, J. Insights into structural features of HDAC1 and its selectivity inhibition elucidated by Molecular dynamic simulation and Molecular Docking. *J. Biomol. Struct. Dyn.* **2018**, *37*, 584–610. [CrossRef]

69. Brindisi, M.; Cavella, C.; Brogi, S.; Nebbioso, A.; Senger, J.; Maramai, S.; Ciotta, A.; Iside, C.; Butini, S.; Lamponi, S.; et al. Phenylpyrrole-based HDAC inhibitors: Synthesis, molecular modeling and biological studies. *Future Med. Chem.* **2016**, *8*, 1573–1587. [CrossRef]
70. Brindisi, M.; Senger, J.; Cavella, C.; Grillo, A.; Chemi, G.; Gemma, S.; Cucinella, D.M.; Lamponi, S.; Sarno, F.; Iside, C.; et al. Novel spiroindoline HDAC inhibitors: Synthesis, molecular modelling and biological studies. *Eur. J. Med. Chem.* **2018**, *157*, 127–138. [CrossRef]
71. Braga, R.C.; Andrade, C.H. Assessing the Performance of 3D Pharmacophore Models in Virtual Screening: How Good are They? *Curr. Top. Med. Chem.* **2013**, *13*, 1127–1138. [CrossRef] [PubMed]
72. Dror, O.; Schneidman-Duhovny, D.; Inbar, Y.; Nussinov, R.; Wolfson, H.J. Novel Approach for Efficient Pharmacophore-Based Virtual Screening: Method and Applications. *J. Chem. Inf. Model.* **2009**, *49*, 2333–2343. [CrossRef] [PubMed]
73. Krishna, S.; Singh, D.K.; Meena, S.; Datta, D.; Siddiqi, M.I.; Banerjee, D. Pharmacophore-Based Screening and Identification of Novel Human Ligase I Inhibitors with Potential Anticancer Activity. *J. Chem. Inf. Model.* **2014**, *54*, 781–792. [CrossRef] [PubMed]
74. Sakkiah, S.; Thangapandian, S.; John, S.; Lee, K.W. Pharmacophore based virtual screening, molecular docking studies to design potent heat shock protein 90 inhibitors. *Eur. J. Med. Chem.* **2011**, *46*, 2937–2947. [CrossRef]
75. Thangapandian, S.; John, S.; Sakkiah, S.; Lee, K.W. Pharmacophore-based virtual screening and Bayesian model for the identification of potential human leukotriene A4 hydrolase inhibitors. *Eur. J. Med. Chem.* **2011**, *46*, 1593–1603. [CrossRef] [PubMed]
76. Triballeau, N.; Acher, F.; Brabet, I.; Pin, J.-P.; Bertrand, H.-O. Virtual Screening Workflow Development Guided by the "Receiver Operating Characteristic" Curve Approach. Application to High-Throughput Docking on Metabotropic Glutamate Receptor Subtype 4. *J. Med. Chem.* **2005**, *48*, 2534–2547. [CrossRef]
77. Zhao, W.; Hevener, K.E.; White, S.W.; Lee, R.E.; Boyett, J.M. A statistical framework to evaluate virtual screening. *BMC Bioinform.* **2009**, *10*. [CrossRef]
78. *Maestro*; Version 10.1; Schrödinger, LLC: New York, NY, USA, 2015.
79. Andrews, D.M.; Gibson, K.M.; Graham, M.A.; Matusiak, Z.S.; Roberts, C.A.; Stokes, E.S.; Brady, M.C.; Chresta, C.M. Design and campaign synthesis of pyridine-based histone deacetylase inhibitors. *Bioorg. Med. Chem. Lett.* **2008**, *18*, 2525–2529. [CrossRef]
80. Methot, J.L.; Chakravarty, P.K.; Chenard, M.; Close, J.; Cruz, J.C.; Dahlberg, W.K.; Fleming, J.; Hamblett, C.L.; Hamill, J.E.; Harrington, P.; et al. Exploration of the internal cavity of histone deacetylase (HDAC) with selective HDAC1/HDAC2 inhibitors (SHI-1:2). *Bioorg. Med. Chem. Lett.* **2008**, *18*, 973–978. [CrossRef]
81. Kattar, S.D.; Surdi, L.M.; Zabierek, A.; Methot, J.L.; Middleton, R.E.; Hughes, B.; Szewczak, A.A.; Dahlberg, W.K.; Kral, A.M.; Ozerova, N.; et al. Parallel medicinal chemistry approaches to selective HDAC1/HDAC2 inhibitor (SHI-1:2) optimization. *Bioorg. Med. Chem. Lett.* **2009**, *19*, 1168–1172. [CrossRef]
82. Methot, J.L.; Hamblett, C.L.; Mampreian, D.M.; Jung, J.; Harsch, A.; Szewczak, A.A.; Dahlberg, W.K.; Middleton, R.E.; Hughes, B.; Fleming, J.C.; et al. SAR profiles of spirocyclic nicotinamide derived selective HDAC1/HDAC2 inhibitors (SHI-1:2). *Bioorg. Med. Chem. Lett.* **2008**, *18*, 6104–6109. [CrossRef]
83. Li, Y.; Wang, Y.; Xie, N.; Xu, M.; Qian, P.; Zhao, Y.; Li, S. Design, synthesis and antiproliferative activities of novel benzamides derivatives as HDAC inhibitors. *Eur. J. Med. Chem.* **2015**, *100*, 270–276. [CrossRef] [PubMed]
84. Li, Y.; Zhou, Y.; Qian, P.; Wang, Y.; Jiang, F.; Yao, Z.; Hu, W.; Zhao, Y.; Li, S. Design, synthesis and bioevalution of novel benzamides derivatives as HDAC inhibitors. *Bioorg. Med. Chem. Lett.* **2013**, *23*, 179–182. [CrossRef] [PubMed]
85. Siliphaivanh, P.; Harrington, P.; Witter, D.J.; Otte, K.; Tempest, P.; Kattar, S.; Kral, A.M.; Fleming, J.C.; Deshmukh, S.V.; Harsch, A.; et al. Design of novel histone deacetylase inhibitors. *Bioorg. Med. Chem. Lett.* **2007**, *17*, 4619–4624. [CrossRef] [PubMed]
86. Andrews, D.M.; Stokes, E.S.; Carr, G.R.; Matusiak, Z.S.; Roberts, C.A.; Waring, M.J.; Brady, M.C.; Chresta, C.M.; East, S.J. Design and campaign synthesis of piperidine- and thiazole-based histone deacetylase inhibitors. *Bioorg. Med. Chem. Lett.* **2008**, *18*, 2580–2584. [CrossRef]

87. Hirata, Y.; Hirata, M.; Kawaratani, Y.; Shibano, M.; Taniguchi, M.; Yasuda, M.; Ohmomo, Y.; Nagaoka, Y.; Baba, K.; Uesato, S. Anti-tumor activity of new orally bioavailable 2-amino-5-(thiophen-2-yl)benzamide-series histone deacetylase inhibitors, possessing an aqueous soluble functional group as a surface recognition domain. *Bioorg. Med. Chem. Lett.* **2012**, *22*, 1926–1930. [CrossRef]
88. Kiyokawa, S.; Hirata, Y.; Nagaoka, Y.; Shibano, M.; Taniguchi, M.; Yasuda, M.; Baba, K.; Uesato, S. New orally bioavailable 2-aminobenzamide-type histone deacetylase inhibitor possessing a (2-hydroxyethyl)(4-(thiophen-2-yl)benzyl)amino group. *Bioorg. Med. Chem.* **2010**, *18*, 3925–3933. [CrossRef]
89. Mahboobi, S.; Dove, S.; Sellmer, A.; Winkler, M.; Eichhorn, E.; Pongratz, H.; Ciossek, T.; Baer, T.; Maier, T.; Beckers, T. Design of chimeric histone deacetylase- and tyrosine kinase-inhibitors: A series of imatinib hybrides as potent inhibitors of wild-type and mutant BCR-ABL, PDGF-Rbeta, and histone deacetylases. *J. Med. Chem.* **2009**, *52*, 2265–2279. [CrossRef]
90. Rajak, H.; Kumar, P.; Parmar, P.; Thakur, B.S.; Veerasamy, R.; Sharma, P.C.; Sharma, A.K.; Gupta, A.K.; Dangi, J.S. Appraisal of GABA and PABA as linker: Design and synthesis of novel benzamide based histone deacetylase inhibitors. *Eur. J. Med. Chem.* **2012**, *53*, 390–397. [CrossRef]
91. Valente, S.; Trisciuoglio, D.; De Luca, T.; Nebbioso, A.; Labella, D.; Lenoci, A.; Bigogno, C.; Dondio, G.; Miceli, M.; Brosch, G.; et al. 1,3,4-Oxadiazole-containing histone deacetylase inhibitors: Anticancer activities in cancer cells. *J. Med. Chem.* **2014**, *57*, 6259–6265. [CrossRef]
92. Rusche, J.R.; Peet, N.P.; Hopper, A.T. Compositions Including 6-Aminohexanoic Acid Derivatives as HDAC Inhibitors. U.S. Patent 9,265,734, 23 February 2016.
93. Liu, T.; Lin, Y.; Wen, X.; Jorissen, R.N.; Gilson, M.K. BindingDB: A web-accessible database of experimentally determined protein-ligand binding affinities. *Nucleic Acids Res.* **2007**, *35*, D198–D201. [CrossRef] [PubMed]
94. *LigPrep*; Version 3.3; Schrödinger, LLC: New York, NY, USA, 2015.
95. Sirous, H.; Chemi, G.; Campiani, G.; Brogi, S. An integrated in silico screening strategy for identifying promising disruptors of p53-MDM2 interaction. *Comput. Biol. Chem.* **2019**, *83*, 107105. [CrossRef] [PubMed]
96. Sirous, H.; Chemi, G.; Gemma, S.; Butini, S.; Debyser, Z.; Christ, F.; Saghaie, L.; Brogi, S.; Fassihi, A.; Campiani, G.; et al. Identification of Novel 3-Hydroxy-pyran-4-One Derivatives as Potent HIV-1 Integrase Inhibitors Using in silico Structure-Based Combinatorial Library Design Approach. *Front. Chem.* **2019**, *7*, 574. [CrossRef] [PubMed]
97. Sirous, H.; Fassihi, A.; Brogi, S.; Campiani, G.; Christ, F.; Debyser, Z.; Gemma, S.; Butini, S.; Chemi, G.; Grillo, A.; et al. Synthesis, Molecular Modelling and Biological Studies of 3-hydroxypyrane- 4-one and 3-hydroxy-pyridine-4-one Derivatives as HIV-1 Integrase Inhibitors. *Med. Chem.* **2019**, *15*, 755–770. [CrossRef] [PubMed]
98. Jorgensen, W.L.; Maxwell, D.S.; Tirado-Rives, J. Development and Testing of the OPLS All-Atom Force Field on Conformational Energetics and Properties of Organic Liquids. *J. Am. Chem. Soc.* **1996**, *118*, 11225–11236. [CrossRef]
99. *MacroModel*; Version 10.7; Schrödinger, LLC: New York, NY, USA, 2015.
100. Still, W.C.; Tempczyk, A.; Hawley, R.C.; Hendrickson, T. Semianalytical treatment of solvation for molecular mechanics and dynamics. *J. Am. Chem. Soc.* **1990**, *112*, 6127–6129. [CrossRef]
101. *Phase*; Version 4.2; Schrödinger, LLC: New York, NY, USA, 2015.
102. Todeschini, R.; Ballabio, D.; Grisoni, F. Beware of Unreliable Q2! A Comparative Study of Regression Metrics for Predictivity Assessment of QSAR Models. *J. Chem. Inf. Model.* **2016**, *56*, 1905–1913. [CrossRef]
103. Frechette, S.; Leit, S.; Woo, S.H.; Lapointe, G.; Jeannotte, G.; Moradei, O.; Paquin, I.; Bouchain, G.; Raeppel, S.; Gaudette, F.; et al. 4-(Heteroarylaminomethyl)-N-(2-aminophenyl)-benzamides and their analogs as a novel class of histone deacetylase inhibitors. *Bioorg. Med. Chem. Lett* **2008**, *18*, 1502–1506. [CrossRef]
104. Marson, C.M.; Matthews, C.J.; Atkinson, S.J.; Lamadema, N.; Thomas, N.S. Potent and Selective Inhibitors of Histone Deacetylase-3 Containing Chiral Oxazoline Capping Groups and a N-(2-Aminophenyl)-benzamide Binding Unit. *J. Med. Chem.* **2015**, *58*, 6803–6818. [CrossRef]
105. Zhu, Y.; Chen, X.; Ran, T.; Niu, J.; Zhao, S.; Lu, T.; Tang, W. Design, synthesis and biological evaluation of urea-based benzamides derivatives as HDAC inhibitors. *Med. Chem. Res.* **2017**, *26*, 2879–2888. [CrossRef]
106. Harrington, P.; Kattar, S.; Miller, T.A.; Stanton, M.G.; Tempest, P.; Witter, D.J. 4-Carboxybenzylamino Derivatives as Histone Deacetylase Inhibitors. U.S. Patent 8,389,553, 5 March 2013.

107. Kirchmair, J.; Markt, P.; Distinto, S.; Wolber, G.; Langer, T. Evaluation of the performance of 3D virtual screening protocols: RMSD comparisons, enrichment assessments, and decoy selection—What can we learn from earlier mistakes? *J. Comput. Aided Mol. Des.* **2008**, *22*, 213–228. [CrossRef] [PubMed]
108. Mysinger, M.M.; Carchia, M.; Irwin, J.J.; Shoichet, B.K. Directory of Useful Decoys, Enhanced (DUD-E): Better Ligands and Decoys for Better Benchmarking. *J. Med. Chem.* **2012**, *55*, 6582–6594. [CrossRef] [PubMed]

6

Brassicasterol with Dual Anti-Infective Properties against HSV-1 and *Mycobacterium tuberculosis* and Cardiovascular Protective Effect

Sherif T. S. Hassan

Department of Applied Ecology, Faculty of Environmental Sciences, Czech University of Life Sciences Prague, Kamýcká 129, 6-Suchdol, 16521 Prague, Czech Republic; sherif.hassan@seznam.cz

Abstract: While few studies have revealed the biological properties of brassicasterol, a phytosterol, against some biological and molecular targets, it is believed that there are still many activities yet to be studied. In this work, brassicasterol exerts a therapeutic utility in an in vitro setting against herpes simplex virus type 1 (HSV-1) and *Mycobacterium tuberculosis* (Mtb) as well as a considerable inhibitory property against human angiotensin-converting enzyme (ACE) that plays a dynamic role in regulating blood pressure. The antireplicative effect of brassicasterol against HSV-1 is remarkably detected (50% inhibitory concentration (IC_{50}): 1.2 μM; selectivity index (SI): 41.7), while the potency of its effect is ameliorated through the combination with standard acyclovir with proper SI (IC_{50}: 0.7 μM; SI: 71.4). Moreover, the capacity of this compound to induce an adequate level of antituberculosis activity against all Mtb strains examined (minimum inhibitory concentration values ranging from 1.9 to 2.4 μM) is revealed. The anti-ACE effect (12.3 μg/mL; 91.2% inhibition) is also ascertained. Molecular docking analyses propose that the mechanisms by which brassicasterol induces anti-HSV-1 and anti-Mtb might be related to inhibiting vital enzymes involved in HSV-1 replication and Mtb cell wall biosynthesis. In summary, the obtained results suggest that brassicasterol might be promising for future anti-HSV-1, antituberculosis, and anti-ACE drug design.

Keywords: brassicasterol; phytosterols; HSV; *Mycobacterium tuberculosis*; HSV-1 DNA polymerase; HSV-1 TK; human CDK2; ACE; UDP-galactopyranose mutase

---

1. Introduction

Herpesviruses are one of the major causes of human viral diseases with highly infectious properties. Herpes simplex virus type 1 (HSV-1) is a type of alpha-herpesviruses with double-stranded DNA placed in an icosahedral capsid and a lipidic envelope made by various glycoproteins [1,2]. This pathogen is known to be a thoroughly contagious infection, which is frequent and endemic globally. Most HSV-1 infections are acquired during childhood, and infection is lifelong. Infections with HSV-1 are typically oral herpes but HSV-1 can also be transmitted to the genitals and causes genital herpes [3–5]. Oral herpes infection is commonly asymptomatic, however, in immunocompromised patients with advanced HIV infection, HSV-1 could generate obvious and severe symptoms with regular recurrences [6]. In some cases, complications such as encephalitis or keratitis were observed to be associated with HSV-1 infection [7]. Antiviral drugs, such as acyclovir, famciclovir, and valacyclovir are the best effective medicines to decrease the severity and frequency of HSV symptoms. These medications act as inhibitors of viral replication with reported undesirable effects. With the extensive use of these drugs in therapy, the problem of drug resistance has been established, leading to treatment failure [1,8].

Tuberculosis (TB) is an infectious disease induced by the Gram-negative bacterium *Mycobacterium tuberculosis* (Mtb) that most often infects the lungs and can also affect the brain, kidneys, or spine [9]. Patients infected with HIV, people with a weak immune system, and people with undernutrition are more likely to acquire active TB infection than healthy people [10]. TB infection is typically symptomatic, where the most frequent symptoms of active lung TB are cough with sputum and blood, at times, and fever, chest pains, weight loss, and overall weakness [11]. Although TB is a treatable disease, the extensive and or inappropriate use of anti-TB medications led to developing multidrug-resistant tuberculosis (MDR-TB), where drugs such as isoniazid and rifampicin, the two most potent first-line anti-TB medicines failed to treat the disease [12,13]. In 2018, the World Health Organization declared that MDR-TB continues to be a public health crisis and a health security threat with an increased level of resistance to first-line drugs [14].

Angiotensin-converting enzyme (ACE) is a key enzyme in the regulation of the renin-angiotensin system, with the ability to cleave angiotensin-I to angiotensin-II and hydrolyze several peptides [15]. It is known that angiotensin-II mainly circulates in the blood and triggers the muscles surrounding blood vessels to contract, thus narrowing the vessels, leading to an increase in blood pressure (hypertension) [16]. Therefore, ACE inhibition is an essential therapeutic approach in controlling acute and chronic hypertension, treating left ventricular dysfunction and heart failure, preventing strokes, and preventing and treating kidney disease (nephropathy), especially with patients suffering from hypertension or diabetes [17,18].

Brassicasterol is a natural product that belongs to phytosterols (called plant sterol/stanol esters) and is biosynthesized by various unicellular algae and few terrestrial plants (Figure 1). This compound is a major sterol in rapeseed and canola oil and known to have nutritional value as a food additive [19]. Generally, cholesterol-lowering properties are the major beneficial effects of phytosterols on human health. However, the health benefits of phytosterols on humans have been a subject of debate for years [20]. Recently, a health claim on phytosterols has been clarified and verified by the U.S. Food and Drug Administration (FDA) with a statement: "Foods containing at least 0.65 g per serving of vegetable oil plant sterol esters, eaten twice a day with meals for a daily total intake of at least 1.3 g, as part of a diet low in saturated fat and cholesterol, may reduce the risk of heart disease." [21].

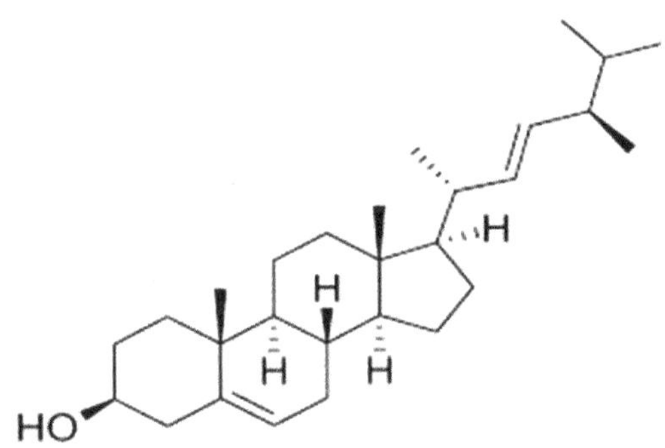

Figure 1. Chemical structure of brassicasterol.

So far, brassicasterol remains a little investigated phytosterol-type molecule with reported few biological activities [19,22,23]. Therefore, in this study, brassicasterol is examined using properly in vitro assay systems for its anti-infective properties against HSV-1 and Mtb along with its cardiovascular protective effect via inhibiting the activity of ACE. Additionally, molecular docking analyses are achieved to predict the mechanisms of action against the molecular targets as well as confirm the results obtained by the in vitro biological assay (for ACE). The investigated molecular targets for HSV-1 are HSV-1 DNA polymerase, HSV-1 thymidine kinase, and human cyclin-dependent kinase 2, while for Mtb it is UDP-galactopyranose mutase.

2. Materials and Methods

Compounds under investigation: Brassicasterol (purity ≥ 98%), standard acyclovir (ACV), and standard rifampicin (European Pharmacopoeia (EP) Reference Standard) were purchased from

Sigma-Aldrich, Berlin, Germany, while standard captopril (EP reference standard) was acquired from Sigma Aldrich, Prague, Czech Republic. The combination of brassicasterol with ACV was prepared as a form of combinatory treatment.

2.1. *Antiherpetic Activity*

2.1.1. Preparation of Vero Cells and the Virus

Vero cells (ATCC: CCL 81™; UK) and an ACV- susceptible strain of HSV-1 (KOS) were collected from Motol University Hospital (MUH; Prague, Czech Republic). Vero cells were prepared and grown following the previously reported protocol [2,6]. HSV-1 stocks were obtained after propagation of the virus in Vero cells. A plaque assay was further used to titrate the HSV-1 stocks on the basis of the plaque-forming unit (PFU) and the HSV-1 stocks were then kept at –80 °C, as previously specified [2,6].

2.1.2. Cell Viability Assay for Determination of Cytotoxicity

The viability of Vero cells was assessed by the neutral red dye-uptake assay, as previously detailed [8]. Briefly, the experiment was initiated by treating Vero cell monolayers grown in 96-well microtiter plates with two-fold serial dilutions of the test compounds (100 μM as a starting concentration) and then exposed to incubation for 48 h at 37 °C in 5% CO_2. After incubation, the treated cells were examined for the morphological changes by an inverted optical microscope (Leitz, Wetzlar, Germany) and the maximum non-toxic concentrations (MNTC) were ascertained. The 50% cytotoxic concentrations (CC_{50}; expressed in μM) of test compounds were calculated as the concentrations that decreased the cell viability by 50% when compared to the untreated control cells.

2.1.3. Plaque Reduction Assay for Determination of Antiherpetic Activity

To evaluate the antiviral activity against the replication of HSV-1, a plaque reduction assay was performed using ACV as a standard antiherpetic drug as earlier detailed [2,6]. The assay was initiated by infecting Vero cell monolayers with the virus (100 PFU) for 1 h at 37 °C. The infected cells were further overlapped with Eagle's minimum essential medium containing carboxymethyl cellulose (1.5%; Sigma-Aldrich, Berlin, Germany) and treated with test compounds at different concentrations. The untreated cells were considered as controls. To determine the plaque reduction, cells were incubated for 72 h at 37 °C and then dyed with naphthol blue-black (Sigma-Aldrich, Berlin, Germany). The concentrations of test molecules that diminished 50% of the number of HSV-1 plaques were assessed in comparison with the untreated control cells and expressed as 50% inhibitory concentration (IC_{50} in μM) values. The ratio CC_{50}/IC_{50} was assigned for each compound to calculate the selectivity index (SI).

2.2. *Antimycobacterial Assay*

2.2.1. Bacterial Strains, Identification protocols, and Culturing Procedures

The anti-Mtb activity was processed using an in vitro microdilution assay with ten Mtb strains (CI1–CI10; bacterial isolates acquired from MUH, Prague, Czech Republic), along with a reference strain (H37Rv; CNCTC My 331-88: ATCC 27294; Czech National Collection of Type Cultures (CNCTC), National Institute of Public Health, Prague, Czech Republic. For identification, all Mtb isolates were subjected to various microbiological, biochemical, and molecular protocols following the accredited guideline of Clinical and Laboratory Standards Institute (CLSI) [24]. All bacterial strains used in this study were identified as rifampicin-susceptible and were cultured and grown as previously described by CLSI guideline [25].

2.2.2. Drug Susceptibility Assay

Minimum inhibitory concentrations (MICs) of test substances (brassicasterol and rifampicin) against mycobacterial strains were investigated by employing a 96-well plate microdilution broth method under optimal assay conditions according to the specified procedure of the CLSI guideline with slight modification [25]. Briefly, the broth Middlebrook OADC (Oleic Albumin Dextrose Catalase) growth supplement was used as a supplement in 7H9 liquid medium to culture Mtb (Sigma-Aldrich, Berlin, Germany) at pH (6.6). Rifampicin was applied as a positive control, while Dimethyl sulfoxide (DMSO; 1%) and the broth were utilized as the negative controls. The test drugs were prepared in DMSO with broth (25 μL of DMSO solution in 4 mL of broth) and an aliquot of 100 μL was placed into microplate wells. An isotonic saline solution was used to suspend Mtb inocula with an adjusted density of 0.5–1.0 McFarland. Further, the suspensions (diluted by 10^{-1}) were employed to inoculate the testing wells with a mixture of suspension (100 μL) and the test drugs (100 μL). After five days of incubation, an aliquot of 30 μL of Alamar Blue solution containing a mixture (1:1) of an aqueous solution of resazurin sodium salt (0.1%) and Tween 80 (10%) was supplemented. Further, the results were finalized after 24 h of incubation and expressed as MIC values that hindered the blue to pink color change.

2.3. Anti-Angiotensin-Converting Enzyme (ACE) Assay

Brassicasterol and standard captopril were investigated for their anti-ACE properties. ACE inhibition activities of test compounds were determined by a spectrophotometric method based on the production of hippuric acid from hippuryl-L-histidyl-L-leucine (HHL; substrate) [15]. Concisely, the assay was performed by incubating the test substances at a fixed concentration of 12.3 μg/mL with 120 mU/mL of human ACE (Sigma-Aldrich, Prague, Czech Republic) prepared in Tris Buffer (50 mM, pH = 8.3) for 80 min at 37 °C. After incubation, ACE activity was initiated by adding 110 μL of HHL (10 mM; Sigma-Aldrich, Prague, Czech Republic) to the mixture. A spectrophotometer (UV–VIS; SPECTROstar^{Nano} BMG Labtech, Ortenberg, Germany) was utilized to detect the hippuric acid from the reaction at λ 228 nm and, subsequently, the degree of inhibition (%) was calculated.

2.4. In Silico Molecular Docking Analyses

The molecular docking studies were performed following the previously described protocol [26] and processed with a PyRx virtual screening tool merged with Autodock VINA software (version 0.8, The Scripps Research Institute, La Jolla, CA, USA). Discovery studio visualizer version v19.1.0.18287 (BIOVIA, San Diego, CA, USA) was further employed to graphically illustrate the docking results.

The three-dimensional (3D) crystal structure of HSV-1 DNA polymerase (PDB ID: 2GV9), the 3D-crystal structure of thymidine kinase from HSV-1 complexed with 5-iododeoxyuridine (HSV-1 TK; PDB ID: 1KI7), the 3D-crystal structure of human cyclin-dependent kinase 2 in complex with roscovitine (CDK2; PDB ID: 2A4L), the 3D-crystal structure of UDP-galactopyranose mutase from Mtb docked with UDP (UGM; PDB ID: 4RPJ), and the 3D-crystal structure of human angiotensin-converting enzyme complexed with captopril (ACE; PDB ID: 1UZF) were obtained from the RCSB Protein Data Bank (www.rcsb.org), while the SDF file of the 3D-structure of brassicasterol (CID: 5281327) was retrieved from PubChem database.

To validate the molecular docking outcomes, 5-iododeoxyuridine, roscovitine, UDP, and captopril were removed from (PDB ID: 1KI7), (PDB ID: 2A4L), (PDB ID: 4RPJ), and (PDB ID: 1UZF), respectively and re-docked back into their receptors. The docking results were expressed as binding energy values (kcal/mol) of ligand-receptor complexes; these are based on hydrogen bond, hydrophobic, and electrostatic interactions. All required docking settings including the preparation of PDBQT files for the receptors and ligands, determination of binding sites, the protonation state, calculations, and the overall charges were established as hitherto described [26].

3. Results and Discussion

3.1. Assessment of Cytotoxicity and Antiherpetic Properties

As shown in Table 1, the cytotoxicity (evaluated by the neutral red dye-uptake assay using Vero cells and expressed as 50% cytotoxic concentration (CC_{50}) value) for brassicasterol, brassicasterol combined with acyclovir (ACV), along with standard ACV was detected to be greater than 50 μM. After the determination of cytotoxicity, Vero cells were infected with HSV-1. Further, the infected cells were treated with the test compounds using an in vitro plaque reduction assay.

Table 1. Antireplicative actions of brassicasterol and brassicasterol in combination with acyclovir against herpes simplex virus type 1 compared to standard acyclovir along with cytotoxicity properties.

Molecules	CC_{50} (μM)	IC_{50} (μM)	SI (CC_{50}/IC_{50})
Brassicasterol	>50	1.2 ± 0.12	>41.7
Brassicasterol combined with ACV	>50	0.7 ± 0.24	>71.4
ACV (standard)	>50	2.1 ± 0.13	>23.8

The acquired values are means ± standard deviation (SD) of three independent measurements assayed in duplicate. CC_{50}: 50% cytotoxic concentration, IC_{50}: 50% inhibitory concentration. CC_{50} and IC_{50} values were determined by nonlinear regressions of concentration-response curves. The differences between treatments with test molecules and the controls were analyzed using a one-way ANOVA test tracked by post-hoc comparison tests (Dunnett and Student–Newman–Kuels), where statistical significance was $p < 0.05$, SI: Selectivity index defined as the ratio CC_{50}/IC_{50}, ACV: Acyclovir. For performing the statistical analyses, PRISM software version 8.0 (GraphPad Software, Inc., La Jolla, CA, USA) was employed.

All test molecules showed obvious antiviral properties against the replication of HSV-1 (expressed as 50% inhibitory concentration (IC_{50}) value), where the treatment with brassicasterol demonstrated greater anti-HSV-1 activity (IC_{50}: 1.2 μM; selectivity index (SI): 41.7) than ACV (IC_{50}: 2.1 μM; SI: 23.8). Additionally, the potency of anti-HSV-1 activity was improved through the combinatory treatment of brassicasterol with ACV (IC_{50}: 0.7 μM; SI: 71.4) compared with that of ACV as a single treatment.

The effective treatment of HSV remains the greatest global challenge in medicine, where the current pharmacological treatment is complicated by the rapid development of drug resistance. Therefore, and to combat and eliminate drug resistance to antiherpetic drugs, new efficient and safe medicines with the ability to provide less resistance are urgently required to enter the clinical practice [1,15].

The acquired results confirmed that brassicasterol has a promising anti-HSV-1 property via inhibiting the viral replication, and its cellular toxicity on Vero cells was observed at a concentration (>50 μM) higher than its IC_{50} value, which means that this compound has an acceptable level of selectivity (expressed as SI) towards the target virus. It has been previously claimed that combinatory treatment with clinically antiherpetic drugs is a valuable option for improving the treatment efficacy of HSV diseases [27]. Hence, the obtained results support this claim by showing the capacity of brassicasterol to increase the anti-HSV activity of standard ACV via a combinatory treatment.

To date, no studies have claimed the antiherpetic properties of brassicasterol. Therefore, the obtained results by this research could be rationalized with other studies in which various natural products have shown in various preclinical investigations the capability of inducing excellent anti-HSV activities with diverse mechanisms of action that could break barriers to novel anti-HSV drug development. This has been documented in a recent review article in which a large number of natural biomolecules extracted from various natural sources with outstanding activities against HSV infections were comprehensively reviewed [28].

3.2. Assessment of Antituberculosis Activity

Brassicasterol was examined for antituberculosis activity by microdilution susceptibility assay. The in vitro susceptibility test was processed with ten clinical isolates of Mtb along with a standard strain. Brassicasterol displayed an adequate level of inhibitory effects on the growth of all Mtb strains tested with MIC values ranging from 1.9 to 2.4 μM (Table 2), while the MIC values for the standard antitubercular drug rifampicin were also recorded.

Table 2. Antituberculosis activity (MIC, μM) of test compounds.

Mycobacterial Strains	MIC (μM)	
	Brassicasterol	**Rifampicin**
Mtb [a]	1.9 ± 0.12	0.1 ± 0.01
Mtb-CI1 [b]	2.0 ± 0.13	0.2 ± 0.02
Mtb-CI2 [b]	2.4 ± 0.15	0.2 ± 0.03
Mtb-CI3 [b]	2.2 ± 0.14	0.3 ± 0.02
Mtb-CI4 [b]	2.1 ± 0.14	0.3 ± 0.02
Mtb-CI5 [b]	1.9 ± 0.13	0.1 ± 0.02
Mtb-CI6 [b]	1.9 ± 0.13	0.3 ± 0.01
Mtb-CI7 [b]	2.1 ± 0.14	0.2 ± 0.01
Mtb-CI8 [b]	1.9 ± 0.11	0.4 ± 0.03
Mtb-CI9 [b]	2.1 ± 0.13	0.3 ± 0.02
Mtb-CI10 [b]	2.0 ± 0.15	0.1 ± 0.01

All recorded values are means ± standard deviation (SD) of three independent experiments assayed in triplicate. [a] Mtb: *Mycobacterium tuberculosis* (reference strain; H37Rv CNCTC My 331-88/ATCC 27294); [b] Mtb: *Mycobacterium tuberculosis* clinical strains; MIC: minimum inhibitory concentration. All presented data were processed by PRISM software (GraphPad Software, Inc., La Jolla, CA, USA; version 8.0).

Although substantial advancements have been achieved during the past few decades in the diagnosis and treatment of TB, the problem of antibiotic resistance remains a challenge [29]. In the present study, brassicasterol showed apparent antitubercular properties via inhibiting the growth of all Mtb strains tested, while no bactericidal effect was observed. In further investigation, and to improve the anti-Mtb activity of brassicasterol, combinatory treatment with standard drug rifampicin was performed. Unfortunately, no positive outcomes were detected to reveal any synergy, additive, or even antagonistic effects.

While several phytosterols derived from marine algae and plants were observed with a slight to moderate degree of antimicrobial actions on Mtb [30–33], their mechanisms of action remain poorly examined. This could be related to their low potency as antitubercular agents, which in turn limits performing further investigations to unveil the mechanisms of action. To the best of the author's knowledge, this research reports the first finding on the anti-Mtb effect of brassicasterol.

3.3. *Evaluation of Anti-Angiotensin-Converting Enzyme Activity*

The inhibition of human ACE activity by brassicasterol was measured by the release of hippuric acid from the enzyme reaction. The activity of ACE was markedly diminished by brassicasterol at a concentration of 12.3 μg/mL with 91.2% inhibition compared with that of standard captopril (99.1% at a concentration of 12.3 μg/mL) (Table 3).

Table 3. Inactivation properties of test compounds against the human angiotensin-converting enzyme.

Compounds	% Inhibition
Brassicasterol	91.2 ± 0.43
Captopril (standard)	99.1 ± 0.12
ACE-catalyzed reaction (no inhibition)	-

All exhibited values are the mean ± standard deviation (SD) (n = 3). ACE: Angiotensin-converting enzyme. The presented data were processed by PRISM software version 8.0 (GraphPad Software, Inc., La Jolla, CA, USA).

ACE inhibitors are known to decrease the production of angiotensin-II, leading to lowering blood pressure, and hence are essential for curing hypertension, heart failure, and other cardiovascular and renal diseases [15]. The re-emerging interest in finding new ACE inhibitors has become urgent, due to the occurrence of undesirable side effects associated with treatment with clinically ACE inhibitors such as captopril, lisinopril, and benazepril [34]. Phytosterols have previously been claimed for their ability to control ACE levels without direct inhibition of ACE. For instance, fucosterol was observed to reduce the ACE levels in endothelial cells by impeding the synthesis of glucocorticoid receptors involved in the regulation of enzyme levels [35]. On the other hand, the current study documents the first investigation on brassicasterol as a direct inhibitor of ACE activity.

3.4. Molecular Docking Evaluation

3.4.1. Brassicasterol with Enzymes Involved in Viral Replication

As depicted in Figure 2, the docking results revealed the substantial ability of brassicasterol to suitably bind to the active sites of HSV-1 DNA polymerase, HSV-1 thymidine kinase (HSV-1 TK) and human cyclin-dependent kinase 2 (CDK2) with detected binding energy values –8.0, –3.3, and –6.5 kcal/mol, respectively. The molecular interactions have been established by forming several fundamental interactions with functional groups of brassicasterol and the interacting amino acid residues of the active sites of target enzymes. These interactions were observed to be hydrogen bond, carbon-hydrogen bond, and hydrophobic (alkyl hydrophobic) along with van der Waals contacts.

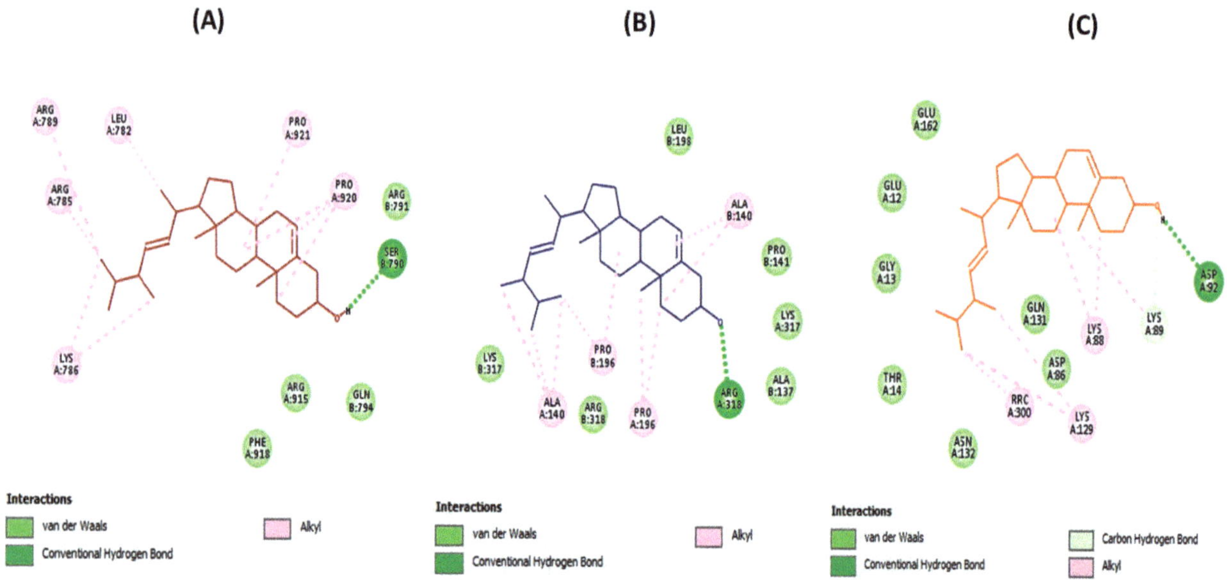

Figure 2. Molecular docking analyses show the molecular interactions and the binding modes of brassicasterol with the active sites of HSV-1 DNA polymerase (**A**), HSV-1 thymidine kinase (**B**), and human cyclin-dependent kinase 2 (**C**), where interactions (hydrogen bond, carbon-hydrogen bond, alkyl hydrophobic, and van der Waals interactions) are presented in a two-dimensional model. Interacting amino acid residues of enzymes active sites with the key functional groups of brassicasterol are shown.

Targeting viral and cellular enzymes that perform significant functions during the HSV-1 replication cycle could help the development of effective broad-spectrum antiherpetic drugs. For instance, HSV-1 DNA polymerase was reported to be an essential enzyme required for viral replication [3], while HSV-1 TK is an important enzyme that catalyzes the transfer of the gamma-phospho group of ATP to thymidine to generate dTMP in the salvage pathway of pyrimidine synthesis, and hence the dTMP serves as a substrate for DNA polymerase during viral DNA replication [36].

It has also been reported that cellular proteins are potential targets for antiviral therapy since most viruses depend on specific cellular proteins for replication. Particularly, CDK2 has been described as a potential target for designing novel anti-HSV-1 drugs [37,38]. According to the currently available evidence, CDK2 was observed to be involved in viral replication and its inhibitors displayed notable anti-HSV-1 activities [39–41]. An additional study unveiled that HSV-1 reactivated in neurons expressing CDK2, and the level of this protein is implicated in the reactivation process [42]. Given together the available data, CDK2 was therefore selected as a target for performing the molecular docking investigations. On the other hand, additional in vitro and in silico studies are necessary to be performed against all CDK families to verify the selectivity of brassicasterol against CDK2.

Unlike the critical role in the viral infection cycle, CDK2 belongs to protein kinases that play a vital role in the eukaryotic cell division cycle. Inhibition of this protein poses a central role in DNA damage-induced cell cycle arrest and DNA repair; however, some negative effects could also be generated [43]. CDK2 is one of the most significant molecular targets identified for cancer-drug discovery and inhibitors of this protein are considered promising chemotherapeutics to combat various types of cancer [44].

3.4.2. Brassicasterol with UDP-Galactopyranose Mutase

UDP-galactopyranose mutase (UGM) is a critical enzyme implicated in the metabolism of galactofuranose, which is known to be a key component of the Mtb cell wall [45]. The docking result of the brassicasterol-UGM complex revealed notable binding mode (Figure 3) with binding energy (–8.1 kcal/mol). The molecular interaction was revealed, where the functional groups of brassicasterol have formed with the interacting amino acid residues of UGM active site several crucial interactions such as hydrogen bond, hydrophobic (alkyl hydrophobic), and van der Waals interactions.

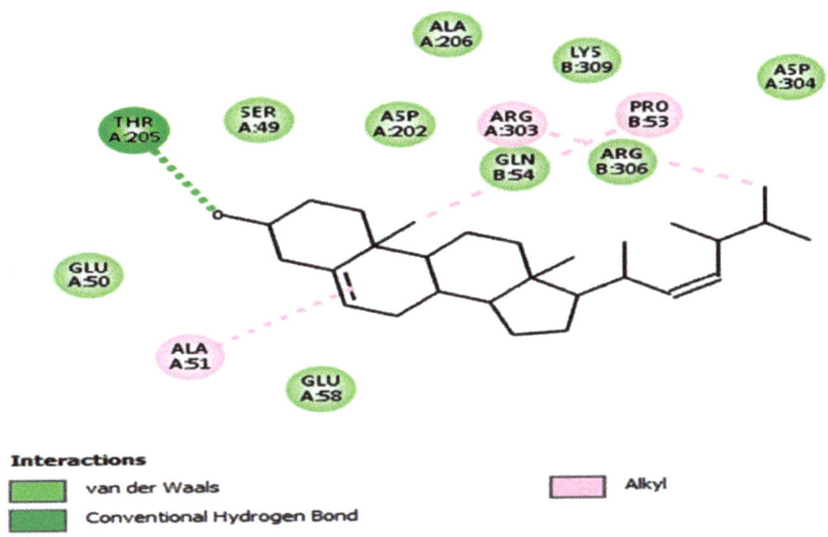

Figure 3. Molecular docking analysis reveals the molecular interaction and the binding mode of brassicasterol with the active site of UDP-galactopyranose mutase (UGM; from *Mycobacterium tuberculosis*), where interactions (hydrogen bond, alkyl hydrophobic, and van der Waals interactions) are shown in a two-dimensional model. Interacting amino acid residues of UGM active site with the key functional groups of brassicasterol are displayed.

Inhibition of mycobacterial cell wall biosynthesis is one of the most effective mechanisms of action of various antibiotics. Mycobacterial cell wall contains a variety of enzymes that play a significant role in its biosynthesis. Therefore, targeting these enzymes is a striking approach for designing effective anti-Mtb drugs [46].

3.4.3. Brassicasterol with Angiotensin-Converting Enzyme

The molecular interaction of brassicasterol with the active site of the angiotensin-converting enzyme (ACE) was explored (Figure 4). The brassicasterol-ACE complex was created with a binding energy value of –9.9 kcal/mol by establishing important hydrogen bond, hydrophobic, and van der Waals interactions. It has been ascertained that zinc is important to the catalytic action of ACE [47], however, brassicasterol was observed to bind to different active pockets than the zinc active-site. Such an outcome may indicate that this compound has a specific type of inhibition that needs to be disclosed in further in vitro investigation.

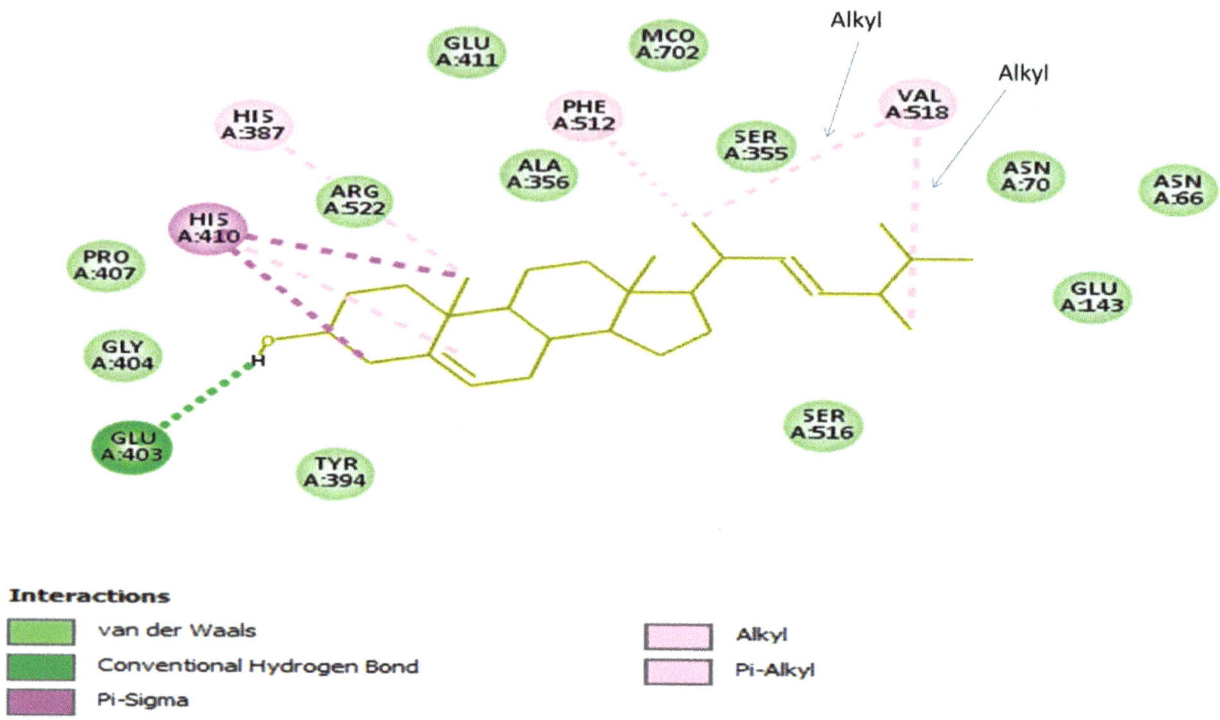

Figure 4. Molecular docking analysis discloses the molecular interaction and the binding mode of brassicasterol with the active site of human angiotensin-converting enzyme (ACE), where interactions (hydrogen bond, alkyl, Pi-alkyl, and Pi-sigma hydrophobic, and van der Waals interactions) are displayed in a two-dimensional model. Interacting amino acid residues of ACE active site with the key functional groups of brassicasterol are shown.

4. Conclusions

In addition to the nutritional and biological values induced by brassicasterol, the outcome of this work has drawn attention to the novel biological properties of this compound, in which anti-infective actions against HSV-1 and Mtb along with cardiovascular protective effects (through inhibition of ACE activity) were ascertained by in vitro and in silico molecular docking studies. Although brassicasterol showed in vitro promising therapeutic values against the investigated targets, further in-depth in vivo investigations are required to validate the obtained results and to unveil the mechanisms of action along with integrated pharmacokinetic and pharmacodynamic studies. Moreover, additional in vitro studies are also necessary to confirm the findings achieved by molecular docking studies.

References

1. Hassan, S.T.; Masarčíková, R.; Berchová, K. Bioactive natural products with anti-herpes simplex virus properties. *J. Pharm. Pharmacol.* **2015**, *67*, 1325–1336. [CrossRef] [PubMed]
2. Brezáni, V.; Leláková, V.; Hassan, S.T.S.; Berchová-Bímová, K.; Nový, P.; Klouček, P.; Maršík, P.; Dall'Acqua, S.; Hošek, J.; Šmejkal, K. Anti-Infectivity against Herpes Simplex Virus and Selected Microbes and Anti-Inflammatory Activities of Compounds Isolated from *Eucalyptus globulus* Labill. *Viruses* **2018**, *10*, 360. [CrossRef] [PubMed]

3. Hassan, S.T.S.; Šudomová, M.; Berchová-Bímová, K.; Šmejkal, K.; Echeverría, J. Psoromic Acid, a Lichen-Derived Molecule, Inhibits the Replication of HSV-1 and HSV-2, and Inactivates HSV-1 DNA Polymerase: Shedding Light on Antiherpetic Properties. *Molecules* **2019**, *24*, 2912. [CrossRef] [PubMed]
4. Čulenová, M.; Sychrová, A.; Hassan, S.T.S.; Berchová-Bímová, K.; Svobodová, P.; Helclová, A.; Michnová, H.; Hošek, J.; Vasilev, H.; Suchý, P.; et al. Multiple In vitro biological effects of phenolic compounds from *Morus alba* root bark. *J. Ethnopharmacol.* **2020**, *248*, 112296. [CrossRef] [PubMed]
5. Hassan, S.T.S.; Šudomová, M.; Masarčíková, R. Herpes simplex virus infection: An overview of the problem, pharmacologic therapy and dietary measures. *Ceska Slov. Farm.* **2017**, *66*, 95–102.
6. Hassan, S.T.S.; Berchová-Bímová, K.; Petráš, J.; Hassan, K.T.S. Cucurbitacin B interacts synergistically with antibiotics against *Staphylococcus aureus* clinical isolates and exhibits antiviral activity against HSV-1. *S. Afr. J. Bot.* **2017**, *108*, 90–94. [CrossRef]
7. Widener, R.W.; Whitley, R.J. Herpes simplex virus. *Handb. Clin. Neurol.* **2014**, *123*, 251–263.
8. Hassan, S.T.S.; Švajdlenka, E.; Berchová-Bímová, K. *Hibiscus sabdariffa* L. and Its Bioactive Constituents Exhibit Antiviral Activity against HSV-2 and Anti-enzymatic Properties against Urease by an ESI-MS Based Assay. *Molecules* **2017**, *22*, 722. [CrossRef]
9. Šudomová, M.; Shariati, M.A.; Echeverría, J.; Berindan-Neagoe, I.; Nabavi, S.M.; Hassan, S.T.S. A Microbiological, Toxicological, and Biochemical Study of the Effects of Fucoxanthin, a Marine Carotenoid, on *Mycobacterium tuberculosis* and the Enzymes Implicated in Its Cell Wall: A Link Between Mycobacterial Infection and Autoimmune Diseases. *Mar. Drugs* **2019**, *17*, 641. [CrossRef]
10. Bell, L.C.K.; Noursadeghi, M. Pathogenesis of HIV-1 and *Mycobacterium tuberculosis* co-infection. *Nat. Rev. Microbiol.* **2018**, *16*, 80–90. [CrossRef]
11. Shingadia, D. The diagnosis of tuberculosis. *Pediatr. Infect. Dis. J.* **2012**, *31*, 302–305. [CrossRef] [PubMed]
12. Hassan, S.T.S.; Šudomová, M.; Berchová-Bímová, K.; Gowrishankar, S.; Rengasamy, K.R.R. Antimycobacterial, Enzyme Inhibition, and Molecular Interaction Studies of Psoromic Acid in *Mycobacterium tuberculosis*: Efficacy and Safety Investigations. *J. Clin. Med.* **2018**, *7*, 226. [CrossRef] [PubMed]
13. Dookie, N.; Rambaran, S.; Padayatchi, N.; Mahomed, S.; Naidoo, K. Evolution of drug resistance in *Mycobacterium tuberculosis*: A review on the molecular determinants of resistance and implications for personalized care. *J. Antimicrob. Chemother.* **2018**, *73*, 1138–1151. [CrossRef] [PubMed]
14. World Health Organization. Fact Sheet on Tuberculosis (2020). Available online: https://www.who.int/news-room/fact-sheets/detail/tuberculosis (accessed on 25 March 2020).
15. Hassan, S.T.S.; Berchová-Bímová, K.; Šudomová, M.; Malaník, M.; Šmejkal, K.; Rengasamy, K.R.R. In Vitro Study of Multi-Therapeutic Properties of *Thymus bovei* Benth. Essential Oil and Its Main Component for Promoting Their Use in Clinical Practice. *J. Clin. Med.* **2018**, *7*, 283. [CrossRef]
16. Li, X.; Chang, P.; Wang, Q.; Hu, H.; Bai, F.; Li, N.; Yu, J. Effects of Angiotensin-Converting Enzyme Inhibitors on Arterial Stiffness: A Systematic Review and Meta-Analysis of Randomized Controlled Trials. *Cardiovasc. Ther.* **2020**, *2020*, 7056184. [CrossRef]
17. Peng, H.; Carretero, O.A.; Vuljaj, N.; Liao, T.D.; Motivala, A.; Peterson, E.L.; Rhaleb, N.E. Angiotensin-converting enzyme inhibitors: A new mechanism of action. *Circulation* **2005**, *112*, 2436–2445. [CrossRef]
18. Izzo, J.L., Jr.; Weir, M.R. Angiotensin-converting enzyme inhibitors. *J. Clin. Hypertens. (Greenwich)* **2011**, *13*, 667–675. [CrossRef]
19. Vanmierlo, T.; Popp, J.; Kölsch, H.; Friedrichs, S.; Jessen, F.; Stoffel-Wagner, B.; Bertsch, T.; Hartmann, T.; Maier, W.; von Bergmann, K.; et al. The plant sterol brassicasterol as additional CSF biomarker in Alzheimer's disease. *Acta Psychiatr. Scand.* **2011**, *124*, 184–192. [CrossRef]
20. Bianconi, V.; Mannarino, M.R.; Sahebkar, A.; Cosentino, T.; Pirro, M. Cholesterol-Lowering Nutraceuticals Affecting Vascular Function and Cardiovascular Disease Risk. *Curr. Cardiol. Rep.* **2018**, *20*, 53. [CrossRef]
21. CFR-Code Federal Regulations: Title 21 (2019). Available online: https://www.accessdata.fda.gov/scripts/cdrh/cfdocs/cfcfr/CFRSearch.cfm?fr=101.83 (accessed on 25 March 2020).
22. Liland, N.S.; Pittman, K.; Whatmore, P.; Torstensen, B.E.; Sissener, N.H. Fucosterol Causes Small Changes in Lipid Storage and Brassicasterol Affects some Markers of Lipid Metabolism in Atlantic Salmon Hepatocytes. *Lipids* **2018**, *53*, 737–747. [CrossRef]

23. Liland, N.S.; Espe, M.; Rosenlund, G.; Waagbø, R.; Hjelle, J.I.; Lie, Ø.; Fontanillas, R.; Torstensen, B.E. High levels of dietary phytosterols affect lipid metabolism and increase liver and plasma TAG in Atlantic salmon (*Salmo salar* L.). *Br. J. Nutr.* **2013**, *110*, 1958–1967. [CrossRef] [PubMed]
24. Clinical and Laboratory Standards Institute. *Laboratory Detection and Identification of Mycobacteria*, 1st ed.; Approved Guideline; CLSI Document M48-A.; Clinical and Laboratory Standards Institute: Wayne, PA, USA, 2008.
25. Clinical and Laboratory Standards Institute. *Susceptibility Testing of Mycobacteria, Nocardiae, and Other Aerobic Actinomycetes*, 2nd ed.; Approved Standard M24-A2; CLSI: Wayne, PA, USA, 2011.
26. Hassan, S.T.S.; Švajdlenka, E. Biological Evaluation and Molecular Docking of Protocatechuic Acid from *Hibiscus sabdariffa* L. as a Potent Urease Inhibitor by an ESI-MS Based Method. *Molecules* **2017**, *22*, 1696. [CrossRef] [PubMed]
27. Field, H.J.; Vere Hodge, R.A. Recent developments in anti-herpesvirus drugs. *Br. Med. Bull.* **2013**, *106*, 213–249. [CrossRef] [PubMed]
28. Treml, J.; Gazdová, M.; Šmejkal, K.; Šudomová, M.; Kubatka, P.; Hassan, S.T.S. Natural Products-Derived Chemicals: Breaking Barriers to Novel Anti-HSV Drug Development. *Viruses* **2020**, *12*, 154. [CrossRef] [PubMed]
29. Jung, Y.E.G.; Schluger, N.W. Advances in the diagnosis and treatment of latent tuberculosis infection. *Curr. Opin. Infect. Dis.* **2020**, *33*, 166–172. [CrossRef]
30. Wächter, G.A.; Franzblau, S.G.; Montenegro, G.; Hoffmann, J.J.; Maiese, W.M.; Timmermann, B.N. Inhibition of *Mycobacterium tuberculosis* growth by saringosterol from *Lessonia nigrescens*. *J. Nat. Prod.* **2001**, *64*, 1463–1464. [CrossRef]
31. Tan, M.A.; Takayama, H.; Aimi, N.; Kitajima, M.; Franzblau, S.G.; Nonato, M.G. Antitubercular triterpenes and phytosterols from *Pandanus tectorius* Soland. var. laevis. *J. Nat. Med.* **2008**, *62*, 232–235. [CrossRef]
32. Olugbuyiro, J.A.; Moody, J.O.; Hamann, M.T. Phytosterols from *Spondias mombin* Linn with Antimycobacterial Activities. *Afr. J. Biomed. Res.* **2013**, *16*, 19–24.
33. Chinsembu, K.C. Tuberculosis and nature's pharmacy of putative anti-tuberculosis agents. *Acta Trop.* **2016**, *153*, 46–56. [CrossRef]
34. Šudomová, M.; Hassan, S.T.S.; Khan, H.; Rasekhian, M.; Nabavi, S.M. A Multi-Biochemical and In Silico Study on Anti-Enzymatic Actions of Pyroglutamic Acid against PDE-5, ACE, and Urease Using Various Analytical Techniques: Unexplored Pharmacological Properties and Cytotoxicity Evaluation. *Biomolecules* **2019**, *9*, 392. [CrossRef]
35. Hagiwara, H.; Wakita, K.; Inada, Y.; Hirose, S. Fucosterol decreases angiotensin converting enzyme levels with reduction of glucocorticoid receptors in endothelial cells. *Biochem. Biophys. Res. Commun.* **1986**, *139*, 348–352. [CrossRef]
36. Xie, Y.; Wu, L.; Wang, M.; Cheng, A.; Yang, Q.; Wu, Y.; Jia, R.; Zhu, D.; Zhao, X.; Chen, S.; et al. Alpha-Herpesvirus Thymidine Kinase Genes Mediate Viral Virulence and Are Potential Therapeutic Targets. *Front. Microbiol.* **2019**, *10*, 941. [CrossRef] [PubMed]
37. Schang, L.M.; St Vincent, M.R.; Lacasse, J.J. Five years of progress on cyclin-dependent kinases and other cellular proteins as potential targets for antiviral drugs. *Antivir. Chem. Chemother.* **2006**, *17*, 293–320. [CrossRef] [PubMed]
38. Viegas, D.J.; Edwards, T.G.; Bloom, D.C.; Abreu, P.A. Virtual screening identified compounds that bind to cyclin dependent kinase 2 and prevent herpes simplex virus type 1 replication and reactivation in neurons. *Antiviral. Res.* **2019**, *172*, 104621. [CrossRef] [PubMed]
39. Schang, L.M. The cell cycle, cyclin-dependent kinases, and viral infections: New horizons and unexpected connections. *Prog. Cell. Cycle Res.* **2003**, *5*, 103–124.
40. Schang, L.M.; Phillips, J.; Schaffer, P.A. Requirement for cellular cyclin-dependent kinases in herpes simplex virus replication and transcription. *J. Virol.* **1998**, *72*, 5626–5637. [CrossRef]
41. Davido, D.J.; Leib, D.A.; Schaffer, P.A. The cyclin-dependent kinase inhibitor roscovitine inhibits the transactivating activity and alters the posttranslational modification of herpes simplex virus type 1 ICP0. *J. Virol.* **2002**, *76*, 1077–1088. [CrossRef]
42. Schang, L.M.; Bantly, A.; Schaffer, P.A. Explant-induced reactivation of herpes simplex virus occurs in neurons expressing nuclear cdk2 and cdk4. *J. Virol.* **2002**, *76*, 7724–7735. [CrossRef]

43. Wang, H.; Kim, N.H. CDK2 Is Required for the DNA Damage Response During Porcine Early Embryonic Development. *Biol. Reprod.* **2016**, *95*, 31. [CrossRef]
44. Tadesse, S.; Caldon, E.C.; Tilley, W.; Wang, S. Cyclin-Dependent Kinase 2 Inhibitors in Cancer Therapy: An Update. *J. Med. Chem.* **2019**, *62*, 4233–4251. [CrossRef]
45. Soltero-Higgin, M.; Carlson, E.E.; Gruber, T.D.; Kiessling, L.L. A unique catalytic mechanism for UDP-galactopyranose mutase. *Nat. Struct. Mol. Biol.* **2004**, *11*, 539–543. [CrossRef] [PubMed]
46. Abrahams, K.A.; Besra, G.S. Mycobacterial cell wall biosynthesis: A multifaceted antibiotic target. *Parasitology* **2018**, *145*, 116–133. [CrossRef] [PubMed]
47. Natesh, R.; Schwager, S.L.; Evans, H.R.; Sturrock, E.D.; Acharya, K.R. Structural details on the binding of antihypertensive drugs captopril and enalaprilat to human testicular angiotensin I-converting enzyme. *Biochemistry* **2004**, *43*, 8718–8724. [CrossRef] [PubMed]

7

Modulation of TRP Channel Activity by Hydroxylation and its Therapeutic Potential

Yagnesh Nagarajan [1], Grigori Y. Rychkov [2,3] and Daniel J. Peet [1,*]

1 School of Biological Sciences, University of Adelaide, Adelaide 5005, SA, Australia; yagnesh.nagarajan@adelaide.edu.au
2 School of Medicine, University of Adelaide, Adelaide 5005, SA, Australia; grigori.rychkov@adelaide.edu.au
3 South Australian Health and Medical Research Institute (SAHMRI), Adelaide 5005, SA, Australia
* Correspondence: daniel.peet@adelaide.edu.au

Academic Editors: Arpad Szallasi and Susan M. Huang

Abstract: Two transient receptor potential (TRP) channels—TRPA1 and TRPV3—are post-translationally hydroxylated, resulting in oxygen-dependent regulation of channel activity. The enzymes responsible are the HIF prolyl hydroxylases (PHDs) and the asparaginyl hydroxylase factor inhibiting HIF (FIH). The PHDs and FIH are well characterized for their hydroxylation of the hypoxic inducible transcription factors (HIFs), mediating their hypoxic regulation. Consequently, these hydroxylases are currently being targeted therapeutically to modulate HIF activity in anemia, inflammation, and ischemic disease. Modulating the HIFs by targeting these hydroxylases may result in both desirable and undesirable effects on TRP channel activity, depending on the physiological context. For the best outcomes, these hydroxylases could be therapeutically targeted in pathologies where activation of both the HIFs and the relevant TRP channels are predicted to independently achieve positive outcomes, such as wound healing and obesity.

Keywords: TRPA1; TRPV3; hydroxylation; PHD; FIH; HIF; oxygen; hypoxia

---

1. Introduction

The transient receptor potential (TRP) channels are non-selective cation channels broadly expressed in most tissues in the body. TRP channels play a role as cellular sensors which respond to a diverse range of extracellular and intracellular stimuli, including second messengers, chemicals, temperature, redox state, mechanical stimulation, and osmolality [1–4]. Recent research suggests that abnormal activity of some members of the TRP super-family contributes to human pathologies such as cancer, diabetes, lung and liver fibrosis, chronic pain, ischemia-reperfusion injury, pulmonary hypertension, irritable bowel disease, drug toxicity, and others [2,5–9].

TRP channels are formed by homo- or hetero-tetramers of TRP proteins, with each a TRP monomer comprised of six transmembrane domains flanked by intracellular N- and C-terminal domains. Similar to voltage-gated channels, a conserved pore-forming loop between transmembrane domains 5 and 6 in TRP proteins is responsible for cation permeability. Although most TRP channels under physiological conditions conduct more Na^+ than Ca^{2+}, the Ca^{2+} permeability of TRP channels is considered to be important for the maintenance of intracellular Ca^{2+} signaling and homeostasis.

Apart from specific stimuli that gate TRP channels, TRP channel activity can be further controlled by a range of post-translational modifications, including phosphorylation and glycosylation (reviewed in [10]). Two specific TRP channels—TRPA1 and TRPV3—are modified post-translationally by hydroxylation (an oxygen-dependent modification), which mediates a characteristic response to hypoxia [11,12]. The hydroxylases responsible for these modifications have emerged as key therapeutic targets for a range of human diseases due to their direct regulation of the hypoxia-inducible factors

(HIFs, the central transcription factors that mediate the genomic response to hypoxia), with important therapeutic implications for TRP channels.

2. Hydroxylation-Dependent Regulation of Hypoxic Gene Expression

The prolyl hydroxylase containing enzymes (PHDs) and the asparaginyl hydroxylase factor inhibiting HIF (FIH) belong to a conserved family of 2-oxoglutarate-dependent dioxygenases, and act as cellular oxygen sensors [13]. These oxygen-sensing enzymes catalyze the addition of hydroxyl (OH) groups to specific prolyl or asparaginyl residues on target proteins, altering their activity. The three closely related PHD enzymes (PHD1, 2, and 3, also referred to in the literature as EGLN2, 1, and 3) were originally characterized through their oxygen-dependent hydroxylation of two proline residues within the HIFα subunit of the heterodimeric HIF transcription factors. HIFα hydroxylation occurs in normoxia and promotes ubiquitination and rapid proteosomal-mediated degradation (reviewed in [14]). In hypoxia the activity of the PHDs decreases, allowing the HIFα subunits to avoid hydroxylation, ubiquitylation and subsequent degradation, and consequently the stabilized HIFα mediates robust gene induction in response to hypoxia (Figure 1). Thus, the PHDs act as the essential oxygen sensors in this pathway and are the primary regulators of the HIF-driven genomic response to hypoxia. FIH was subsequently characterized as a related hydroxylase that hydroxylates a single asparaginyl residue in a transactivation domain of the HIFα subunit, resulting in transcriptional repression in hypoxia (reviewed in [15]). As with the PHDs, hypoxia results in the loss of efficient oxygen-dependent hydroxylation, and alleviates the transcriptional repression, contributing to increased hypoxic gene induction mediated by the HIFs. However, the role of FIH in modulating oxygen-dependent gene regulation via the HIFs is modest compared to the PHDs, and its physiological importance less well characterized.

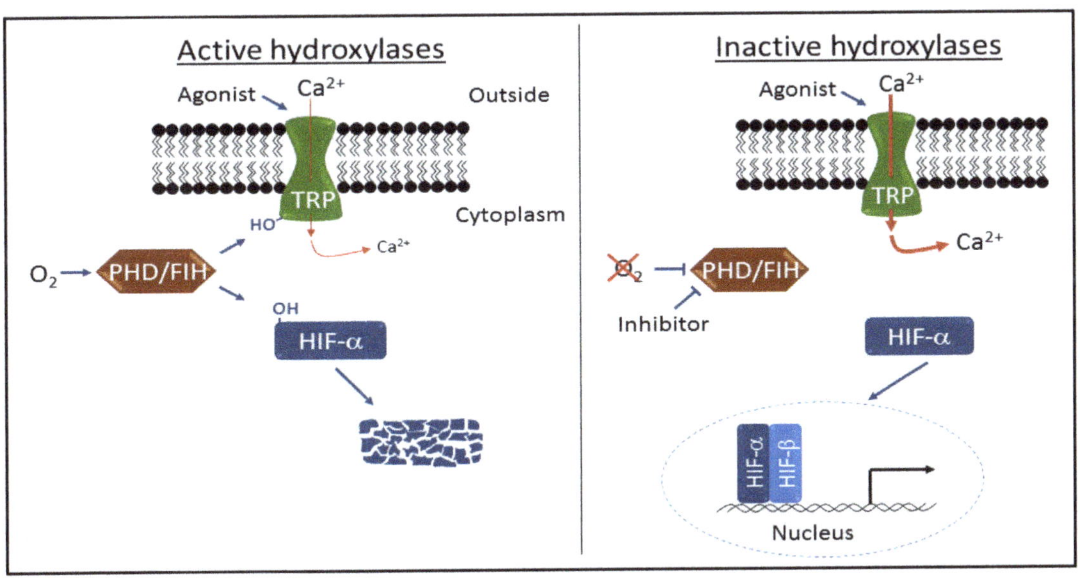

Figure 1. Schematic representation of transient receptor potential (TRP) channel and hypoxia-inducible factor (HIF) regulation by the prolyl hydroxylase containing enzymes (PHD) and asparaginyl hydroxylase factor inhibiting HIF (FIH) hydroxylases. Oxygen-dependent hydroxylation (-OH) of TRPA1 and TRPV3 channels inhibits cation entry through activated channels, and hydroxylation of HIFα proteins leads to proteolytic degradation and transcriptional repression. Inhibition of hydroxylase activity by hypoxia or specific inhibitors leads to increased cation entry and robust HIF-dependent gene activation.

The PHDs and FIH also have a number of substrates in addition to the HIF proteins, although the physiological consequence of hydroxylation on these substrates has not been well established. Other substrates for the PHDs include pyruvate kinase M2, RNA polymerase II, erythropoietin receptor, eukaryotic elongation factor 2, and beta(2)-adrenergic receptor [16]. FIH has been shown to hydroxylate a number of proteins containing ankyrin repeat domains (ARDs), although in most cases there is no obvious effect on the function of the hydroxylated substrate [17]. However, two more recently identified ARD substrates and one non-ARD substrate show some hydroxylation-dependent changes in activity [11,18,19].

3. Hydroxylation-Dependent Regulation of TRP Channel Activity

TRPA1 is activated by a range of chemical agonists (both endogenous and exogenous), mechanical stimulation, and cold temperature (reviewed in [20]). It has been implicated in a number of pathologies, including acute inflammation and cartilage degeneration in osteoarthritis [21], urinary bladder pain in cystitis [22], neuropathic and inflammatory pain, migraine, and familial episodic pain syndrome [23,24]. Takahashi and colleagues reported that TRPA1 is also sensitive to changes in oxygen, undergoing oxygen-dependent hydroxylation on a single proline residue within the ARD by the PHDs in normoxia [12]. Their data supported hydroxylation-dependent inhibition of channel activity that was rapidly reversed in hypoxia, when the oxygen-sensing PHDs have greatly diminished activity, leading to an increase in activity of the unmodified channel. Furthermore, they demonstrated that TRPA1 channels also respond to oxygen through the oxidation in hyperoxia of specific cysteine residues located within the seventeenth ARD (Cys 633 and Cys 856). A recent study proposes a role for TRPA1 hydroxylation in the hypoxic ventilator response [25]. In addition, this oxygen-dependent hydroxylation has been implicated in mediating the response to cold temperature through the production of reactive oxygen species [26]. Of interest, TRPA1 also responds to ischemia in oligodendrocytes, mediating Ca^{2+} entry and subsequent damage to myelin, although the role of hydroxylation in this response has not been explored [27].

TRPV3 was originally characterized as a warm temperature sensing channel [28–30], and is also activated by endogenous and exogenous chemical ligands. It plays roles in the maintenance of epidermal barrier function, hair growth, and nociception, and has been implicated in pathologies associated with dermatitis, pruritus, inflammation, ischemia, and wound healing [31,32]. The TRPV3 channel has also been shown to be hydroxylated, but on a single asparaginyl residue within the ARD, by FIH [11]. In common with the PHD-mediated hydroxylation of TRPA1, FIH-dependent hydroxylation of TRPV3 in normoxia inhibits channel activity, but is rapidly reversed in hypoxia, leading to increased hypoxic TRPV3 activity (Figure 1).

In the case of both TRPA1 and TRPV3, the mechanism by which hydroxylation modulates channel activity has not been determined. For example, hydroxylation may influence the physical structure of the channels and consequently influence gating, or may affect agonist binding, multimerisation with other TRP channels, or the recruitment of accessory proteins that modulate function. In addition, while the evidence for TRPA1 and TRPV3 hydroxylation is strong, as with other non-HIF substrates, the physiological role for these hydroxylation events remains poorly defined.

Whether other TRP channels are regulated by hydroxylation, mediated by the PHDs, FIH, or other hydroxylases remains unclear. In addition to TRPA1 and TRPV3, it has also been reported that peptides from the ARD of TRPV4 can be hydroxylated in vitro by FIH [33]. We have investigated the hydroxylation of nine other TRP channels predicted using bioinformatics to be substrates of FIH (TRPC1, C3, C4, C5, C6, V2, V5, V6), but found no evidence for hydroxylation using in vitro hydroxylation assays (unpublished data). Furthermore, other than TRPA1, none of the nine other TRP channels analyzed by Takahashi et al. displayed hypoxic induction, including TRPV3. However, it is important to note that these experiments were performed in 10% oxygen, which is relatively mild hypoxia and unlikely to influence FIH-mediated hydroxylation [12,34]. A recent report of interest implicated mouse TRPC2 in sensing low oxygen within olfactory epithelium [35]. While it is unclear whether this response involves hydroxylation (and TRPC2 is only a pseudogene in humans), it does support the hypothesis that other TRP channels may also be regulated in a similar manner to TRPA1 and TRPV3. The formation of heterotetramers with other channels may also cause the modification of one channel to influence the activity of another. For example, TRPV3 is known to form functional heterotetramers with TRPV1 [29,36], hence regulation of TRPV3 via hydroxylation may indirectly influence the activity of a TRPV1/V3 heterotetramer where V1 is activated.

Although the body of literature on TRP-hydroxylation is clearly very limited and more research is required to ascertain the physiological relevance, these studies establish that the oxygen-dependent hydroxylation of at least two members of the TRP superfamily confers hypoxic responsiveness to these channels. These findings have important implications regarding the potential for novel therapeutic manipulation of the activity of these specific TRP channels via altered hydroxylation, either directly or as a consequence of the therapeutic targeting of the PHDs and FIH to regulate other substrates.

4. Therapeutic Targeting of PHDs and FIH to Activate HIF

Given that hypoxia contributes to the pathophysiology of most major diseases, including myocardial and cerebral ischemia, vascular disease, and cancer, it is not surprising that therapeutic manipulation of the ubiquitous HIF pathway has become a highly sought after goal. The PHDs and FIH are attractive therapeutic targets, as they are well characterized functionally and structurally [37–40], can be expressed recombinantly [41,42], and inhibition results in HIF activation, with the PHDs of particular interest as the primary regulators of the HIFs [43]. However, specificity is an important issue when targeting PHDs or FIH in human pathologies, given the large family of related 2-oxoglutarate-dependent oxygenases, the hundreds of target genes directly regulated by the HIFs that influence diverse biological processes including erythropoiesis, angiogenesis, metabolism, cell migration and survival, and the other less well characterized substrates of the PHDs and FIH, including the TRP channels.

To date, numerous PHD inhibitors have been developed, with a number in pre-clinical and clinical trials (reviewed in [43]). The initial focus has been on the treatment of anemia, as erythropoietin is a direct target gene of HIF, with two PHD inhibitors currently in Phase 3 clinical trials showing considerable promise. Additional clinical and preclinical trials have also targeted ischemia and inflammation, with other pathologies also under investigation. Specificity for different HIF-mediated outcomes is achieved through the use of inhibitors that display selectivity for one or more of the PHDs (the three different PHDs show some specificity for different HIFα proteins, and consequently regulate distinct target gene responses), as well as distinct delivery and treatment regimes. Little is known regarding the consequence of these treatments on non-HIF targets of the PHDs, including TRPA1.

Preliminary screens have also been performed to identify specific inhibitors of FIH [44,45], but given the modest effects on HIF activity mediated by FIH, it has not been a focus of pharmaceutical research. However, one potential advantage of targeting FIH is that additional specificity may be achieved compared with the PHDs, as FIH only influences the expression of a discrete subset of HIF target genes, and shows some specificity for different HIF isoforms [34,46].

5. Therapeutic Targeting of PHDs and FIH to Modulate TRP Channel Activity

Therapeutic manipulation of the PHDs and FIH is likely to modulate the activity of TRPA1 and TRPV3, respectively. Importantly, inhibition of hydroxylase activity—which has been the focus of therapeutic manipulation to achieve HIF activation—has the potential to increase TRPA1 and TRPV3 activity through abrogation of hydroxylation. However, given the key role of the hydroxylases—specifically the PHDs—in regulating the ubiquitously expressed HIFs, specificity is likely to be a major issue. Importantly, while specific inhibitors of the PHDs and FIH should theoretically also modulate TRPA1 and TRPV3 activity, respectively, through altered hydroxylation, this needs to be determined experimentally. This characterization should include inhibitors that show specificity for each of the hydroxylases, including those currently in clinical trials, and their consequence on both hydroxylation and activity. In the case of both TRPA1 and TRPV3, loss of hydroxylation does not appear to independently activate the channels, but rather the limited data are consistent with an increase in the activity of an already active channel. Hence therapeutic targeting of the PHDs or FIH might only modulate the activity of an already active channel. Physiologically, this would depend on the presence of endogenous chemical agonists, mechanical stimuli, or temperature to activate the channels.

The knowledge that TRPA1 is also regulated by PHD-mediated hydroxylation should also inform the current clinical and preclinical trials using PHD inhibitors to activate the HIFs. For example, a number of pre-clinical studies have targeted inflammation in mouse models of colitis with mostly positive outcomes [43]. However, in similar models of colitis, TRPA1 channels are shown to contribute to disease pathology [47], with TRPA1 antagonists being designed and trialed for treatment of inflammation and pain [48]. Consequently, the activation of TRPA1 achieved with PHD inhibitors is likely to promote rather than inhibit disease pathology and associated pain.

Targeting TRPV3 activity via FIH should be more specific, given the modest role for FIH in HIF regulation and the apparent lack of an effect of hydroxylation on the activity of most characterized ARD substrates [17]. However, this is complicated by the metabolic phenotype of FIH null mice, which are viable and display hypermetabolism, hyperventilation, lowered body mass and adiposity, resistance to weight gain when fed a high fat diet, and insulin hypersensitivity. This phenotype is not readily explained by the known roles for FIH in regulating the HIFs or other characterized ARD substrates, and supports the existence of one or more additional substrates involved in controlling metabolism [49].

A more prudent strategy to therapeutically target the PHDs or FIH to modulate TRP channel activity would focus on pathologies where activation of both the HIFs and the relevant TRP channels are predicted to independently achieve positive outcomes. For example, both TRPV3 and HIF have been implicated in wound healing [50,51], hence the therapeutic inhibition of FIH may promote wound healing through two independent pathways, via activation of both HIF and TRPV3. The targeted deletion of FIH in mice and mice treated with activators of TRPV3 channels both display similar metabolic effects, including decreased adiposity and resistance to weight gain on a high fat diet [49,52]. So, the therapeutic inhibition of FIH in the context of obesity or diabetes may also result in beneficial outcomes through two independent pathways.

6. Conclusions

The recent identification of hydroxylation-mediated changes in TRPA1 and TRPV3 channel activity—although based on a limited number of highly focused studies—has expanded our understanding of the role of channel post-translational modifications, and the oxygen-dependent modulation of these channels. It has also uncovered new therapeutic strategies to modulate the activity of these specific channels by targeting the PHDs and FIH, while identifying potential TRP channel-mediated side effects as a consequence of targeting these hydroxylases to therapeutically regulate HIF activity.

Acknowledgments: This work was supported by a grant from the Australian Research Council (DP150102860).

Author Contributions: Yagnesh Nagarajan, Grigori Y. Rychkov and Daniel J. Peet all contributed to the planning and writing of this manuscript.

References

1. Brierley, S.M.; Hughes, P.A.; Page, A.J.; Kwan, K.Y.; Martin, C.M.; O'Donnell, T.A.; Cooper, N.J.; Harrington, A.M.; Adam, B.; Liebregts, T.; et al. The ion channel TRPA1 is required for normal mechanosensation and is modulated by algesic stimuli. *Gastroenterology* **2009**, *137*, 2084–2095. [CrossRef] [PubMed]
2. Darby, W.G.; Grace, M.S.; Baratchi, S.; McIntyre, P. Modulation of TRPV4 by diverse mechanisms. *Int. J. Biochem. Cell Biol.* **2016**, *78*, 217–228. [CrossRef] [PubMed]

3. Ogawa, N.; Kurokawa, T.; Mori, Y. Sensing of redox status by TRP channels. *Cell Calcium* **2016**, *60*, 115–122. [CrossRef] [PubMed]
4. Vrenken, K.S.; Jalink, K.; van Leeuwen, F.N.; Middelbeek, J. Beyond ion-conduction: Channel-dependent and -independent roles of TRP channels during development and tissue homeostasis. *Biochim. Biophys. Acta* **2016**, *1863*, 1436–1446. [CrossRef] [PubMed]
5. Dai, Y. TRPs and pain. *Semin. Immunopathol.* **2016**, *38*, 277–291. [CrossRef] [PubMed]
6. De Logu, F.; Patacchini, R.; Fontana, G.; Geppetti, P. TRP functions in the broncho-pulmonary system. *Semin. Immunopathol.* **2016**, *38*, 321–329. [CrossRef] [PubMed]
7. Derbenev, A.V.; Zsombok, A. Potential therapeutic value of TRPV1 and TRPA1 in diabetes mellitus and obesity. *Semin. Immunopathol.* **2016**, *38*, 397–406. [CrossRef] [PubMed]
8. Shapovalov, G.; Ritaine, A.; Skryma, R.; Prevarskaya, N. Role of TRP ion channels in cancer and tumorigenesis. *Semin. Immunopathol.* **2016**, *38*, 357–369. [CrossRef] [PubMed]
9. Xu, T.; Wu, B.M.; Yao, H.W.; Meng, X.M.; Huang, C.; Ni, M.M.; Li, J. Novel insights into TRPM7 function in fibrotic diseases: A potential therapeutic target. *J. Cell. Physiol.* **2015**, *230*, 1163–1169. [PubMed]
10. Voolstra, O.; Huber, A. Post-translational modifications of TRP channels. *Cells* **2014**, *3*, 258–287. [CrossRef] [PubMed]
11. Karttunen, S.; Duffield, M.; Scrimgeour, N.R.; Squires, L.; Lim, W.L.; Dallas, M.L.; Scragg, J.L.; Chicher, J.; Dave, K.A.; Whitelaw, M.L.; et al. Oxygen-dependent hydroxylation by FIH regulates the TRPV3 ion channel. *J. Cell Sci.* **2015**, *128*, 225–231. [CrossRef] [PubMed]
12. Takahashi, N.; Kuwaki, T.; Kiyonaka, S.; Numata, T.; Kozai, D.; Mizuno, Y.; Yamamoto, S.; Naito, S.; Knevels, E.; Carmeliet, P.; et al. TRPA1 underlies a sensing mechanism for O_2. *Nat. Chem. Biol.* **2011**, *7*, 701–711. [CrossRef] [PubMed]
13. Loenarz, C.; Schofield, C.J. Physiological and biochemical aspects of hydroxylations and demethylations catalyzed by human 2-oxoglutarate oxygenases. *Trends Biochem. Sci.* **2011**, *36*, 7–18. [CrossRef] [PubMed]
14. Kaelin, W.G., Jr.; Ratcliffe, P.J. Oxygen sensing by metazoans: The central role of the HIF hydroxylase pathway. *Mol. Cell* **2008**, *30*, 393–402. [CrossRef] [PubMed]
15. Peet, D.; Linke, S. Regulation of HIF: Asparaginyl hydroxylation. *Novartis Found. Symp.* **2006**, *272*, 37–49. [PubMed]
16. Nguyen, T.L.; Duran, R.V. Prolyl hydroxylase domain enzymes and their role in cell signaling and cancer metabolism. *Int. J. Biochem. Cell Biol.* **2016**, *80*, 71–80. [CrossRef] [PubMed]
17. Cockman, M.E.; Webb, J.D.; Ratcliffe, P.J. FIH-dependent asparaginyl hydroxylation of ankyrin repeat domain-containing proteins. *Ann. N. Y. Acad. Sci.* **2009**, *1177*, 9–18. [CrossRef] [PubMed]
18. Janke, K.; Brockmeier, U.; Kuhlmann, K.; Eisenacher, M.; Nolde, J.; Meyer, H.E.; Mairbaurl, H.; Metzen, E. Factor inhibiting HIF-1 (FIH-1) modulates protein interactions of apoptosis-stimulating p53 binding protein 2 (ASPP2). *J. Cell Sci.* **2013**, *126*, 2629–2640. [CrossRef] [PubMed]
19. Scholz, C.C.; Rodriguez, J.; Pickel, C.; Burr, S.; Fabrizio, J.A.; Nolan, K.A.; Spielmann, P.; Cavadas, M.A.; Crifo, B.; Halligan, D.N.; et al. FIH regulates cellular metabolism through hydroxylation of the deubiquitinase OTUB1. *PLoS Biol.* **2016**, *14*, e1002347. [CrossRef] [PubMed]
20. Laursen, W.J.; Bagriantsev, S.N.; Gracheva, E.O. TRPA1 channels: Chemical and temperature sensitivity. *Curr. Top. Membr.* **2014**, *74*, 89–112. [PubMed]
21. Moilanen, L.J.; Hamalainen, M.; Nummenmaa, E.; Ilmarinen, P.; Vuolteenaho, K.; Nieminen, R.M.; Lehtimaki, L.; Moilanen, E. Monosodium iodoacetate-induced inflammation and joint pain are reduced in trpa1 deficient mice-potential role of TRPA1 in osteoarthritis. *Osteoarthr. Cartil.* **2015**, *23*, 2017–2026. [CrossRef] [PubMed]
22. DeBerry, J.J.; Schwartz, E.S.; Davis, B.M. TRPA1 mediates bladder hyperalgesia in a mouse model of cystitis. *Pain* **2014**, *155*, 1280–1287. [CrossRef] [PubMed]
23. Kremeyer, B.; Lopera, F.; Cox, J.J.; Momin, A.; Rugiero, F.; Marsh, S.; Woods, C.G.; Jones, N.G.; Paterson, K.J.; Fricker, F.R.; et al. A gain-of-function mutation in TRPA1 causes familial episodic pain syndrome. *Neuron* **2010**, *66*, 671–680. [CrossRef] [PubMed]
24. Nassini, R.; Materazzi, S.; Benemei, S.; Geppetti, P. The TRPA1 channel in inflammatory and neuropathic pain and migraine. *Rev. Physiol. Biochem. Pharmacol.* **2014**, *167*, 1–43. [PubMed]
25. Pokorski, M.; Takeda, K.; Sato, Y.; Okada, Y. The hypoxic ventilatory response and TRPA1 antagonism in conscious mice. *Acta Physiol.* **2014**, *210*, 928–938. [CrossRef] [PubMed]

26. Miyake, T.; Nakamura, S.; Zhao, M.; So, K.; Inoue, K.; Numata, T.; Takahashi, N.; Shirakawa, H.; Mori, Y.; Nakagawa, T.; et al. Cold sensitivity of TRPA1 is unveiled by the prolyl hydroxylation blockade-induced sensitization to ROS. *Nat. Commun.* **2016**, *7*, 12840. [CrossRef] [PubMed]
27. Hamilton, N.B.; Kolodziejczyk, K.; Kougioumtzidou, E.; Attwell, D. Proton-gated Ca(2+)-permeable TRP channels damage myelin in conditions mimicking ischaemia. *Nature* **2016**, *529*, 523–527. [CrossRef] [PubMed]
28. Peier, A.M.; Reeve, A.J.; Andersson, D.A.; Moqrich, A.; Earley, T.J.; Hergarden, A.C.; Story, G.M.; Colley, S.; Hogenesch, J.B.; McIntyre, P.; et al. A heat-sensitive TRP channel expressed in keratinocytes. *Science* **2002**, *296*, 2046–2049. [CrossRef] [PubMed]
29. Smith, G.D.; Gunthorpe, M.J.; Kelsell, R.E.; Hayes, P.D.; Reilly, P.; Facer, P.; Wright, J.E.; Jerman, J.C.; Walhin, J.P.; Ooi, L.; et al. TRPV3 is a temperature-sensitive vanilloid receptor-like protein. *Nature* **2002**, *418*, 186–190. [CrossRef] [PubMed]
30. Xu, H.; Ramsey, I.S.; Kotecha, S.A.; Moran, M.M.; Chong, J.A.; Lawson, D.; Ge, P.; Lilly, J.; Silos-Santiago, I.; Xie, Y.; et al. TRPV3 is a calcium-permeable temperature-sensitive cation channel. *Nature* **2002**, *418*, 181–186. [CrossRef] [PubMed]
31. Broad, L.M.; Mogg, A.J.; Eberle, E.; Tolley, M.; Li, D.L.; Knopp, K.L. TRPV3 in drug development. *Pharmaceuticals* **2016**, *9*, 55. [CrossRef] [PubMed]
32. Luo, J.; Hu, H. Thermally activated TRPV3 channels. *Curr. Top. Membr.* **2014**, *74*, 325–364. [PubMed]
33. Yang, M.; Chowdhury, R.; Ge, W.; Hamed, R.B.; McDonough, M.A.; Claridge, T.D.; Kessler, B.M.; Cockman, M.E.; Ratcliffe, P.J.; Schofield, C.J. Factor-inhibiting hypoxia-inducible factor (FIH) catalyses the post-translational hydroxylation of histidinyl residues within ankyrin repeat domains. *FEBS J.* **2011**, *278*, 1086–1097. [CrossRef] [PubMed]
34. Bracken, C.P.; Fedele, A.O.; Linke, S.; Balrak, W.; Lisy, K.; Whitelaw, M.L.; Peet, D.J. Cell-specific regulation of hypoxia-inducible factor (HIF)-1alpha and HIF-2alpha stabilization and transactivation in a graded oxygen environment. *J. Biol. Chem.* **2006**, *281*, 22575–22585. [CrossRef] [PubMed]
35. Bleymehl, K.; Perez-Gomez, A.; Omura, M.; Moreno-Perez, A.; Macias, D.; Bai, Z.; Johnson, R.S.; Leinders-Zufall, T.; Zufall, F.; Mombaerts, P. A sensor for low environmental oxygen in the mouse main olfactory epithelium. *Neuron* **2016**, *92*, 1196–1203. [CrossRef] [PubMed]
36. Cheng, W.; Yang, F.; Liu, S.; Colton, C.K.; Wang, C.; Cui, Y.; Cao, X.; Zhu, M.X.; Sun, C.; Wang, K.; et al. Heteromeric heat-sensitive transient receptor potential channels exhibit distinct temperature and chemical response. *J. Biol. Chem.* **2012**, *287*, 7279–7288. [CrossRef] [PubMed]
37. Dann, C.E., 3rd; Bruick, R.K.; Deisenhofer, J. Structure of factor-inhibiting hypoxia-inducible factor 1: An asparaginyl hydroxylase involved in the hypoxic response pathway. *Proc. Natl. Acad. Sci. USA* **2002**, *99*, 15351–15356. [CrossRef] [PubMed]
38. Elkins, J.M.; Hewitson, K.S.; McNeill, L.A.; Seibel, J.F.; Schlemminger, I.; Pugh, C.W.; Ratcliffe, P.J.; Schofield, C.J. Structure of factor-inhibiting hypoxia-inducible factor (HIF) reveals mechanism of oxidative modification of HIF-1 alpha. *J. Biol. Chem.* **2003**, *278*, 1802–1806. [CrossRef] [PubMed]
39. Lee, C.; Kim, S.J.; Jeong, D.G.; Lee, S.M.; Ryu, S.E. Structure of human FIH-1 reveals a unique active site pocket and interaction sites for HIF-1 and von hippel-lindau. *J. Biol. Chem.* **2003**, *278*, 7558–7563. [CrossRef] [PubMed]
40. McDonough, M.A.; Li, V.; Flashman, E.; Chowdhury, R.; Mohr, C.; Lienard, B.M.; Zondlo, J.; Oldham, N.J.; Clifton, I.J.; Lewis, J.; et al. Cellular oxygen sensing: Crystal structure of hypoxia-inducible factor prolyl hydroxylase (PHD2). *Proc. Natl. Acad. Sci. USA* **2006**, *103*, 9814–9819. [CrossRef] [PubMed]
41. Hewitson, K.S.; Schofield, C.J.; Ratcliffe, P.J. Hypoxia-inducible factor prolyl-hydroxylase: Purification and assays of PHD2. *Methods Enzymol.* **2007**, *435*, 25–42. [PubMed]
42. Linke, S.; Hampton-Smith, R.J.; Peet, D.J. Characterization of ankyrin repeat-containing proteins as substrates of the asparaginyl hydroxylase factor inhibiting hypoxia-inducible transcription factor. *Methods Enzymol.* **2007**, *435*, 61–85. [PubMed]
43. Chan, M.C.; Holt-Martyn, J.P.; Schofield, C.J.; Ratcliffe, P.J. Pharmacological targeting of the HIF hydroxylases—A new field in medicine development. *Mol. Asp. Med.* **2016**, *47–48*, 54–75. [CrossRef] [PubMed]
44. Flagg, S.C.; Martin, C.B.; Taabazuing, C.Y.; Holmes, B.E.; Knapp, M.J. Screening chelating inhibitors of HIF-prolyl hydroxylase domain 2 (PHD2) and factor inhibiting hif (FIH). *J. Inorg. Biochem.* **2012**, *113*, 25–30. [CrossRef] [PubMed]

45. McDonough, M.A.; McNeill, L.A.; Tilliet, M.; Papamicael, C.A.; Chen, Q.Y.; Banerji, B.; Hewitson, K.S.; Schofield, C.J. Selective inhibition of factor inhibiting hypoxia-inducible factor. *J. Am. Chem. Soc.* **2005**, *127*, 7680–7681. [CrossRef] [PubMed]
46. Dayan, F.; Roux, D.; Brahimi-Horn, M.C.; Pouyssegur, J.; Mazure, N.M. The oxygen sensor factor-inhibiting hypoxia-inducible factor-1 controls expression of distinct genes through the bifunctional transcriptional character of hypoxia-inducible factor-1alpha. *Cancer Res.* **2006**, *66*, 3688–3698. [CrossRef] [PubMed]
47. Engel, M.A.; Leffler, A.; Niedermirtl, F.; Babes, A.; Zimmermann, K.; Filipovic, M.R.; Izydorczyk, I.; Eberhardt, M.; Kichko, T.I.; Mueller-Tribbensee, S.M.; et al. TRPA1 and substance p mediate colitis in mice. *Gastroenterology* **2011**, *141*, 1346–1358. [CrossRef] [PubMed]
48. Kaneko, Y.; Szallasi, A. Transient receptor potential (TRP) channels: A clinical perspective. *Br. J. Pharmacol.* **2014**, *171*, 2474–2507. [PubMed]
49. Zhang, N.; Fu, Z.; Linke, S.; Chicher, J.; Gorman, J.J.; Visk, D.; Haddad, G.G.; Poellinger, L.; Peet, D.J.; Powell, F.; et al. The asparaginyl hydroxylase factor inhibiting HIF-1alpha is an essential regulator of metabolism. *Cell Metab.* **2010**, *11*, 364–378. [CrossRef] [PubMed]
50. Aijima, R.; Wang, B.; Takao, T.; Mihara, H.; Kashio, M.; Ohsaki, Y.; Zhang, J.Q.; Mizuno, A.; Suzuki, M.; Yamashita, Y.; et al. The thermosensitive TRPV3 channel contributes to rapid wound healing in oral epithelia. *FASEB J.* **2015**, *29*, 182–192. [CrossRef] [PubMed]
51. Hong, W.X.; Hu, M.S.; Esquivel, M.; Liang, G.Y.; Rennert, R.C.; McArdle, A.; Paik, K.J.; Duscher, D.; Gurtner, G.C.; Lorenz, H.P.; et al. The role of hypoxia-inducible factor in wound healing. *Adv. Wound Care* **2014**, *3*, 390–399. [CrossRef] [PubMed]
52. Cheung, S.Y.; Huang, Y.; Kwan, H.Y.; Chung, H.Y.; Yao, X. Activation of transient receptor potential vanilloid 3 channel suppresses adipogenesis. *Endocrinology* **2015**, *156*, 2074–2086. [CrossRef] [PubMed]

8

TRP Channels in Skin Biology and Pathophysiology

Michael J. Caterina * and Zixuan Pang

Departments of Neurosurgery, Biological Chemistry and Neuroscience, Neurosurgery Pain Research Institute, Johns Hopkins School of Medicine, 725 N. Wolfe St., Baltimore, MD 21205, USA; punfilict@gmail.com
* Correspondence: caterina@jhmi.edu

Academic Editors: Arpad Szallasi and Susan M. Huang

Abstract: Ion channels of the Transient Receptor Potential (TRP) family mediate the influx of monovalent and/or divalent cations into cells in response to a host of chemical or physical stimuli. In the skin, TRP channels are expressed in many cell types, including keratinocytes, sensory neurons, melanocytes, and immune/inflammatory cells. Within these diverse cell types, TRP channels participate in physiological processes ranging from sensation to skin homeostasis. In addition, there is a growing body of evidence implicating abnormal TRP channel function, as a product of excessive or deficient channel activity, in pathological skin conditions such as chronic pain and itch, dermatitis, vitiligo, alopecia, wound healing, skin carcinogenesis, and skin barrier compromise. These diverse functions, coupled with the fact that many TRP channels possess pharmacologically accessible sites, make this family of proteins appealing therapeutic targets for skin disorders.

Keywords: transient receptor potential; skin; pain; itch; dermatitis; epidermis

---

1. Introduction to TRP Channels

Transient Receptor Potential (TRP) channels constitute a large family of ion channels expressed across vertebrate and invertebrate animal species. Mammals express at least 28 different TRP channels that can be divided into six subfamilies, based on their primary amino acid structures: TRPA (ankyrin), TRPC (canonical), TRPM (melastatin), TRPML (mucolipin), TRPP (polycystin) and TRPV (vanilloid) [1–3]. TRP channels are widely distributed across tissues, such that every cell in the body likely expresses one or more subtypes. Furthermore, TRP channels can be gated by an astonishingly diverse array of physical and chemical stimuli, ranging from ions and small molecules to heat, cold, and mechanical force [1–3]. Consequently, TRP channels are important for many aspects of health and disease [4].

Functional TRP channels consist of four subunits surrounding a central channel pore. In most cases, TRP channels are homotetramers of a given subunit, while in others, subunits of two different TRP channel subtypes contribute to a heterotetrameric channel. Although there are some exceptions, as described later in this chapter, each TRP channel subunit possesses six transmembrane domains, interconnected by relatively short loops, plus a relatively long N terminal domain and a somewhat shorter C terminal domain, with the latter two both extending into the cytoplasm (Figure 1). In some, but not all subfamilies, the N terminal domain contains multiple copies of a motif known as the ankyrin repeat that contributes to channel assembly and gating [2]. Recent cryo-electron microscopy studies of TRPV [5–9] and TRPA [10] family members have provided a high-resolution view of the structures of these channels, as well as insights into how their pores can be gated by their respective activators. All known TRP channels are selective for cations, with little or no anion permeability. However, their relative selectivity among cations can vary. Whereas most TRP channels are so-called nonselective cation channels that show permeability to both monovalent cations such as sodium and divalent cations such as calcium and magnesium, a few are highly selective for either calcium or sodium ions [3].

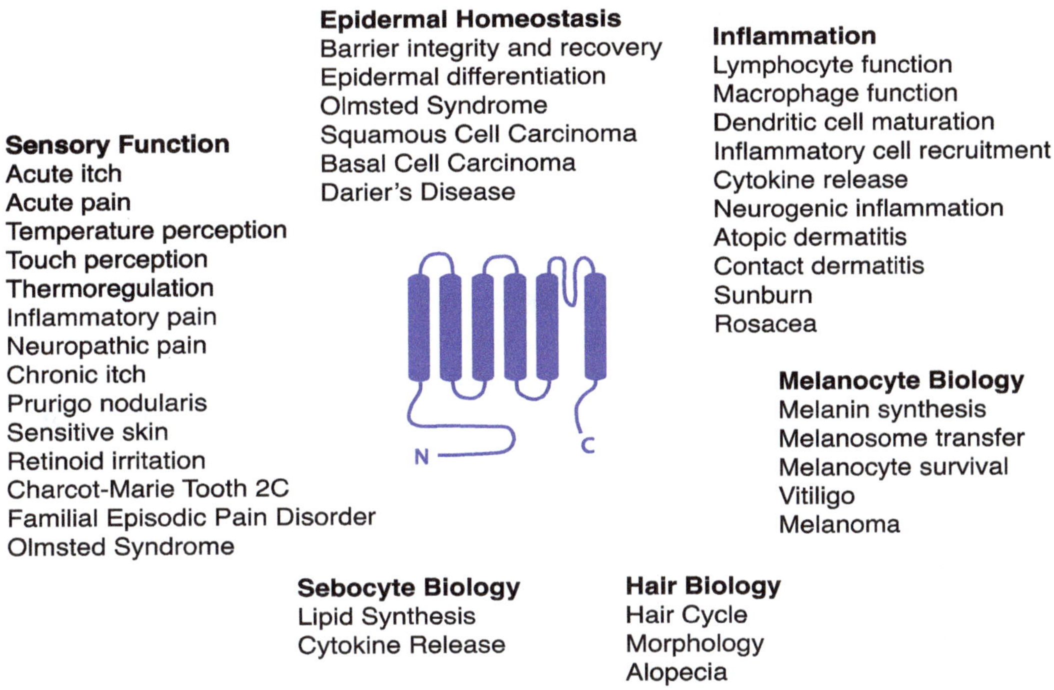

Figure 1. Summary of physiological (black) and pathophysiological (red) processes to which Transient Receptor Potential (TRP) channels contribute in various skin cell types. Topological diagram of a TRP channel subunit is shown at center, with amino (N) and carboxyl (C) termini labeled. Extracellular domain is at top.

Like other tissues, the skin expresses an abundance of TRP channel subtypes that significantly affect its development, integrity, and function under healthy conditions and in disease states [11,12]. There are a number of fundamental mechanisms, described in greater detail throughout this review, through which this occurs. Most notably, the ability of many TRP channels to mediate calcium influx into cutaneous neurons, keratinocytes, melanocytes, or immune cells provides a mechanism by which these channels influence cellular proliferation, differentiation, secretion of paracrine/autocrine factors, cytotoxicity, cell migration, and a host of other processes relevant to skin health and disease. Calcium is of particular importance to keratinocytes, since the skin exhibits a gradient of extracellular calcium from relatively low levels in the basal epidermis to relatively high levels in more mature epidermal layers. This gradient, in part, helps to drive the progressive differentiation of epidermal keratinocytes as they are displaced apically by proliferating basal cells [13]. Dysregulation of calcium homeostasis, as occurs in conditions such as Hailey-Hailey disease [14] or Darier's disease [15], results in abnormal epidermal differentiation, keratosis, poor adhesion between keratinocytes, and other abnormalities. Another important output of TRP channels is membrane depolarization. In cutaneous sensory neurons, TRP channel-mediated depolarization in response to a host of chemical, thermal, and mechanical stimuli triggers action potential firing, eventually leading to sensations of temperature, pain, or itch [16]. The effects of TRP channel-mediated depolarization, moreover, are not confined to neurons, since membrane depolarization in nonexcitable cells like keratinocytes or lymphocytes can affect cellular processes such as ATP release [17] or calcium flux through Orai family channels [18]. Finally, a growing list of protein interactors has been identified for TRP channels, further expanding the potential signaling repertoire of these molecules [19,20]. In this chapter, we will provide an overview of TRP channel expression in various cell types in the skin, as well as the physiological and pathological cutaneous processes to which they contribute. A summary of these diverse processes is presented in Figure 1, highlighting multiple opportunities for therapeutic targeting of TRP channels in skin.

2. Contributions of TRP Channels to Skin Biology and Pathophysiology

2.1. TRPC Channels and Skin

2.1.1. TRPC Channels and Keratinocyte Differentiation

Expression of nearly every TRPC channel subtype, including TRPC1, TRPC3, TRPC4, TRPC5, and TRPC6, has been reported in human keratinocytes. TRPC1 and TRPC4 are both upregulated during keratinocyte differentiation in vitro. This expression level change appears to be functionally important, since knockdown of either TRPC1 or TRPC4 in keratinocytes in vitro was shown to reduce the level of store-operated calcium entry and to inhibit keratinocyte differentiation [21,22]. TRPC6 has also been shown to be required for normal human keratinocyte differentiation in vitro [23]. In addition, small molecules of the triterpine family have been shown to promote keratinocyte differentiation both in vitro and in vivo through a mechanism that appears to involve TRPC6 [24].

2.1.2. TRPC Channels in Darier's Disease

Darier's Disease, also known as Darier-White disease, is a rare autosomal dominant dermatological disease initially discovered by the French dermatologist Ferdinard-Jean Darier in 1889. It is characterized by keratotic papules that may occur throughout the body [25]. Darier's Disease is caused by heterozygous loss of the endoplasmic reticulum calcium pump protein SERCA2b, which is encoded by the gene ATP2A2 located on 12q23-24.1 [26]. In addition to skin papules, patients with this disorder often suffer from neuropsychiatric symptoms [27]. There have also been reports of bone cysts [28]. Because SERCA2b is the only SERCA pump expressed in keratinocytes, this defect results in failure to sequester calcium in the ER lumen and the consequent accumulation of excess cytoplasmic calcium. Interestingly, examination of TRP channel expression in keratinocytes from heterozygous SERCA knockout mice revealed a compensatory upregulation of TRPC1 [29]. Although this change might a priori be predicted to worsen calcium overload in these cells, it was found that TRPC1 upregulation somehow enhanced keratinocyte resistance to apoptosis [29]. Whether compensatory TRPC1 expression ameliorates or exacerbates the Darier's Disease phenotype in intact skin, however, remains unclear. It also remains to be determined whether other syndromic features of Darier's disease involve alterations in TRP channel-mediated calcium signaling in skeletal or nervous tissues similar to those proposed for keratinocytes.

2.1.3. TRPC Channels and Sensory Function

There are numerous connections between TRPC channels and cutaneous sensory function. Although TRPC channels are expressed in most cell types, TRPC1, TRPC3, TRPC5 and TRPC6 are the subfamily members characterized most extensively in sensory neurons. Based on pharmacological studies with the relatively nonselective TRPC channel antagonist, SKF-96365, TRPC channels might also contribute to pain and hyperalgesia caused by the bee venom component, mellitin [30]. TRPC3 is expressed in small- to medium-diameter nociceptors [31–33], and has been shown to be important for store-operated calcium entry responses downstream of G protein-coupled receptors for purines and proteases [32], providing a potential mechanism for the involvement of this channel in some forms of inflammatory hyperalgesia. TRPC3 has further been implicated in nociceptor activation by IgG immune complexes and thus might be a contributor to pain in allergic contact dermatitis [34]. It has also been shown that TRPC1 and TRPC6, which are co-expressed in sensory neurons with TRPV4, facilitate hyperalgesic responses mediated by the latter channel, through mechanisms that have not been clearly resolved [31]. Further evidence for a role for TRPC1 in sensory function comes from the observation that this channel is required for normal mechanically evoked responses in two subpopulations of mechanosensory cutaneous neurons (Aδ-low threshold mechanoreceptors and slowly-adapting Aβ-low threshold mechanoreceptors) and for behavioral responses to very gentle mechanical stimuli [35]. Finally, TRPC5, which is also expressed in a subpopulation of peripheral sensory neurons that innervate the skin, can be activated by mildly cold temperatures. However, no obvious defects in cold detection were observed in mice lacking this channel [33].

2.2. *TRPV1 and Skin*

TRPV1 is among the most extensively characterized mammalian TRP channels. Upon gating, this channel produces multiple cellular signals, including membrane depolarization and an increase in cytoplasmic calcium. TRPV1 is expressed at the highest level in a subpopulation of peptidergic peripheral sensory neurons involved in the perception of pain. When overexpressed recombinantly in cell lines, TRPV1 can be activated by capsaicin, the major pungent ingredient in chili peppers, or by related chemical compounds that share a vanilloid chemical group, thus providing the "transient receptor vanilloid" subfamily its name [1]. TRPV1 can alternatively be activated by extracellular protons, by certain small lipophilic molecules, including endogenous cannabinoid lipids such as anandamide and N-arachidonoyl dopamine [1], or by a number of other chemical agonists such as 2-aminoethoxydiphenyl borate (2-APB), which had previously been recognized as a dose dependent activator and inhibitor of IP3 receptors and store-operated calcium channels [36]. In addition, TRPV1 was the first recognized molecular thermoreceptor, as it can be activated in the absence of chemical ligands by painfully hot temperatures (>42 °C) [1]. This polymodal chemo-thermo sensitivity likely accounts for the perception of "heat" experienced during consumption of chili peppers, and has led TRPV1 to receive substantial attention as a candidate target for pain control [37].

2.2.1. TRPV1 in Pain, Itch, and Neurogenic Inflammation

Gene knockout studies in mice, as well as administration of TRPV1 antagonists to mice, rats, and humans, have confirmed roles for this channel in pain sensation. For example, mice lacking TRPV1 are insensitive to capsaicin and show partially diminished heat-evoked pain at baseline and a virtual absence of inflammation-induced thermal hyperalgesia [38,39]. Reductions in heat pain [40], inflammatory pain [41,42] and cancer pain [43,44] sensitivity have also been observed in rodents and/or human treated with TRPV1-selective antagonists. Furthermore, a number of phase I and II clinical trials of TRPV1 antagonists have been conducted to examine their potential analgesic utility [45,46]. Studies using TRPV1 antagonists have also provided evidence for a role of TRPV1 molecules located at the central terminals of primary sensory neurons in certain forms of mechanical hypersensitivity, though the cellular mechanisms underlying such roles remain to be elucidated [47].

Beyond the perception of pain, TRPV1 has been shown to participate in other neuronal functions relevant to the skin. For example, TRPV1 null mice exhibit reduced itch-related scratching behavior in response to interleukin 31 (IL31) [48] or histamine [49]. TRPV1 also facilitates the function of TRPV4 in itch perception [50]. In addition, capsaicin-induced neurogenic inflammation (i.e., inflammation produced by the neuronal release of vasoactive peptides) is suppressed in the absence of TRPV1 [1,51]. Therefore, the interaction of neuronally-expressed TRPV1 with the skin is bidirectional, involving both sensory and efferent activities.

2.2.2. TRPV1 Expression in Keratinocytes

Aside from the functional importance of neuronally-expressed TRPV1, there is considerable evidence to suggest that TRPV1 may participate more directly in epidermal biology by virtue of its expression in keratinocytes. Evidence for such expression is strongest in human keratinocytes. Inoue et al. [52] first reported the existence of TRPV1-like immunoreactivity and TRPV1 mRNA in cultured human keratinocytes. They also showed that in these keratinocyte cell cultures, capsaicin or protons could evoke an influx of calcium that was inhibited by the TRPV1 antagonist, capsazepine. In contrast, whereas primary neonatal mouse keratinocytes and the mouse 308 keratinocyte cell line were shown to express TRPV1 mRNA, they did not respond to capsaicin in physiological assays [53,54]. Immunological, mRNA, and calcium imaging-based evidence for TRPV1 expression was also reported in the human HaCaT keratinocyte cell line [55]. In these cells, capsaicin could evoke the release of IL8 and prostaglandin E2 (PGE2) and upregulate the expression of cyclooxygenase 2 (COX2), providing evidence for potential proinflammatory activities. TRPV1 agonist-mediated calcium influx was also observed in human NHEK keratinocytes, and these responses, as well, could be blocked by either capsazepine or another TRPV1 antagonist, PAC-14028 [56]. Furthermore, heat shock was shown to trigger matrix metalloproteinase 1 (MMP-1) transcription in both HaCaT and NHK keratinocytes, in a manner apparently dependent on TRPV1 [57]. There is additional evidence that TRPV1 may be expressed in keratinocytes in intact healthy human skin. For example, Stander et al. [58] observed TRPV1-like immunoreactivity in keratinocytes of the stratum basalis and stratum granularis, as well as in dermal mast cells, hair follicles, sebaceous gland epithelial cells, and cutaneous sensory nerve terminals. A common problem with many human skin immunostaining studies is the absence of definitive controls for antibody specificity. However, the possibility of intrinsic cutaneous TRPV1 expression in that same study was corroborated by polymerase chain reaction detection of TRPV1 mRNA.

2.2.3. TRPV1 in Epidermal Homeostasis and Dermatitis

Despite the challenges of definitive demonstration of TRPV1 expression in rodent keratinocytes, multiple studies in rodents have suggested TRPV1 involvement in epidermal barrier function and the regulation of dermatitis. In hairless mice, capsaicin delays epidermal barrier recovery following tape-stripping and the TRPV1 antagonist capsazepine accelerates such recovery [59]. A potential role for heat as a mediator of this effect arose indirectly from the observation that barrier recovery is accelerated at relatively warm skin temperatures (36 °C–40 °C), compared with cooler temperatures. Agonists of two other warmth-sensitive TRP channels found in keratinocytes, TRPV3 and TRPV4 (see below), failed to recapitulate the effects of heat. In a series of studies [56,60,61], a TRPV1 antagonist, PAC-14028, was shown to accelerate skin barrier recovery either following tape stripping or in two models of atopic dermatitis: *Dermatophagoides farina* (Df) challenge in a susceptible mouse strain and challenge with the small molecule hapten oxazolone in previously sensitized mice. PAC-14028 also reduced rises in serum immunoglobulins, skin thickening, mast cell degranulation, and scratching behavior following repetitive Df administration. However, the apparent direction of TRPV1 effects on epidermal homeostasis and dermatitis has not been uniform across studies. In one study, oxazolone induced ear edema was increased in mice lacking TRPV1 or in wild-type mice in which TRPV1-expressing neurons were desensitized with vanilloid compounds [62]. The authors of that study postulated that anti-inflammatory agents released by TRPV1 expressing neurons accounted for the apparently anti-dermatitic effects of this channel. Although the reasons for discrepancies among these studies remain unclear, they might include the use of immunologically distinct mouse strains or off-target effects of some of the TRPV1 modulating agents used. Furthermore, a definitive dissection of the functions of neuronal vs. non-neuronal TRPV1 function in these models remains to be performed.

2.2.4. TRPV1 and Ultraviolet Radiation

Lee et al. [63] demonstrated that ultraviolet B (UVB) light could induce a calcium influx in HaCaT cells that was sensitive to TRPV1 antagonists, as well as an increase in MMP1 expression that was suppressed by TRPV1 antagonists and TRPV1 siRNA knockdown and facilitated by capsaicin. This study also reported a UVB-induced increase in TRPV1 western blot signal in HaCaT cells and a UVB induced increase in TRPV1 immunostaining in human skin. Based on their findings, the authors of this study speculated on a potential role for TRPV1 in UVB induced skin aging. Consistent with human keratinocyte studies, in hairless mice, the TRPV1 antagonist, iodo-resiniferatoxin, could suppress UVB induced skin thickening and expression of MMP, COX2, and p53 [64]. However, whether that effect was keratinocyte-intrinsic or neuronally mediated was again not definitively established.

2.2.5. TRPV1 Epidermal Upregulation in Human Skin Diseases

Elevations in either epidermal TRPV1-like immunostaining or skin TRPV1 mRNA expression have been reported in several different human skin diseases, including prurigo nodularis [58], rosacea [65], and herpes zoster infection [66]. In addition, there may be a link between TRPV1 and sensitive skin, as defined by augmented sensitivity in the lactic acid stinging test [67]. TRPV1 mRNA and keratinocyte TRPV1-like immunostaining were elevated in patients with positive responses in this psychophysical test [67]. These patients are presumed to have either an impaired skin barrier and/or alterations in their neurovascular responsiveness [67]. Interestingly, TRPV1 immunoreactivity was lower in individuals with darker skin, suggesting that melanin might interfere with those factors that promote TRPV1 upregulation [67]. Perhaps related to these findings, the skin irritant phenoxyethanol was found to increase calcium influx into HaCaT cells in a manner inhibitable by TRPV1 antagonists [68]. Furthermore, it has been shown that retinoids evoke pain behavior in rodents by acting at TRPV1, presumably in neurons. This might explain the burning sensation reported for these compounds in humans [69].

2.2.6. TRPV1 and Skin Cancer

Some studies have provided evidence suggestive of a connection between TRPV1 and skin cancer. However, these findings have often been indirect and relied upon pharmacological tools. For example, capsaicin was shown to be co-carcinogenic in rodent skin [70] and the TRPV1 antagonist AMG9810 was shown to act as a tumor promoter [71] However, in the former study, the effects of capsaicin turned out to be mediated by EGFR signaling, independent of TRPV1, while in the latter study, the TRPV1 dependence of the AMG9810 effects, which also somehow involved EGFR signaling, was not directly addressed. Thus, no role for TRPV1 in skin cancer has yet been definitively established.

2.2.7. TRPV1 in Skin Appendages

In human hair follicles, TRPV1-like immunoreactivity was observed in specific epithelial subcompartments, including the outer root sheath and hair matrix [58,72]. In organ cultures of these hair follicles, activation of TRPV1 suppressed epithelial proliferation and hair shaft elongation and promoted hair follicle regression [72]. TRPV1-like immunoreactivity has also been reported in epithelial compartments of mouse hair follicles, and examination of hair cycle in TRPV1 knockout mice revealed a delayed catagen phase [73].

There is also evidence for TRPV1 expression in human sebocytes, the major constituents of cutaneous sebaceous glands. In these cells, TRPV1 stimulation with capsaicin suppresses lipid synthesis and the release of proinflammatory cytokines [74].

2.3. *TRPV2 and Skin*

TRPV2 was originally discovered as a calcium-permeable channel that could be regulated by insulin-like growth factor I signaling [75], and in parallel, as a channel that could be activated by extremely high temperatures (>52 °C) [76]. TRPV2 was subsequently found to be capable of being activated by a range of stimuli, including PI3 kinase signaling [77], certain cannabinoid compounds (Δ9-tetrahydrocannabinol, cannabidiol) [78], probenecid [79], 2-APB [36], hypoosmolarity [80], and mechanical cell stretch [81]. In the skin, TRPV2 is most highly expressed in two categories of cells: sensory neurons and immune/inflammatory cells.

2.3.1. TRPV2 and Sensory Function

The contribution of TRPV2 to sensory function remains enigmatic. Although rodent TRPV2 has been shown to be activated by heat [76], mice lacking TRPV2 showed no detectable defects in noxious heat sensation, even if the potentially confounding activity of TRPV1 was eliminated [82]. Furthermore, heat sensitivity appears not to be conserved in human TRPV2 [83]. There is evidence that TRPV2 plays a role in neurite outgrowth, particularly in response to mechanical stretch of neurons [81] or nerve growth factor stimulation [84]. Whether this has implications for nerve regeneration in the skin has yet to be explored.

2.3.2. TRPV2 and Immune Cell Function

TRPV2 expression has been reported in a range of immune/inflammatory cell types, including macrophages, mast cells, natural killer cells, dendritic cells and lymphocytes [85]. Within these cell types, TRPV2 has been implicated in regulating diverse functions that include cytokine release [86], chemotaxis [87,88], phagocytosis [87], endocytosis [89], inflammasome activity [90], and podosome assembly [91]. In human skin, elevated TRPV2-like immunoreactivity was observed in both macrophages and mast cells in the setting of rosacea [65]. Aberrant TRPV2 expression has also been reported in hematological tumors and cell lines, including those derived from mantle cell lymphoma, multiple myeloma, Burkitt lymphoma, acute myeloid leukemia, and myelodysplastic syndrome [92,93].

2.4. TRPV3 and Skin

The cloning of TRPV3 was reported almost simultaneously by three groups [94–96]. TRPV3 mRNA and protein were shown to be expressed prominently in skin keratinocytes [94,96]. Like several other TRPV channels, TRPV3 can be activated by thermal or chemical stimuli. TRPV3 exhibits a temperature-dependent rise in activity at temperatures exceeding 33 °C–39 °C, with the specific apparent threshold varying among studies [94–96]. Reported chemical agonists of TRPV3 include 2-APB [36,97], farnesyl Pyrophosphate [98], and various plant-derived compounds, including camphor [99], carvacrol, eugenol, and thymol [100]. TRPV3 responses agonist stimulation can be further potentiated by several factors, including unsaturated fatty acids [101], repetitive heat stimulation [96], or cholesterol [102]. Conversely, factors that suppress TRPV3 activity include oxygen-dependent hydroxylation of TRPV3 by Factor-inhibiting-hypoxia inducible factor [103].

2.4.1. TRPV3 and Cutaneous Temperature Sensation

The robust expression of TRPV3 in keratinocytes, as well as this channel's heat-responsiveness, led a number of labs to investigate potential roles for this channel in skin temperature sensation. In vitro experiments in both the mouse 308 keratinocyte cell line and primary keratinocytes demonstrated warmth-evoked currents that resembled those mediated by recombinantly expressed TRPV3 [54]. Accordingly, these TRPV3-like currents were lost in keratinocytes isolated from TRPV3 knock out mice [99]. In contrast, TRPV3 protein proved difficult to detect in sensory neurons [99]. Together, these findings suggested that TRPV3 might participate in an "indirect" mechanism of heat sensation involving skin keratinocyte communication with sensory neurons. Consistent with this notion, TRPV3 was shown to mediate the heat-evoked release of a number of mediators with the capability to influence neuronal activity. For example, in keratinocyte-sensory neuron cocultures, heat activation was reported to produce a rise in keratinocyte calcium levels, followed by a delayed calcium influx response in the neurons, an effect that was apparently mediated by ATP signaling and dependent on keratinocyte TRPV3 [104]. It was also demonstrated that in keratinocytes, heat evokes the release of nitric oxide through a mechanism that is independent of nitric oxide synthase, and that this response is dependent on TRPV3 [105]. Similarly, keratinocytes cultured from mice overexpressing TRPV3 selectively in keratinocytes showed augmented release of prostaglandin E2 (PGE2) in response to both heat and 2-APB stimulation [106]. Together, these findings provided evidence that TRPV3 may serve as an important role in keratinocyte-neuron communication.

At the whole-animal level, there is also evidence that TRPV3 might contribute, under some circumstances, to heat perception. The original description of TRPV3 knockout mice reported that these mice exhibited deficits in both thermal preference behavior and heat-evoked nociception [99]. However, subsequent studies of these behaviors in TRPV3 knockout mice on more homogeneous genetic backgrounds yielded a more complex picture. Although the absence of TRPV3 on a pure C57Bl6 background produced no detectable change in thermally-evoked behavior, in two separate studies, TRPV3 knockout on the 129/S6 [107], or 129S1/SvImJ [105] backgrounds resulted in subtle alterations in thermal preference behavior. Interestingly, in one of these studies [105], the TRPV3 phenotype was sex dependent, occurring only in females. It should be noted that all these observations were made in global TRPV3 knockout mice, in which the channel was absent from all tissues throughout life. It is possible that a more definitive conclusion about the role of TRPV3 might be obtained from analysis of inducible keratinocyte- or neuron-selective TRPV3 knockout in adults. Mice lacking both TRPV3 and TRPV4 (see below) exhibited virtually normal thermal preference behavior and only a slight deficit in heat-evoked nociception [107]. However, in another study, it was demonstrated that while in mice lacking TRPV1 alone, a dynamic hotplate evoked an unusual escape behavior, this phenotype was abolished in mice lacking both TRPV1 and TRPV3 [108]. Thus, while TRPV3 might be a partial contributor to heat sensation under specific conditions, these genetic studies suggest that it is not a major participant in this process.

2.4.2. TRPV3 and Epidermal Homeostasis and Hair Development

A number of studies have implicated TRPV3 in epidermal homeostasis and hair growth. Global TRPV3 knockout in mice was originally reported to produce transient alterations in abdominal hair morphology [99]. Subsequently, selective knockout of TRPV3 in mouse keratinocytes was found to produce several skin phenotypes, including perinatal skin barrier defects and abnormal epidermal maturation that appeared to resolve spontaneously and curly body hair and whiskers [109]. Similarities to reported effects of perturbations in EGFR signaling led the investigators of this latter paper to explore a potential relationship between these two signaling proteins. Indeed, they found that activation of TRPV3 in keratinocytes triggers the protease-mediated shedding of the EGFR ligand, TGF-α. They also found that TRPV3 could promote transglutaminase activity in keratinocytes, providing a potential explanation for the skin barrier defects in TRPV3 knockout mice. At least one human study also implicated TRPV3 in the regulation of hair growth [110]. These authors showed that application of the TRPV3 agonists eugenol or 2-APB to either cultured human hair follicles or outer root sheath (ORS) keratinocytes, produced a dose-dependent suppression of proliferation and induction of apoptosis in both systems.

2.4.3. TRPV3 and Skin Pathology

There is also a growing body of evidence suggesting that TRPV3 is a key contributor to epidermal homeostasis and skin sensory function in certain pathological conditions. For example, although published studies are limited, there are reports in the patent literature that TRPV3 antagonists can suppress certain forms of mechanical hypersensitivity in rats after nerve injury [111]. In addition, it was reported that, in the mouse acetone-ether-water model of chronic dry skin, the genetic absence of TRPV3 resulted in reduced scratching behavior [112]. TRPV3-like immunoreactivity was also noted to be upregulated in the skin of breast surgery patients who reported postsurgical pain [113]. Similarly, TRPV3 mRNA was found to be upregulated in keratinocytes derived from patients with hypertrophic post burn scars who also reported itching [114]. Moreover, mouse studies have linked TRPV3 to epithelial wound healing in skin and oral mucosa [105,115].

The most compelling association between TRPV3 and skin pathology has come from the study of naturally occurring mutations in the gene encoding this channel. The earliest indications of this link came from rodent studies, where two TRPV3 mutations at the same residue (Gly573Ser and Gly573Cys, respectively) were found to be the causes of alopecia in two different rodent lines, the DS-Nh mouse and the WBN/Kob-Ht rat [116]. Further research by the same group [117] indicated that epidermal sheets derived from Ds-Nh mice exhibited elevated intracellular calcium levels. This finding is consistent with the subsequent finding that both the Gly573Ser and Gly 573Cys mutations confer a high level of constitutive activity on recombinant TRPV3 [118]. Additional examination of the in vivo consequences of these same TRPV3 mutations, resulted in additional skin phenotypes that included enhanced predilection towards evoked allergic contact dermatitis or, in some cases, spontaneous dermatitis [116,119]. The development of these dermatitis phenotypes was quite variable between studies and even within a study, between mice crossed onto different genetic backgrounds or housed under different conditions. This variable penetrance suggests the existence of both intrinsic and environmental modifiers of the dermatitis phenotype.

It is especially noteworthy that pathological gain-of-function mutations in TRPV3 are not confined to rodents. In 2012, whole-exome sequencing of six patients with Olmsted Syndrome revealed a TRPV3 mutation is strongly associated with this disease [120]. Olmsted Syndrome is a severe dermatological disease characterized by bilateral palmoplantar and periorificial keratoderma as well as severe itching or pain. Remarkably, the mutations discovered in Olmsted patients were homologous to those observed previously the Ds-Nh mice. The discovery of the link between Olmsted Syndrome and TRPV3 led to additional genetic studies in this condition. As a result, an increasing number of Olmsted patients were found to have TRPV3 mutations. Thus far, 10 TRPV3 mutations have been associated with approximately 20 Olmsted patients [121]. In addition, investigators recently discovered a gain-of-function mutation in a Chinese family that appears to be the cause of focal palmoplantar keratoderma [122] and another that was linked to another form of hereditary palmoplantar keratoderma without associated perioreficial lesions [121].

2.5. TRPV4 and Skin

TRPV4 was originally identified as a widely-expressed TRP channel that could be activated by changes in extracellular osmolarity [123–125]. Subsequently, it was shown that this channel could be activated by a range of physical and chemical stimuli, including cytochrome P450 metabolites of arachidonic acid [126], and warm temperatures [127]. Consistent with its expression pattern and wide range of activators, TRPV4 has been implicated in numerous processes in health and disease, many of which involve the skin.

2.5.1. TRPV4 and Epidermal Barrier Function

TRPV4 is abundantly expressed in skin keratinocytes [127]. A role for this channel in epidermal barrier homeostasis comes from the observations that activation of this channel increases intracellular calcium in human keratinocytes and promotes cell-cell junction formation between these cells, and that knockdown of TRPV4 expression impairs development of high transepithelial resistance in cultured human keratinocytes [128]. Furthermore, warm temperatures and chemical agonists of TRPV4 accelerate barrier recovery in explanted human skin tissues after stratum corneum removal [129].

2.5.2. TRPV4 and Skin Cancer

TRPV4 mRNA and immunohistochemical staining are reduced in premalignant skin lesions and in basal and squamous cell carcinomas [130]. Whether there is a functional role for TRPV4 in tumorigenesis has yet to be determined.

2.5.3. TRPV4 and Sensory Function

Multiple studies have provided evidence for roles for TRPV4 in sensory processes. In some cases, these functions are attributable to keratinocyte-expressed TRPV4, while in others TRPV4 channels expressed in neurons may be the more relevant pool. TRPV4 has been shown to participate in osmotically-evoked pain behaviors [131,132] and also in acute mechanical nociception [133,134] and in mechanical hyperalgesia in certain models of inflammatory [135–137] and neuropathic [138–140] pain. In some chemotherapy induced neuropathy models, mechanical hyperalgesia appears to involve alterations in the interactions between TRPV4, $\alpha 2\beta 1$ integrin, and src kinase [138]. Certain pro-algesic agents, such as agonists of the protease-activate receptor PAR2, also produce mechanical hyperalgesia through a process that involves TRPV4 [141]. TRPV4 has also been implicated in sunburn-associated hyperalgesia. TRPV4 mediates the release of the nociceptive/pruriceptive peptide, endothelin-1 from keratinocytes in response to UVB irradiation [142]. Moreover, mice lacking TRPV4 or treated with TRPV4 antagonists exhibited reduced UVB induced inflammation and mechanical and thermal hyperalgesia [142]. This effect is partially keratinocyte-autonomous, since it was observed in keratinocyte conditional TRPV4 knockout animals, and since TRPV4 mediates calcium entry into cultured mouse keratinocytes upon UVB exposure [142]. Consistent with these findings in mouse, TRPV4-like immunoreactivity was found to be elevated in human skin following UVB exposure [142].

There is a growing body of evidence implicating TRPV4 in itch perception. TRPV4 appears to play a role in itch perception in response to some, but not all pruritogens [143,144]. This is attributable at least in part to TRPV4 function in keratinocytes, where calcium influx through this channel triggers ERK phosphorylation. Scratching behaviors evoked by several pruritogens, including histamine, compound 48/80, and endothelin-1, but not that evoked by chloroquine, were partially suppressed in mice in which TRPV4 was deleted from keratinocytes [144]. However, contributions from sensory neuron-expressed TRPV4 to itch perception cannot be excluded. In both histaminergic and non-histaminergic itch, the contribution of TRPV4 appears to be facilitated by TRPV1 [50].

TRPV4 has also been implicated in innocuous warmth sensation, although the effect of TRPV4 knockout on this function is modest and condition-dependent. For example, whereas mice lacking TRPV4 were originally reported to show a shift in thermal preference on a thermal gradient towards slightly warmer temperatures [145], in later studies, as indicated above, mice lacking both TRPV4 and TRPV3 showed apparently normal thermal selection behavior, with only a slightly delayed withdrawal response to painful heat [107].

Numerous point mutations in TRPV4 have been shown to produce Charcot Marie Tooth disease type 2C [146–148]. Although not a skin disease per se, CMT2C is a sensorimotor degenerative disease that can include mild sensory loss.

2.6. *TRPV6 and Skin*

TRPV6 and Keratinocyte Differentiation

TRPV6, one of the most calcium-selective of mammalian TRP channels, is expressed in keratinocytes, where it plays important roles in epidermal differentiation [23]. Two different stimuli that are known to promote keratinocyte differentiation, elevations in extracellular calcium and 1, 25, dihydroxyvitamin D3, both upregulate transcription of TRPV6 [23]. This channel, in turn, mediates calcium influx to elevate basal intracellular levels [23]. As evidence of the importance of this process, in vitro siRNA silencing of TRPV6 suppresses the differentiation of keratinocytes in response to a calcium switch [23]. Moreover, one form of thermal spring water was shown to augment human keratinocyte differentiation in vitro through a mechanism that appeared to involve TRPV6 [149]. In addition, mice lacking TRPV6 exhibit an abnormally thin stratum corneum and a defective epidermal calcium gradient [150]. Although elevated TRPV6 expression has been associated with increased aggressiveness of prostate cancer [151], a potential link between TRPV6 and skin cancer has not been explored.

2.7. *TRPA1 and Skin*

TRPA1 is a nonselective cation channel that is abundantly expressed in a subpopulation of nociceptive sensory neurons, in addition to numerous other cell types. This channel is noteworthy for its direct and indirect responsiveness to an astoundingly diverse range of chemical, thermal, and mechanical stimuli. One large class of chemical TRPA1 activators includes electrophillic agents such as allyl isothiocyanate (mustard oil), cinnamaldehyde, acrolein, tear gas constituents, formaldehyde, and certain prostaglandins such as 15-deoxy-Δ12,14-prostaglandin J2. These electrophiles activate TRPA1 by covalent modification of specific cysteine residues located in the channel's cytoplasmic N-terminus. Many non-electrophillic chemicals, including certain anesthetics (e.g., propophol, isofluorane, lidocaine), fenamate nonsteroidal anti-inflammatory drugs, cannabinoids (e.g., Δ(9)-Tetrahydrocannabinol), cooling agents (e.g., icillin), and intracellular calcium ions can also activate TRPA1, presumably via more conventional ligand-receptor interactions. Its regulation by intracellular Ca^{2+} makes TRPA1 an effective integrator of other excitatory signaling pathways [152]. TRPA1 also exhibits a complex and species-specific pattern of thermosensitivity. In certain invertebrate and reptile species, TRPA1 can be activated directly or indirectly by warm temperatures and is essential for the detection of these temperatures in vivo [153–155]. Massive overexpression of TRPA1 in trigeminal sensory neurons likely accounts for the exquisite sensitivity of pit vipers to their warm prey [156]. In mammals, conversely, TRPA1 was originally reported to be activated by intense cold [157], a phenomenon that was recapitulated in some [158] but not all subsequent studies. Warm temperatures were shown to suppress and desensitize rat TRPA1 [159]. However, it was also recently shown that human TRPA1 exhibits a U-shaped temperature-response profile, with activation by both cold and heat. The complexity of this thermosensory behavior may in part be a consequence of strong TRPA1 regulation by modulating factors such as redox state [160]. TRPA1 proline hydroxylation analogously mediates changes in TRPA1 cold sensitivity in response to intracellular oxygen concentrations [161]. TRPA1 can also be activated in response to certain pathogen-associated molecular patterns and host-derived damage-associated molecular patterns. These effects can be either direct (e.g., lipopolysaccharide [162]) or indirect (e.g., let-7 miRNA acting via TLR7 [163]). Finally, TRPA1 has been implicated in mechanosensory processes [164–166]. However, this may reflect indirect mechanisms, rather than direct mechanical activation of the channel. Indeed, whereas classical mechanically-activated currents have not been reported in excised patches from cells expressing TRPA1, hypertonic stimuli can activate this channel in heterologous expression systems [167].

2.7.1. TRPA1 and Cutaneous Pain Sensation

The complex pattern of direct and indirect response characteristics described above renders TRPA1 an active participant in a host of sensory and non-sensory processes in both health and disease, many of which involve the skin. For example, studies employing knockout mice or TRPA1 selective antagonists have revealed essential functions for TRPA1 in multiple aspects of cutaneous pain sensation, including pain evoked by electrophilic chemicals (e.g., mustard oil, formalin) or mechanical stimulation [165,168,169]. In the case of cold-evoked pain, the importance of TRPA1 is less evident under baseline conditions, but becomes exaggerated in the setting of tissue injury or inflammation [170]. TRPA1 is also a key participant in two common models of pathological chronic pain, streptozotocin-induced diabetic neuropathy [171] and chemotherapy-induced neuropathy [172]. At least part of the acute pain component in the former model is attributable to activation of TRPA1 by streptozotocin-generated peroxynitrite [173]. However, even later stages of neuropathic pain, including the loss of peripheral nerve fibers, are inhibited by the inhibition of TRPA1 [174]. Moreover, methylglyoxal, a metabolic byproduct of diabetic hyperglycemia, is an electrophillic TRPA1 activator [171]. In the case of chemotherapy-induced neuropathy, TRPA1 appears to be activated indirectly by platin-induced alteration of redox state [172]. Mutations or polymorphisms in TRPA1 have also been linked to human pain. Patients bearing an N855S gain-of-function mutation in this channel are afflicted with Familial Episodic Pain Disorder, a condition associated with upper body pain that can be triggered by stressful stimuli such as fatigue, cold, or fasting [175]. Reactive oxygen species acting at TRPA1 may also be responsible for the augmented cutaneous sensitivity to ambient light in patients with porphyria, a potential contributor to pain in that condition [176].

2.7.2. TRPA1 and Itch

Multiple studies have shown that TRPA1 is also an important mediator of acute and chronic itch perception. Acute responses to non-histaminergic pruritogens (e.g., chloroquine, endothelin-1, compound 48/80) in the mouse are defective in the absence of TRPA1, owing to the positioning of this channel downstream of signaling by two pruritogen-sensing G protein-coupled receptors, MrgA3 and MrgC11 [177]. Endogenous pruritogens can also produce scratching behavior through TRPA1. For example, thymic stromal lymphopoietin (TSLP), which is released by keratinocytes in response to histaminergic signaling, activates neuronal TRPA1 downstream of the TSLP receptor [178]. Similarly, itch produced in response to bile acids, as might occur in the context of biliary obstruction, appears to be TRPA1 dependent, with the channel acting downstream of G protein-coupled bile receptors such as TGR5 [179]. The absence of TRPA1 has also been shown to reduce scratching behaviors in the acetone-ether-water mouse model of dry skin and chronic itch [180]. In addition, TRPA1 was upregulated in sensory neurons and TRPA1 antagonists reduced itch behavior in an interleukin 13-overexpressing transgenic model of atopic dermatitis [181]. Consistent with this observation, IL31 receptors were found to be colocalized with both TRPA1 and TRPV1 in sensory neurons, and genetic elimination of either channel reduced IL31-induced itch [48]. TRPA1 has also been shown to be an important contributor to the pruritis associated with contact dermatitis evoked by any of several different haptens [182]. This latter role might involve, among other mechanisms, direct action of TRPA1 by haptens, since 2,4-dinitrochlorobenzene and oxazolone, commonly used haptens for contact hypersensitivity experiments, have been shown to activate recombinant TRPA1 [182,183].

2.7.3. TRPA1 and Inflammation

As a nonselective cation channel expressed in nociceptive and pruriceptive sensory neurons, TRPA1 is ideally suited to trigger the membrane depolarization necessary for the pain and itch sensations ascribed to it in the previous sections. However, evidence from a variety of studies indicates that the participation of TRPA1 in pathological processes related to itch and pain extends beyond its sensory function to include an active role in inflammation. For example, in the acetone-ether-water model of chronic dry skin [180] and in several different models of contact hypersensitivity [182], mice lacking TRPA1 showed reduced epidermal thickening, a suppressed cytokine response, and reductions in other hallmarks of inflammation. A similar proinflammatory role for TRPA1 has also been observed in other tissues, such as the lungs of mice with allergen-induced asthma [184].

2.7.4. TRPA1 and Barrier Function

Although TRPA1 knockout mice have not been reported to exhibit any alterations in epidermal barrier function, there is pharmacological data to suggest that this channel can modulate barrier restoration. In hairless mice, cinnamaldehyde, mustard oil, and bradykinin all accelerated barrier recovery following tape stripping, and these effects could be blocked by a selective TRPA1 antagonist. Similarly, cooling of skin could accelerate barrier recovery, again in a manner inhibitable by the TRPA1 antagonist [185]. Given that TRPA1 and TRPV1 produce similar effects of cellular depolarization and calcium influx, it is interesting to compare these effects of TRPA1 activation with those described above for TRPV1, where channel activation appears to delay barrier recovery. Whether the apparently opposite consequences of activating these functionally similar channels relates to differential coupling to downstream signaling pathways, differential expression patterns, a complex consequence of channel activation and desensitization, or some other distinction remains to be determined.

2.7.5. Loci of TRPA1 Action in Its Cutaneous Functions

Within neurons, the apparent sites at which TRPA1 might mediate its sensory functions include not only the peripheral terminals, where TRPA1 triggers action potential firing, but also their cell bodies and their central terminals in the spinal cord dorsal horn, where TRPA1 can modulate neurotransmitter release onto spinal circuits [186]. At least a component of the pro-inflammatory roles of TRPA1 in skin and in other tissues such as lung might also be attributable to its expression in sensory neurons. When stimulated, many of the sensory neurons expressing TRPA1 release pro-inflammatory neuropeptides such as substance P (SP) and calcitonin gene-related polypeptide (CGRP) into their target tissues, with consequent vasodilation and plasma extravasation [51]. Moreover, pharmacological or genetic blockade of SP signaling was shown to attenuate the inflammatory response associated with contact dermatitis [182]. However, the relationship between neuronal peptide release and inflammation is not entirely straightforward, since the neurogenic release of SP and CGRP has been shown to paradoxically suppress recruitment of immune cells to sites of bacterial infection [187] and since these neurons might also release anti-inflammatory peptides such as somatostatin [188].

As with many other TRP channels, TRPA1 expression in the skin is not confined to neurons. For example, expression of this channel has also been observed in cutaneous mast cells, where it is upregulated in the interleukin 13 overexpression mouse model of atopic dermatitis [181].

There is also evidence for TRPA1 expression in keratinocytes, although again this finding might differ between species. While it was originally reported that TRPA1 is expressed directly in mouse keratinocytes, a recent study, called this finding into question [189]. Although this leaves the function of TRPA1 in mouse keratinocytes unclear, transient expression of TRPA1 in keratin 14-lineage cells and consequent roles in the establishment of mechanosensory circuits cannot be excluded as a possibility. By comparison, TRPA1 expression in human keratinocytes is more strongly supported. In human scalp skin-derived cultures, TRPA1 mRNA and a TRPA1-like Western blot band were observed in primary keratinocytes. TRPA1-like immunoreactivity was also observed in basal epidermal and hair follicle keratinocytes in skin biopsies [181].

TRPA1 mRNA and protein were also detected in human scalp skin-derived melanocytes, and fibroblasts [181]. Moreover, by means of its responsiveness to ROS, TRPA1 mediates the earliest component of the bimodal hyperpigmentation response of melanocytes to Ultraviolet A (UVA) irradiation [190]. Several human melanoma-derived cell lines were also shown to express TRPA1 and to exhibit calcium responses to TRPA1 agonists that could be suppressed by a TRPA1 selective antagonist. However, in the same study, TRPA1 agonist-induced changes in cellular proliferation were insensitive to this same antagonist, potentially arguing against a clear role for this channel as a target of melanoma therapy [191]. Given these findings, additional tools and experiments will be required to precisely define the sites at which TRPA1 produces its effects on skin biology and the mechanisms by which it does so.

2.8. TRPM1 and Skin

2.8.1. TRPM1 and Melanocytes

TRPM1 is prominently expressed in melanocytes, where it appears to participate in the generation of the photoprotective pigment, melanin, presumably by increasing intracellular Ca^{2+} levels [192]. Regulation of TRPM1 in melanocytes occurs at multiple levels, including transcription of TRPM1 mRNA [193], generation of different TRPM1 splice variants [194], TRPM1 activation downstream of G protein-coupled receptors such as metabotropic glutamate receptor 6 [195], and, possibly, miRNA regulation of TRPM1 mRNA stability or translation [196]. An early clue that TRPM1 was functionally important in melanogenesis came from the observation that mutations in the TRPM1 gene with incomplete dominance results in so-called "leopard spotting", the patchy loss of pigmentation in the skin of Apalloosa horses [197]. In humans, TRPM1 expression levels are correlated with melanin content, with greater levels of TRPM1 in populations with more heavily pigmented skin [198]. The contribution of TRPM1 to pigmentation might be relevant to the pathogenesis of human vitiligo. Lesional skin in patients with either localized or generalized vitiligo shows significantly reduced levels of TRPM1 mRNA expression [196]. Within melanocytic nevii, TRPM1 expression drops as the melanocytes progress towards a less-differentiated melanoblast phenotype that does not produce melanin [194]. TRPM1 might also be involved in UV induced changes in skin pigmentation, though this link has not been explicitly confirmed [192]. One barrier to better defining the biological functions of TRPM1 in this process is that mice lack epidermal melanocytes, and thus do not exhibit UVB induced pigmentation changes. However, experiments involving humanized mouse skin might help overcome this limitation [199].

2.8.2. TRPM1 and Melanoma

TRPM1 has also long been linked to melanoma, where reduced levels of TRPM1 expression and the appearance of alternatively spliced forms of TRPM1 mRNA are correlated with a less differentiated and more malignant phenotype [192,194]. While it is possible that TRPM1 activity, per se, contributes to melanoma progression and invasiveness, a more likely mechanism arises from the fact that miRNA 211, a tumor suppressor miRNA, is encoded in one of the introns of the TRPM1 gene and its transcription is co-regulated with that of TRPM1 [200].

2.9. TRPM2 and Skin

2.9.1. TRPM2 and Cutaneous Pain Sensation

TRPM2 is a widely expressed channel that can be activated by two types of stimuli: reactive oxygen species (e.g., H_2O_2) and warm temperatures. It was recently demonstrated that this channel is required for normal behavioral responses of mice to innocuous warm temperatures [201]. Consistent with this requirement, TRPM2 is expressed in a subpopulation of peripheral sensory neurons, and genetic elimination of TRPM2 results in an apparent reduction in the proportion of sensory neurons responsive to warm temperatures but not to other chemical agonists of heat-sensitive TRP channels. Curiously, however, the proportion of cells that express TRPM2 mRNA is far greater than that responsive to warmth. The basis of this discrepancy is unclear, but it might reflect inefficient translation or trafficking of TRPM2 protein or a requirement for other components for full thermal responsiveness.

2.9.2. TRPM2 and Melanoma

TRPM2 is also expressed in melanocytes and its activity can be suppressed by an endogenous dominant negative splice variant, TRPM2-TE. This splice variant is upregulated in melanoma, and either prevention of its synthesis or exogenous overexpression of full-length TRPM2 renders melanoma cells more susceptible to apoptosis and necrosis [194].

2.10. TRPM3 and Skin

TRPM3 and Cutaneous Pain Sensation

TRPM3 is expressed in a wide range of cell types, including a subpopulation of small to medium diameter sensory neurons. Like several other TRP channels expressed in this latter cell type, TRPM3 can be activated by painfully hot temperatures. It can alternatively be activated by chemical agonists, including the neurosteroid, pregnenolone sulfate and sphingolipids such as D-erythro-sphingosine [202]. Another curious feature of TRPM3 is that, in addition to a conventional nonselective cation pore, when this channel is stimulated with a combination of PS and clotrimazole, it exhibits a second, parallel ion permeation path, selective for small monovalent cations [203]. The physiological significance of this secondary conduction pathway, which resembles the "omega current" observed in some mutant voltage-gated sodium channels, has yet to be determined. Nevertheless, there is strong evidence supporting the physiological importance of TRPM3 to cutaneous sensory function. Neurons derived from mice lacking TRPM3 show defects in acute responsiveness to either PS or painful heat. Accordingly, these mice show behavioral deficits in response to these agonists, as well as defective heat hyperalgesia following inflammation with complete Freund's adjuvant [202].

2.11. TRPM4 and Skin

TRPM4 and Lymphocytes

Although TRPM4 expression has not been demonstrated in either keratinocytes or sensory neurons, it is expressed in various immune cell populations, including T lymphocytes. Comparison of TH2 and TH1 cells has revealed a higher TRPM4 expression level in the former cells [18]. Inhibition of

TRPM4 expression in TH2 cells leads to an elevation in intracellular calcium levels, with associated alterations in cytokine release profile. This seemingly paradoxical finding likely stems from the fact that TRPM4 is monovalent cation-selective, and activation of this channel depolarizes the membrane without associated calcium flux. That depolarization, moreover, reduces the electrochemical driving force for calcium influx through Orai channels. Thus, TRPM4 is poised to regulate T cell polarization and inflammatory responses in the skin.

2.12. TRPM7 and Skin

TRPM7 and Melanocytes

Although TRPM7 has not been studied extensively in mammalian skin, studies in zebrafish illustrate an important role for this channel in melanocytes. Melanocytes in mutant zebrafish lacking TRPM7 undergo death by necrosis [204]. This phenotype could be ameliorated by prevention of melanin synthesis, suggesting that the importance of TRPM7 is to facilitate chemical detoxification of intermediates of melanin synthesis.

2.13. TRPM8 and Skin

2.13.1. TRPM8 and Cutaneous Cold and Pain Sensation

TRPM8 was originally identified as a protein differentially expressed in prostate cancer cell lines. However, it was subsequently "rediscovered" as a receptor for cold-mimetic compounds such as menthol and icilin, as well as a channel that could be gated by mildly cold temperatures, themselves. TRPM8 is robustly expressed by a subpopulation of primary sensory neurons that are responsive to these same stimuli. Consistent with this expression pattern, genetic knockout experiments have shown convincingly that TRPM8 is required for normal responsiveness of sensory neurons to mild cold and, even more strikingly, for mouse behavioral avoidance of uncomfortably cool temperatures [205–207]. By comparison, the relationship of TRPM8 to pain is more complex. On the one hand, TRPM8 expression in a population of nociceptive neurons that also express TRPV1 appears to contribute to hypersensitivity to cold under conditions of inflammation or nerve injury. On the other hand, behavioral avoidance of intense cold is largely unaffected in TRPM8 knockout mice and under certain circumstances, TRPM8 stimulation (presumably in TRPM8-only neurons) actually suppresses pain sensitivity [208]. This cross-modal suppression is analogous to that observed between cold and itch perception [209], and is probably mediated by central nervous system circuits. At the same time, within sensory neurons, activation of mu opiate receptors leads to internalization of TRPM8 protein, providing a possible mechanism for opioid induced cold analgesia [210].

Another, recently identified TRPM8 activator is testosterone [211,212]. Androgen-dependent upregulation of TRPM8 gene expression has long been recognized in androgen-dependent prostate tumors [213]. However, in addition to its conventional transcription-mediated mechanisms of action, testosterone appears to activate TRPM8 by directly binding to the extracellular domain of the channel. In a recent human psychophysical study, testosterone application to the skin produced a cooling sensation, followed by a mild stinging sensation. This dual response was greater in female subjects than in males. Based on these findings, the authors speculated that testosterone acts as a natural cold-mimetic agent, but that high endogenous testosterone levels in males might desensitize TRPM8 over time. If true, this might account, in part, for the enhanced sensitivity of females to cold. Further experiments will be necessary to evaluate this provocative notion.

2.13.2. TRPM8 and Epidermal Homeostasis

With respect to non-thermosensory cutaneous functions for TRPM8, the earliest studies of TRPM8 knockout mice yielded no obvious epidermal phenotypes [205–207]. However, according to a more recent study [214], this lack of phenotype might have been a consequence of the specific strategies used to generate those mice, since those early strategies were based on disrupting exons encoding the TRPM8 amino terminus. Full-length TRPM8, which contains this domain, is not prominently expressed in keratinocytes. However, the authors of this recent study found that both human and mouse keratinocytes express an N terminally truncated TRPM8 splice variant lacking the N terminus and the first two transmembrane domains. They named this splice variant epithelial TRPM8 (eTRPM8). Genetically ablating the pore region shared by all TRPM8 isoforms, including eTRPM8, resulted in mice with an epidermal homeostasis phenotype. Specifically, these "pan-TRPM8 knockouts" exhibited a reduced proliferative cell number in the basal epidermis, an increase in superficial, late stage epidermal differentiation, and a reduction in the thickness of the stratum corneum. Unlike full-length TRPM8, eTRPM8 protein is confined to the endoplasmic reticulum, where it functions as a calcium release channel that facilitates elevations in calcium within adjacent mitochondria in response to canonical TRPM8 stimuli such as icilin, menthol, or cold. The authors of this study outlined two potential mechanisms by which this response might alter keratinocyte biology. First, mitochondrial calcium influx enhances synthesis of adenosine triphosphate, which when released from keratinocytes might alter their proliferation and differentiation in an autocrine manner. Second, in response to mildly cold stimuli, eTRPM8 augments production of superoxide, another candidate modulator of epidermal proliferation/differentiation. While these are certainly plausible explanations for the pan-TRPM8 knockout epidermal phenotype, additional cell type-specific knockout experiments will be required to determine whether the phenotype is truly a keratinocyte-autonomous phenomenon, or whether neuronal TRPM8 is also a contributor.

Other studies have provided additional links between TRPM8 and epidermal homeostasis. For example, TRPM8 agonists, like TRPA1 agonists, have been shown to accelerate barrier recovery following tape stripping of the skin and to reduce the epithelial proliferation response of the skin to barrier disruption [215]. It has also been reported that either chemical or thermal TRPM8 activation can reduce PGE2 release from human keratinocytes in response to UVB irradiation [216]. Whether these effects are mediated by full-length TRPM8 and/or eTRPM8 has not yet been established.

2.13.3. TRPM8 and Melanoma

TRPM8 expression has been observed in human melanoma cells, where its activation results in elevations in intracellular calcium and reduced cell viability [217,218]. This finding suggests that TRPM8 agonists might serve as candidate therapeutics for melanoma.

2.14. TRPML3 and Skin

TRPML3 and Melanocytes

Members of the TRP-mucolipin (TRPML) channel subfamily are most notable for their functions not at the plasma membrane, but rather within intracellular organelles. One member of this family, TRPML3, has been shown to be especially important for normal melanocyte differentiation [219]. TRPML3 is highly expressed in healthy melanocytes. However, a gain-of-function mutation in the TRPML3 gene is responsible for the phenotypic traits of varitint-waddler mutant mice, which exhibit a combination of a vestibular defect and coat pigmentation defects. The pigmentation defect appears to result from the constitutive elevation of intracellular calcium in the melanocytes of these animals, and their subsequent cell death.

3. Conclusions

In summary, numerous TRP channels are expressed in the cell types that constitute the skin, and they contribute in multiple ways to skin physiology under healthy conditions and to the pathological changes that occur in the setting of skin disease. Consequently, strategies aimed at this functionally diverse family of ion channels might provide useful means of combatting disorders of cutaneous homeostasis, sensation, and neoplasia.

Acknowledgments: Supported by the Neurosurgery Pain Research Institute at Johns Hopkins School of Medicine.

Author Contributions: Z.P. and M.J.C. both contributed to the writing of the manuscript.

References

1. Caterina, M.J.; Julius, D. The vanilloid receptor: A molecular gateway to the pain pathway. *Annu. Rev. Neurosci.* **2001**, *24*, 487–517. [CrossRef] [PubMed]
2. Montell, C.; Birnbaumer, L.; Flockerzi, V.; Bindels, R.J.; Bruford, E.A.; Caterina, M.J.; Clapham, D.E.; Harteneck, C.; Heller, S.; Julius, D.; et al. A unified nomenclature for the superfamily of TRP cation channels. *Mol. Cell* **2002**, *9*, 229–231. [CrossRef]
3. Ramsey, I.S.; Delling, M.; Clapham, D.E. An introduction to TRP channels. *Annu. Rev. Physiol.* **2006**, *68*, 619–647. [CrossRef] [PubMed]
4. Nilius, B.; Owsianik, G.; Voets, T.; Peters, J.A. Transient receptor potential cation channels in disease. *Physiol. Rev.* **2007**, *87*, 165–217. [CrossRef] [PubMed]
5. Agarwala, M.K.; George, R.; Pramanik, R.; McGrath, J.A. Olmsted syndrome in an Indian male with a new de novo mutation in TRPV3. *Br. J. Dermatol.* **2016**, *174*, 209–211. [CrossRef] [PubMed]
6. Cao, E.; Liao, M.; Cheng, Y.; Julius, D. TRPV1 structures in distinct conformations reveal activation mechanisms. *Nature* **2013**, *504*, 113–118. [CrossRef] [PubMed]
7. Huynh, K.W.; Cohen, M.R.; Jiang, J.; Samanta, A.; Lodowski, D.T.; Zhou, Z.H.; Moiseenkova-Bell, V.Y. Structure of the full-length TRPV2 channel by cryo-EM. *Nat. Commun.* **2016**, *7*, 11130. [CrossRef] [PubMed]
8. Liao, M.; Cao, E.; Julius, D.; Cheng, Y. Structure of the TRPV1 ion channel determined by electron cryo-microscopy. *Nature* **2013**, *504*, 107–112. [CrossRef] [PubMed]
9. Zubcevic, L.; Herzik, M.A., Jr.; Chung, B.C.; Liu, Z.; Lander, G.C.; Lee, S.Y. Cryo-electron microscopy structure of the TRPV2 ion channel. *Nat. Struct. Mol. Biol.* **2016**, *23*, 180–186. [CrossRef] [PubMed]
10. Paulsen, C.E.; Armache, J.P.; Gao, Y.; Cheng, Y.; Julius, D. Structure of the TRPA1 ion channel suggests regulatory mechanisms. *Nature* **2015**, *525*, 552. [CrossRef] [PubMed]
11. Caterina, M.J. TRP channel cannabinoid receptors in skin sensation, homeostasis, and inflammation. *ACS Chem. Neurosci.* **2014**, *5*, 1107–1116. [CrossRef] [PubMed]
12. Lumpkin, E.A.; Caterina, M.J. Mechanisms of sensory transduction in the skin. *Nature* **2007**, *445*, 858–865. [CrossRef] [PubMed]
13. Yuspa, S.H.; Hennings, H.; Tucker, R.W.; Jaken, S.; Kilkenny, A.E.; Roop, D.R. Signal transduction for proliferation and differentiation in keratinocytes. *Ann. N. Y. Acad. Sci.* **1988**, *548*, 191–196. [CrossRef] [PubMed]
14. Hu, Z.; Bonifas, J.M.; Beech, J.; Bench, G.; Shigihara, T.; Ogawa, H.; Ikeda, S.; Mauro, T.; Epstein, E.H., Jr. Mutations in ATP2C1, encoding a calcium pump, cause Hailey-Hailey disease. *Nat. Genet.* **2000**, *24*, 61–65. [CrossRef] [PubMed]
15. Sakuntabhai, A.; Dhitavat, J.; Burge, S.; Hovnanian, A. Mosaicism for ATP2A2 mutations causes segmental darier's disease. *J. Investig. Dermatol.* **2000**, *115*, 1144–1147. [CrossRef] [PubMed]
16. Basbaum, A.I.; Bautista, D.M.; Scherrer, G.; Julius, D. Cellular and molecular mechanisms of pain. *Cell* **2009**, *139*, 267–284. [CrossRef] [PubMed]
17. Zhao, P.; Barr, T.P.; Hou, Q.; Dib-Hajj, S.D.; Black, J.A.; Albrecht, P.J.; Petersen, K.; Eisenberg, E.; Wymer, J.P.; Rice, F.L.; et al. Voltage-gated sodium channel expression in rat and human epidermal keratinocytes: Evidence for a role in pain. *Pain* **2008**, *139*, 90–105. [CrossRef] [PubMed]
18. Weber, K.S.; Hildner, K.; Murphy, K.M.; Allen, P.M. TRPM4 differentially regulates Th1 and Th2 function by altering calcium signaling and NFAT localization. *J. Immunol.* **2010**, *185*, 2836–2846. [CrossRef] [PubMed]
19. Hanack, C.; Moroni, M.; Lima, W.C.; Wende, H.; Kirchner, M.; Adelfinger, L.; Schrenk-Siemens, K.; Tappe-Theodor, A.; Wetzel, C.; Kuich, P.H.; et al. GABA blocks pathological but not acute TRPV1 pain signals. *Cell* **2015**, *160*, 759–770. [CrossRef] [PubMed]

20. Kiselyov, K.; Shin, D.M.; Kim, J.Y.; Yuan, J.P.; Muallem, S. TRPC channels: Interacting proteins. *Handb. Exp. Pharmacol.* **2007**, 559–574. [CrossRef]
21. Beck, B.; Lehen'kyi, V.; Roudbaraki, M.; Flourakis, M.; Charveron, M.; Bordat, P.; Polakowska, R.; Prevarskaya, N.; Skryma, R. TRPC channels determine human keratinocyte differentiation: New insight into basal cell carcinoma. *Cell Calcium* **2008**, *43*, 492–505. [CrossRef] [PubMed]
22. Cai, S.; Fatherazi, S.; Presland, R.B.; Belton, C.M.; Izutsu, K.T. TRPC channel expression during calcium-induced differentiation of human gingival keratinocytes. *J. Dermatol. Sci.* **2005**, *40*, 21–28. [CrossRef] [PubMed]
23. Lehen'kyi, V.; Beck, B.; Polakowska, R.; Charveron, M.; Bordat, P.; Skryma, R.; Prevarskaya, N. TRPV6 is a Ca^{2+} entry channel essential for Ca^{2+}-induced differentiation of human keratinocytes. *J. Biol. Chem.* **2007**, *282*, 22582–22591. [CrossRef] [PubMed]
24. Woelfle, U.; Laszczyk, M.N.; Kraus, M.; Leuner, K.; Kersten, A.; Simon-Haarhaus, B.; Scheffler, A.; Martin, S.F.; Muller, W.E.; Nashan, D.; et al. Triterpenes promote keratinocyte differentiation in vitro, ex vivo and in vivo: A role for the transient receptor potential canonical (subtype) 6. *J. Investig. Dermatol.* **2010**, *130*, 113–123. [CrossRef] [PubMed]
25. Takagi, A.; Kamijo, M.; Ikeda, S. Darier disease. *J. Dermatol.* **2016**, *43*, 275–279. [CrossRef] [PubMed]
26. Sakuntabhai, A.; Ruiz-Perez, V.; Carter, S.; Jacobsen, N.; Burge, S.; Monk, S.; Smith, M.; Munro, C.S.; O'Donovan, M.; Craddock, N.; et al. Mutations in ATP2A2, encoding a Ca^{2+} pump, cause darier disease. *Nat. Genet.* **1999**, *21*, 271–277. [PubMed]
27. Gordon-Smith, K.; Jones, L.A.; Burge, S.M.; Munro, C.S.; Tavadia, S.; Craddock, N. The neuropsychiatric phenotype in darier disease. *Br. J. Dermatol.* **2010**, *163*, 515–522. [CrossRef] [PubMed]
28. Castori, M.; Barboni, L.; Duncan, P.J.; Paradisi, M.; Laino, L.; De Bernardo, C.; Robinson, D.O.; Grammatico, P. Darier disease, multiple bone cysts, and aniridia due to double de novo heterozygous mutations in ATP2A2 and PAX6. *Am. J. Med. Genet. A* **2009**, *149A*, 1768–1772. [CrossRef] [PubMed]
29. Pani, B.; Cornatzer, E.; Cornatzer, W.; Shin, D.M.; Pittelkow, M.R.; Hovnanian, A.; Ambudkar, I.S.; Singh, B.B. Up-regulation of transient receptor potential canonical 1 (TRPC1) following sarco(endo)plasmic reticulum Ca^{2+} ATPase 2 gene silencing promotes cell survival: A potential role for TRPC1 in darier's disease. *Mol. Biol. Cell* **2006**, *17*, 4446–4458. [CrossRef] [PubMed]
30. Ding, J.; Zhang, J.R.; Wang, Y.; Li, C.L.; Lu, D.; Guan, S.M.; Chen, J. Effects of a non-selective TRPC channel blocker, SKF-96365, on melittin-induced spontaneous persistent nociception and inflammatory pain hypersensitivity. *Neurosci. Bull.* **2012**, *28*, 173–181. [CrossRef] [PubMed]
31. Alessandri-Haber, N.; Dina, O.A.; Chen, X.; Levine, J.D. TRPC1 and TRPC6 channels cooperate with TRPV4 to mediate mechanical hyperalgesia and nociceptor sensitization. *J. Neurosci.* **2009**, *29*, 6217–6228. [CrossRef] [PubMed]
32. Alkhani, H.; Ase, A.R.; Grant, R.; O'Donnell, D.; Groschner, K.; Seguela, P. Contribution of TRPC3 to store-operated calcium entry and inflammatory transductions in primary nociceptors. *Mol. Pain* **2014**, *10*, 43. [CrossRef] [PubMed]
33. Zimmermann, K.; Lennerz, J.K.; Hein, A.; Link, A.S.; Kaczmarek, J.S.; Delling, M.; Uysal, S.; Pfeifer, J.D.; Riccio, A.; Clapham, D.E. Transient receptor potential cation channel, subfamily C, member 5 (TRPC5) is a cold-transducer in the peripheral nervous system. *Proc. Natl. Acad. Sci. USA* **2011**, *108*, 18114–18119. [CrossRef] [PubMed]
34. Qu, L.; Li, Y.; Pan, X.; Zhang, P.; LaMotte, R.H.; Ma, C. Transient receptor potential canonical 3 (TRPC3) is required for IgG immune complex-induced excitation of the rat dorsal root ganglion neurons. *J. Neurosci.* **2012**, *32*, 9554–9562. [CrossRef] [PubMed]
35. Garrison, S.R.; Dietrich, A.; Stucky, C.L. TRPC1 contributes to light-touch sensation and mechanical responses in low-threshold cutaneous sensory neurons. *J. Neurophysiol.* **2012**, *107*, 913–922. [CrossRef] [PubMed]
36. Hu, H.Z.; Gu, Q.; Wang, C.; Colton, C.K.; Tang, J.; Kinoshita-Kawada, M.; Lee, L.Y.; Wood, J.D.; Zhu, M.X. 2-aminoethoxydiphenyl borate is a common activator of TRPV1, TRPV2, and TRPV3. *J. Biol. Chem.* **2004**, *279*, 35741–35748. [CrossRef] [PubMed]
37. Gunthorpe, M.J.; Chizh, B.A. Clinical development of TRPV1 antagonists: Targeting a pivotal point in the pain pathway. *Drug Discov. Today* **2009**, *14*, 56–67. [CrossRef] [PubMed]

38. Caterina, M.J.; Leffler, A.; Malmberg, A.B.; Martin, W.J.; Trafton, J.; Petersen-Zeitz, K.R.; Koltzenburg, M.; Basbaum, A.I.; Julius, D. Impaired nociception and pain sensation in mice lacking the capsaicin receptor. *Science* **2000**, *288*, 306–313. [CrossRef] [PubMed]
39. Davis, J.B.; Gray, J.; Gunthorpe, M.J.; Hatcher, J.P.; Davey, P.T.; Overend, P.; Harries, M.H.; Latcham, J.; Clapham, C.; Atkinson, K.; et al. Vanilloid receptor-1 is essential for inflammatory thermal hyperalgesia. *Nature* **2000**, *405*, 183–187. [CrossRef] [PubMed]
40. Chizh, B.A.; O'Donnell, M.B.; Napolitano, A.; Wang, J.; Brooke, A.C.; Aylott, M.C.; Bullman, J.N.; Gray, E.J.; Lai, R.Y.; Williams, P.M.; et al. The effects of the TRPV1 antagonist SB-705498 on TRPV1 receptor-mediated activity and inflammatory hyperalgesia in humans. *Pain* **2007**, *132*, 132–141. [CrossRef] [PubMed]
41. Gavva, N.R.; Tamir, R.; Qu, Y.; Klionsky, L.; Zhang, T.J.; Immke, D.; Wang, J.; Zhu, D.; Vanderah, T.W.; Porreca, F.; et al. AMG 9810 [(*E*)-3-(4-*t*-butylphenyl)-*N*-(2,3-dihydrobenzo[b][1,4] dioxin-6-yl)acrylamide], a novel vanilloid receptor 1 (TRPV1) antagonist with antihyperalgesic properties. *J. Pharmacol. Exp. Ther.* **2005**, *313*, 474–484. [CrossRef] [PubMed]
42. Puttfarcken, P.S.; Han, P.; Joshi, S.K.; Neelands, T.R.; Gauvin, D.M.; Baker, S.J.; Lewis, L.G.; Bianchi, B.R.; Mikusa, J.P.; Koenig, J.R.; et al. A-995662 [(*R*)-8-(4-methyl-5-(4-(trifluoromethyl)phenyl)oxazol-2-ylamino)-1,2,3,4-tetrahydr onaphthalen-2-ol], a novel, selective TRPV1 receptor antagonist, reduces spinal release of glutamate and CGRP in a rat knee joint pain model. *Pain* **2010**, *150*, 319–326. [CrossRef] [PubMed]
43. Ghilardi, J.R.; Rohrich, H.; Lindsay, T.H.; Sevcik, M.A.; Schwei, M.J.; Kubota, K.; Halvorson, K.G.; Poblete, J.; Chaplan, S.R.; Dubin, A.E.; et al. Selective blockade of the capsaicin receptor TRPV1 attenuates bone cancer pain. *J. Neurosci.* **2005**, *25*, 3126–3131. [CrossRef] [PubMed]
44. Niiyama, Y.; Kawamata, T.; Yamamoto, J.; Furuse, S.; Namiki, A. SB366791, a TRPV1 antagonist, potentiates analgesic effects of systemic morphine in a murine model of bone cancer pain. *Br. J. Anaesth.* **2009**, *102*, 251–258. [CrossRef] [PubMed]
45. Lee, Y.; Hong, S.; Cui, M.; Sharma, P.K.; Lee, J.; Choi, S. Transient receptor potential vanilloid type 1 antagonists: A patent review (2011–2014). *Expert Opin. Ther. Pat.* **2015**, *25*, 291–318. [CrossRef] [PubMed]
46. Rami, H.K.; Gunthorpe, M.J. The therapeutic potential of TRPV1 (VR1) antagonists: Clinical answers await. *Drug Disc. Today Ther. Strateg.* **2004**. [CrossRef]
47. McGaraughty, S.; Chu, K.L.; Faltynek, C.R.; Jarvis, M.F. Systemic and site-specific effects of a-425619, a selective TRPV1 receptor antagonist, on wide dynamic range neurons in CFA-treated and uninjured rats. *J. Neurophysiol.* **2006**, *95*, 18–25. [CrossRef] [PubMed]
48. Cevikbas, F.; Wang, X.; Akiyama, T.; Kempkes, C.; Savinko, T.; Antal, A.; Kukova, G.; Buhl, T.; Ikoma, A.; Buddenkotte, J.; et al. A sensory neuron-expressed IL-31 receptor mediates T helper cell-dependent itch: Involvement of TRPV1 and TRPA1. *J. Allergy Clin. Immunol.* **2014**, *133*, 448–460. [CrossRef] [PubMed]
49. Shim, W.S.; Tak, M.H.; Lee, M.H.; Kim, M.; Kim, M.; Koo, J.Y.; Lee, C.H.; Kim, M.; Oh, U. TRPV1 mediates histamine-induced itching via the activation of phospholipase A2 and 12-lipoxygenase. *J. Neurosci.* **2007**, *27*, 2331–2337. [CrossRef] [PubMed]
50. Kim, S.; Barry, D.M.; Liu, X.Y.; Yin, S.; Munanairi, A.; Meng, Q.T.; Cheng, W.; Mo, P.; Wan, L.; Liu, S.B.; et al. Facilitation of TRPV4 by TRPV1 is required for itch transmission in some sensory neuron populations. *Sci. Signal.* **2016**, *9*, ra71. [CrossRef] [PubMed]
51. Geppetti, P.; Nassini, R.; Materazzi, S.; Benemei, S. The concept of neurogenic inflammation. *BJU Int.* **2008**, *101* (Suppl. 3), 2–6. [CrossRef] [PubMed]
52. Inoue, K.; Koizumi, S.; Fuziwara, S.; Denda, S.; Inoue, K.; Denda, M. Functional vanilloid receptors in cultured normal human epidermal keratinocytes. *Biochem. Biophys. Res. Commun.* **2002**, *291*, 124–129. [CrossRef] [PubMed]
53. Chung, M.K.; Lee, H.; Caterina, M.J. Warm temperatures activate TRPV4 in mouse 308 keratinocytes. *J. Biol. Chem.* **2003**, *278*, 32037–32046. [CrossRef] [PubMed]
54. Chung, M.K.; Lee, H.; Mizuno, A.; Suzuki, M.; Caterina, M.J. TRPV3 and TRPV4 mediate warmth-evoked currents in primary mouse keratinocytes. *J. Biol. Chem.* **2004**, *279*, 21569–21575. [CrossRef] [PubMed]
55. Southall, M.D.; Li, T.; Gharibova, L.S.; Pei, Y.; Nicol, G.D.; Travers, J.B. Activation of epidermal vanilloid receptor-1 induces release of proinflammatory mediators in human keratinocytes. *J. Pharmacol. Exp. Ther.* **2003**, *304*, 217–222. [CrossRef] [PubMed]

56. Yun, J.W.; Seo, J.A.; Jeong, Y.S.; Bae, I.H.; Jang, W.H.; Lee, J.; Kim, S.Y.; Shin, S.S.; Woo, B.Y.; Lee, K.W.; et al. TRPV1 antagonist can suppress the atopic dermatitis-like symptoms by accelerating skin barrier recovery. *J. Dermatol. Sci* **2011**, *62*, 8–15. [CrossRef] [PubMed]
57. Li, W.H.; Lee, Y.M.; Kim, J.Y.; Kang, S.; Kim, S.; Kim, K.H.; Park, C.H.; Chung, J.H. Transient receptor potential vanilloid-1 mediates heat-shock-induced matrix metalloproteinase-1 expression in human epidermal keratinocytes. *J. Investig. Dermatol.* **2007**, *127*, 2328–2335. [CrossRef] [PubMed]
58. Stander, S.; Moormann, C.; Schumacher, M.; Buddenkotte, J.; Artuc, M.; Shpacovitch, V.; Brzoska, T.; Lippert, U.; Henz, B.M.; Luger, T.A.; et al. Expression of vanilloid receptor subtype 1 in cutaneous sensory nerve fibers, mast cells, and epithelial cells of appendage structures. *Exp. Dermatol.* **2004**, *13*, 129–139. [CrossRef] [PubMed]
59. Denda, M.; Sokabe, T.; Fukumi-Tominaga, T.; Tominaga, M. Effects of skin surface temperature on epidermal permeability barrier homeostasis. *J. Investig. Dermatol.* **2007**, *127*, 654–659. [CrossRef] [PubMed]
60. Lim, K.M.; Park, Y.H. Development of PAC-14028, a novel transient receptor potential vanilloid type 1 (TRPV1) channel antagonist as a new drug for refractory skin diseases. *Arch. Pharm. Res.* **2012**, *35*, 393–396. [CrossRef] [PubMed]
61. Yun, J.W.; Seo, J.A.; Jang, W.H.; Koh, H.J.; Bae, I.H.; Park, Y.H.; Lim, K.M. Antipruritic effects of TRPV1 antagonist in murine atopic dermatitis and itching models. *J. Investig. Dermatol.* **2011**, *131*, 1576–1579. [CrossRef] [PubMed]
62. Banvolgyi, A.; Palinkas, L.; Berki, T.; Clark, N.; Grant, A.D.; Helyes, Z.; Pozsgai, G.; Szolcsanyi, J.; Brain, S.D.; Pinter, E. Evidence for a novel protective role of the vanilloid TRPV1 receptor in a cutaneous contact allergic dermatitis model. *J. Neuroimmunol.* **2005**, *169*, 86–96. [CrossRef] [PubMed]
63. Lee, Y.M.; Kim, Y.K.; Kim, K.H.; Park, S.J.; Kim, S.J.; Chung, J.H. A novel role for the TRPV1 channel in UV-induced matrix metalloproteinase (MMP)-1 expression in HaCaT cells. *J. Cell. Physiol.* **2009**, *219*, 766–775. [CrossRef] [PubMed]
64. Lee, Y.M.; Kang, S.M.; Lee, S.R.; Kong, K.H.; Lee, J.Y.; Kim, E.J.; Chung, J.H. Inhibitory effects of TRPV1 blocker on UV-induced responses in the hairless mice. *Arch. Dermatol. Res.* **2011**, *303*, 727–736. [CrossRef] [PubMed]
65. Sulk, M.; Seeliger, S.; Aubert, J.; Schwab, V.D.; Cevikbas, F.; Rivier, M.; Nowak, P.; Voegel, J.J.; Buddenkotte, J.; Steinhoff, M. Distribution and expression of non-neuronal transient receptor potential (TRPV) ion channels in rosacea. *J. Investig. Dermatol.* **2012**, *132*, 1253–1262. [CrossRef] [PubMed]
66. Han, S.B.; Kim, H.; Cho, S.H.; Lee, J.D.; Chung, J.H.; Kim, H.S. Transient receptor potential vanilloid-1 in epidermal keratinocytes may contribute to acute pain in herpes zoster. *Acta Derm. Venereol.* **2016**, *96*, 319–322. [CrossRef] [PubMed]
67. Ehnis-Perez, A.; Torres-Alvarez, B.; Cortes-Garcia, D.; Hernandez-Blanco, D.; Fuentes-Ahumada, C.; Castanedo-Cazares, J.P. Relationship between transient receptor potential vanilloid-1 expression and the intensity of sensitive skin symptoms. *J. Cosmet. Dermatol.* **2016**, *15*, 231–237. [CrossRef] [PubMed]
68. Li, D.G.; Du, H.Y.; Gerhard, S.; Imke, M.; Liu, W. Inhibition of TRPV1 prevented skin irritancy induced by phenoxyethanol. A preliminary in vitro and in vivo study. *Int. J. Cosmet. Sci.* **2016**. [CrossRef]
69. Yin, S.; Luo, J.; Qian, A.; Du, J.; Yang, Q.; Zhou, S.; Yu, W.; Du, G.; Clark, R.B.; Walters, E.T.; et al. Retinoids activate the irritant receptor TRPV1 and produce sensory hypersensitivity. *J. Clin. Investig.* **2013**, *123*, 3941–3951. [CrossRef] [PubMed]
70. Hwang, M.K.; Bode, A.M.; Byun, S.; Song, N.R.; Lee, H.J.; Lee, K.W.; Dong, Z. Cocarcinogenic effect of capsaicin involves activation of EGFR signaling but not TRPV1. *Cancer Res.* **2010**, *70*, 6859–6869. [CrossRef] [PubMed]
71. Li, S.; Bode, A.M.; Zhu, F.; Liu, K.; Zhang, J.; Kim, M.O.; Reddy, K.; Zykova, T.; Ma, W.Y.; Carper, A.L.; et al. TRPV1-antagonist AMG9810 promotes mouse skin tumorigenesis through EGFR/akt signaling. *Carcinogenesis* **2011**, *32*, 779–785. [CrossRef] [PubMed]
72. Bodo, E.; Biro, T.; Telek, A.; Czifra, G.; Griger, Z.; Toth, B.I.; Mescalchin, A.; Ito, T.; Bettermann, A.; Kovacs, L.; et al. A hot new twist to hair biology: Involvement of vanilloid receptor-1 (VR1/TRPV1) signaling in human hair growth control. *Am. J. Pathol.* **2005**, *166*, 985–998. [CrossRef]
73. Biro, T.; Bodo, E.; Telek, A.; Geczy, T.; Tychsen, B.; Kovacs, L.; Paus, R. Hair cycle control by vanilloid receptor-1 (TRPV1): Evidence from TRPV1 knockout mice. *J. Investig. Dermatol.* **2006**, *126*, 1909–1912. [CrossRef] [PubMed]

74. Toth, B.I.; Benko, S.; Szollosi, A.G.; Kovacs, L.; Rajnavolgyi, E.; Biro, T. Transient receptor potential vanilloid-1 signaling inhibits differentiation and activation of human dendritic cells. *FEBS Lett.* **2009**, *583*, 1619–1624. [CrossRef] [PubMed]
75. Kanzaki, M.; Zhang, Y.Q.; Mashima, H.; Li, L.; Shibata, H.; Kojima, I. Translocation of a calcium-permeable cation channel induced by insulin-like growth factor-i. *Nat. Cell Biol.* **1999**, *1*, 165–170. [PubMed]
76. Caterina, M.J.; Rosen, T.A.; Tominaga, M.; Brake, A.J.; Julius, D. A capsaicin receptor homologue with a high threshold for noxious heat. *Nature* **1999**, *398*, 436–441. [PubMed]
77. Penna, A.; Juvin, V.; Chemin, J.; Compan, V.; Monet, M.; Rassendren, F.A. Pi3-kinase promotes TRPV2 activity independently of channel translocation to the plasma membrane. *Cell Calcium* **2006**, *39*, 495–507. [CrossRef] [PubMed]
78. Qin, N.; Neeper, M.P.; Liu, Y.; Hutchinson, T.L.; Lubin, M.L.; Flores, C.M. TRPV2 is activated by cannabidiol and mediates CGRP release in cultured rat dorsal root ganglion neurons. *J. Neurosci.* **2008**, *28*, 6231–6238. [CrossRef] [PubMed]
79. Bang, S.; Kim, K.Y.; Yoo, S.; Lee, S.H.; Hwang, S.W. Transient receptor potential V2 expressed in sensory neurons is activated by probenecid. *Neurosci. Lett.* **2007**, *425*, 120–125. [CrossRef] [PubMed]
80. Muraki, K.; Iwata, Y.; Katanosaka, Y.; Ito, T.; Ohya, S.; Shigekawa, M.; Imaizumi, Y. TRPV2 is a component of osmotically sensitive cation channels in murine aortic myocytes. *Circ. Res.* **2003**, *93*, 829–838. [CrossRef] [PubMed]
81. Shibasaki, K.; Murayama, N.; Ono, K.; Ishizaki, Y.; Tominaga, M. TRPV2 enhances axon outgrowth through its activation by membrane stretch in developing sensory and motor neurons. *J. Neurosci.* **2010**, *30*, 4601–4612. [CrossRef] [PubMed]
82. Park, U.; Vastani, N.; Guan, Y.; Raja, S.N.; Koltzenburg, M.; Caterina, M.J. TRP vanilloid 2 knock-out mice are susceptible to perinatal lethality but display normal thermal and mechanical nociception. *J. Neurosci.* **2011**, *31*, 11425–11436. [CrossRef] [PubMed]
83. Neeper, M.P.; Liu, Y.; Hutchinson, T.L.; Wang, Y.; Flores, C.M.; Qin, N. Activation properties of heterologously expressed mammalian TRPV2: Evidence for species dependence. *J. Biol. Chem.* **2007**, *282*, 15894–15902. [CrossRef] [PubMed]
84. Cohen, M.R.; Johnson, W.M.; Pilat, J.M.; Kiselar, J.; DeFrancesco-Lisowitz, A.; Zigmond, R.E.; Moiseenkova-Bell, V.Y. Nerve growth factor regulates transient receptor potential vanilloid 2 via extracellular signal-regulated kinase signaling to enhance neurite outgrowth in developing neurons. *Mol. Cell. Biol.* **2015**, *35*, 4238–4252. [CrossRef] [PubMed]
85. Santoni, G.; Farfariello, V.; Liberati, S.; Morelli, M.B.; Nabissi, M.; Santoni, M.; Amantini, C. The role of transient receptor potential vanilloid type-2 ion channels in innate and adaptive immune responses. *Front. Immunol.* **2013**, *4*, 34. [CrossRef] [PubMed]
86. Yamashiro, K.; Sasano, T.; Tojo, K.; Namekata, I.; Kurokawa, J.; Sawada, N.; Suganami, T.; Kamei, Y.; Tanaka, H.; Tajima, N.; et al. Role of transient receptor potential vanilloid 2 in LPS-induced cytokine production in macrophages. *Biochem. Biophys. Res. Commun.* **2010**, *398*, 284–289. [CrossRef] [PubMed]
87. Link, T.M.; Park, U.; Vonakis, B.M.; Raben, D.M.; Soloski, M.J.; Caterina, M.J. TRPV2 has a pivotal role in macrophage particle binding and phagocytosis. *Nat. Immunol.* **2010**, *11*, 232–239. [CrossRef] [PubMed]
88. Nagasawa, M.; Nakagawa, Y.; Tanaka, S.; Kojima, I. Chemotactic peptide fmetleuphe induces translocation of the TRPV2 channel in macrophages. *J. Cell. Physiol.* **2007**, *210*, 692–702. [CrossRef] [PubMed]
89. Szollosi, A.G.; Olah, A.; Toth, I.B.; Papp, F.; Czifra, G.; Panyi, G.; Biro, T. Transient receptor potential vanilloid-2 mediates the effects of transient heat shock on endocytosis of human monocyte-derived dendritic cells. *FEBS Lett.* **2013**, *587*, 1440–1445. [CrossRef] [PubMed]
90. Compan, V.; Baroja-Mazo, A.; Lopez-Castejon, G.; Gomez, A.I.; Martinez, C.M.; Angosto, D.; Montero, M.T.; Herranz, A.S.; Bazan, E.; Reimers, D.; et al. Cell volume regulation modulates NLRP3 inflammasome activation. *Immunity* **2012**, *37*, 487–500. [CrossRef] [PubMed]
91. Nagasawa, M.; Kojima, I. Translocation of calcium-permeable TRPV2 channel to the podosome: Its role in the regulation of podosome assembly. *Cell Calcium* **2012**, *51*, 186–193. [CrossRef] [PubMed]
92. Liberati, S.; Morelli, M.B.; Amantini, C.; Farfariello, V.; Santoni, M.; Conti, A.; Nabissi, M.; Cascinu, S.; Santoni, G. Loss of TRPV2 homeostatic control of cell proliferation drives tumor progression. *Cells* **2014**, *3*, 112–128. [CrossRef] [PubMed]

93. Morelli, M.B.; Liberati, S.; Amantini, C.; Nabiss, M.; Santoni, M.; Farfariello, V.; Santoni, G. Expression and function of the transient receptor potential ion channel family in the hematologic malignancies. *Curr. Mol. Pharmacol.* **2013**, *6*, 137–148. [CrossRef] [PubMed]
94. Peier, A.M.; Reeve, A.J.; Andersson, D.A.; Moqrich, A.; Earley, T.J.; Hergarden, A.C.; Story, G.M.; Colley, S.; Hogenesch, J.B.; McIntyre, P.; et al. A heat-sensitive TRP channel expressed in keratinocytes. *Science* **2002**, *296*, 2046–2049. [CrossRef] [PubMed]
95. Smith, G.D.; Gunthorpe, M.J.; Kelsell, R.E.; Hayes, P.D.; Reilly, P.; Facer, P.; Wright, J.E.; Jerman, J.C.; Walhin, J.P.; Ooi, L.; et al. TRPV3 is a temperature-sensitive vanilloid receptor-like protein. *Nature* **2002**, *418*, 186–190. [CrossRef] [PubMed]
96. Xu, H.; Ramsey, I.S.; Kotecha, S.A.; Moran, M.M.; Chong, J.A.; Lawson, D.; Ge, P.; Lilly, J.; Silos-Santiago, I.; Xie, Y.; et al. TRPV3 is a calcium-permeable temperature-sensitive cation channel. *Nature* **2002**, *418*, 181–186. [CrossRef] [PubMed]
97. Chung, M.K.; Lee, H.; Mizuno, A.; Suzuki, M.; Caterina, M.J. 2-aminoethoxydiphenyl borate activates and sensitizes the heat-gated ion channel TRPV3. *J. Neurosci.* **2004**, *24*, 5177–5182. [CrossRef] [PubMed]
98. Bang, S.; Yoo, S.; Yang, T.J.; Cho, H.; Hwang, S.W. Farnesyl pyrophosphate is a novel pain-producing molecule via specific activation of TRPV3. *J. Biol. Chem.* **2010**, *285*, 19362–19371. [CrossRef] [PubMed]
99. Moqrich, A.; Hwang, S.W.; Earley, T.J.; Petrus, M.J.; Murray, A.N.; Spencer, K.S.; Andahazy, M.; Story, G.M.; Patapoutian, A. Impaired thermosensation in mice lacking TRPV3, a heat and camphor sensor in the skin. *Science* **2005**, *307*, 1468–1472. [CrossRef] [PubMed]
100. Xu, H.; Delling, M.; Jun, J.C.; Clapham, D.E. Oregano, thyme and clove-derived flavors and skin sensitizers activate specific TRP channels. *Nat. Neurosci.* **2006**, *9*, 628–635. [CrossRef] [PubMed]
101. Hu, H.Z.; Xiao, R.; Wang, C.; Gao, N.; Colton, C.K.; Wood, J.D.; Zhu, M.X. Potentiation of TRPV3 channel function by unsaturated fatty acids. *J. Cell. Physiol.* **2006**, *208*, 201–212. [CrossRef] [PubMed]
102. Klein, A.S.; Tannert, A.; Schaefer, M. Cholesterol sensitises the transient receptor potential channel TRPV3 to lower temperatures and activator concentrations. *Cell Calcium* **2014**, *55*, 59–68. [CrossRef] [PubMed]
103. Karttunen, S.; Duffield, M.; Scrimgeour, N.R.; Squires, L.; Lim, W.L.; Dallas, M.L.; Scragg, J.L.; Chicher, J.; Dave, K.A.; Whitelaw, M.L.; et al. Oxygen-dependent hydroxylation by fih regulates the TRPV3 ion channel. *J. Cell Sci.* **2015**, *128*, 225–231. [CrossRef] [PubMed]
104. Mandadi, S.; Sokabe, T.; Shibasaki, K.; Katanosaka, K.; Mizuno, A.; Moqrich, A.; Patapoutian, A.; Fukumi-Tominaga, T.; Mizumura, K.; Tominaga, M. TRPV3 in keratinocytes transmits temperature information to sensory neurons via atp. *Pflugers Arch.* **2009**, *458*, 1093–1102. [CrossRef] [PubMed]
105. Miyamoto, T.; Petrus, M.J.; Dubin, A.E.; Patapoutian, A. TRPV3 regulates nitric oxide synthase-independent nitric oxide synthesis in the skin. *Nat. Commun.* **2011**, *2*, 369. [CrossRef] [PubMed]
106. Huang, S.M.; Lee, H.; Chung, M.K.; Park, U.; Yu, Y.Y.; Bradshaw, H.B.; Coulombe, P.A.; Walker, J.M.; Caterina, M.J. Overexpressed transient receptor potential vanilloid 3 ion channels in skin keratinocytes modulate pain sensitivity via prostaglandin E2. *J. Neurosci.* **2008**, *28*, 13727–13737. [CrossRef] [PubMed]
107. Huang, S.M.; Li, X.; Yu, Y.; Wang, J.; Caterina, M.J. TRPV3 and TRPV4 ion channels are not major contributors to mouse heat sensation. *Mol. Pain* **2011**, *7*, 37. [CrossRef] [PubMed]
108. Marics, I.; Malapert, P.; Reynders, A.; Gaillard, S.; Moqrich, A. Acute heat-evoked temperature sensation is impaired but not abolished in mice lacking TRPV1 and TRPV3 channels. *PLoS ONE* **2014**, *9*, e99828. [CrossRef] [PubMed]
109. Cheng, X.; Jin, J.; Hu, L.; Shen, D.; Dong, X.P.; Samie, M.A.; Knoff, J.; Eisinger, B.; Liu, M.L.; Huang, S.M.; et al. TRP channel regulates EGFR signaling in hair morphogenesis and skin barrier formation. *Cell* **2010**, *141*, 331–343. [CrossRef] [PubMed]
110. Borbiro, I.; Lisztes, E.; Toth, B.I.; Czifra, G.; Olah, A.; Szollosi, A.G.; Szentandrassy, N.; Nanasi, P.P.; Peter, Z.; Paus, R.; et al. Activation of transient receptor potential vanilloid-3 inhibits human hair growth. *J. Investig. Dermatol.* **2011**, *131*, 1605–1614. [CrossRef] [PubMed]
111. Broad, L.M.; Mogg, A.J.; Eberle, E.; Tolley, M.; Li, D.L.; Knopp, K.L. TRPV3 in drug development. *Pharmaceuticals* **2016**, *9*. [CrossRef] [PubMed]
112. Yamamoto-Kasai, E.; Imura, K.; Yasui, K.; Shichijou, M.; Oshima, I.; Hirasawa, T.; Sakata, T.; Yoshioka, T. TRPV3 as a therapeutic target for itch. *J. Investig. Dermatol.* **2012**, *132*, 2109–2112. [CrossRef] [PubMed]

113. Gopinath, P.; Wan, E.; Holdcroft, A.; Facer, P.; Davis, J.B.; Smith, G.D.; Bountra, C.; Anand, P. Increased capsaicin receptor TRPV1 in skin nerve fibres and related vanilloid receptors TRPV3 and TRPV4 in keratinocytes in human breast pain. *BMC Womens Health* **2005**, *5*, 2. [CrossRef] [PubMed]
114. Kim, H.O.; Cho, Y.S.; Park, S.Y.; Kwak, I.S.; Choi, M.G.; Chung, B.Y.; Park, C.W.; Lee, J.Y. Increased activity of TRPV3 in keratinocytes in hypertrophic burn scars with postburn pruritus. *Wound Repair Regen.* **2016**, *24*, 841–850. [CrossRef] [PubMed]
115. Aijima, R.; Wang, B.; Takao, T.; Mihara, H.; Kashio, M.; Ohsaki, Y.; Zhang, J.Q.; Mizuno, A.; Suzuki, M.; Yamashita, Y.; et al. The thermosensitive TRPV3 channel contributes to rapid wound healing in oral epithelia. *FASEB J.* **2015**, *29*, 182–192. [CrossRef] [PubMed]
116. Asakawa, M.; Yoshioka, T.; Matsutani, T.; Hikita, I.; Suzuki, M.; Oshima, I.; Tsukahara, K.; Arimura, A.; Horikawa, T.; Hirasawa, T.; et al. Association of a mutation in TRPV3 with defective hair growth in rodents. *J. Investig. Dermatol.* **2006**, *126*, 2664–2672. [CrossRef] [PubMed]
117. Imura, K.; Yoshioka, T.; Hikita, I.; Tsukahara, K.; Hirasawa, T.; Higashino, K.; Gahara, Y.; Arimura, A.; Sakata, T. Influence of TRPV3 mutation on hair growth cycle in mice. *Biochem. Biophys. Res. Commun.* **2007**, *363*, 479–483. [CrossRef] [PubMed]
118. Xiao, R.; Tian, J.; Tang, J.; Zhu, M.X. The TRPV3 mutation associated with the hairless phenotype in rodents is constitutively active. *Cell Calcium* **2008**, *43*, 334–343. [CrossRef] [PubMed]
119. Imura, K.; Yoshioka, T.; Hirasawa, T.; Sakata, T. Role of TRPV3 in immune response to development of dermatitis. *J. Inflamm. (Lond.)* **2009**, *6*, 17. [CrossRef] [PubMed]
120. Lin, Z.; Chen, Q.; Lee, M.; Cao, X.; Zhang, J.; Ma, D.; Chen, L.; Hu, X.; Wang, H.; Wang, X.; et al. Exome sequencing reveals mutations in TRPV3 as a cause of olmsted syndrome. *Am. J. Hum. Genet.* **2012**, *90*, 558–564. [CrossRef] [PubMed]
121. Wilson, N.J.; Cole, C.; Milstone, L.M.; Kiszewski, A.E.; Hansen, C.D.; O'Toole, E.A.; Schwartz, M.E.; McLean, W.H.; Smith, F.J. Expanding the phenotypic spectrum of olmsted syndrome. *J. Investig. Dermatol.* **2015**, *135*, 2879–2883. [CrossRef] [PubMed]
122. He, Y.; Zeng, K.; Zhang, X.; Chen, Q.; Wu, J.; Li, H.; Zhou, Y.; Glusman, G.; Roach, J.; Etheridge, A.; et al. A gain-of-function mutation in TRPV3 causes focal palmoplantar keratoderma in a Chinese family. *J. Investig. Dermatol.* **2015**, *135*, 907–909. [CrossRef] [PubMed]
123. Liedtke, W.; Choe, Y.; Marti-Renom, M.A.; Bell, A.M.; Denis, C.S.; Sali, A.; Hudspeth, A.J.; Friedman, J.M.; Heller, S. Vanilloid receptor-related osmotically activated channel (VR-OAC), a candidate vertebrate osmoreceptor. *Cell* **2000**, *103*, 525–535. [CrossRef]
124. Strotmann, R.; Harteneck, C.; Nunnenmacher, K.; Schultz, G.; Plant, T.D. OTRPC4, a nonselective cation channel that confers sensitivity to extracellular osmolarity. *Nat. Cell Biol.* **2000**, *2*, 695–702. [PubMed]
125. Wissenbach, U.; Bodding, M.; Freichel, M.; Flockerzi, V. TRP12, a novel TRP related protein from kidney. *FEBS Lett.* **2000**, *485*, 127–134. [CrossRef]
126. Watanabe, H.; Vriens, J.; Prenen, J.; Droogmans, G.; Voets, T.; Nilius, B. Anandamide and arachidonic acid use epoxyeicosatrienoic acids to activate TRPV4 channels. *Nature* **2003**, *424*, 434–438. [CrossRef] [PubMed]
127. Guler, A.D.; Lee, H.; Iida, T.; Shimizu, I.; Tominaga, M.; Caterina, M. Heat-evoked activation of the ion channel, TRPV4. *J. Neurosci.* **2002**, *22*, 6408–6414. [PubMed]
128. Kida, N.; Sokabe, T.; Kashio, M.; Haruna, K.; Mizuno, Y.; Suga, Y.; Nishikawa, K.; Kanamaru, A.; Hongo, M.; Oba, A.; et al. Importance of transient receptor potential vanilloid 4 (TRPV4) in epidermal barrier function in human skin keratinocytes. *Pflugers Arch.* **2012**, *463*, 715–725. [CrossRef] [PubMed]
129. Akazawa, Y.; Yuki, T.; Yoshida, H.; Sugiyama, Y.; Inoue, S. Activation of TRPV4 strengthens the tight-junction barrier in human epidermal keratinocytes. *Skin Pharmacol. Physiol.* **2013**, *26*, 15–21. [CrossRef] [PubMed]
130. Fusi, C.; Materazzi, S.; Minocci, D.; Maio, V.; Oranges, T.; Massi, D.; Nassini, R. Transient receptor potential vanilloid 4 (TRPV4) is downregulated in keratinocytes in human non-melanoma skin cancer. *J. Investig. Dermatol.* **2014**, *134*, 2408–2417. [CrossRef] [PubMed]
131. Alessandri-Haber, N.; Joseph, E.; Dina, O.A.; Liedtke, W.; Levine, J.D. TRPV4 mediates pain-related behavior induced by mild hypertonic stimuli in the presence of inflammatory mediator. *Pain* **2005**, *118*, 70–79. [CrossRef] [PubMed]
132. Alessandri-Haber, N.; Yeh, J.J.; Boyd, A.E.; Parada, C.A.; Chen, X.; Reichling, D.B.; Levine, J.D. Hypotonicity induces TRPV4-mediated nociception in rat. *Neuron* **2003**, *39*, 497–511. [CrossRef]

133. Liedtke, W.; Friedman, J.M. Abnormal osmotic regulation in TRPV4 −/− mice. *Proc. Natl. Acad. Sci. USA* **2003**, *100*, 13698–13703. [CrossRef] [PubMed]
134. Suzuki, M.; Mizuno, A.; Kodaira, K.; Imai, M. Impaired pressure sensation in mice lacking TRPV4. *J. Biol. Chem.* **2003**, *278*, 22664–22668. [CrossRef] [PubMed]
135. Chen, Y.; Kanju, P.; Fang, Q.; Lee, S.H.; Parekh, P.K.; Lee, W.; Moore, C.; Brenner, D.; Gereau, R.W.T.; Wang, F.; et al. TRPV4 is necessary for trigeminal irritant pain and functions as a cellular formalin receptor. *Pain* **2014**, *155*, 2662–2672. [CrossRef] [PubMed]
136. Chen, Y.; Williams, S.H.; McNulty, A.L.; Hong, J.H.; Lee, S.H.; Rothfusz, N.E.; Parekh, P.K.; Moore, C.; Gereau, R.W., IV; Taylor, A.B.; et al. Temporomandibular joint pain: A critical role for TRPV4 in the trigeminal ganglion. *Pain* **2013**, *154*, 1295–1304. [CrossRef] [PubMed]
137. Segond von Banchet, G.; Boettger, M.K.; Konig, C.; Iwakura, Y.; Brauer, R.; Schaible, H.G. Neuronal IL-17 receptor upregulates TRPV4 but not TRPV1 receptors in DRG neurons and mediates mechanical but not thermal hyperalgesia. *Mol. Cell. Neurosci.* **2013**, *52*, 152–160. [CrossRef] [PubMed]
138. Alessandri-Haber, N.; Dina, O.A.; Yeh, J.J.; Parada, C.A.; Reichling, D.B.; Levine, J.D. Transient receptor potential vanilloid 4 is essential in chemotherapy-induced neuropathic pain in the rat. *J. Neurosci.* **2004**, *24*, 4444–4452. [CrossRef] [PubMed]
139. Chen, Y.; Yang, C.; Wang, Z.J. Proteinase-activated receptor 2 sensitizes transient receptor potential vanilloid 1, transient receptor potential vanilloid 4, and transient receptor potential ankyrin 1 in paclitaxel-induced neuropathic pain. *Neuroscience* **2011**, *193*, 440–451. [CrossRef] [PubMed]
140. Ding, X.L.; Wang, Y.H.; Ning, L.P.; Zhang, Y.; Ge, H.Y.; Jiang, H.; Wang, R.; Yue, S.W. Involvement of TRPV4-NO-cGMP-PKG pathways in the development of thermal hyperalgesia following chronic compression of the dorsal root ganglion in rats. *Behav. Brain Res.* **2010**, *208*, 194–201. [CrossRef] [PubMed]
141. Grant, A.D.; Cottrell, G.S.; Amadesi, S.; Trevisani, M.; Nicoletti, P.; Materazzi, S.; Altier, C.; Cenac, N.; Zamponi, G.W.; Bautista-Cruz, F.; et al. Protease-activated receptor 2 sensitizes the transient receptor potential vanilloid 4 ion channel to cause mechanical hyperalgesia in mice. *J. Physiol.* **2007**, *578 Pt 3*, 715–733. [CrossRef] [PubMed]
142. Moore, C.; Cevikbas, F.; Pasolli, H.A.; Chen, Y.; Kong, W.; Kempkes, C.; Parekh, P.; Lee, S.H.; Kontchou, N.A.; Yeh, I.; et al. Uvb radiation generates sunburn pain and affects skin by activating epidermal TRPV4 ion channels and triggering endothelin-1 signaling. *Proc. Natl. Acad. Sci. USA* **2013**, *110*, E3225–3234. [CrossRef] [PubMed]
143. Akiyama, T.; Ivanov, M.; Nagamine, M.; Davoodi, A.; Carstens, M.I.; Ikoma, A.; Cevikbas, F.; Kempkes, C.; Buddenkotte, J.; Steinhoff, M.; et al. Involvement of TRPV4 in serotonin-evoked scratching. *J. Investig. Dermatol.* **2016**, *136*, 154–160. [CrossRef] [PubMed]
144. Chen, Y.; Fang, Q.; Wang, Z.; Zhang, J.Y.; MacLeod, A.S.; Hall, R.P.; Liedtke, W.B. Transient receptor potential vanilloid 4 ion channel functions as a pruriceptor in epidermal keratinocytes to evoke histaminergic itch. *J. Biol. Chem.* **2016**, *291*, 10252–10262. [CrossRef] [PubMed]
145. Lee, H.; Iida, T.; Mizuno, A.; Suzuki, M.; Caterina, M.J. Altered thermal selection behavior in mice lacking transient receptor potential vanilloid 4. *J. Neurosci.* **2005**, *25*, 1304–1310. [CrossRef] [PubMed]
146. Auer-Grumbach, M.; Olschewski, A.; Papic, L.; Kremer, H.; McEntagart, M.E.; Uhrig, S.; Fischer, C.; Frohlich, E.; Balint, Z.; Tang, B.; et al. Alterations in the ankyrin domain of TRPV4 cause congenital distal SMA, scapuloperoneal SMA and HMSN2C. *Nat. Genet.* **2010**, *42*, 160–164. [CrossRef] [PubMed]
147. Deng, H.X.; Klein, C.J.; Yan, J.; Shi, Y.; Wu, Y.; Fecto, F.; Yau, H.J.; Yang, Y.; Zhai, H.; Siddique, N.; et al. Scapuloperoneal spinal muscular atrophy and CMT2C are allelic disorders caused by alterations in TRPV4. *Nat. Genet.* **2010**, *42*, 165–169. [CrossRef] [PubMed]
148. Landoure, G.; Zdebik, A.A.; Martinez, T.L.; Burnett, B.G.; Stanescu, H.C.; Inada, H.; Shi, Y.; Taye, A.A.; Kong, L.; Munns, C.H.; et al. Mutations in TRPV4 cause charcot-marie-tooth disease type 2C. *Nat. Genet.* **2010**, *42*, 170–174. [CrossRef] [PubMed]
149. Lehen'kyi, V.; Vandenberghe, M.; Belaubre, F.; Julie, S.; Castex-Rizzi, N.; Skryma, R.; Prevarskaya, N. Acceleration of keratinocyte differentiation by transient receptor potential vanilloid (TRPV6) channel activation. *J. Eur. Acad. Dermatol. Venereol.* **2011**, *25* (Suppl. 1), 12–18. [CrossRef] [PubMed]
150. Bianco, S.D.; Peng, J.B.; Takanaga, H.; Suzuki, Y.; Crescenzi, A.; Kos, C.H.; Zhuang, L.; Freeman, M.R.; Gouveia, C.H.; Wu, J.; et al. Marked disturbance of calcium homeostasis in mice with targeted disruption of the TRPV6 calcium channel gene. *J. Bone Miner. Res.* **2007**, *22*, 274–285. [CrossRef] [PubMed]

151. Peng, J.B.; Zhuang, L.; Berger, U.V.; Adam, R.M.; Williams, B.J.; Brown, E.M.; Hediger, M.A.; Freeman, M.R. CAT1 expression correlates with tumor grade in prostate cancer. *Biochem. Biophys. Res. Commun.* **2001**, *282*, 729–734. [CrossRef] [PubMed]
152. Nilius, B.; Appendino, G.; Owsianik, G. The transient receptor potential channel TRPA1: From gene to pathophysiology. *Pflugers Arch.* **2012**, *464*, 425–458. [CrossRef] [PubMed]
153. Kwon, Y.; Shim, H.S.; Wang, X.; Montell, C. Control of thermotactic behavior via coupling of a TRP channel to a phospholipase C signaling cascade. *Nat. Neurosci.* **2008**, *11*, 871–873. [CrossRef] [PubMed]
154. Rosenzweig, M.; Brennan, K.M.; Tayler, T.D.; Phelps, P.O.; Patapoutian, A.; Garrity, P.A. The Drosophila ortholog of vertebrate TRPA1 regulates thermotaxis. *Genes Dev.* **2005**, *19*, 419–424. [CrossRef] [PubMed]
155. Viswanath, V.; Story, G.M.; Peier, A.M.; Petrus, M.J.; Lee, V.M.; Hwang, S.W.; Patapoutian, A.; Jegla, T. Opposite thermosensor in fruitfly and mouse. *Nature* **2003**, *423*, 822–823. [CrossRef] [PubMed]
156. Gracheva, E.O.; Ingolia, N.T.; Kelly, Y.M.; Cordero-Morales, J.F.; Hollopeter, G.; Chesler, A.T.; Sanchez, E.E.; Perez, J.C.; Weissman, J.S.; Julius, D. Molecular basis of infrared detection by snakes. *Nature* **2010**, *464*, 1006–1011. [CrossRef] [PubMed]
157. Story, G.M.; Peier, A.M.; Reeve, A.J.; Eid, S.R.; Mosbacher, J.; Hricik, T.R.; Earley, T.J.; Hergarden, A.C.; Andersson, D.A.; Hwang, S.W.; et al. ANKTM1, a TRP-like channel expressed in nociceptive neurons, is activated by cold temperatures. *Cell* **2003**, *112*, 819–829. [CrossRef]
158. Moparthi, L.; Survery, S.; Kreir, M.; Simonsen, C.; Kjellbom, P.; Hogestatt, E.D.; Johanson, U.; Zygmunt, P.M. Human TRPA1 is intrinsically cold- and chemosensitive with and without its N-terminal ankyrin repeat domain. *Proc. Natl. Acad. Sci. USA* **2014**, *111*, 16901–16906. [CrossRef] [PubMed]
159. Wang, S.; Lee, J.; Ro, J.Y.; Chung, M.K. Warmth suppresses and desensitizes damage-sensing ion channel TRPA1. *Mol. Pain* **2012**, *8*, 22. [CrossRef] [PubMed]
160. Moparthi, L.; Kichko, T.I.; Eberhardt, M.; Hogestatt, E.D.; Kjellbom, P.; Johanson, U.; Reeh, P.W.; Leffler, A.; Filipovic, M.R.; Zygmunt, P.M. Human TRPA1 is a heat sensor displaying intrinsic u-shaped thermosensitivity. *Sci. Rep.* **2016**, *6*, 28763. [CrossRef] [PubMed]
161. Miyake, T.; Nakamura, S.; Zhao, M.; So, K.; Inoue, K.; Numata, T.; Takahashi, N.; Shirakawa, H.; Mori, Y.; Nakagawa, T.; et al. Cold sensitivity of TRPA1 is unveiled by the prolyl hydroxylation blockade-induced sensitization to ROS. *Nat. Commun.* **2016**, *7*, 12840. [CrossRef] [PubMed]
162. Meseguer, V.; Alpizar, Y.A.; Luis, E.; Tajada, S.; Denlinger, B.; Fajardo, O.; Manenschijn, J.A.; Fernandez-Pena, C.; Talavera, A.; Kichko, T.; et al. TRPA1 channels mediate acute neurogenic inflammation and pain produced by bacterial endotoxins. *Nat. Commun.* **2014**, *5*, 3125. [CrossRef] [PubMed]
163. Park, C.K.; Xu, Z.Z.; Berta, T.; Han, Q.; Chen, G.; Liu, X.J.; Ji, R.R. Extracellular micrornas activate nociceptor neurons to elicit pain via TLR7 and TRPA1. *Neuron* **2014**, *82*, 47–54. [CrossRef] [PubMed]
164. Kerstein, P.C.; del Camino, D.; Moran, M.M.; Stucky, C.L. Pharmacological blockade of TRPA1 inhibits mechanical firing in nociceptors. *Mol. Pain* **2009**, *5*, 19. [CrossRef] [PubMed]
165. Kwan, K.Y.; Glazer, J.M.; Corey, D.P.; Rice, F.L.; Stucky, C.L. TRPA1 modulates mechanotransduction in cutaneous sensory neurons. *J. Neurosci.* **2009**, *29*, 4808–4819. [CrossRef] [PubMed]
166. Lennertz, R.C.; Kossyreva, E.A.; Smith, A.K.; Stucky, C.L. TRPA1 mediates mechanical sensitization in nociceptors during inflammation. *PLoS ONE* **2012**, *7*, e43597. [CrossRef] [PubMed]
167. Zhang, X.F.; Chen, J.; Faltynek, C.R.; Moreland, R.B.; Neelands, T.R. Transient receptor potential A1 mediates an osmotically activated ion channel. *Eur. J. Neurosci.* **2008**, *27*, 605–611. [CrossRef] [PubMed]
168. Bautista, D.M.; Jordt, S.E.; Nikai, T.; Tsuruda, P.R.; Read, A.J.; Poblete, J.; Yamoah, E.N.; Basbaum, A.I.; Julius, D. TRPA1 mediates the inflammatory actions of environmental irritants and proalgesic agents. *Cell* **2006**, *124*, 1269–1282. [CrossRef] [PubMed]
169. McNamara, C.R.; Mandel-Brehm, J.; Bautista, D.M.; Siemens, J.; Deranian, K.L.; Zhao, M.; Hayward, N.J.; Chong, J.A.; Julius, D.; Moran, M.M.; et al. TRPA1 mediates formalin-induced pain. *Proc. Natl. Acad. Sci. USA* **2007**, *104*, 13525–13530. [CrossRef] [PubMed]
170. del Camino, D.; Murphy, S.; Heiry, M.; Barrett, L.B.; Earley, T.J.; Cook, C.A.; Petrus, M.J.; Zhao, M.; D'Amours, M.; Deering, N.; et al. TRPA1 contributes to cold hypersensitivity. *J. Neurosci.* **2010**, *30*, 15165–15174. [CrossRef] [PubMed]
171. Andersson, D.A.; Gentry, C.; Light, E.; Vastani, N.; Vallortigara, J.; Bierhaus, A.; Fleming, T.; Bevan, S. Methylglyoxal evokes pain by stimulating TRPA1. *PLoS ONE* **2013**, *8*, e77986. [CrossRef]

172. Nassini, R.; Gees, M.; Harrison, S.; De Siena, G.; Materazzi, S.; Moretto, N.; Failli, P.; Preti, D.; Marchetti, N.; Cavazzini, A.; et al. Oxaliplatin elicits mechanical and cold allodynia in rodents via TRPA1 receptor stimulation. *Pain* **2011**, *152*, 1621–1631. [CrossRef] [PubMed]
173. Andersson, D.A.; Filipovic, M.R.; Gentry, C.; Eberhardt, M.; Vastani, N.; Leffler, A.; Reeh, P.; Bevan, S. Streptozotocin stimulates the ion channel TRPA1 directly: Involvement of peroxynitrite. *J. Biol. Chem.* **2015**, *290*, 15185–15196. [CrossRef] [PubMed]
174. Koivisto, A.; Hukkanen, M.; Saarnilehto, M.; Chapman, H.; Kuokkanen, K.; Wei, H.; Viisanen, H.; Akerman, K.E.; Lindstedt, K.; Pertovaara, A. Inhibiting TRPA1 ion channel reduces loss of cutaneous nerve fiber function in diabetic animals: Sustained activation of the TRPA1 channel contributes to the pathogenesis of peripheral diabetic neuropathy. *Pharmacol. Res.* **2012**, *65*, 149–158. [CrossRef] [PubMed]
175. Kremeyer, B.; Lopera, F.; Cox, J.J.; Momin, A.; Rugiero, F.; Marsh, S.; Woods, C.G.; Jones, N.G.; Paterson, K.J.; Fricker, F.R.; et al. A gain-of-function mutation in TRPA1 causes familial episodic pain syndrome. *Neuron* **2010**, *66*, 671–680. [CrossRef] [PubMed]
176. Babes, A.; Sauer, S.K.; Moparthi, L.; Kichko, T.I.; Neacsu, C.; Namer, B.; Filipovic, M.; Zygmunt, P.M.; Reeh, P.W.; Fischer, M.J. Photosensitization in porphyrias and photodynamic therapy involves TRPA1 and TRPV1. *J. Neurosci.* **2016**, *36*, 5264–5278. [CrossRef] [PubMed]
177. Wilson, S.R.; Gerhold, K.A.; Bifolck-Fisher, A.; Liu, Q.; Patel, K.N.; Dong, X.; Bautista, D.M. TRPA1 is required for histamine-independent, Mas-related G protein-coupled receptor-mediated itch. *Nat. Neurosci.* **2011**, *14*, 595–602. [CrossRef] [PubMed]
178. Wilson, S.R.; The, L.; Batia, L.M.; Beattie, K.; Katibah, G.E.; McClain, S.P.; Pellegrino, M.; Estandian, D.M.; Bautista, D.M. The epithelial cell-derived atopic dermatitis cytokine TSLP activates neurons to induce itch. *Cell* **2013**, *155*, 285–295. [CrossRef] [PubMed]
179. Lieu, T.; Jayaweera, G.; Zhao, P.; Poole, D.P.; Jensen, D.; Grace, M.; McIntyre, P.; Bron, R.; Wilson, Y.M.; Krappitz, M.; et al. The bile acid receptor TGR5 activates the TRPA1 channel to induce itch in mice. *Gastroenterology* **2014**, *147*, 1417–1428. [CrossRef] [PubMed]
180. Wilson, S.R.; Nelson, A.M.; Batia, L.; Morita, T.; Estandian, D.; Owens, D.M.; Lumpkin, E.A.; Bautista, D.M. The ion channel TRPA1 is required for chronic itch. *J. Neurosci.* **2013**, *33*, 9283–9294. [CrossRef] [PubMed]
181. Oh, M.H.; Oh, S.Y.; Lu, J.; Lou, H.; Myers, A.C.; Zhu, Z.; Zheng, T. TRPA1-dependent pruritus in IL-13-induced chronic atopic dermatitis. *J. Immunol.* **2013**, *191*, 5371–5382. [CrossRef] [PubMed]
182. Liu, B.; Escalera, J.; Balakrishna, S.; Fan, L.; Caceres, A.I.; Robinson, E.; Sui, A.; McKay, M.C.; McAlexander, M.A.; Herrick, C.A.; et al. TRPA1 controls inflammation and pruritogen responses in allergic contact dermatitis. *FASEB J.* **2013**, *27*, 3549–3563. [CrossRef] [PubMed]
183. Saarnilehto, M.; Chapman, H.; Savinko, T.; Lindstedt, K.; Lauerma, A.I.; Koivisto, A. Contact sensitizer 2,4-dinitrochlorobenzene is a highly potent human TRPA1 agonist. *Allergy* **2014**, *69*, 1424–1427. [CrossRef] [PubMed]
184. Caceres, A.I.; Brackmann, M.; Elia, M.D.; Bessac, B.F.; del Camino, D.; D'Amours, M.; Witek, J.S.; Fanger, C.M.; Chong, J.A.; Hayward, N.J.; et al. A sensory neuronal ion channel essential for airway inflammation and hyperreactivity in asthma. *Proc. Natl. Acad. Sci. USA* **2009**, *106*, 9099–9104. [CrossRef] [PubMed]
185. Denda, M.; Tsutsumi, M.; Goto, M.; Ikeyama, K.; Denda, S. Topical application of TRPA1 agonists and brief cold exposure accelerate skin permeability barrier recovery. *J. Investig. Dermatol.* **2010**, *130*, 1942–1945. [CrossRef] [PubMed]
186. Uta, D.; Furue, H.; Pickering, A.E.; Rashid, M.H.; Mizuguchi-Takase, H.; Katafuchi, T.; Imoto, K.; Yoshimura, M. TRPA1-expressing primary afferents synapse with a morphologically identified subclass of substantia gelatinosa neurons in the adult rat spinal cord. *Eur. J. Neurosci.* **2010**, *31*, 1960–1973. [CrossRef] [PubMed]
187. Chiu, I.M.; Heesters, B.A.; Ghasemlou, N.; Von Hehn, C.A.; Zhao, F.; Tran, J.; Wainger, B.; Strominger, A.; Muralidharan, S.; Horswill, A.R.; et al. Bacteria activate sensory neurons that modulate pain and inflammation. *Nature* **2013**, *501*, 52–57. [CrossRef] [PubMed]
188. Pinter, E.; Helyes, Z.; Szolcsanyi, J. Inhibitory effect of somatostatin on inflammation and nociception. *Pharmacol. Ther.* **2006**, *112*, 440–456. [CrossRef] [PubMed]
189. Zappia, K.J.; Garrison, S.R.; Palygin, O.; Weyer, A.D.; Barabas, M.E.; Lawlor, M.W.; Staruschenko, A.; Stucky, C.L. Mechanosensory and atp release deficits following keratin14-cre-mediated TRPA1 deletion despite absence of TRPA1 in murine keratinocytes. *PLoS ONE* **2016**, *11*, e0151602. [CrossRef] [PubMed]

190. Bellono, N.W.; Kammel, L.G.; Zimmerman, A.L.; Oancea, E. Uv light phototransduction activates transient receptor potential a1 ion channels in human melanocytes. *Proc. Natl. Acad. Sci. USA* **2013**, *110*, 2383–2388. [CrossRef] [PubMed]
191. Oehler, B.; Scholze, A.; Schaefer, M.; Hill, K. TRPA1 is functionally expressed in melanoma cells but is not critical for impaired proliferation caused by allyl isothiocyanate or cinnamaldehyde. *Naunyn Schmiedebergs Arch. Pharmacol.* **2012**, *385*, 555–563. [CrossRef] [PubMed]
192. Oancea, E.; Wicks, N.L. TRPM1: New trends for an old TRP. *Adv. Exp. Med. Biol.* **2011**, *704*, 135–145. [PubMed]
193. Miller, A.J.; Du, J.; Rowan, S.; Hershey, C.L.; Widlund, H.R.; Fisher, D.E. Transcriptional regulation of the melanoma prognostic marker melastatin (TRPM1) by MITF in melanocytes and melanoma. *Cancer Res.* **2004**, *64*, 509–516. [CrossRef] [PubMed]
194. Guo, H.; Carlson, J.A.; Slominski, A. Role of TRPM in melanocytes and melanoma. *Exp. Dermatol.* **2012**, *21*, 650–654. [CrossRef] [PubMed]
195. Devi, S.; Markandeya, Y.; Maddodi, N.; Dhingra, A.; Vardi, N.; Balijepalli, R.C.; Setaluri, V. Metabotropic glutamate receptor 6 signaling enhances TRPM1 calcium channel function and increases melanin content in human melanocytes. *Pigment Cell Melanoma Res.* **2013**, *26*, 348–356. [CrossRef] [PubMed]
196. Mansuri, M.S.; Singh, M.; Begum, R. miRNA signatures and transcriptional regulation of their target genes in vitiligo. *J. Dermatol. Sci* **2016**, *84*, 50–58. [CrossRef] [PubMed]
197. Bellone, R.R.; Brooks, S.A.; Sandmeyer, L.; Murphy, B.A.; Forsyth, G.; Archer, S.; Bailey, E.; Grahn, B. Differential gene expression of TRPM1, the potential cause of congenital stationary night blindness and coat spotting patterns (LP) in the Appaloosa horse (Equus caballus). *Genetics* **2008**, *179*, 1861–1870. [CrossRef] [PubMed]
198. Oancea, E.; Vriens, J.; Brauchi, S.; Jun, J.; Splawski, I.; Clapham, D.E. TRPM1 forms ion channels associated with melanin content in melanocytes. *Sci. Signal.* **2009**, *2*, ra21. [CrossRef] [PubMed]
199. Kunisada, T.; Lu, S.Z.; Yoshida, H.; Nishikawa, S.; Nishikawa, S.; Mizoguchi, M.; Hayashi, S.; Tyrrell, L.; Williams, D.A.; Wang, X.; et al. Murine cutaneous mastocytosis and epidermal melanocytosis induced by keratinocyte expression of transgenic stem cell factor. *J. Exp. Med.* **1998**, *187*, 1565–1573. [CrossRef] [PubMed]
200. Levy, C.; Khaled, M.; Iliopoulos, D.; Janas, M.M.; Schubert, S.; Pinner, S.; Chen, P.H.; Li, S.; Fletcher, A.L.; Yokoyama, S.; et al. Intronic miR-211 assumes the tumor suppressive function of its host gene in melanoma. *Mol. Cell* **2010**, *40*, 841–849. [CrossRef] [PubMed]
201. Tan, C.H.; McNaughton, P.A. The TRPM2 ion channel is required for sensitivity to warmth. *Nature* **2016**, *536*, 460–463. [CrossRef] [PubMed]
202. Held, K.; Voets, T.; Vriens, J. TRPM3 in temperature sensing and beyond. *Temperature (Austin)* **2015**, *2*, 201–213. [CrossRef] [PubMed]
203. Vriens, J.; Held, K.; Janssens, A.; Toth, B.I.; Kerselaers, S.; Nilius, B.; Vennekens, R.; Voets, T. Opening of an alternative ion permeation pathway in a nociceptor TRP channel. *Nat. Chem. Biol.* **2014**, *10*, 188–195. [CrossRef] [PubMed]
204. McNeill, M.S.; Paulsen, J.; Bonde, G.; Burnight, E.; Hsu, M.Y.; Cornell, R.A. Cell death of melanophores in zebrafish TRPM7 mutant embryos depends on melanin synthesis. *J. Investig. Dermatol.* **2007**, *127*, 2020–2030. [CrossRef] [PubMed]
205. Bautista, D.M.; Siemens, J.; Glazer, J.M.; Tsuruda, P.R.; Basbaum, A.I.; Stucky, C.L.; Jordt, S.E.; Julius, D. The menthol receptor TRPM8 is the principal detector of environmental cold. *Nature* **2007**, *448*, 204–208. [CrossRef] [PubMed]
206. Colburn, R.W.; Lubin, M.L.; Stone, D.J., Jr.; Wang, Y.; Lawrence, D.; D'Andrea, M.R.; Brandt, M.R.; Liu, Y.; Flores, C.M.; Qin, N. Attenuated cold sensitivity in TRPM8 null mice. *Neuron* **2007**, *54*, 379–386. [CrossRef] [PubMed]
207. Dhaka, A.; Murray, A.N.; Mathur, J.; Earley, T.J.; Petrus, M.J.; Patapoutian, A. TRPM8 is required for cold sensation in mice. *Neuron* **2007**, *54*, 371–378. [CrossRef] [PubMed]
208. Chung, M.K.; Caterina, M.J. TRP channel knockout mice lose their cool. *Neuron* **2007**, *54*, 345–347. [CrossRef] [PubMed]
209. Bromm, B.; Scharein, E.; Darsow, U.; Ring, J. Effects of menthol and cold on histamine-induced itch and skin reactions in man. *Neurosci. Lett.* **1995**, *187*, 157–160. [CrossRef]

210. Shapovalov, G.; Gkika, D.; Devilliers, M.; Kondratskyi, A.; Gordienko, D.; Busserolles, J.; Bokhobza, A.; Eschalier, A.; Skryma, R.; Prevarskaya, N. Opiates modulate thermosensation by internalizing cold receptor TRPM8. *Cell Rep.* **2013**, *4*, 504–515. [CrossRef] [PubMed]
211. Asuthkar, S.; Demirkhanyan, L.; Sun, X.; Elustondo, P.A.; Krishnan, V.; Baskaran, P.; Velpula, K.K.; Thyagarajan, B.; Pavlov, E.V.; Zakharian, E. The TRPM8 protein is a testosterone receptor: II. Functional evidence for an ionotropic effect of testosterone on TRPM8. *J. Biol. Chem.* **2015**, *290*, 2670–2688. [CrossRef] [PubMed]
212. Asuthkar, S.; Elustondo, P.A.; Demirkhanyan, L.; Sun, X.; Baskaran, P.; Velpula, K.K.; Thyagarajan, B.; Pavlov, E.V.; Zakharian, E. The TRPM8 protein is a testosterone receptor: I. Biochemical evidence for direct TRPM8-testosterone interactions. *J. Biol. Chem.* **2015**, *290*, 2659–2669. [CrossRef] [PubMed]
213. Zhang, L.; Barritt, G.J. Evidence that TRPM8 is an androgen-dependent Ca^{2+} channel required for the survival of prostate cancer cells. *Cancer Res.* **2004**, *64*, 8365–8373. [CrossRef] [PubMed]
214. Bidaux, G.; Borowiec, A.S.; Gordienko, D.; Beck, B.; Shapovalov, G.G.; Lemonnier, L.; Flourakis, M.; Vandenberghe, M.; Slomianny, C.; Dewailly, E.; et al. Epidermal TRPM8 channel isoform controls the balance between keratinocyte proliferation and differentiation in a cold-dependent manner. *Proc. Natl. Acad. Sci. USA* **2015**, *112*, E3345–E3354. [CrossRef] [PubMed]
215. Denda, M.; Tsutsumi, M.; Denda, S. Topical application of TRPM8 agonists accelerates skin permeability barrier recovery and reduces epidermal proliferation induced by barrier insult: Role of cold-sensitive TRP receptors in epidermal permeability barrier homoeostasis. *Exp. Dermatol.* **2010**, *19*, 791–795. [CrossRef] [PubMed]
216. Park, N.H.; Na, Y.J.; Choi, H.T.; Cho, J.C.; Lee, H.K. Activation of transient receptor potential melastatin 8 reduces ultraviolet B-induced prostaglandin E2 production in keratinocytes. *J. Dermatol.* **2013**, *40*, 919–922. [CrossRef] [PubMed]
217. Mergler, S.; Derckx, R.; Reinach, P.S.; Garreis, F.; Bohm, A.; Schmelzer, L.; Skosyrski, S.; Ramesh, N.; Abdelmessih, S.; Polat, O.K.; et al. Calcium regulation by temperature-sensitive transient receptor potential channels in human uveal melanoma cells. *Cell Signal.* **2014**, *26*, 56–69. [CrossRef] [PubMed]
218. Yamamura, H.; Ugawa, S.; Ueda, T.; Morita, A.; Shimada, S. TRPM8 activation suppresses cellular viability in human melanoma. *Am. J. Physiol. Cell Physiol.* **2008**, *295*, C296–C301. [CrossRef] [PubMed]
219. Xu, H.; Delling, M.; Li, L.; Dong, X.; Clapham, D.E. Activating mutation in a mucolipin transient receptor potential channel leads to melanocyte loss in varitint-waddler mice. *Proc. Natl. Acad. Sci. USA* **2007**, *104*, 18321–18326. [CrossRef] [PubMed]

9

Detailed Characterization of the Cooperative Binding of Piperine with Heat Shock Protein 70 by Molecular Biophysical Approaches

Gabriel Zazeri [1], Ana Paula Ribeiro Povinelli [1], Marcelo de Freitas Lima [2] and Marinônio Lopes Cornélio [1,*]

1 Departamento de Física, Instituto de Biociências, Letras e Ciências Exatas (IBILCE), UNESP, Rua Cristovão Colombo 2265, CEP 15054-000 São José do Rio Preto, SP, Brazil; gabriel.zazeri@unesp.br (G.Z.); ana.povinelli@unesp.br (A.P.R.P.)

2 Departamento de Química, Instituto de Biociências, Letras e Ciências Exatas (IBILCE), UNESP, Rua Cristovão Colombo 2265, CEP 15054-000 São José do Rio Preto, SP, Brazil; marcelo.f.lima@unesp.br

* Correspondence: m.cornelio@unesp.br

Abstract: In this work, for the first time, details of the complex formed by heat shock protein 70 (HSP70) independent nucleotide binding domain (NBD) and piperine were characterized through experimental and computational molecular biophysical methods. Fluorescence spectroscopy results revealed positive cooperativity between the two binding sites. Circular dichroism identified secondary conformational changes. Molecular dynamics along with molecular mechanics Poisson Boltzmann surface area (MM/PBSA) reinforced the positive cooperativity, showing that the affinity of piperine for NBD increased when piperine occupied both binding sites instead of one. The spontaneity of the complexation was demonstrated through the Gibbs free energy ($\Delta G < 0$ kJ/mol) for different temperatures obtained experimentally by van't Hoff analysis and computationally by umbrella sampling with the potential of mean force profile. Furthermore, the mean forces which drove the complexation were disclosed by van't Hoff and MM/PBSA as being the non-specific interactions. In conclusion, the work revealed characteristics of NBD and piperine interaction, which may support further drug discover studies.

Keywords: heat shock protein 70; Hsp70; piperine; fluorescence spectroscopy; molecular docking; molecular dynamics; molecular biophysics

---

1. Introduction

Heat shock proteins (HSPs) constitute the first line of protection for cells exposed to stressful conditions [1]. HSPs belong to the family of intracellular molecular chaperones, which are involved in many cellular processes including protein folding, prevention of protein aggregation, modulation of protein complexes and protein transport between cellular compartments [2].

The comprehension of HSPs functions was very accepted by the scientific community until Asea et al. [3] initiated a paradigm in the understanding of the function of one of the heat shock proteins (HSP70), revealing that this protein may be found in the extracellular medium acting as an inflammatory cytokine that stimulates innate immune response through the activation of Nuclear Factor-κB (NF-κB) [4–6], which in turn is responsible for the transcription of more than 150 inflammatory cytokines genes including TNF-α, IL-1β and IL6 [6].

HSP70 is a 70 kDa protein that consists of an independent conserved N-terminal nucleotide binding domain (NBD ≈ 40 kDa) with ATPase activity, a substrate binding domain (SBD ≈ 25 kDa) and a weakly conserved C-terminal domain [2]. The NBD and SBD are linked by a short inter-domain linker [7]. The NBD consists of two subdomains, I and II, which are further divided into regions a and b. The Ia and IIa regions interact with ATP [7]. The interaction with ATP leads the NBD structure to conformational changes that affect the affinity of HSP70 for its receptors (TLRs), revealing the plasticity of this protein [8]. Cheeseman et al. [9] and Jones et al. [2] identified some ligands that caused conformational changes in NBD, reinforcing the plasticity of the domain. Moreover, the authors highlighted the need to find small ligands with the potential to inhibit HSP70. Considering the NBD structural flexibility, the key to inhibit the cytokine function of HSP70 may be the search for small molecules able to induce conformational changes that reduce the affinity for the receptors.

Studies reported in the literature showed by means of biological assays that piperine, a bioactive natural product (inset of Figure 1) [10], inhibited IL-1β-mediated activation of NF-κB, leading to the downregulation of pro-inflammatory proteins in human osteoarthritis chondrocyte [11], in human interleukin 1β-stimulated fibroblast-like synoviocytes and in rat arthritis models [12]. Further, it was reported that piperine also inhibited the LPS-mediated activation of NF-κB in RAW 264.7, not allowing the expression of inflammatory mediators [13]. Although it was recently reported in the literature that HSP70 also triggers the NF-κB activation pathway playing a similar role to IL-1β and LPS, there are no studies either at a cellular level or at a molecular level regarding the interaction of the anti-inflammatory molecule piperine and HSP70.

From this perspective, the present work comes to describe a detailed biophysical characterization of the interaction between NDB and piperine to point out the main features of the interaction, supporting drug discovery teams in order to give them an insight into the possible inhibitory role of piperine. Fluorescence spectroscopy and circular dichroism spectroscopic methods were employed to disclose the number of binding sites, the cooperativity, the binding affinity, the thermodynamic parameters of interaction and the protein conformational changes due to the interactions. To have a complete description of the complex, molecular docking and dynamics were employed to predict and confirm the binding sites, to disclose the molecular interactions involved and to calculate the binding free energy.

2. Materials and Methods

2.1. Reagents

Piperine (>97%) was purchased from Sigma-Aldrich Chemical Co. (Schnelldorf, Bavaria, Germany), as dibasic sodium phosphate (>99%) reagents, anhydrous citric acid (>99%) and sodium chloride (>99%). Lyophilised NBD (>97%) was purchased from GenScript. Methanol alcohol was purchased from Dynamics Química Contemporânea LTDA (Indaiatuba, SP, Brazil). Ultrapure water was prepared by a Millipore water purification system—Direct-Q UV-3 (Merck KGaA, Darmstadt, Germany). Lyophilized NBD was reconstituted in 50 mM phosphate buffer containing 150 mM of sodium chloride, and the pH was adjusted to 7.4 with anhydrous citric acid. Stock solutions of piperine were prepared in pure methanol. The concentrations of piperine and NBD solutions were determined by UV-VIS experiments performed on a Biospectro spectrophotometer (Biospectro, Curitiba, PR, Brazil), using the extinction coefficient at 16,500 $M^{-1}cm^{-1}$ at 345 nm for piperine and 20,525 $M^{-1}cm^{-1}$ at 280 nm for NBD.

2.2. Steady-State Fluorescence Spectroscopy

Fluorescence experiments were performed on the Lumina (Thermo Fisher Scientific, Waltham, MA, USA) stationary state spectrofluorimeter equipped with a thermal bath and Xenon lamp. A 100 μL quartz cuvette with a 10 × 2 mm optical path was used in the experiments. The widths of the excitation and the emission slits were adjusted to 10 nm. A wavelength of 295 nm was used to excite the single tryptophan residue of NBD (Trp90). The emission spectra were obtained in the range of 305 to 570 nm with a resolution of 1.0 ± 5.0 nm. Each emission point collected was the average of 15 accumulations. The software ScanWave was used to collect the measured data.

In the binding equilibrium experiments, aliquots of piperine (increment of 0.5 μM) were added in NBD solution at 4 μM. Measurements were performed at 288, 298 and 308 K. In the interaction density function analysis, small aliquots of piperine (increments of 1 μM) were added to NBD solutions at 4 μM, 6 μM and 8 μM at a fixed temperature (288 K). In all experiments, the final volume of methanol in the buffer was less than 1.0%.

The correction of the inner filter effects was performed with Equation (1), where F_{corr} and F_{obs} are corrected and observed fluorescence intensities, and A_{ex} and A_{em} are the absorbance at the excitation and the emission wavelengths, respectively, considering a cuvette of 10 × 10 mm of optical path [14].

$$F_{corr} = F_{obs} \cdot 10^{\frac{(5 \cdot A_{ex} + A_{em})}{10}} \tag{1}$$

2.3. Time-Resolved Fluorescence

Fluorescence lifetime measurements were performed using a mini-tau filter-based fluorescence lifetime spectrometer coupled to a time-correlated single-photon counting (TCSPC) system (Edinburgh Instruments, Livingston, UK). Aliquots of piperine were added in the NBD solution at 4 μM. The piperine concentration varied from 0 to 20 μM. Experiments were carried out at 298 K.

The sample was excited at 295 nm using a picosecond pulsed light emitting diode (LED), and fluorescence decay was collected using a 340 nm filter. The fluorescence decay profile (Figure S1) was fitted using multiexponential decay (Equation (2)), where τ_i is the lifetime of each component, and α_i is the contribution of each component to total fluorescence decay. The average lifetime $<\tau_{avg}>$ was calculated using Equation (3) (Table S1).

$$I_T = \sum_{i=1}^{n} \alpha_i \cdot e^{\frac{-T}{\tau_i}} \tag{2}$$

$$\tau_{avg} = \frac{\alpha_1 {\tau_1}^2 + \alpha_2 {\tau_2}^2}{\alpha_1 \tau_1 + \alpha_2 \tau_2} \tag{3}$$

2.4. Circular Dichroism

Circular dichroism spectra were recorded at 288, 298 and 308 K on a Jasco J-815 spectropolarimeter model DRC-H (Jasco, Easton, MD, USA) equipped with a demountable quartz cell with a 0.01 cm optical path length. The CD spectra were recorded from the 200 to 260 nm range with a scan rate of 20 nm/min and a spectral resolution of 0.1 nm. For each spectrum, 15 accumulations were performed. The molar ratios of NBD and piperine were 1:0, 1:2.5, 1:5, 1:7.5, 1:10 and 1:12.5, and the buffer spectrum was subtracted. The ellipticity θ collected in millidegrees was converted to mean residue ellipticity [θ] ($deg.cm^2.dmol^{-1}$) using Equation (4).

$$[\theta] = \frac{\theta(mdeg)}{10 \cdot [P] \cdot l \cdot n} \tag{4}$$

The secondary structures' percentages were calculated with CDPro, applying the CONTIN method with the SP43 protein library [15].

2.5. Molecular Docking

The piperine structures used in the molecular docking were obtained from ab initio calculations from our previous work [16]. The NBD structure used in the molecular docking was extracted from PDB (1S3X). AutoDockTools [17] software of the MGL program Tools 1.5.4 was used to prepare the NBD by adding polar hydrogen atoms and Gasteiger charges. The maps were generated by the AutoGrid 4.2 program [18] with a spacing of 0.541 Å, a dimension of 126 × 126 × 126 points and grid center coordinates of 51.315, 43.754 and 48.905 for x, y and z coordinates, respectively. The AutoDock 4.2 program [17] was used to investigate the NBD binding sites using the Lamarckian genetic algorithm (LGA) with a population size of 150, a maximum number of generations of 27,000 and energy evaluations equal to 2.5×10^6. The other parameters were selected as software defaults. To generate different conformations, the total number of runs was set to 100. The final conformations were chosen among the most negative energies and belonging to the most representative cluster (Figure S2). The final conformations were visualized on VMD [19]. The binding microenvironment was generated by LigPlot [20].

2.6. Molecular Dynamics

The simulations of the complex NBD/piperine were performed with the GROMOS54a6 force field [21] by Gromacs v.5.1.4 [22]. The complex was placed in a rectangular box, solvated with simple point charge water (SPC) [23] and neutralized with NaCl in a concentration of 150 mM. The energy minimization was performed with the steepest descent. The first step of equilibration was performed in an NVT ensemble for 100 ps. The system was coupled to a V-rescale thermostat [24] at 298 K. All bonds were constrained with the LINCS algorithm [25], the cut-off for short-range non-bonded interactions was set at 1.4 nm and long-range electrostatics were calculated using the particle mesh ewald (PME) algorithm [26]. The second step of equilibration was performed in the NPT ensemble coupled to a Parrinello-Rahman barostat [27] to isotropically regulate the pressure for 100 ps. The pulling of piperine from the NBD pocket was performed without restraints to allow the protein conformational changes. The reaction coordinate ξ was chosen as being the distance between the Thr14 oxygen atom (O index 97) and piperine carbon atom (CAA 3802) for piperine into binding site 1 (Figure S3a) and between the Leu309 carbon atom (CA index 3073) and piperine carbon atom (CAL index 3800) for piperine into binding site 2 (Figure S3b). Piperine was pulled away from the NBD binding site in a Z direction until the reaction coordinate reached 7 nm for binding site 1 and 6 nm for binding site 2, using a spring constant of 1000 kJ/mol^{-1}nm^{-2} and a pull rate of 0.01 nm/ns (Figure S4). A sampling of the pullings was analyzed to guarantee a good sampling (Figure S5). The potential of mean force (PMF) profile [28] along the reaction coordinate was calculated with the WHAM method [29]. Statistical errors were estimated with a bootstrap analysis, with 1000 bootstraps properly autocorrelated.

The free energy of the binding process of piperine toward NBD was calculated by a G_mmpbsa tool [30], using the molecular mechanics Poisson Boltzmann surface area (MM/PBSA) method applied to the snapshots obtained from the molecular dynamics simulations. The snapshots were extracted from the trajectory after the system reached equilibrium, which was verified by the root mean square deviation (RMSD) obtained by the program *gmx rms* from Gromacs (Figure S6). The snapshots were extracted in intervals of 250 ps. The coarse grid-box (cfac) was set as 2 and the finner grid-box (fadd) was set as 20. The concentration of positive and negative ions was set as 0.150, being the positive and negative radii set as 0.95 and 1.81 Å, which correspond to sodium and chloride atoms, respectively. The values for the vacuum (vdie) and solvent (sdie) dielectric constants were set as 1 and 80, respectively. The solute dielectric constant (pdie) was set as 4.

3. Results and Discussions

3.1. Fluorescence Spectroscopy

Figure 1 shows the effect in the NBD Trp90 fluorescence caused by the addition of piperine in the solution. According to the spectra, there are two fluorescent bands centered at 330 nm and at 485 nm. The first one refers to protein Trp90 fluorescence emission while the second one refers to piperine fluorescence emission. The full-width half maximum (FWHM) for the band at 330 is ±30 nm and for the band at 480 is ±46 nm, which guarantees that the bands do not overlap and allows the fluorescence intensity at 330 nm to be handled accurately. Figure 1 also shows the fluorescence intensity of tryptophan decreased while piperine was added to the solution, which evidenced that Trp90 was quenched. Another characteristic observed is that the Trp90 fluorescence band remained centered at 330 nm during the piperine titration, which showed the fluorophore was not exposed to an environment with a different polarity [31].

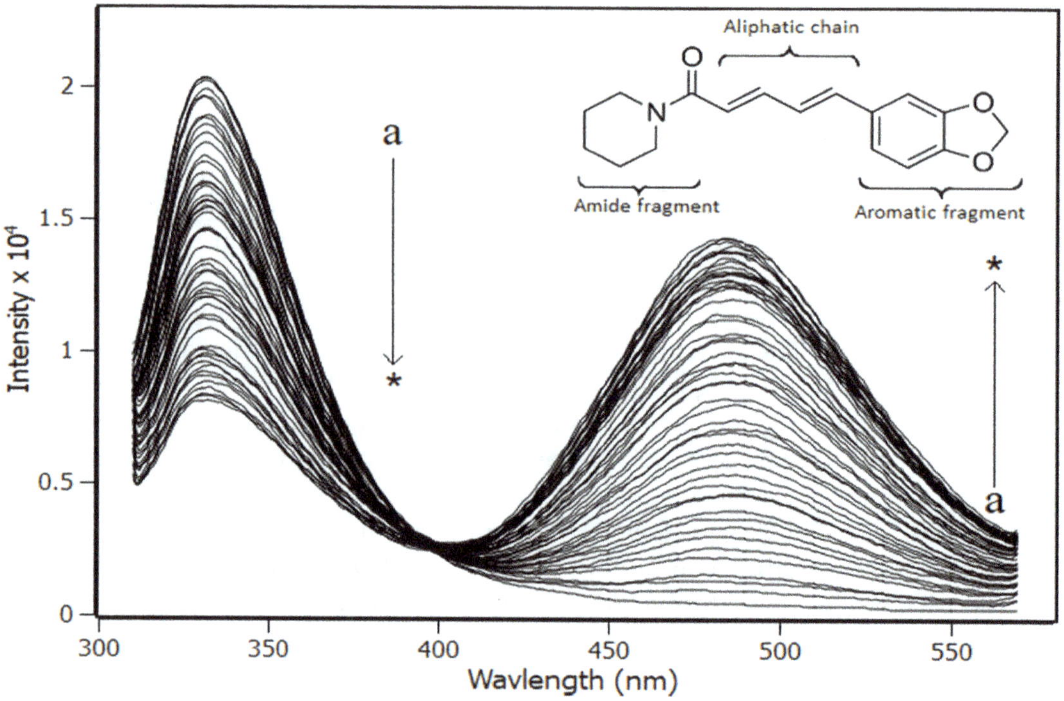

Figure 1. Spectra of fluorescence emission of nucleotide binding domain (NBD) obtained from titration experiments with increments in the concentration of piperine (pH 7.4, T = 288 K, λ_{exc} = 295 nm). (NBD) = 4.0 μM; piperine titrations with increment of 0.5 μM (a → * = 0 μM → 20 μM).

There are two possible different quenching mechanisms. One is dynamic quenching, when the ligand deactivates the excited form of the protein fluorophore by collisions. Another is static quenching, when there is a complex formation between the protein and the ligand. A simple way to distinguish the quenching mechanisms is by analyzing the Stern-Volmer constants (K_{SV}) at different temperatures [14] obtained by Equation (5). If the K_{SV} decreases with the rise in temperature, it is evidence of static quenching. On the other hand, if the K_{SV} increases with the rise in temperature, the quenching mechanism is not directly determined because the increase of K_{SV} may be an effect of either a complex formation drove by entropic factors or an effect of collisions.

A complementary method to determine the quenching mechanism is the association of the steady-state and time-resolved fluorescence data [32]. If the fluorophore is quenched by collisions, the ratio of fluorescence intensities F_0/F is equivalent to the ratio of fluorophore lifetime τ_0/τ, e.g.,: $F_0/F = \tau_0/\tau$. On the other hand, if such equivalence is not verified, static quenching is occurring. In addition, the combination of steady-state and time-resolved fluorescence data can result in a constant known as bimolecular quenching rate constant (k_q), which can be obtained through Equation (5). This constant is related to processes of diffusion, and in the case that the system is under collisions between the fluorophore and the ligand, the constant cannot exceed the order of 10^{10} $M^{-1}{\cdot}s^{-1}$ [32]; otherwise the quenching is static.

$$\frac{F_0}{F} = 1 + K_{SV}\cdot[\text{piperine}] = 1 + k_q\cdot\tau_0\cdot[\text{piperine}] \quad (5)$$

The Stern-Volmer plots (Figure 2) exhibited a linear response under piperine titration, indicating a single class of fluorophore in the protein and therefore the presence of one quenching mechanism process [33]. According to the results obtained for the K_{SV} constants presented in Table 1, the increase in temperature also caused the values of the constants to follow it. Figure 2 also shows that piperine poorly affected the Trp90 lifetime, once τ_0/τ remained close to the unity. Further, according to the plots, no equivalence is found between the ratios of fluorescence intensities and the lifetime values ($F_0/F \neq \tau_0/\tau$). The set of these results indicated that the system is under static quenching. To reinforce this indication, an analysis of the bimolecular constant at different temperatures was carried out (Table 1). It was found that for the three temperatures, k_q magnitude was of the order of 10^{12} $M^{-1} \cdot s^{-1}$, which is two orders of magnitude greater than that observed for collisional quenching (10^{10} $M^{-1} \cdot s^{-1}$). In conclusion, all these results revealed that the quenching mechanism is undoubtedly static and therefore a complex is formed by NBD and piperine.

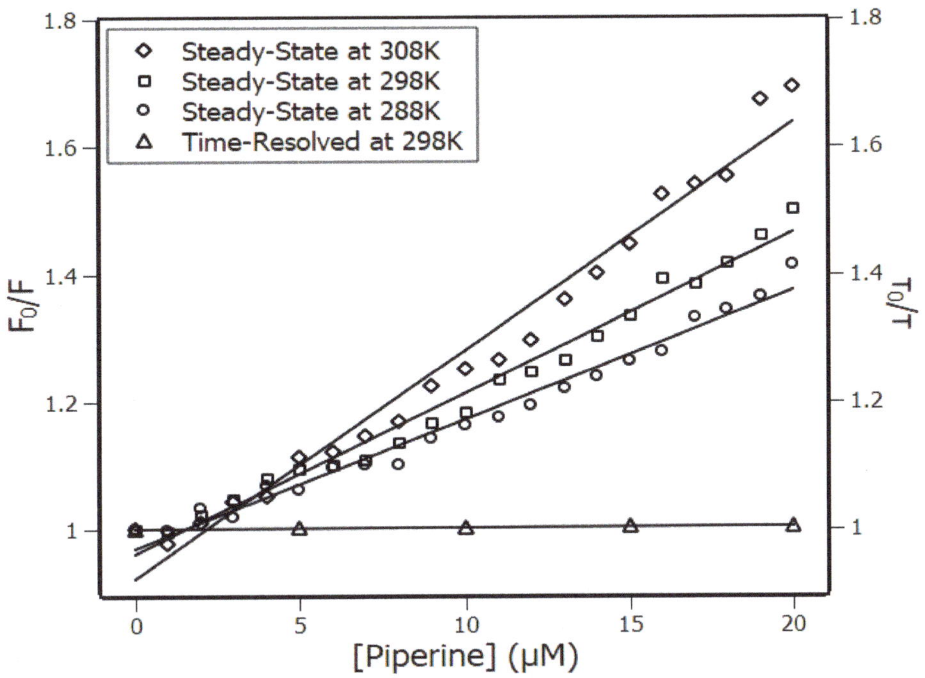

Figure 2. Left ordinate Stern–Volmer plots at three temperatures, 288 K, 298 K and 308 K, and right ordinate time-resolved fluorescence lifetime plot at 298 K; (NBD) = 4 μM, (piperine) = 0–20 μM. $R^2 > 0.98$.

Table 1. Stern-Volmer constant (K_{SV}), bimolecular constants (k_q) and binding constant (K_a) for the complex NBD and piperine at 288, 298 and 308 K.

Temperature (K)	Stern-Volmer (K_{SV}) $\times 10^4$ M^{-1}	Bimolecular (K_q) $\times 10^{12}$ $M^{-1} \cdot s^{-1}$	Binding (K_a) $\times 10^5$ M^{-1}
288	2.02 ± 0.07	9.18 ± 0.01	8.82 ± 0.07
298	2.52 ± 0.08	11.45 ± 0.01	44.60 ± 0.10
308	3.58 ± 0.1	16.27 ± 0.01	301.37 ± 1.1

Once the complex formation is proven, the next step was to obtain the binding constant (K_a), applying the binding equilibrium model. The K_a was obtained from the plot of Figure 3 using the double-logarithm equation (Equation (6)), which relates the quenching fluorescence intensities with the total concentration of piperine.

$$\log\left(\frac{F_0 - F}{F}\right) = \log K_a - n \cdot \log[\text{piperine}] \tag{6}$$

The results of K_a at different temperatures for the first order model ($n \approx 1$) are presented in Table 1. The binding constants found at different temperatures have a magnitude order of 10^5 M^{-1}, however their values differ at each temperature, meaning that it is under the direct influence of the available thermal energy.

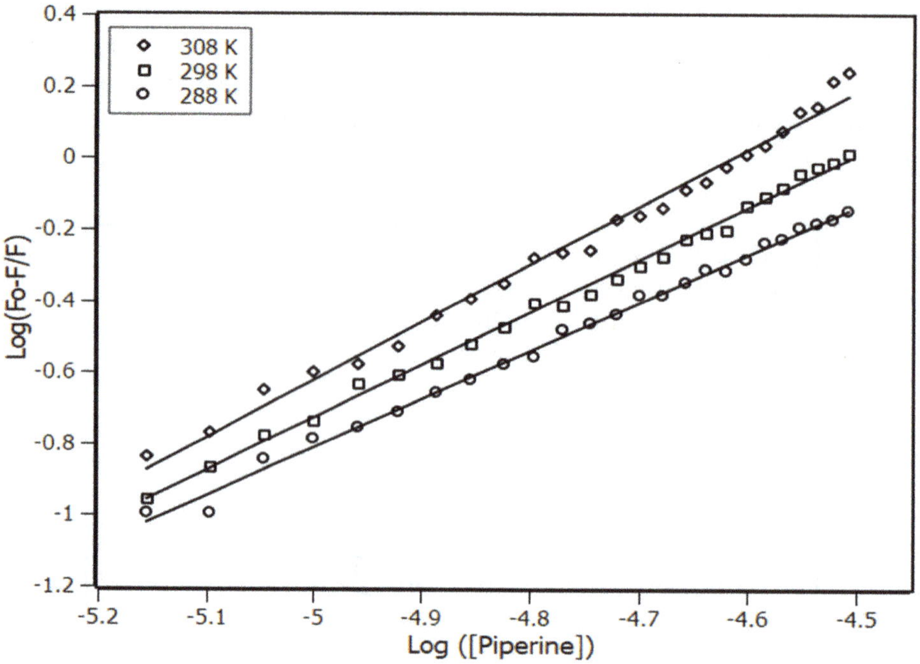

Figure 3. Double-log plots for the fluorescence quenching of NBD (4 μM) in the presence of piperine at 288 K, 298 K and 308 K. $R^2 > 0.99$.

3.2. *Thermodynamic Parameters*

Based on thermodynamic parameters such as ΔS (entropy variation), ΔH (enthalpy variation) and ΔG (Gibbs free variation) it is possible to gain more information about the complex formation and the forces that drive the process [34]. The parameters ΔS and ΔH are obtained from the van't Hoff plot (Figure 4) according to Equation (7) and ΔG is calculated from Equation (8).

$$\ln K_a = -\frac{\Delta H}{R \cdot T} + \frac{\Delta S}{R} \tag{7}$$

$$\Delta G = \Delta H - T\Delta S \tag{8}$$

The results of ΔS, ΔH and ΔG are shown in Table 2. Regarding the results, ΔG values were negative at the range of the applied temperatures, indicating that the complexation was a spontaneous process. Furthermore, the values of ΔG moved to more negative values with the rise in temperature due to the influence of the entropic factor, which favored the complex formation. Moreover, both terms T.ΔS and ΔH are positive, which indicated the non-specific interactions as the main contributor for the complexation. In addition, the entropic term is higher than the enthalpic, which reinforced the non-specific characteristic of the interactions.

Table 2. Thermodynamic parameters of the complex NBD-piperine at temperatures of 288 K, 298 K and 308 K.

T (K)	ΔG (kJ/mol)	ΔH (kJ/mol)	T.ΔS (kJ/mol)
288	−32.65 ± 1.31	130.13 ± 8.69	162.78 ± 8.4
298	−38.3 ± 1.94	130.13 ± 8.69	168.43 ± 8.69
308	−43.95 ± 2.06	130.13 ± 8.69	174.01 ± 8.98

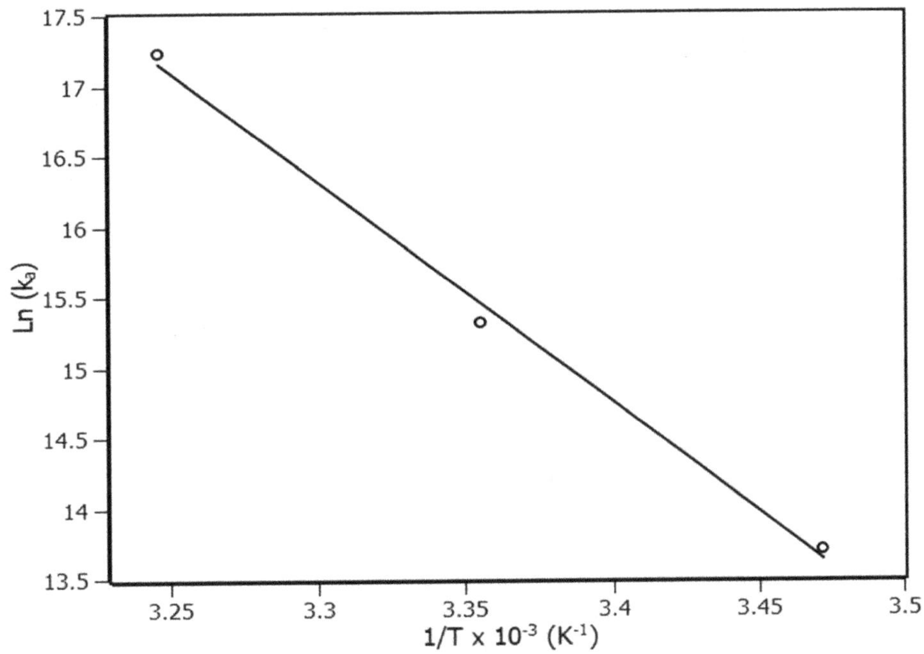

Figure 4. van't Hoff plot for the complex NBD-piperine at 288 K, 298 K and 308 K. $R^2 > 0.99$.

3.3. Interaction Density Function (IDF)

Considering the need to understand the way in which an NBD domain accommodates piperine in its sites, the IDF method was applied to the system as an alternative method in comparison to the binding equilibrium model in order to obtain a more complete description of the system. Interaction density function is a methodology used to treat experimental data, but it is different from the binding equilibrium model, as IDF does not make use of any model a priori and it is based on mass conservation law [35]. The advantage of applying IDF is the possibility of determining the real number of binding sites and identifying any matching factor between the sites. IDF considers that, if the free ligand concentration ($(\text{piperine})_{\text{free}}$) is the same for two or more solutions at different concentrations of total protein ((NBD)), the average interaction density ($\Sigma\upsilon_i$) will also be the same and consequently the system will have the same variation on the percentage of quenching (ΔF). The percentage of fluorescence quenching is given by Equation (9), where F and F_0 are the observed fluorescence signal with and without piperine, respectively. Figure 5 shows the plot of ΔF against the log [piperine] for three concentrations of NBD adjusted by a sigmoidal function.

$$\Delta F = \frac{|F - F_0|}{F_0} \cdot 100\% \tag{9}$$

Free ligand concentration and the average interaction density are related to each other through the expression of mass conservation (Equation (10)).

$$[\text{piperine}] = [\text{piperine}]_{\text{free}} + \left(\sum \nu_i\right) \cdot [\text{NBD}] \tag{10}$$

By means of the plot shown in Figure 5, the values of (NBD) and (piperine) for each ΔF was obtained. The inset of Figure 5 shows an example of 3 datasets of the plot of (piperine) versus (NBD) for each ΔF, in which $\Sigma\nu_i$ is obtained from the slope, and $(\text{piperine})_{\text{free}}$ is obtained from the y-intercept of the linear function.

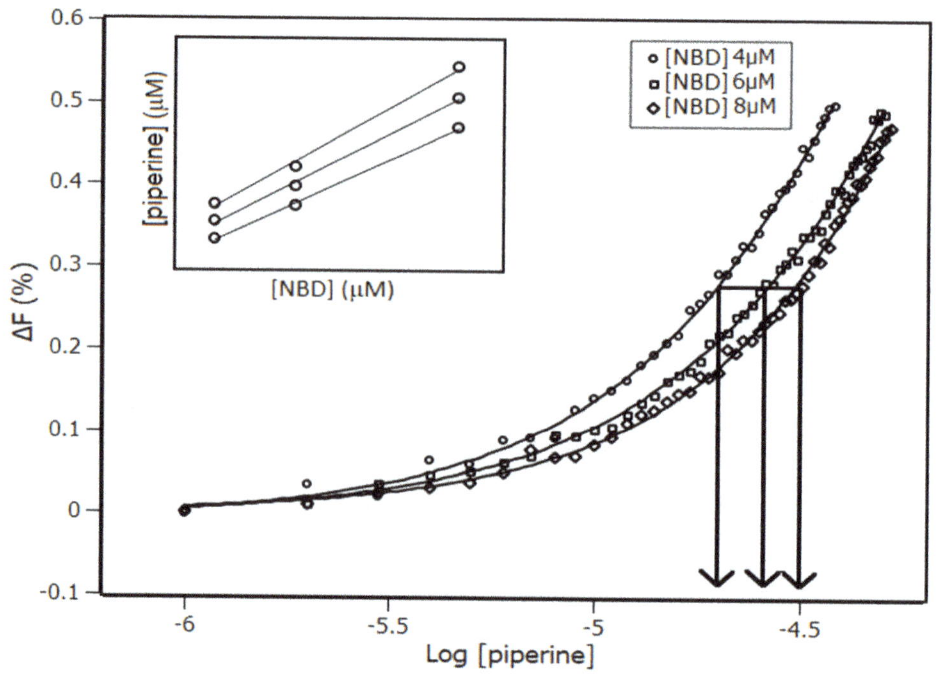

Figure 5. Plot of ΔF versus the log (piperine) obtained from piperine titration experiments with NBD concentrations of 4 μM, 6 μM and 8 μM at 288 K. The inset contains 3 datasets of (piperine) and (NBD) as an example of using Equation (5) to obtain the values of $\Sigma\nu_i$ and $(\text{piperine})_{free}$.

With the parameters $\Sigma\nu_i$ and $(\text{piperine})_{free}$ obtained from IDF, a Scatchard plot was built (Figure 6a), an important source of information about cooperativity. It may reveal if the binding sites of the protein are equivalents or non-equivalents, if there is cooperativity among them as well as if the cooperativity is positive or negative [36,37]. Figure 6a shows a line profile with negative concavity, pointing out positive cooperativity. Although Scatchard's plot reveals the occurrence of cooperativity, it does not identify the number of sites that NBD has. To complement this information, it is necessary to use the Hill's plot to disclose additional features such as the number of binding sites (n) and the binding constants (K_b) [38,39]. The Hill's plot is shown in Figure 6b, whose parameters n and K_b were obtained by Equation (11). The parameter h is called the Hill coefficient, which indicates the type of cooperativity. The Hill coefficient can assume values of >1, <1 and =1 indicating positive cooperativity, negative cooperativity and non-cooperativity, respectively.

$$\sum \nu_i = \sum_j \frac{n.(k_b \cdot [\text{piperine}]_{free}])^h}{1 + (k_b \cdot [\text{piperine}]_{free}])^h} \tag{11}$$

Regarding the results obtained by the Hill equation, the protein has two equivalent binding sites with $K_b = (2.67 \pm 0.12) \times 10^5\ M^{-1}$ and positive cooperativity (h = 2.4). The results show that both methods (Scatchard and Hill) are in full agreement, revealing a positive cooperativity system. Further, the binding constant found with Hill's method is in the magnitude order of $10^5\ M^{-1}$, which is in agreement with that found by the binding equilibrium method. Both methods (the binding equilibrium and Hill methods) differed somewhat in terms of the absolute value of the binding constant. This difference found is due to the fact that the binding equilibrium method uses a first order chemical reaction model while the Hill method does not, as discussed previously in the literature [16,31,40].

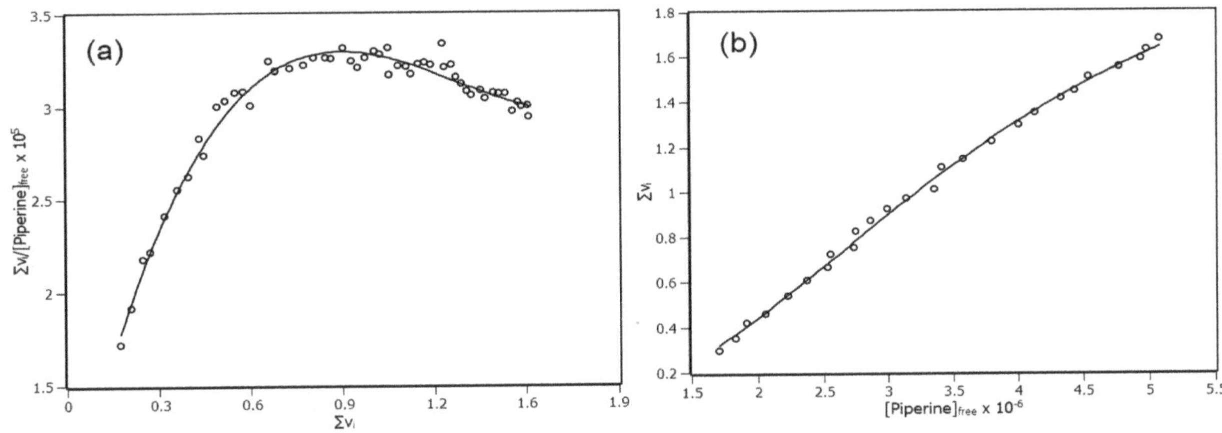

Figure 6. (**a**) Scatchard plot for the interaction of NBD and piperine obtained at 288 K based on interaction density function (IDF) data. (**b**) Hill plot for the interaction of NBD and piperine obtained at 288 K based on IDF data. $R^2 > 0.99$.

3.4. Circular Dichroism

A protein that presents cooperativity when interacting with a ligand may be susceptible to conformational changes, adjusting its structure. To have a complete description about the influence of piperine in NBD structure, circular dichroism experiments were performed (Figure 7).

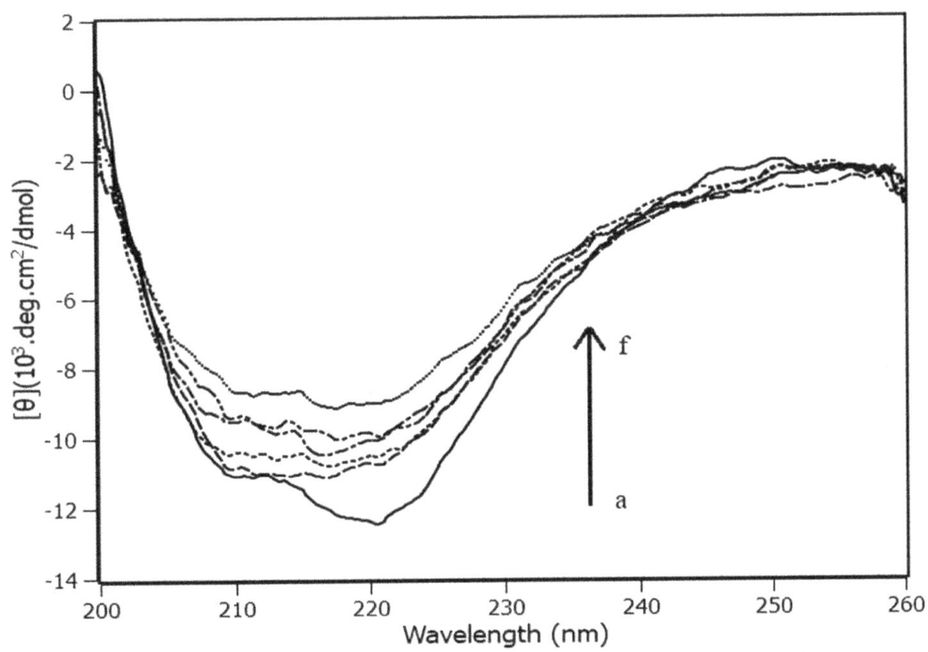

Figure 7. NBD circular dichroism experiments at 298 K in the presence and absence of piperine. Aliquots of piperine were added to the solution from a → f = 1:0 → 1:12.5.

The circular dichroism spectrum of NBD in solution has well-defined bands at 208 nm and 222 nm, which is characteristic of an alpha-helices secondary structure. In order to obtain more details about the secondary structures, the protein spectra were deconvolved by CDPro software aided by the CONTINNL algorithm with 43 soluble proteins spectra deposited in its library. According to the analyses, NBD has 34% of alpha-helices, 16% of beta sheet, 20% of turns and 30% of coil. These results are in good agreement with the data reported in the literature for the same protein using CDNN software [41].

According to the results presented in Figure 7, the protein underwent structural changes during the titration. At the highest concentration of piperine and NDB (1:12.5), its secondary structure was composed 25% of alpha-helices, 21% of beta-sheet, 22% of turn and 32% of coil. Turn and coil content results did not undergo significant secondary structural changes (≈2%). In the meantime, alpha-helices dropped from 34% to 26% and beta sheet content rose from 16% to 31%. These results revealed that the positive cooperativity found by the Scatchard and Hill methods are followed by the NBD structural changes.

3.5. Molecular Modeling

3.5.1. Molecular Docking

Molecular docking was applied to predict the two binding sites found experimentally. The binding environment of the two sites is shown in Figure 8 and according to the results, the predominant molecular interactions are non-specific, with just one hydrogen bond with 2.79 Å of length performed by piperine and His89. This result is in agreement with the experimental van't Hoff analysis that indicated the non-specific interactions were predominant. The binding site 1 is composed of the non-polar amino acids Pro91, Phe68, Phe92, Phe150 and Trp90, by the polar amino acids Gln154, Asn151, Tyr149, Thr13 and His89, by amino acids charged positively, Arg76, Lys71, Arg72 and His89, and a negative Asp69.

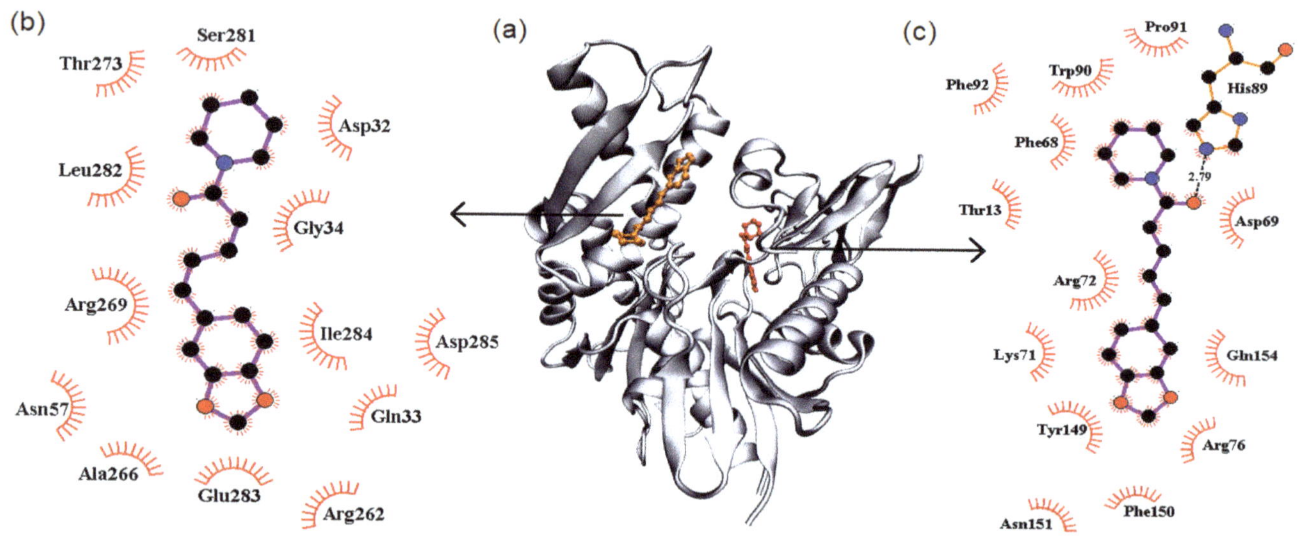

Figure 8. The central picture represents the molecular docking (**a**) in a general view. In red is piperine in binding site 1, in orange in site 2. Pose (**b**) binding environment of site 2, and (**c**) site 1 with a dotted line indicating the hydrogen bonds.

Binding site 2 is composed of the non-polar amino acids Gly34, Ile284, Ala266 and Leu282, by the polar amino acids Ser281, Gln33, Asn57 and Thr273, by amino acids charged positively, Arg262 and Arg269, and by amino acids charged negatively, Asp32, Asp285 and Glu283.

3.5.2. Molecular Dynamics

The two most promising binding sites predicted by molecular docking were explored by the umbrella sampling method. Figure 9 shows the potential of mean force profiles resulting from the complex dissociation obtained for the two binding sites. According to the results, both binding site profiles presented the minimum of energy at the configuration predicted by molecular docking, which indicated that the two configurations are stable. Potential of mean force (PMF) profiles also revealed that the energetic barrier to unbind piperine from the binding sites is higher in site 1 than in site 2. The standard free energy for the binding sites (ΔG_{pred}) was determined from WHAM analyses, with (−45 ± 5) kJ/mol for binding site 1 and (−41.8 ± 4) kJ/mol for binding site 2. Although the PMF profiles revealed that the binding sites are distinct in terms of the energetic barrier profile to dissociate piperine, the binding free energy values determined with WHAM analyses are very close considering the statistical errors, corroborating the results obtained from Hill's plot that showed equivalence between the binding affinities of both sites.

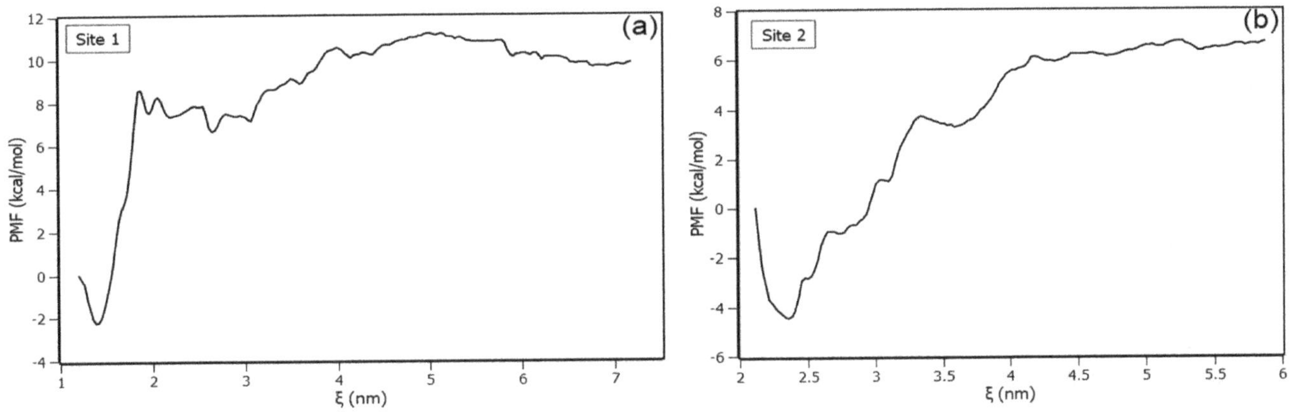

Figure 9. Potential of mean force (PMF) for the dissociation of piperine from NBD, (**a**) for binding site 1 and for (**b**) binding site 2.

The lower computational time consuming method MM/PBSA was employed to highlight the effect on binding free energy caused by piperine into the two binding sites (Table 3). It is an advantageous method to compare binding energies and comprehend which interaction has the highest binding affinity. The binding free energy calculations were performed in two steps. The first step consisted of calculating the binding free energy of the complex with one binding site occupied. The second step consisted of calculating the binding free energy of the complex with both binding sites occupied. According to the results summarized in Table 3, the binding free energy when both binding sites were accessed (columns 4 and 5) is more negative than when just one site is accessed by piperine (columns 2 and 3), with approximately 10 kJ/mol of difference. These results showed a higher binding affinity of piperine for NBD accessing both sites than a single site, which is evidence of cooperativity, in agreement with the experimental fluorescence analyses of the interaction.

Table 3. Energies obtained from molecular mechanics Poisson Boltzmann surface area (MM/PBSA) for piperine occupying both sites and for piperine occupying just one site. Van der Waals, Electrostatic, polar solvation and SASA were obtained from a PBSA calculation.

Energies (kJ/mol)	**Site 1**	**Site 2**	**Both Sites Occupied**	
			Site 1	**Site 2**
Binding free energy ΔG	−35.22 ± 2.45	−34.59 ± 2.60	−49.92 ± 3.01	−46.15 ± 2.03
van der Waals	−97.63 ± 1.86	−119.61 ± 2.25	−73.74 ± 1.98	−96.12 ± 1.45
Electrostatic	−11.76 ± 0.85	−25.23 ± 0.95	−2.80 ± 1.73	−12.31 ± 1.17
Polar solvation	86.80 ± 2.89	124.32 ± 3.52	36.25 ± 3.34	73.88 ± 2.1
SASA	−12.64 ± 0.24	−14.07 ± 0.23	−9.64 ± 0.25	−11.59 ± 0.12

The root mean square fluctuation (RMSF) of NBD simulated in the absence of ligand disclosed the dynamic of the protein residues, indicating that NBD presented some specific regions with high fluctuation (>0.25 nm). The RMSF of NBD simulated with site 1 and 2 occupied by piperine showed that the interaction with ligand induced a decrease in the fluctuation of some regions that was previously high; such regions where marked with blue dots in Figure S7a. According to the results, most of the amino acids that exhibited expressive changes in RMSF surround piperine in binding site 2 (blue new cartoon regions of Figure S7b,c), while it was noted that there were few fluctuation changes for residues surrounding piperine in binding site 1.

4. Conclusions

In the present work, the interaction between piperine and NBD was investigated by means of experimental and computational molecular biophysical tools. Steady-state and time-resolved fluorescence showed that NBD in the presence of piperine presented a static-quenching process, which means that a complex was formed. Fluorescence spectroscopy revealed with a Scatchard plot and Hill's method an important feature about the interaction of NBD and piperine, which was the presence of positive cooperativity between the two binding sites. In addition, the thermodynamic parameters were disclosed, showing the spontaneity of a complex formation ($\Delta G < 0$ kJ/mol) for the three temperatures. Circular dichroism revealed that the protein underwent conformational changes due to the interaction with piperine. The binding sites were unveiled by molecular docking and molecular dynamics, which reinforced the binding free energy found experimentally. Molecular dynamics along with MM/PBSA reinforced the positive cooperativity found experimentally, showing that the binding free energy was more negative when both binding sites were occupied by piperine. In other words, the affinity was higher under this condition than when just one binding site was occupied. A multispectroscopic evaluation aided by molecular docking and dynamics elucidated in detail the NBD/piperine molecular interaction, which may support further drug discovery studies.

Supplementary Materials:
Figure S1: Time-resolved fluorescence decay of (a) NBD with Piperine (→e) from 0 to 20 μM. [IL-1β] = 10 μM, T = 298 K and λex = 295 nm, Figure S2: Molecular docking clusters with their respectives energy scores, Figure S3: The atoms picked to define the reaction coordinate (ξ) for (a) binding site 1 and (b) binding site 2, Figure S4: Pulling profile during the pulling simulation. Y-axis is the value of reaction coordinate (ξ) and x-axis is the time of simulation, Figure S5: Configuration histograms of the pulling in z-axis with the windows distance as being 0.1 nm for (a) binding site 1 and (b) binding site 2, Figure S6: Root mean square deviation (RMSD) of (a) NBD in the presence of piperine and (b) piperine occupying the binding sites, Figure S7: (a) Root mean square fluctuation (RMSF) of NBD residues in the absence and presence of piperine in both binding sites (red and black, respectively), blue dots represent the residues that altered the fluctuation from high to low when the ligands were inserted in the binding sites. (b) and (c) Blue cartoon represents the regions that altered the fluctuation from high to low when the ligands were inserted in the binding sites. Red and Orange represent piperine in site 1 and in site 2, respectively, Table S1: Tryptophan lifetime in different stoichiometries NBD: Piperine.

Author Contributions: Experimental data acquisition: G.Z. and A.P.R.P. Theoretical models: G.Z., A.P.R.P. and M.d.F.L. Data analysis: G.Z., A.P.R.P., M.d.F.L. and M.L.C. Manuscript writing: G.Z., A.P.R.P. and M.L.C. Project Administration and Supervision: M.L.C. All authors have read and agreed to the published version of the manuscript.

Acknowledgments: Molecular Dynamics simulations were performed at the Center for Scientific Computing (NCC/GridUNESP) of São Paulo State University (UNESP), Brazil. The authors thank João Ruggiero Neto for availability of spectropolarimeter and Valdecir Ximenes for availability of fluorescence lifetime spectrometer.

References

1. Dubrez, L.; Causse, S.; Bonan, N.B.; Dumetier, B.; Garrido, C. Heat-shock proteins: Chaperoning DNA repair. *Oncogene* **2019**, *39*, 1–14. [CrossRef] [PubMed]
2. Jones, A.M.; Westwood, I.M.; Osborne, J.D.; Matthews, T.P.; Cheeseman, M.D.; Rowlands, M.G.; Jeganathan, F.; Burke, R.; Lee, D.; Kadi, N. A fragment-based approach applied to a highly flexible target: Insights and challenges towards the inhibition of HSP70 isoforms. *Sci. Rep.* **2016**, *6*, 34701. [CrossRef] [PubMed]

3. Asea, A.; Kraeft, S.-K.; Kurt-Jones, E.A.; Stevenson, M.A.; Chen, L.B.; Finberg, R.W.; Koo, G.C.; Calderwood, S.K. HSP70 stimulates cytokine production through a CD14-dependant pathway, demonstrating its dual role as a chaperone and cytokine. *Nat. Med.* **2000**, *6*, 435–442. [CrossRef] [PubMed]
4. Asea, A.; Rehli, M.; Kabingu, E.; Boch, J.A.; Baré, O.; Auron, P.E.; Stevenson, M.A.; Calderwood, S.K. Novel signal transduction pathway utilized by extracellular HSP70 role of Toll-like receptor (TLR) 2 and TLR4. *J. Biol. Chem.* **2002**, *277*, 15028–15034. [CrossRef] [PubMed]
5. Somensi, N.; Brum, P.O.; de Miranda Ramos, V.; Gasparotto, J.; Zanotto-Filho, A.; Rostirolla, D.C.; da Silva Morrone, M.; Moreira, J.C.F.; Gelain, D.P. Extracellular HSP70 activates ERK1/2, NF-kB and pro-inflammatory gene transcription through binding with RAGE in A549 human lung cancer cells. *Cell. Physiol. Biochem.* **2017**, *42*, 2507–2522. [CrossRef]
6. Pahl, H.L. Activators and target genes of Rel/NF-κB transcription factors. *Oncogene* **1999**, *18*, 6853–6866. [CrossRef]
7. Evans, C.G.; Chang, L.; Gestwicki, J.E. Heat shock protein 70 (hsp70) as an emerging drug target. *J. Med. Chem.* **2010**, *53*, 4585–4602. [CrossRef]
8. de Oliveira, A.A.; Faustino, J.; de Lima, M.E.; Menezes, R.; Nunes, K.P. Unveiling the interplay between the TLR4/MD2 complex and HSP70 in the human cardiovascular system: A computational approach. *Int. J. Mol. Sci.* **2019**, *20*, 3121. [CrossRef]
9. Cheeseman, M.D.; Westwood, I.M.; Barbeau, O.; Rowlands, M.; Dobson, S.; Jones, A.M.; Jeganathan, F.; Burke, R.; Kadi, N.; Workman, P. Exploiting protein conformational change to optimize adenosine-derived inhibitors of HSP70. *J. Med. Chem.* **2016**, *59*, 4625–4636. [CrossRef]
10. Zazeri, G.; Povinelli, A.P.R.; Le Duff, C.S.; Tang, B.; Cornelio, M.L.; Jones, A.M. Synthesis and Spectroscopic Analysis of Piperine-and Piperlongumine-Inspired Natural Product Scaffolds and Their Molecular Docking with IL-1β and NF-κB Proteins. *Molecules* **2020**, *25*, 2841. [CrossRef]
11. Ying, X.; Chen, X.; Cheng, S.; Shen, Y.; Peng, L.; Xu, H. Piperine inhibits IL-β induced expression of inflammatory mediators in human osteoarthritis chondrocyte. *Int. Immunopharmacol.* **2013**, *17*, 293–299. [CrossRef] [PubMed]
12. Bang, J.S.; Choi, H.M.; Sur, B.-J.; Lim, S.-J.; Kim, J.Y.; Yang, H.-I.; Yoo, M.C.; Hahm, D.-H.; Kim, K.S. Anti-inflammatory and antiarthritic effects of piperine in human interleukin 1β-stimulated fibroblast-like synoviocytes and in rat arthritis models. *Arthritis Res. Ther.* **2009**, *11*, R49. [CrossRef] [PubMed]
13. Ying, X.; Yu, K.; Chen, X.; Chen, H.; Hong, J.; Cheng, S.; Peng, L. Piperine inhibits LPS induced expression of inflammatory mediators in RAW 264.7 cells. *Cell. Immunol.* **2013**, *285*, 49–54. [CrossRef] [PubMed]
14. Lakowicz, J.R. *Principles of Fluorescence Spectroscopy*; Springer Science & Business Media: Berlin/Heidelberg, Germany, 2004.
15. Sreerama, N.; Woody, R.W. Estimation of protein secondary structure from circular dichroism spectra: Comparison of CONTIN, SELCON, and CDSSTR methods with an expanded reference set. *Anal. Biochem.* **2000**, *287*, 252–260. [CrossRef]
16. Zazeri, G.; Povinelli, A.P.R.; de Lima, M.F.; Cornélio, M.L. Experimental Approaches and Computational Modeling of Rat Serum Albumin and Its Interaction with Piperine. *Int. J. Mol. Sci.* **2019**, *20*, 2856. [CrossRef]
17. Morris, G.M.; Huey, R.; Lindstrom, W.; Sanner, M.F.; Belew, R.K.; Goodsell, D.S.; Olson, A.J. AutoDock4 and AutoDockTools4: Automated docking with selective receptor flexibility. *J. Comput. Chem.* **2009**, *30*, 2785–2791. [CrossRef]
18. Morris, G.M.; Goodsell, D.S.; Pique, M.E.; Lindstrom, W.; Huey, R.; Forli, S.; Hart, W.E.; Halliday, S.; Belew, R.; Olson, A.J. *User Guide AutoDock Version 4.2. Automated Docking of Flexible Ligands to Flexible Receptors*; AutoGrid: Redwood City, CA, USA, 2010.
19. Humphrey, W.; Dalke, A.; Schulten, K. VMD: Visual molecular dynamics. *J. Mol. Graph.* **1996**, *14*, 33–38. [CrossRef]
20. Wallace, A.C.; Laskowski, R.A.; Thornton, J.M. LIGPLOT: A program to generate schematic diagrams of protein-ligand interactions. *Protein Eng. Des. Sel.* **1995**, *8*, 127–134. [CrossRef]
21. Oostenbrink, C.; Villa, A.; Mark, A.E.; Van Gunsteren, W.F. A biomolecular force field based on the free enthalpy of hydration and solvation: The GROMOS force-field parameter sets 53A5 and 53A6. *J. Comput. Chem.* **2004**, *25*, 1656–1676. [CrossRef]
22. Van Der Spoel, D.; Lindahl, E.; Hess, B.; Groenhof, G.; Mark, A.E.; Berendsen, H.J.C. GROMACS: Fast, flexible, and free. *J. Comput. Chem.* **2005**, *26*, 1701–1718. [CrossRef]

23. Wu, Y.; Tepper, H.L.; Voth, G.A. Flexible simple point-charge water model with improved liquid-state properties. *J. Chem. Phys.* **2006**, *124*, 24503. [CrossRef] [PubMed]
24. Bussi, G.; Donadio, D.; Parrinello, M. Canonical sampling through velocity rescaling. *J. Chem. Phys.* **2007**, *126*, 14101. [CrossRef] [PubMed]
25. Hess, B.; Bekker, H.; Berendsen, H.J.C.; Fraaije, J.G.E.M. LINCS: A linear constraint solver for molecular simulations. *J. Comput. Chem.* **1997**, *18*, 1463–1472. [CrossRef]
26. Batcho, P.F.; Case, D.A.; Schlick, T. Optimized particle-mesh Ewald/multiple-time step integration for molecular dynamics simulations. *J. Chem. Phys.* **2001**, *115*, 4003–4018. [CrossRef]
27. Parrinello, M.; Rahman, A. Polymorphic transitions in single crystals: A new molecular dynamics method. *J. Appl. Phys.* **1981**, *52*, 7182–7190. [CrossRef]
28. Roux, B. The calculation of the potential of mean force using computer simulations. *Comput. Phys. Commun.* **1995**, *91*, 275–282. [CrossRef]
29. Kumar, S.; Rosenberg, J.M.; Bouzida, D.; Swendsen, R.H.; Kollman, P.A. The weighted histogram analysis method for free-energy calculations on biomolecules. I. The method. *J. Comput. Chem.* **1992**, *13*, 1011–1021. [CrossRef]
30. Kumari, R.; Kumar, R.; Consortium, O.S.D.D.; Lynn, A. g_mmpbsa A GROMACS tool for high-throughput MM-PBSA calculations. *J. Chem. Inf. Model.* **2014**, *54*, 1951–1962. [CrossRef]
31. Povinelli, A.P.R.; Zazeri, G.; de Freitas Lima, M.; Cornélio, M.L. Details of the cooperative binding of piperlongumine with rat serum albumin obtained by spectroscopic and computational analyses. *Sci. Rep.* **2019**, *9*, 1–11. [CrossRef]
32. Lakowicz, J.R.; Weber, G. Quenching of fluorescence by oxygen. Probe for structural fluctuations in macromolecules. *Biochemistry* **1973**, *12*, 4161–4170. [CrossRef]
33. Soares, S.; Mateus, N.; De Freitas, V. Interaction of different polyphenols with bovine serum albumin (BSA) and human salivary α-amylase (HSA) by fluorescence quenching. *J. Agric. Food Chem.* **2007**, *55*, 6726–6735. [CrossRef] [PubMed]
34. Ross, P.D.; Subramanian, S. Thermodynamics of protein association reactions: Forces contributing to stability. *Biochemistry* **1981**, *20*, 3096–3102. [CrossRef] [PubMed]
35. Lohman, T.M.; Bujalowski, W. Thermodynamic methods for model-independent determination of equilibrium binding isotherms for protein-DNA interactions: Spectroscopic approaches to monitor binding. *Methods Enzymol.* **1991**, *208*, 258–290. [PubMed]
36. Scatchard, G. The attractions of proteins for small molecules and ions. *Ann. N. Y. Acad. Sci.* **1949**, *51*, 660–672. [CrossRef]
37. Povinelli, A.P.R.; Zazeri, G.; Cornélio, M.L. Molecular Mechanism of Flavonoids Using Fluorescence Spectroscopy and Computational Tools. In *Flavonoids-A Coloring Model For Cheering Up Life*; IntechOpen: Rijeka, Croatia, 2019.
38. Bordbar, A.K.; Saboury, A.A.; Moosavi-Movahedi, A.A. The shapes of Scatchard plots for systems with two sets of binding sites. *Biochem. Educ.* **1996**, *24*, 172–175. [CrossRef]
39. Barcroft, J.; Hill, A.V. The nature of oxyhaemoglobin, with a note on its molecular weight. *J. Physiol.* **1910**, *39*, 411. [CrossRef]
40. Zazeri, G.; Povinelli, A.P.R.; de Freitas Lima, M.; Cornélio, M.L. The Cytokine IL-1β and Piperine Complex Surveyed by Experimental and Computational Molecular Biophysics. *Biomolecules* **2020**, *10*, 1337. [CrossRef]
41. Borges, J.C.; Ramos, C.H.I. Spectroscopic and thermodynamic measurements of nucleotide-induced changes in the human 70-kDa heat shock cognate protein. *Arch. Biochem. Biophys.* **2006**, *452*, 46–54. [CrossRef]

10

Differential Activation of TRP Channels in the Adult Rat Spinal Substantia Gelatinosa by Stereoisomers of Plant-Derived Chemicals

Eiichi Kumamoto * and Tsugumi Fujita

Department of Physiology, Saga Medical School, 5-1-1 Nabeshima, Saga 849-8501, Japan; fujitat@cc.saga-u.ac.jp
* Correspondence: kumamote@cc.saga-u.ac.jp

Academic Editors: Arpad Szallasi, Susan M. Huang and Jean Jacques Vanden Eynde

Abstract: Activation of TRPV1, TRPA1 or TRPM8 channel expressed in the central terminal of dorsal root ganglion (DRG) neuron increases the spontaneous release of L-glutamate onto spinal dorsal horn lamina II (substantia gelatinosa; SG) neurons which play a pivotal role in regulating nociceptive transmission. The TRP channels are activated by various plant-derived chemicals. Although stereoisomers activate or modulate ion channels in a distinct manner, this phenomenon is not fully addressed for TRP channels. By applying the whole-cell patch-clamp technique to SG neurons of adult rat spinal cord slices, we found out that all of plant-derived chemicals, carvacrol, thymol, carvone and cineole, increase the frequency of spontaneous excitatory postsynaptic current, a measure of the spontaneous release of L-glutamate from nerve terminals, by activating TRP channels. The presynaptic activities were different between stereoisomers (carvacrol and thymol; (−)-carvone and (+)-carvone; 1,8-cineole and 1,4-cineole) in the extent or the types of TRP channels activated, indicating that TRP channels in the SG are activated by stereoisomers in a distinct manner. This result could serve to know the properties of the central terminal TRP channels that are targets of drugs for alleviating pain.

Keywords: TRPV1; TRPA1; TRPM8; plant-derived chemical; L-glutamate release; spinal dorsal horn; patch-clamp; rat

---

1. TRP Channels Involved in Nociceptive Transmission through Dorsal Root Ganglion Neurons

Cation-permeable transient receptor potential (TRP) channels expressed in dorsal root ganglion (DRG) neurons are involved in nociceptive transmission from the periphery (for a review see [1]). TRP channels, which are synthesized in the cell body of the DRG neuron, are transported to the peripheral and central terminals of the neuron by axonal transport. Among TRP channels involved in the nociceptive transmission, there are TRP vanilloid-1 (TRPV1), TRP ankyrin-1 (TRPA1) and TRP melastatin-8 (TRPM8) channels. The TRPA1 channel is found in a subset of rat DRG neurons in which it is co-expressed with the TRPV1, but not the TRPM8 channel [2,3]. They are activated by chemical substances and temperature (for reviews see [4,5]). For instance, in the peripheral terminal of the DRG neuron, the TRPV1 channel is activated by capsaicin (a natural pungent ingredient contained in red peppers), protons and noxious heat (>43 °C; [6]; for review see [7]); the TRPA1 channel by pungent compounds in mustard, cinnamon and garlic (allyl isothiocyanate (AITC), cinnamaldehyde and allicin, respectively), and noxious cold temperature (<17 °C; [2,8–10]); and the TRPM8 channel by menthol (a secondary alcohol contained in peppermint or other mint) and mild temperature (<25 °C; [11,12]). Such an activation depolarizes the membrane of the peripheral terminal, resulting in the production of action potentials. As a result, the nociceptive or temperature information is transferred to the spinal dorsal horn.

On the other hand, TRP channels in the central terminal of the DRG neuron are expressed in the superficial laminae of the dorsal horn, especially the substantia gelatinosa (SG; lamina II of Rexed; [13,14]). In support of this idea about TRP activation in the SG, many of plant-derived chemicals increase in SG neurons the frequency of spontaneous excitatory postsynaptic current (sEPSC), a measure of the spontaneous release of L-glutamate from nerve terminals, by activating TRPV1 channel [15–18], TRPA1 channel [19,20] and TRPM8 channel [21,22] (for a review see [23]). The SG neurons play a pivotal role in modulating nociceptive transmission from the periphery [24–26] and thus TRP channels in the SG are involved in its modulation. Their expressions in the SG have been shown by immunohistochemistry [27].

2. Spinal Substantia Gelatinosa Involved in Regulating Nociceptive Transmission

Nociceptive transmission in the SG is in origin not only monosynaptic from glutamatergic DRG neurons but also polysynaptic from glutamate-, GABA- and/or glycine-containing interneurons [28]. In support of the involvement of the SG in nociceptive transmission, a plastic change in glutamatergic inputs to SG neurons through DRG neurons occurred in hyperalgesic rats that were subject to either an intraplantar injection of complete Freund's adjuvant [29] or ovariectomy [30]. Endogenous and exogenous analgesics, which exhibit antinociception when administrated intrathecally, hyperpolarize membranes of SG neurons and reduce the release of L-glutamate onto SG neurons from nerve terminals, both of which actions reduce the membrane excitability of the SG neurons [31]. For example, opioids ([32]; for a review see [33]), nociceptin [34,35], a $GABA_B$-receptor agonist baclofen [36,37], a μ-opioid receptor agonist tramadol [38], norepinephrine [39], serotonin [30,40], adenosine ([41,42]; for review see [43]), somatostatin [44,45], dopamine [46,47] and galanin [48] hyperpolarized membranes of rat SG neurons. Inhibition of the release of L-glutamate from nerve terminals onto rat SG neurons was produced by opioids ([49]; for review see [33]), nociceptin [50,51], baclofen [36,52,53], the endocannabinoid anandamide [16,54], norepinephrine [55], serotonin [30,40], adenosine ([41,56,57]; for a review see [43]) and galanin [48,58].

3. TRP Channels in Nociception

Much evidence demonstrates that TRP channels play a role in transferring nociceptive information. For example, neuropathic pain and hyperalgesia developed following excessive or ectopical expression of TRPV1 channel in the central nervous system (CNS) and peripheral nervous system, in both animals and humans [59–62]. Hyperalgesia in inflammatory pain models was reduced in TRPV1-knockout mice [63]. Nerve growth factor, which mediates inflammatory pain, upregulated the expression of TRPV1 channel in rat DRG neurons by an action of the small GTPase Ras [64]. Excessive expression of TRPV1 channel in primary-afferent fibers occurred in disease states including inflammatory disease and irritable bowel syndrome [65,66]. Peripheral inflammation upregulated TRPV1 channel involved in the enhancement of spontaneous excitatory transmission in rat SG neurons [67]. When intrathecally administrated, a powerful TRPV1 agonist resiniferatoxin (RTX, a component contained in the dried latex of the cactus-like plant; [68]) produced a prolonged antinociceptive response in dogs with bone cancer [69], possibly owing to a desensitization of TRPV1 channel. Selective inhibition of TRPV1 channel attenuated bone cancer pain in the mouse [70]. TRPV1 channel, which is a potential treatment target for cancer pain, was expressed in neurons that transfer information of this type of pain (for a review see [71]). Intrathecal application of a TRPV1 antagonist AS1928370 resulted in an inhibition of mechanical allodynia in a mouse model of neuropathic pain [72].

The TRPA1 agonist cinnamaldehyde evoked spontaneous pain, and induced mechanical hyperalgesia and cold hypoalgesia following its application to the forearm skin of human volunteers [73]. Moreover, TRPA1 channel was over-expressed in rat DRG neurons following peripheral inflammation and nerve injury, and cold hyperalgesia produced by inflammation and nerve injury was accompanied by the activation of the TRPA1 but not the TRPM8 channel [74]. Alternatively, TRPA1 channel was excessively expressed in the mouse spinal cord and DRG after peripheral inflammation occurred as a result of intraplantar injection of complete Freund's adjuvant; intrathecally-applied TRPA1 antagonist reversed hyperalgesia that occurred in mouse models of neuropathic pain [75].

TRPM8 channel is also involved in nociceptive transmission. Proudfoot et al. [76] have proposed the idea that TRPM8 activation in both peripheral and central terminals of adult rat DRG neurons produces the release of L-glutamate from its central terminal onto dorsal horn neurons expressing group II/III metabotropic glutamate receptors, the activation of which results in antinociception. In chronic constrictive nerve injury rat models, which exhibited cold allodynia in hindlimbs, compared with the sham group, TRPM8-immunoreactive DRG neurons increased in number, menthol-sensitive DRG neurons increased in number in neurons that responded to capsaicin, and membrane currents produced by menthol in DRG neurons enhanced in amplitude [77]. Kono et al. [78] have suggested an involvement of TRPM8 channel in acute peripheral hypersensitivity to cold in oxaliplatin (a third-generation platinum analog)-treated cancer patients. In adult mice, (−)-menthol and its derivative WS-12 (which activated TRPM8 channel in DRG neurons) inhibited acute thermal, capsaicin- and acrolein-induced nociceptive behavior in a manner sensitive to a nonselective opioid-receptor antagonist naloxone, suggesting an involvement of endogenous opioids in antinociception produced by TRPM8 activation [79].

In conclusion, the effects of the activation of TRPV1, TRPA1 or TRPM8 channel on nociceptive transmission appear to depend on the location of the TRP channels activated, i.e., the peripheral or central terminal of DRG neuron, or both of them. When antinociceptive drugs are administrated intrathecally, it would be necessary to consider the activation of TRP channels located in not only primary-afferent central terminal but also neuronal and glial cells in the CNS, because their expressions in the CNS have been reported [80,81].

4. Actions of Plant-Derived Stereoisomers on Spontaneous Excitatory Transmission in Substantia Gelatinosa Neurons

It is well-known that there is a difference among stereoisomers in their actions on voltage-gated ion channels and neurotransmitter receptors (see [82,83] for reviews). Activation of TRPA1 channel expressed in Chinese hamster ovary cells differs in efficacy between stereoisomers such as (+)-menthol and (−)-menthol [84]. In order to know whether such a difference between stereoisomers is seen in the SG, we examined the actions of plant-derived stereoisomers on spontaneous excitatory transmission in SG neurons with a focus on TRP activation by using transverse slice preparations dissected from the adult rat spinal cord [85].

4.1. *Actions of Thymol and Carvacrol*

Thymol (5-methyl-2-isopropylphenol, a compound where the cyclohexane ring of menthol is replaced by a benzene ring) differs only in the position of the -OH in the benzene ring from carvacrol (5-isopropyl-2-methylphenol; Figure 1A,B). Thymol and carvacrol are contained in thyme and oregano, respectively, and exhibit antinociception [86,87]. In all SG neurons tested, bath-applied thymol (1 mM) for 3 min increased the frequency of sEPSC with a small increase in its amplitude. The sEPSC frequency increase averaged to be 326% around 5 min (when a maximal effect was obtained) after the onset of thymol superfusion. Such a sEPSC frequency increase was concentration-dependent with the half-maximal effective concentration (EC_{50}) value of 0.18 mM (Figure 1C). In 77% of the neurons tested, thymol (1 mM) produced an outward current having the averaged peak amplitude of 16 pA at the V_H of −70 mV (see Figure 1E); remaining neurons had no outward currents [88].

Carvacrol exhibited similar actions to those of thymol. In 22% of the SG neurons tested, carvacrol (1 mM) superfused for 2 min produced an outward current, which was not accompanied by a change in sEPSC frequency, at −70 mV. On the other hand, 11% of the SG neurons produced no change in holding currents while exhibiting sEPSC frequency increase (see Figure 1Fa). In 63% of the neurons, both of the outward current and sEPSC frequency increase were produced [89].

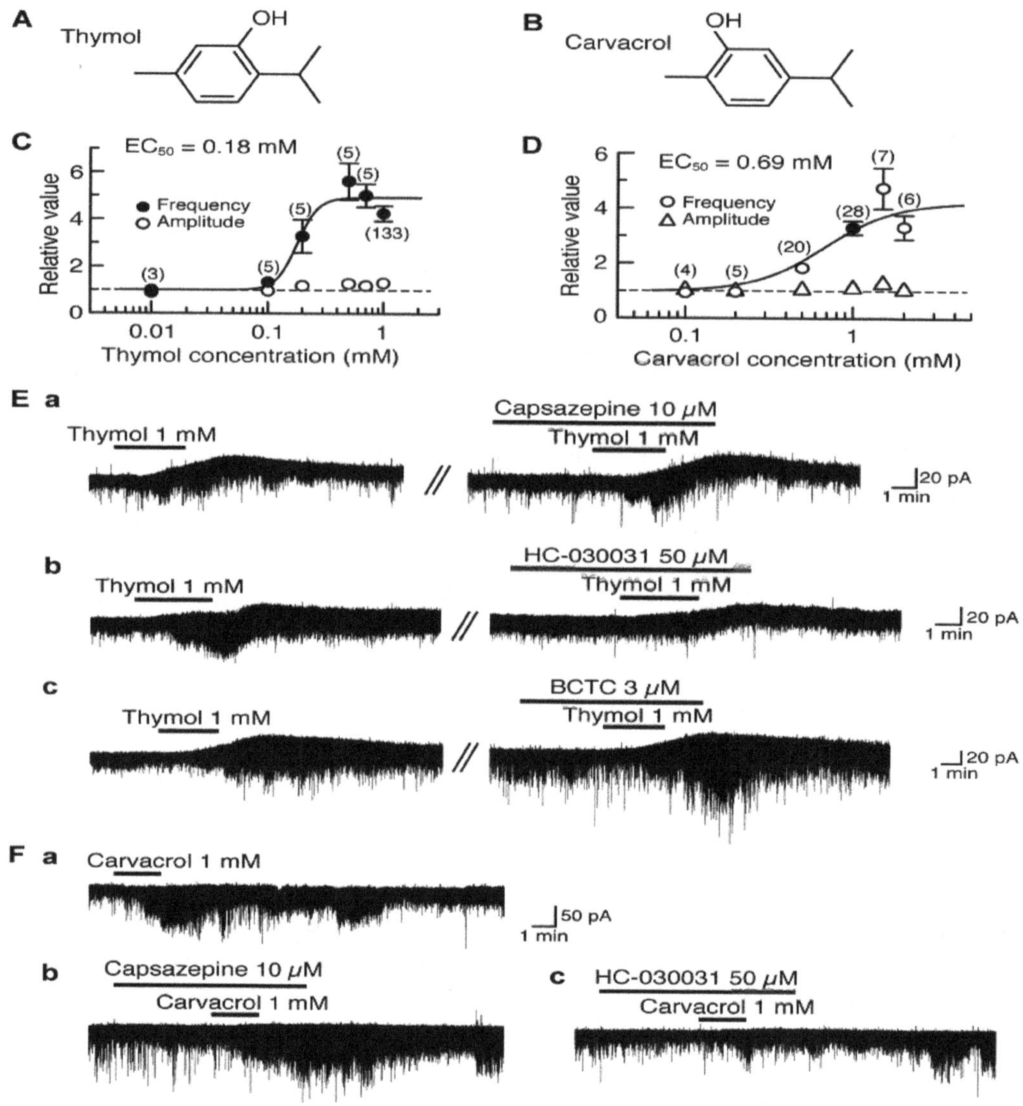

Figure 1. Effects of thymol and carvacrol on glutamatergic spontaneous excitatory transmission in rat substantia gelatinosa (SG) neurons. (**A**,**B**) The chemical structures of thymol (**A**) and carvacrol (**B**). (**C**,**D**) The frequency and amplitude of sEPSC under the action of thymol (**C**) or carvacrol (**D**), relative to those before drug superfusion, which were plotted against the logarithm of drug concentration. This thymol (carvacrol) effect was measured for 0.5 min around 5 min (3.5 min) after the beginning of its superfusion. The results in (**C**) were obtained from all neurons tested, while those in (**D**) were obtained from neurons where carvacrol (1 mM) increased sEPSC frequency > 5%. The continuous curves in (**C**) and (**D**) were drawn according to the Hill equation [half-maximal effective concentration (EC_{50}) and Hill coefficient (n_H) in (**C**) and (**D**): 0.18 mM, 4.9 and 0.69 mM, 2.1, respectively]. (**Ea–c**) Chart recordings showing sEPSCs and holding currents in the absence and presence of thymol in Krebs solution without (left) or with a TRPV1 antagonist capsazepine (**Ea**), a TRPA1 antagonist HC-030031 (**Eb**) or a TRPM8 antagonist BCTC (**Ec**; right). In each of (**Ea–c**), the right recording was obtained about 30 min after the left one from the same neuron. (**Fa–c**) Chart recordings showing sEPSCs in the absence and presence of carvacrol in Krebs solution without (**Fa**) and with capsazepine (**Fb**) or HC-030031 (**Fc**); these recordings were obtained from the same neuron at an interval of 30 min. In this and subsequent figures, value in parentheses indicates the number of neurons tested; each point with vertical bars represents the mean values and standard error of the mean (SEM); if the SEM of the values is less than the size of symbol, the vertical bar is not shown; control level (1) is indicated by horizontal dotted line; the duration of drug superfusion is shown by a horizontal bar above the chart recording. Holding potential (V_H) = −70 mV. This research was originally published in [88,89].

sEPSC frequency increase around 3.5 min (when a maximal effect was obtained) after the beginning of carvacrol superfusion averaged to be 262% with a small increase in its amplitude and the outward current had the averaged peak amplitude of 26 pA. Such a sEPSC frequency increase was concentration-dependent with the EC_{50} value of 0.69 mM (Figure 1D; [89]), a value larger than that of thymol. Thymol has an ability to activate TRP vanilloid-3 (TRPV3; [90]), TRPA1 [91] and TRPM8 channels [92] expressed in heterologous cells. On the other hand, carvacrol has been reported to activate TRPV3 and TRPA1 channels but not TRPV1 channel expressed in human embryonic kidney (HEK) or *Xenopus laevis* oocyte cells [90,91,93,94]. We next examined what types of TRP channel mediate the sEPSC frequency increases produced by thymol and carvacrol. The thymol activity was inhibited by a TRPA1 antagonist HC-030031 (50 μM; [95]) but not a TRPV1 antagonist capsazepine (10 μM; [96]) and a TRPM8 antagonist (4-(3-chloro- 2-pyridinyl)-*N*-[4-(1,1-dimethyl-ethyl)phenyl]-1-piperazinecarboxamide, BCTC, 3 μM; [97]; Figure 1E). BCTC at this concentration was effective in inhibiting sEPSC frequency increase produced by menthol in adult rat SG neurons [27]. As with thymol, the carvacrol activity was resistant to capsazepine (10 μM) while being depressed by HC-030031 (50 μM; Figure 1F). These results indicate an involvement of TRPA1 channel in the presynaptic activities of thymol and carvacrol. As distinct from these presynaptic actions, the outward currents produced by thymol and carvacrol were insensitive to capsazepine (10 μM), BCTC (3 μM) and HC-030031 (50 μM), indicating no involvement of TRP channels ([88,89]; for example see Figure 1E). The carvacrol current was inhibited in 10 mM-K^+ but not K^+-channel blockers (5 mM tetraethylammonium and 0.1 mM Ba^{2+})-containing and 11.0 mM-Cl^- Krebs solution, indicating an involvement of tetraethylammonium- and Ba^{2+}-insensitive K^+ channels [89]. It remains to be examined what types of ion channel are involved in the thymol current.

4.2. *Actions of (−)-Carvone and (+)-Carvone*

(−)-Carvone [(−)-2-methyl-5-(1-methylethenyl)-2-cyclohexenone; Figure 2A] contained in spearmint increased intracellular Ca^{2+} concentration in rat DRG neurons in a manner sensitive to capsazepine, indicating an involvement of TRPV1 channel [98]. A similar action of (−)-carvone was observed in HEK293 cells expressing human TRPV1 channel [98]. (+)-Carvone (a stereoisomer of (−)-carvone; Figure 2B) contained in caraway has been shown to have actions different from those of (−)-carvone in mouse locomotive [99] and anticonvulsive activities [100]. We examined the effects of (−)-carvone and (+)-carvone on glutamatergic spontaneous excitatory transmission with a focus on TRP activation. (−)-Carvone and (+)-carvone (each 1 mM) superfused for 2 min increased the frequency of sEPSC with a slight increase in its amplitude. Their sEPSC frequency increases averaged to be 299% and 284%, respectively, around 3 min (when a maximal effect was obtained) after the beginning of its superfusion. Such presynaptic activities of (−)-carvone and (+)-carvone were concentration-dependent with the EC_{50} values of 0.70 mM and 0.72 mM, respectively (Figure 2C,D).

(−)-Carvone and (+)-carvone (each 1 mM) did not produce any outward currents, as different from thymol and carvacrol. About 40% of the SG neurons tested produced a small inward current following the application of (−)-carvone or (+)-carvone [101], as seen by many kinds of TRPV1 agonists (capsaicin and RTX; [15,18]) and TRPA1 agonists (AITC, cinnamaldehyde and allicin; [19]).

The sEPSC frequency increase produced by (−)-carvone was resistant to HC-030031 (50 μM) while being inhibited by capsazepine (10 μM; Figure 2Ea,b). On the other hand, the sEPSC frequency increase produced by (+)-carvone was inhibited by HC-030031 (50 μM) while being resistant to capsazepine (10 μM; Figure 2Fa,b). These results indicate that (−)-carvone and (+)-carvone activate TRPV1 and TRPA1 channels, respectively, in the SG [101].

4.3. *Actions of 1,8-Cineole and 1,4-Cineole*

1,8-Cineole (1,3,3-trimethyl-2-oxabicylo[2.2.2]octane; Figure 3A), which is present in eucalyptus and rosemary, has various actions including antinociception [102]. As a minor component of plant extracts containing 1,8-cineole, there is its stereoisomer 1,4-cineole (1-methyl-4-(1-methylethyl)-

7-oxabicyclo[2.2.1]heptane; Figure 3B), which has on plant species an action which is different from that of 1,8-cineole [103].

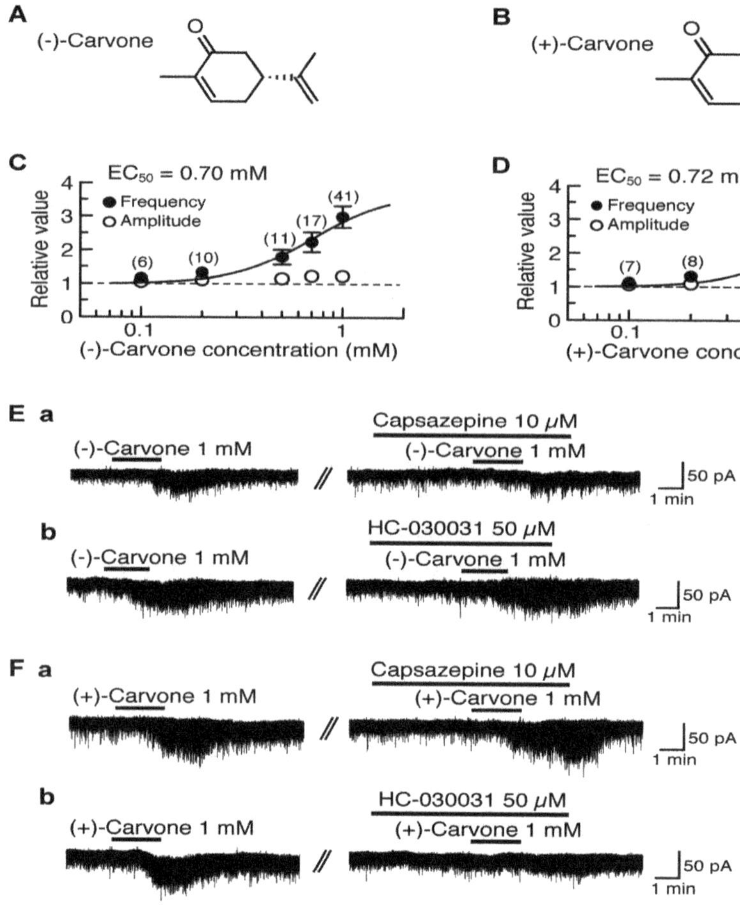

Figure 2. Effects of (−)-carvone and (+)-carvone on glutamatergic spontaneous excitatory transmission in rat SG neurons. (**A**,**B**) The chemical structures of (−)-carvone (**A**) and (+)-carvone (**B**). (**C**,**D**) The frequency and amplitude of sEPSC under the action of (−)-carvone (**C**) or (+)-carvone (**D**), relative to those before drug superfusion, which were plotted against the logarithm of drug concentration. This carvone effect was measured for 0.5 min around 3 min after the beginning of its superfusion. The continuous curves in (**C**) and (**D**) were drawn according to the Hill equation (EC_{50} and n_H in (**C**) and (**D**): 0.70 mM, 2.2 and 0.72 mM, 2.4, respectively). (**Ea**,**b**,**Fa**,**b**) Chart recordings showing sEPSCs in the absence and presence of (−)-carvone (**E**) or (+)-carvone (**F**) in Krebs solution without (left) and with capsazepine (**Ea**,**Fa**) or HC-030031 (**Eb**,**Fb**; right). In each of (**Ea**,**b**,**Fa**,**b**), the right recording was obtained about 20 min after the left one from the same neuron. $V_H = -70$ mV. This research was originally published in [101].

1,8-Cineole and 1,4-cineole have an ability to activate TRPM8 channel expressed heterologously in *Xenopus* oocytes [11] or HEK293 cells [104,105], although their efficacies are much less than that of the TRPM8 agonist menthol. We examined the effects of 1,8-cineole and 1,4-cineole on glutamatergic spontaneous excitatory transmission with a focus on TRP activation. As with (−)-carvone and (+)-carvone, bath-applied 1,8-cineole and 1,4-cineole for 3 min increased the frequency of sEPSC with a small increase in its amplitude. The sEPSC frequency increases produced by 1,8-cineole and 1,4-cineole (5 mM and 0.5 mM, respectively) averaged to be 159% and 226%, respectively, around 3.5 min (when a maximal effect was obtained) after the beginning of its superfusion. Such presynaptic actions of 1,8-cineole and 1,4-cineole were concentration-dependent with the EC_{50} values of 3.2 mM and 0.42 mM, respectively (Figure 3C,D).

The presynaptic activities of 1,8-cineole and 1,4-cineole were not accompanied by the production of outward current, as different from those of thymol and carvacrol. As with many kinds of TRPV1 and TRPA1 agonists [15,18,19] including (−)-carvone and (+)-carvone, 1,8-cineole and 1,4-cineole produced a small inward current (Figure 3E,F; [27]).

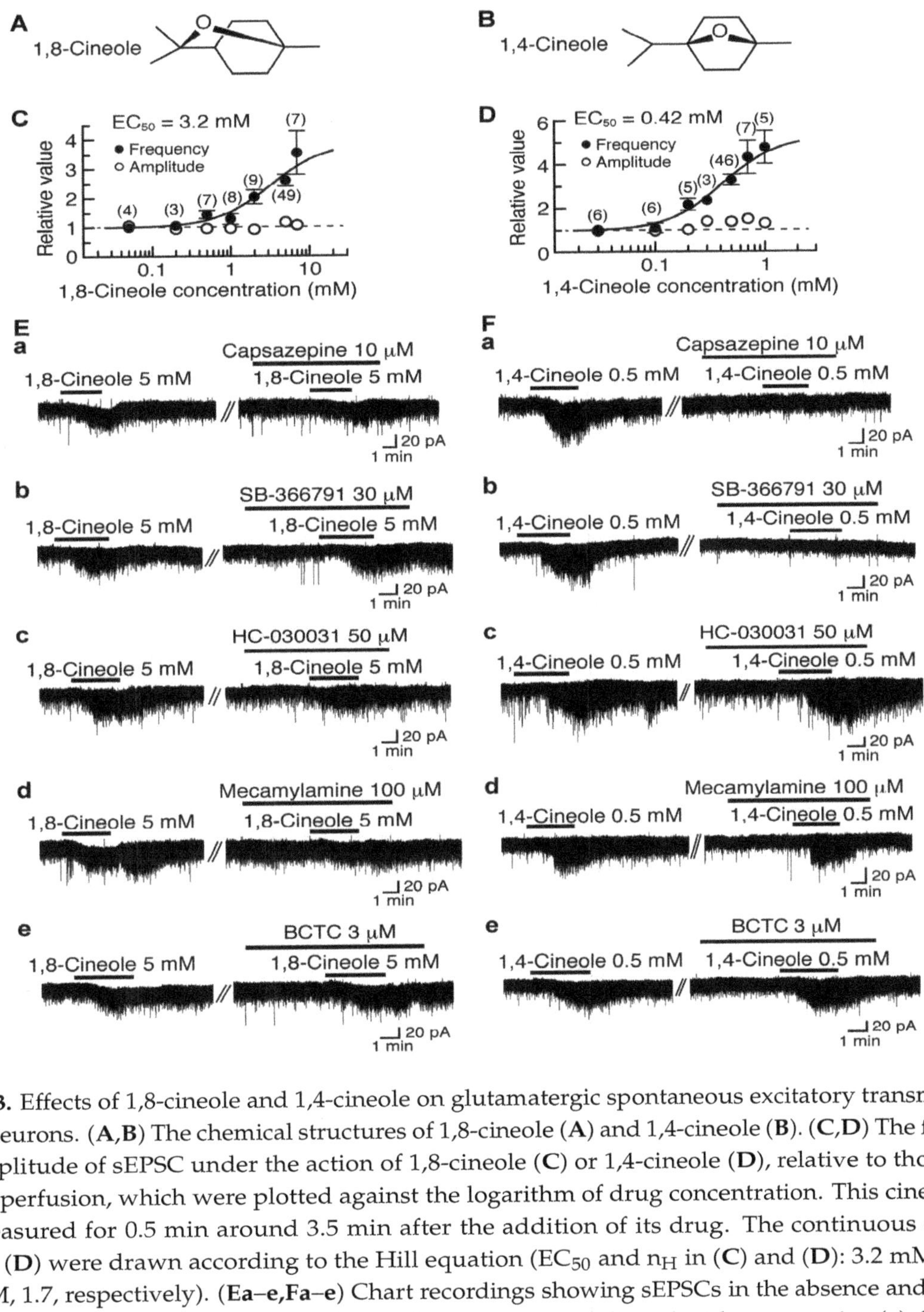

Figure 3. Effects of 1,8-cineole and 1,4-cineole on glutamatergic spontaneous excitatory transmission in rat SG neurons. (**A,B**) The chemical structures of 1,8-cineole (**A**) and 1,4-cineole (**B**). (**C,D**) The frequency and amplitude of sEPSC under the action of 1,8-cineole (**C**) or 1,4-cineole (**D**), relative to those before drug superfusion, which were plotted against the logarithm of drug concentration. This cineole effect was measured for 0.5 min around 3.5 min after the addition of its drug. The continuous curves in (**C**) and (**D**) were drawn according to the Hill equation (EC_{50} and n_H in (**C**) and (**D**): 3.2 mM, 1.3 and 0.42 mM, 1.7, respectively). (**Ea–e,Fa–e**) Chart recordings showing sEPSCs in the absence and presence of 1,8-cineole (**E**) or 1,4-cineole (**F**) in Krebs solution without (left) and with capsazepine (**a**), SB-366791 (**b**), HC-030031 (**c**), mecamylamine (**d**) or BCTC (**e**; right). In each of (**Ea–e,Fa–e**), the right recording was obtained about 20 min after the left one from the same neuron. $V_H = -70$ mV. This research was originally published in [27].

The presynaptic action of 1,8-cineole was inhibited by HC-030031 (50 μM) and another TRPA1 antagonist mecamylamine (100 μM; which is known to be also a nicotinic acetylcholine-receptor antagonist [106]) while being resistant to capsazepine (10 μM) and another TRPV1 antagonist SB-366791 (30 μM; [67]; Figure 3Ea–d). On the contrary, 1,4-cineole's one was depressed by capsazepine (10 μM) and SB-366791 (30 μM) while being insensitive to HC-030031 (50 μM) and mecamylamine (100 μM; Figure 3Fa–d). BCTC (3 μM) did not affect the activities of 1,8-cineole and 1,4-cineole (Figure 3Ee,Fe). These results indicate that 1,8-cineole and 1,4-cineole activate TRPA1 and TRPV1 channels, respectively, in the SG.

5. Activation by Plant-Derived Stereoisomers of TRP Channels in the Substantia Gelatinosa in a Different Manner

Thymol and carvacrol, which are distinct only in the position of the -OH in the benzene ring (Figure 1A,B), activated the TRPA1 channel with EC_{50} values which differ four-fold from each other. Optic isomers, (–)-carvone and (+)-carvone (Figure 2A,B), activated TRPV1 and TRPA1 channels, respectively, with almost the same EC_{50} value. 1,8-Cineole and 1,4-cineole, which are different in the placement of the oxygen bridge (Figure 3A,B; where there is a free dimethyl side chain in 1,4-cineole but not 1,8-cineole [103]), activated TRPA1 and TRPV1 channels, respectively, with EC_{50} values eight-fold different from each other. The TRPV1 and TRPA1 activations resulted in an increase in spontaneous L-glutamate release from nerve terminals onto SG neurons. These results indicate that TRP channels in the SG have an ability to discriminate plant-derived stereoisomers from each other.

The stereoisomers mentioned in this review article are not endogenous ones that act on TRP channels located in the central terminals of DRG neurons under physiological conditions. There are several candidates for endogenous substances that activate TRP channels. For example, endogenous agonists for TRPV1 channel include endocannabinoids such as anandamide and lipoxygenase metabolites, which have structures similar to that of capsaicin which is not produced endogenously ([107,108]; for reviews see [7,109]). TRPV1 channel in the SG did not appear to be activated by anandamide [54] while anandamide-transport inhibitor AM404 activated the SG TRPV1 channel [110]. As candidates of endogenous TRPA1 activators, there is a potent and systemically active inhibitor of fatty acid amide hydrolase, 3′-carbamoylbiphenyl-3-yl cyclohexylcarbamate (URB597; [111]), a cyclopentane prostaglandin D_2 metabolite (15-deoxy-$\Delta^{12,14}$-prostaglandin J_2; [112]) or bradykinin [113]. To our knowledge, endogenous agonists for TRPM8 channel do not appear to be surely identified. Testosterone (a steroid hormone from the androgen group) has been recently reported to activate TRPM8 channel [114,115]. Although endogenous stereoisomers for TRP activation do not appear to be available, our findings about stereoisomers could serve to know the properties of the central terminal TRP channels.

Many of the properties of the TRP channels have been examined in the cell body of the primary-afferent neuron and in heterologous cell expressing the TRP channels. We have found out that a local anesthetic lidocaine, which acts on TRPV1 channel [116] and by a less extent on TRPA1 channel [117] in the cell body of primary-afferent neuron, activates TRPA1 but not TRPV1 channel in its central terminal [118]. The central terminal TRPV1 channel was activated by piperine (a pungent component of black pepper; [119]) but not olvanil (the synthetic oleic acid homologue of capsaicin; [120]), both of which compounds activated TRPV1 channel in the cell body of primary-afferent neuron [121,122]. Vanilloid compounds, eugenol (contained in clove) and zingerone (a pungent component of ginger), that reportedly activated TRPV1 channel in the cell body of primary-afferent neuron [121,123] were shown to activate the central terminal TRPA1 but not TRPV1 channel [124,125]. Based on their findings, we have proposed the idea that TRP channels located in the cell body and central terminal of the primary-afferent neuron have properties different from each other [23]. Such a difference may be due to a distinction between cell body and central terminal TRPA1 channels in terms of a functional interaction of TRPA1 channel and toll-like receptor-7 ([126]; see [125] for the other possibilities). It remains to be examined whether TRP channels in the cell body of DRG neuron are activated by plant-derived stereoisomers in a distinct manner.

TRPA1 channel in the central terminal of DRG neuron in the SG is activated by many plant-derived chemicals. Very recently, we have reported that citral, a mixture of geranial and neral, which is contained in lemongrass, activates TRPA1 channel in the SG [127]. Table 1 summarizes available values of EC_{50} for plant-derived chemicals in activating TRPV1 and TRPA1 channels in the adult rat SG. Their efficacy sequence for the TRPA1 activation was thymol (EC_{50} = 0.18 mM) > citral (0.58 mM) ⩾ carvacrol (0.69 mM) ⩾ (+)-carvone (0.72 mM) > zingerone (1.3 mM) > 1,8-cineole (3.2 mM) ⩾ eugenol (3.8 mM). This result could serve to know the property of central terminal TRPA1 channel that is a target of drugs for alleviating pain together with the above-mentioned results of stereoisomers.

Table 1. EC_{50} values for plant-derived chemicals in activating TRPV1 and TRPA1 channels in the adult rat SG.

Plant-Derived Chemicals	TRPV1 (mM)	TRPA1 (mM)	References
Resiniferatoxin	2.1×10^{-4}	–	[18]
Piperine	0.052	–	[120]
Eugenol	–	3.8	[124]
Zingerone	–	1.3	[125]
(−)-Carvone	0.70	–	[101]
(+)-Carvone	–	0.72	[101]
Carvacrol	–	0.69	[89]
Thymol	–	0.18	[88]
1,8-Cineole	–	3.2	[27]
1,4-Cineole	0.42	–	[27]
Cital	–	0.58	[127]

TRP activation in the SG is generally thought to be involved in nociception [1], because the enhancement of the spontaneous release of L-glutamate from nerve terminals onto SG neurons as a result of the TRP activation increases an excitability of the SG neurons, an action different from those of analgesic substances (see Section 2). However, antinociception produced by the intrathecal administration of acetaminophen has been attributed to TRPA1 activation in the superficial spinal dorsal horn [128]. AITC inhibited current responses recorded from SG neurons by using the in vivo patch-clamp technique [129] in response to pinch stimuli given to the skin [130]. It remains to be addressed whether TRPA1 activation in the SG results in nociception or antinociception.

Although the present review article mentions the actions of plant-derived stereoisomers on excitatory transmission, the regulation of nociceptive transmission in the SG is due to a modulation of not only excitatory but also GABAergic and/or glycinergic inhibitory transmissions [25,131,132]. It is possible that a modulation of inhibitory transmission by TRP activation is involved in nociceptive transmission. There is much evidence supporting the idea that inhibitory transmission enhancement in the spinal dorsal horn results in antinociception. First, the lack of GABA-synthesizing enzyme [133,134] and also reduction in the expression of K^+-Cl^- exporter KCC2, which causes inhibitory synaptic response to be excitatory [135], in the rat spinal dorsal horn leaded to nociception. Second, peripheral inflammation resulted in a reduced glycinergic transmission in rat spinal lamina I neurons [136]. Third, an increase in endogenous glycine due to glycine transporter-1 blockade produced an inhibitory effect on spinal nociceptive transmission ([137]; for reviews see [138,139]). Fourth, endogenous analgesics, acetylcholine, norepinephrine and serotonin, enhanced GABAergic and glycinergic inhibitory transmissions [140–145]. It appears to depend on the agonists used to activate TRP channels how TRP activation affects spontaneous inhibitory transmission in SG neurons. AITC and zingerone enhanced inhibitory transmission [19,125] while capsaicin and cinnamaldehyde did not [15,20]. It remains to be examined how plant-derived stereoisomers affect spontaneous inhibitory transmission.

Itch is partly similar to pain in the neuronal pathway and receptors involved, although they are distinct from each other in many points of neuronal transmissions. There is much evidence supporting the idea that TRPV1 and TRPA1 channels are involved in itch. For instance, a topical application of capsaicin to the skin produced itch [146,147]. It is thus likely that TRP channels located in the central terminal of a pruriceptive primary-afferent neuron are involved in the modulation of itch sensation. Although proteinase-activated receptor (PAR)-2 in the peripheral terminal of a primary-afferent neuron is involved in the production of itch [148,149], other types of PAR may play a role in modulating pruriceptive transmission in the spinal dorsal horn. Fujita et al. [150] have reported that PAR-1 activation presynaptically increases spontaneous excitatory transmission in adult rat SG neurons. The findings about plant-derived stereoisomers, mentioned in this review article, may serve to know how to modulate itch transmission in the spinal dorsal horn.

There are known to be species differences on the pharmacology of TRP channels. For example, Jordt and Julius [151] have found out that chicken TRPV1 channel has a much less sensitivity to capsaicin than rat one. Rat and human TRPV1 channels were about 100-fold more sensitive to capsaicin than rabbit one [152]. 4-Methyl-*N*-[2,2,2-trichloro-1-(4-nitro-phenylsulfanyl)-ethyl]-benzamide activated rat TRPA1 channel while blocking human TRPA1 activation by reactive and nonreactive agonists [153]. Caffeine inhibited human TRPA1 channel but activated mouse TRPA1 channel [154]. A967079 blocked mammalian TRPA1 channel [155], but failed to inhibit chicken TRPA1 channel [156]. It remains to be investigated whether a difference in TRP activation among plant-derived stereoisomers is seen in animal species other than rats.

6. Conclusions

Plant-derived chemical stereoisomers, i.e., thymol and carvacrol, (−)-carvone and (+)-carvone, or 1,8-cineole and 1,4-cineole, activated TRP channels in the SG in a manner different from each other in the extent and the types of TRP channels activated. TRP channels expressed in the central terminals of DRG neurons are thus suggested to have an ability to discriminate stereoisomers.

Acknowledgments: This study was partly supported by JSPS KAKENHI Grant Number 15K08673.

References

1. Patapoutian, A.; Tate, S.; Woolf, C.J. Transient receptor potential channels: Targeting pain at the source. *Nat. Rev. Drug Discov.* **2009**, *8*, 55–68. [CrossRef] [PubMed]
2. Story, G.M.; Peier, A.M.; Reeve, A.J.; Eid, S.R.; Mosbacher, J.; Hricik, T.R.; Earley, T.J.; Hergarden, A.C.; Andersson, D.A.; Hwang, S.W.; et al. ANKTM1, a TRP-like channel expressed in nociceptive neurons, is activated by cold temperatures. *Cell* **2003**, *112*, 819–829. [CrossRef]
3. Kobayashi, K.; Fukuoka, T.; Obata, K.; Yamanaka, H.; Dai, Y.; Tokunaga, A.; Noguchi, K. Distinct expression of TRPM8, TRPA1, and TRPV1 mRNAs in rat primary afferent neurons with Aδ/C-fibers and colocalization with Trk receptors. *J. Comp. Neurol.* **2005**, *493*, 596–606. [CrossRef] [PubMed]
4. Tominaga, M. TRP channels and nociception. In *Cellular and Molecular Mechanisms for the Modulation of Nociceptive Transmission in the Peripheral and Central Nervous Systems*; Kumamoto, E., Ed.; Research Signpost: Kelara, India, 2007; pp. 23–40.
5. Julius, D. TRP channels and pain. *Annu. Rev. Cell Dev. Biol.* **2013**, *29*, 355–384. [CrossRef] [PubMed]
6. Caterina, M.J.; Schumacher, M.A.; Tominaga, M.; Rosen, T.A.; Levine, J.D.; Julius, D. The capsaicin receptor: a heat-activated ion channel in the pain pathway. *Nature* **1997**, *389*, 816–824. [PubMed]
7. Caterina, M.J.; Julius, D. The vanilloid receptor: a molecular gateway to the pain pathway. *Annu. Rev. Neurosci.* **2001**, *24*, 487–517. [CrossRef] [PubMed]
8. Bandell, M.; Story, G.M.; Hwang, S.W.; Viswanath, V.; Eid, S.R.; Petrus, M.J.; Earley, T.J.; Patapoutian, A. Noxious cold ion channel TRPA1 is activated by pungent compounds and bradykinin. *Neuron* **2004**, *41*, 849–857. [CrossRef]
9. Jordt, S.E.; Bautista, D.M.; Chuang, H.H.; McKemy, D.D.; Zygmunt, P.M.; Högestätt, E.D.; Meng, I.D.; Julius, D. Mustard oils and cannabinoids excite sensory nerve fibres through the TRP channel ANKTM1. *Nature* **2004**, *427*, 260–265. [CrossRef] [PubMed]

10. Nilius, B.; Voets, T. TRP channels: a TR(I)P through a world of multifunctional cation channels. *Pflügers Arch.* **2005**, *451*, 1–10. [CrossRef] [PubMed]
11. McKemy, D.D.; Neuhausser, W.M.; Julius, D. Identification of a cold receptor reveals a general role for TRP channels in thermosensation. *Nature* **2002**, *416*, 52–58. [CrossRef] [PubMed]
12. Peier, A.M.; Moqrich, A.; Hergarden, A.C.; Reeve, A.J.; Andersson, D.A.; Story, G.M.; Earley, T.J.; Dragoni, I.; McIntyre, P.; Bevan, S.; et al. A TRP channel that senses cold stimuli and menthol. *Cell* **2002**, *108*, 705–715. [CrossRef]
13. Kumazawa, T.; Perl, E.R. Excitation of marginal and substantia gelatinosa neurons in the primate spinal cord: indications of their place in dorsal horn functional organization. *J. Comp. Neurol.* **1978**, *177*, 417–434. [CrossRef] [PubMed]
14. Sugiura, Y.; Lee, C.L.; Perl, E.R. Central projections of identified, unmyelinated (C) afferent fibers innervating mammalian skin. *Science* **1986**, *234*, 358–361. [CrossRef] [PubMed]
15. Yang, K; Kumamoto, E.; Furue, H.; Yoshimura, M. Capsaicin facilitates excitatory but not inhibitory synaptic transmission in substantia gelatinosa of the rat spinal cord. *Neurosci. Lett.* **1998**, *255*, 135–138. [CrossRef]
16. Morisset, V.; Urbán, L. Cannabinoid-induced presynaptic inhibition of glutamatergic EPSCs in substantia gelatinosa neurons of the rat spinal cord. *J. Neurophysiol.* **2001**, *86*, 40–48. [PubMed]
17. Baccei, M.L.; Bardoni, R.; Fitzgerald, M. Development of nociceptive synaptic inputs to the neonatal rat dorsal horn: glutamate release by capsaicin and menthol. *J. Physiol.* **2003**, *549*, 231–242. [CrossRef] [PubMed]
18. Jiang, C.-Y.; Fujita, T.; Yue, H.-Y.; Piao, L.-H.; Liu, T.; Nakatsuka, T.; Kumamoto, E. Effect of resiniferatoxin on glutamatergic spontaneous excitatory synaptic transmission in substantia gelatinosa neurons of the adult rat spinal cord. *Neuroscience* **2009**, *164*, 1833–1844. [CrossRef] [PubMed]
19. Kosugi, M.; Nakatsuka, T.; Fujita, T.; Kuroda, Y.; Kumamoto, E. Activation of TRPA1 channel facilitates excitatory synaptic transmission in substantia gelatinosa neurons of the adult rat spinal cord. *J. Neurosci.* **2007**, *27*, 4443–4451. [CrossRef] [PubMed]
20. Uta, D.; Furue, H.; Pickering, A.E.; Rashid, M.H.; Mizuguchi-Takase, H.; Katafuchi, T.; Imoto, K.; Yoshimura, M. TRPA1-expressing primary afferents synapse with a morphologically identified subclass of substantia gelatinosa neurons in the adult rat spinal cord. *Eur. J. Neurosci.* **2010**, *31*, 1960–1973. [CrossRef] [PubMed]
21. Suzuki, S.C.; Furue, H.; Koga, K.; Jiang, N.; Nohmi, M.; Shimazaki, Y.; Katoh-Fukui, Y.; Yokoyama, M.; Yoshimura, M.; Takeichi, M. Cadherin-8 is required for the first relay synapses to receive functional inputs from primary sensory afferents for cold sensation. *J. Neurosci.* **2007**, *27*, 3466–3476. [CrossRef] [PubMed]
22. Wrigley, P.J.; Jeong, H.-J.; Vaughan, C.W. Primary afferents with TRPM8 and TRPA1 profiles target distinct subpopulations of rat superficial dorsal horn neurones. *Br. J. Pharmacol.* **2009**, *157*, 371–380. [CrossRef] [PubMed]
23. Kumamoto, E.; Fujita, T.; Jiang, C.-Y. TRP channels involved in spontaneous L-glutamate release enhancement in the adult rat spinal substantia gelatinosa. *Cells* **2014**, *3*, 331–362. [CrossRef] [PubMed]
24. Melzack, R.; Wall, P.D. Pain mechanisms: a new theory. *Science* **1965**, *150*, 971–979. [CrossRef] [PubMed]
25. Willis, W.D., Jr.; Coggeshall, R.E. *Sensory Mechanisms of the Spinal Cord*, 2nd ed.; Plenum: New York, NY, USA, 1991.
26. Todd, A.J. Neuronal circuitry for pain processing in the dorsal horn. *Nat. Rev. Neurosci.* **2010**, *11*, 823–836. [CrossRef] [PubMed]
27. Jiang, C.-Y.; Wang, C.; Xu, N.-X.; Fujita, T.; Murata, Y.; Kumamoto, E. 1,8- and 1,4-cineole enhance spontaneous excitatory transmission by activating different types of transient receptor potential channels in the rat spinal substantia gelatinosa. *J. Neurochem.* **2016**, *136*, 764–777. [CrossRef] [PubMed]
28. Yoshimura, M.; Nishi, S. Blind patch-clamp recordings from substantia gelatinosa neurons in adult rat spinal cord slices: pharmacological properties of synaptic currents. *Neuroscience* **1993**, *53*, 519–526. [CrossRef]
29. Nakatsuka, T.; Park, J.-S.; Kumamoto, E.; Tamaki, T.; Yoshimura, M. Plastic changes in sensory inputs to rat substantia gelatinosa neurons following peripheral inflammation. *Pain* **1999**, *82*, 39–47. [CrossRef]
30. Ito, A.; Kumamoto, E.; Takeda, M.; Takeda, M.; Shibata, K.; Sagai, H.; Yoshimura, M. Mechanisms for ovariectomy-induced hyperalgesia and its relief by calcitonin: participation of 5-HT_{1A}-like receptor on C-afferent terminals in substantia gelatinosa of the rat spinal cord. *J. Neurosci.* **2000**, *20*, 6302–6308. [PubMed]
31. Fürst, S. Transmitters involved in antinociception in the spinal cord. *Brain Res. Bull.* **1999**, *48*, 129–141. [CrossRef]

32. Yoshimura, M.; North, R.A. Substantia gelatinosa neurones hyperpolarized *in vitro* by enkephalin. *Nature* **1983**, *305*, 529–530. [CrossRef] [PubMed]
33. Fujita, T.; Nakatsuka, T.; Kumamoto, E. Opioid receptor activation in spinal dorsal horn. In *Cellular and Molecular Mechanisms for the Modulation of Nociceptive Transmission in the Peripheral and Central Nervous Systems*; Kumamoto, E., Ed.; Research Signpost: Kelara, India, 2007; pp. 87–111.
34. Lai, C.C.; Wu, S.Y.; Dun, S.L.; Dun, N.J. Nociceptin-like immunoreactivity in the rat dorsal horn and inhibition of substantia gelatinosa neurons. *Neuroscience* **1997**, *81*, 887–891. [CrossRef]
35. Luo, C.; Kumamoto, E.; Furue, H.; Yoshimura, M. Nociceptin-induced outward current in substantia gelatinosa neurones of the adult rat spinal cord. *Neuroscience* **2001**, *108*, 323–330. [CrossRef]
36. Kangrga, I.; Jiang, M.; Randić, M. Actions of (−)-baclofen on rat dorsal horn neurons. *Brain Res.* **1991**, *562*, 265–275. [CrossRef]
37. Yang, K.; Kumamoto, E.; Furue, H.; Li, Y.-Q.; Yoshimura, M. Capsaicin induces a slow inward current which is not mediated by substance P in substantia gelatinosa neurons of the rat spinal cord. *Neuropharmacology* **2000**, *39*, 2185–2194. [CrossRef]
38. Koga, A.; Fujita, T.; Totoki, T.; Kumamoto, E. Tramadol produces outward currents by activating μ-opioid receptors in adult rat substantia gelatinosa neurones. *Br. J. Pharmacol.* **2005**, *145*, 602–607. [CrossRef] [PubMed]
39. Sonohata, M.; Furue, H.; Katafuchi, T.; Yasaka, T.; Doi, A.; Kumamoto, E.; Yoshimura, M. Actions of noradrenaline on substantia gelatinosa neurones in the rat spinal cord revealed by *in vivo* patch recording. *J. Physiol.* **2004**, *555*, 515–526. [CrossRef] [PubMed]
40. Abe, K.; Kato, G.; Katafuchi, T.; Tamae, A.; Furue, H.; Yoshimura, M. Responses to 5-HT in morphologically identified neurons in the rat substantia gelatinosa *in vitro*. *Neuroscience* **2009**, *159*, 316–324. [CrossRef] [PubMed]
41. Li, J.; Perl, E.R. Adenosine inhibition of synaptic transmission in the substantia gelatinosa. *J. Neurophysiol.* **1994**, *72*, 1611–1621. [PubMed]
42. Liu, T.; Fujita, T.; Kawasaki, Y.; Kumamoto, E. Regulation by equilibrative nucleoside transporter of adenosine outward currents in adult rat spinal dorsal horn neurons. *Brain Res. Bull.* **2004**, *64*, 75–83. [CrossRef] [PubMed]
43. Kumamoto, E.; Fujita, T. Role of adenosine in regulating nociceptive transmission in the spinal dorsal horn. In *Recent Research Developments in Physiology*; Pandalai, S.G., Ed.; Research Signpost: Kerala, India, 2005; Volume 3, pp. 39–57.
44. Jiang, N.; Furue, H.; Katafuchi, T.; Yoshimura, M. Somatostatin directly inhibits substantia gelatinosa neurons in adult rat spinal dorsal horn in vitro. *Neurosci. Res.* **2003**, *47*, 97–107. [CrossRef]
45. Nakatsuka, T.; Fujita, T.; Inoue, K.; Kumamoto, E. Activation of GIRK channels in substantia gelatinosa neurones of the adult rat spinal cord: a possible involvement of somatostatin. *J. Physiol.* **2008**, *586*, 2511–2522. [CrossRef] [PubMed]
46. Tamae, A.; Nakatsuka, T.; Koga, K.; Kato, G.; Furue, H.; Katafuchi, T.; Yoshimura, M. Direct inhibition of substantia gelatinosa neurones in the rat spinal cord by activation of dopamine D2-like receptors. *J. Physiol.* **2005**, *568*, 243–253. [CrossRef] [PubMed]
47. Taniguchi, W.; Nakatsuka, T.; Miyazaki, N.; Yamada, H.; Takeda, D.; Fujita, T.; Kumamoto, E.; Yoshida, M. *In vivo* patch-clamp analysis of dopaminergic antinociceptive actions on substantia gelatinosa neurons in the spinal cord. *Pain* **2011**, *152*, 95–105. [CrossRef] [PubMed]
48. Yue, H.-Y.; Fujita, T.; Kumamoto, E. Biphasic modulation by galanin of excitatory synaptic transmission in substantia gelatinosa neurons of adult rat spinal cord slices. *J. Neurophysiol.* **2011**, *105*, 2337–2349. [CrossRef] [PubMed]
49. Kohno, T.; Kumamoto, E.; Higashi, H.; Shimoji, K.; Yoshimura, M. Actions of opioids on excitatory and inhibitory transmission in substantia gelatinosa of adult rat spinal cord. *J. Physiol.* **1999**, *518*, 803–813. [CrossRef] [PubMed]
50. Liebel, J.T.; Swandulla, D.; Zeilhofer, H.U. Modulation of excitatory synaptic transmission by nociceptin in superficial dorsal horn neurones of the neonatal rat spinal cord. *Br. J. Pharmacol.* **1997**, *121*, 425–432. [CrossRef] [PubMed]

51. Luo, C.; Kumamoto, E.; Furue, H.; Chen, J.; Yoshimura, M. Nociceptin inhibits excitatory but not inhibitory transmission to substantia gelatinosa neurones of adult rat spinal cord. *Neuroscience* **2002**, *109*, 349–358. [CrossRef]
52. Ataka, T.; Kumamoto, E.; Shimoji, K.; Yoshimura, M. Baclofen inhibits more effectively C-afferent than Aδ-afferent glutamatergic transmission in substantia gelatinosa neurons of adult rat spinal cord slices. *Pain* **2000**, *86*, 273–282. [CrossRef]
53. Iyadomi, M.; Iyadomi, I.; Kumamoto, E.; Tomokuni, K.; Yoshimura, M. Presynaptic inhibition by baclofen of miniature EPSCs and IPSCs in substantia gelatinosa neurons of the adult rat spinal dorsal horn. *Pain* **2000**, *85*, 385–393. [CrossRef]
54. Luo, C.; Kumamoto, E.; Furue, H.; Chen, J.; Yoshimura, M. Anandamide inhibits excitatory transmission to rat substantia gelatinosa neurones in a manner different from that of capsaicin. *Neurosci. Lett.* **2002**, *321*, 17–20. [CrossRef]
55. Kawasaki, Y.; Kumamoto, E.; Furue, H.; Yoshimura, M. α_2 Adrenoceptor-mediated presynaptic inhibition of primary afferent glutamatergic transmission in rat substantia gelatinosa neurons. *Anesthesiology* **2003**, *98*, 682–689. [CrossRef] [PubMed]
56. Lao, L.-J.; Kumamoto, E.; Luo, C.; Furue, H.; Yoshimura, M. Adenosine inhibits excitatory transmission to substantia gelatinosa neurons of the adult rat spinal cord through the activation of presynaptic A_1 adenosine receptor. *Pain* **2001**, *94*, 315–324. [CrossRef]
57. Lao, L.-J.; Kawasaki, Y.; Yang, K.; Fujita, T.; Kumamoto, E. Modulation by adenosine of Aδ and C primary-afferent glutamatergic transmission in adult rat substantia gelatinosa neurons. *Neuroscience* **2004**, *125*, 221–231. [CrossRef] [PubMed]
58. Alier, K.A.; Chen, Y.; Sollenberg, U.E.; Langel, Ü.; Smith, P.A. Selective stimulation of GalR1 and GalR2 in rat *substantia gelatinosa* reveals a cellular basis for the anti- and pro-nociceptive actions of galanin. *Pain* **2008**, *137*, 138–146. [CrossRef] [PubMed]
59. Hudson, L.J.; Bevan, S.; Wotherspoon, G.; Gentry, C.; Fox, A.; Winter, J. VR1 protein expression increases in undamaged DRG neurons after partial nerve injury. *Eur. J. Neurosci.* **2001**, *13*, 2105–2114. [CrossRef] [PubMed]
60. Walker, K.M.; Urbán, L.; Medhurst, S.J.; Patel, S.; Panesar, M.; Fox, A.J.; McIntyre, P. The VR1 antagonist capsazepine reverses mechanical hyperalgesia in models of inflammatory and neuropathic pain. *J. Pharmacol. Exp. Ther.* **2003**, *304*, 56–62. [CrossRef] [PubMed]
61. Gavva, N.R.; Tamir, R.; Qu, Y.; Klionsky, L.; Zhang, T.J.; Immke, D.; Wang, J.; Zhu, D.; Vanderah, T.W.; Porreca, F.; et al. AMG 9810 [(*E*)-3-(4-*t*-butylphenyl)-*N*-(2,3-dihydrobenzo[*b*][1,4] dioxin-6-yl)acrylamide], a novel vanilloid receptor 1 (TRPV1) antagonist with antihyperalgesic properties. *J. Pharmacol. Exp. Ther.* **2005**, *313*, 474–484. [CrossRef] [PubMed]
62. Culshaw, A.J.; Bevan, S.; Christiansen, M.; Copp, P.; Davis, A.; Davis, C.; Dyson, A.; Dziadulewicz, E.K.; Edwards, L.; Eggelte, H.; et al. Identification and biological characterization of 6-aryl-7-isopropylquinazolinones as novel TRPV1 antagonists that are effective in models of chronic pain. *J. Med. Chem.* **2006**, *49*, 471–474. [CrossRef] [PubMed]
63. Davis, J.B.; Gray, J.; Gunthorpe, M.J.; Hatcher, J.P.; Davey, P.T.; Overend, P.; Harries, M.H.; Latcham, J.; Clapham, C.; Atkinson, K.; et al. Vanilloid receptor-1 is essential for inflammatory thermal hyperalgesia. *Nature* **2000**, *405*, 183–187. [CrossRef] [PubMed]
64. Bron, R.; Klesse, L.J.; Shah, K.; Parada, L.F.; Winter, J. Activation of Ras is necessary and sufficient for upregulation of vanilloid receptor type 1 in sensory neurons by neurotrophic factors. *Mol. Cell. Neurosci.* **2003**, *22*, 118–132. [CrossRef]
65. Yiangou, Y.; Facer, P.; Dyer, N.H.C.; Chan, C.L.H.; Knowles, C.; Williams, N.S.; Anand, P. Vanilloid receptor 1 immunoreactivity in inflamed human bowel. *Lancet* **2001**, *357*, 1338–1339. [CrossRef]
66. Chan, C.L.H.; Facer, P.; Davis, J.B.; Smith, G.D.; Egerton, J.; Bountra, C.; Williams, N.S.; Anand, P. Sensory fibres expressing capsaicin receptor TRPV1 in patients with rectal hypersensitivity and faecal urgency. *Lancet* **2003**, *361*, 385–391. [CrossRef]
67. Lappin, S.C.; Randall, A.D.; Gunthorpe, M.J.; Morisset, V. TRPV1 antagonist, SB-366791, inhibits glutamatergic synaptic transmission in rat spinal dorsal horn following peripheral inflammation. *Eur. J. Pharmacol.* **2006**, *540*, 73–81. [CrossRef] [PubMed]

68. Szallasi, A.; Blumberg, P.M. Resiniferatoxin, a phorbol-related diterpene, acts as an ultrapotent analog of capsaicin, the irritant constituent in red pepper. *Neuroscience* **1989**, *30*, 515–520. [CrossRef]
69. Brown, D.C.; Iadarola, M.J.; Perkowski, S.Z.; Erin, H.; Shofer, F.; Laszlo, K.J.; Olah, Z.; Mannes, A.J. Physiologic and antinociceptive effects of intrathecal resiniferatoxin in a canine bone cancer model. *Anesthesiology* **2005**, *103*, 1052–1059. [CrossRef] [PubMed]
70. Ghilardi, J.R.; Röhrich, H.; Lindsay, T.H.; Sevcik, M.A.; Schwei, M.J.; Kubota, K.; Halvorson, K.G.; Poblete, J.; Chaplan, S.R.; Dubin, A.E.; et al. Selective blockade of the capsaicin receptor TRPV1 attenuates bone cancer pain. *J. Neurosci.* **2005**, *25*, 3126–3131. [CrossRef] [PubMed]
71. Prevarskaya, N.; Zhang, L.; Barritt, G. TRP channels in cancer. *Biochim. Biophys. Acta* **2007**, *1772*, 937–946. [CrossRef] [PubMed]
72. Watabiki, T.; Kiso, T.; Tsukamoto, M.; Aoki, T.; Matsuoka, N. Intrathecal administration of AS1928370, a transient receptor potential vanilloid 1 antagonist, attenuates mechanical allodynia in a mouse model of neuropathic pain. *Biol. Pharm. Bull.* **2011**, *34*, 1105–1108. [CrossRef] [PubMed]
73. Namer, B.; Seifert, F.; Handwerker, H.O.; Maihöfner, C. TRPA1 and TRPM8 activation in humans: effects of cinnamaldehyde and menthol. *NeuroReport* **2005**, *16*, 955–959. [CrossRef] [PubMed]
74. Obata, K.; Katsura, H.; Mizushima, T.; Yamanaka, H.; Kobayashi, K.; Dai, Y.; Fukuoka, T.; Tokunaga, A.; Tominaga, M.; Noguchi, K. TRPA1 induced in sensory neurons contributes to cold hyperalgesia after inflammation and nerve injury. *J. Clin. Investig.* **2005**, *115*, 2393–2401. [CrossRef] [PubMed]
75. da Costa, D.S.M.; Meotti, F.C.; Andrade, E.L.; Leal, P.C.; Motta, E.M.; Calixto, J.B. The involvement of the transient receptor potential A1 (TRPA1) in the maintenance of mechanical and cold hyperalgesia in persistent inflammation. *Pain* **2010**, *148*, 431–437. [CrossRef] [PubMed]
76. Proudfoot, C.J.; Garry, E.M.; Cottrell, D.F.; Rosie, R.; Anderson, H.; Robertson, D.C.; Fleetwood-Walker, S.M.; Mitchell, R. Analgesia mediated by the TRPM8 cold receptor in chronic neuropathic pain. *Curr. Biol.* **2006**, *16*, 1591–1605. [CrossRef] [PubMed]
77. Xing, H.; Chen, M.; Ling, J.; Tan, W.; Gu, J.G. TRPM8 mechanism of cold allodynia after chronic nerve injury. *J. Neurosci.* **2007**, *27*, 13680–13690. [CrossRef] [PubMed]
78. Kono, T.; Satomi, M.; Suno, M.; Kimura, N.; Yamazaki, H.; Furukawa, H.; Matsubara, K. Oxaliplatin-induced neurotoxicity involves TRPM8 in the mechanism of acute hypersensitivity to cold sensation. *Brain Behav.* **2012**, *2*, 68–73. [CrossRef] [PubMed]
79. Liu, B.; Fan, L.; Balakrishna, S.; Sui, A.; Morris, J.B.; Jordt, S.-E. TRPM8 is the principal mediator of menthol-induced analgesia of acute and inflammatory pain. *Pain* **2013**, *154*, 2169–2177. [CrossRef] [PubMed]
80. Edwards, J.G. TRPV1 in the central nervous system: synaptic plasticity, function, and pharmacological implications. *Prog. Drug Res.* **2014**, *68*, 77–104. [PubMed]
81. Zygmunt, P.M.; Högestätt, E.D. TRPA1. *Handb. Exp. Pharmacol.* **2014**, *222*, 583–630. [PubMed]
82. Soudijn, W.; van Wijngaarden, I.; IJzerman, A.P. Stereoselectivity of drug-receptor interactions. *IDrugs* **2003**, *6*, 43–56.
83. Valenzuela, C.; Moreno, C.; de la Cruz, A.; Macías, Á.; Prieto, Á.; González, T. Stereoselective interactions between local anesthetics and ion channels. *Chirality* **2012**, *24*, 944–950. [CrossRef] [PubMed]
84. Karashima, Y.; Damann, N.; Prenen, J.; Talavera, K.; Segal, A.; Voets, T.; Nilius, B. Bimodal action of menthol on the transient receptor potential channel TRPA1. *J. Neurosci.* **2007**, *27*, 9874–9884. [CrossRef] [PubMed]
85. Yang, K.; Li, Y.-Q.; Kumamoto, E.; Furue, H.; Yoshimura, M. Voltage-clamp recordings of postsynaptic currents in substantia gelatinosa neurons in vitro and its applications to assess synaptic transmission. *Brain Res. Protoc.* **2001**, *7*, 235–240. [CrossRef]
86. Baser, K.H.C. Biological and pharmacological activities of carvacrol and carvacrol bearing essential oils. *Curr. Pharm. Des.* **2008**, *14*, 3106–3119. [CrossRef] [PubMed]
87. Angeles-López, G.; Pérez-Vásquez, A.; Hernández-Luis, F.; Déciga-Campos, M.; Bye, R.; Linares, E.; Mata, R. Antinociceptive effect of extracts and compounds from *Hofmeisteria schaffneri*. *J. Ethnopharmacol.* **2010**, *131*, 425–432. [CrossRef] [PubMed]
88. Xu, Z.-H.; Wang, C.; Fujita, T.; Jiang, C.-Y.; Kumamoto, E. Action of thymol on spontaneous excitatory transmission in adult rat spinal substantia gelatinosa neurons. *Neurosci. Lett.* **2015**, *606*, 94–99. [CrossRef] [PubMed]

89. Luo, Q.-T.; Fujita, T.; Jiang, C.-Y.; Kumamoto, E. Carvacrol presynaptically enhances spontaneous excitatory transmission and produces outward current in adult rat spinal substantia gelatinosa neurons. *Brain Res.* **2014**, *1592*, 44–54. [CrossRef] [PubMed]
90. Xu, H.; Delling, M.; Jun, J.C.; Clapham, D.E. Oregano, thyme and clove-derived flavors and skin sensitizers activate specific TRP channels. *Nat. Neurosci.* **2006**, *9*, 628–635. [CrossRef] [PubMed]
91. Lee, S.P.; Buber, M.T.; Yang, Q.; Cerne, R.; Cortés, R.Y.; Sprous, D.G.; Bryant, R.W. Thymol and related alkyl phenols activate the hTRPA1 channel. *Br. J. Pharmacol.* **2008**, *153*, 1739–1749. [CrossRef] [PubMed]
92. Ortar, G.; Morera, L.; Moriello, A.S.; Morera, E.; Nalli, M.; Di Marzo, V.; De Petrocellis, L. Modulation of thermo-transient receptor potential (thermo-TRP) channels by thymol-based compounds. *Bioorg. Med. Chem. Lett.* **2012**, *22*, 3535–3539. [CrossRef] [PubMed]
93. Vogt-Eisele, A.K.; Weber, K.; Sherkheli, M.A.; Vielhaber, G.; Panten, J.; Gisselmann, G.; Hatt, H. Monoterpenoid agonists of TRPV3. *Br. J. Pharmacol.* **2007**, *151*, 530–540. [CrossRef] [PubMed]
94. de la Roche, J.; Eberhardt, M.J.; Klinger, A.B.; Stanslowsky, N.; Wegner, F.; Koppert, W.; Reeh, P.W.; Lampert, A.; Fischer, M.J.M.; Leffler, A. The molecular basis for species-specific activation of human TRPA1 protein by protons involves poorly conserved residues within transmembrane domains 5 and 6. *J. Biol. Chem.* **2013**, *288*, 20280–20292. [CrossRef] [PubMed]
95. McNamara, C.R.; Mandel-Brehm, J.; Bautista, D.M.; Siemens, J.; Deranian, K.L.; Zhao, M.; Hayward, N.J.; Chong, J.A.; Julius, D.; Moran, M.M.; et al. TRPA1 mediates formalin-induced pain. *Proc. Natl. Acad. Sci. USA* **2007**, *104*, 13525–13530. [CrossRef] [PubMed]
96. Urban, L.; Dray, A. Capsazepine, a novel capsaicin antagonist, selectively antagonises the effects of capsaicin in the mouse spinal cord in vitro. *Neurosci. Lett.* **1991**, *134*, 9–11. [CrossRef]
97. Madrid, R.; Donovan-Rodríguez, T.; Meseguer, V.; Acosta, M.C.; Belmonte, C.; Viana, F. Contribution of TRPM8 channels to cold transduction in primary sensory neurons and peripheral nerve terminals. *J. Neurosci.* **2006**, *26*, 12512–12525. [CrossRef] [PubMed]
98. Gonçalves, J.C.R.; Silveira, A.L.; de Souza, H.D.N.; Nery, A.A.; Prado, V.F.; Prado, M.A.M.; Ulrich, H.; Araújo, D.A.M. The monoterpene (−)-carvone: a novel agonist of TRPV1 channels. *Cytometry Part A* **2013**, *83*, 212–219. [CrossRef] [PubMed]
99. Buchbauer, G.; Jäger, W.; Gruber, A.; Dietrich, H. *R*-(+)- and *S*-(−)-carvone: influence of chirality on locomotion activity in mice. *Flavour Fragr. J.* **2005**, *20*, 686–689. [CrossRef]
100. de Sousa, D.P.; de Farias Nóbrega, F.F.; de Almeida, R.N. Influence of the chirality of (*R*)-(−)- and (*S*)-(+)-carvone in the central nervous system: a comparative study. *Chirality* **2007**, *19*, 264–268. [CrossRef] [PubMed]
101. Kang, Q.; Jiang, C.-Y.; Fujita, T.; Kumamoto, E. Spontaneous L-glutamate release enhancement in rat substantia gelatinosa neurons by (−)-carvone and (+)-carvone which activate different types of TRP channel. *Biochem. Biophys. Res. Commun.* **2015**, *459*, 498–503. [CrossRef] [PubMed]
102. Liapi, C.; Anifantis, G.; Chinou, I.; Kourounakis, A.P.; Theodosopoulos, S.; Galanopoulou, P. Antinociceptive properties of 1,8-cineole and β-pinene, from the essential oil of *Eucalyptus camaldulensis* leaves, in rodents. *Planta Med.* **2007**, *73*, 1247–1254. [CrossRef] [PubMed]
103. Romagni, J.G.; Allen, S.N.; Dayan, F.E. Allelopathic effects of volatile cineoles on two weedy plant species. *J. Chem. Ecol.* **2000**, *26*, 303–313. [CrossRef]
104. Behrendt, H.-J.; Germann, T.; Gillen, C.; Hatt, H.; Jostock, R. Characterization of the mouse cold-menthol receptor TRPM8 and vanilloid receptor type-1 VR1 using a fluorometric imaging plate reader (FLIPR) assay. *Br. J. Pharmacol.* **2004**, *141*, 737–745. [CrossRef] [PubMed]
105. Takaishi, M.; Fujita, F.; Uchida, K.; Yamamoto, S.; Sawada Shimizu, M.; Hatai Uotsu, C.; Shimizu, M.; Tominaga, M. 1,8-Cineole, a TRPM8 agonist, is a novel natural antagonist of human TRPA1. *Mol. Pain* **2012**, *8*, 86. [CrossRef] [PubMed]
106. Talavera, K.; Gees, M.; Karashima, Y.; Meseguer, V.M.; Vanoirbeek, J.A.J.; Damann, N.; Everaerts, W.; Benoit, M.; Janssens, A.; Vennekens, R.; et al. Nicotine activates the chemosensory cation channel TRPA1. *Nat. Neurosci.* **2009**, *12*, 1293–1299. [CrossRef] [PubMed]
107. Zygmunt, P.M.; Petersson, J.; Andersson, D.A.; Chuang, H.-h.; Sørgård, M.; Di Marzo, V.; Julius, D.; Högestätt, E.D. Vanilloid receptors on sensory nerves mediate the vasodilator action of anandamide. *Nature* **1999**, *400*, 452–457. [PubMed]

108. Hwang, S.W.; Cho, H.; Kwak, J.; Lee, S.-Y.; Kang, C.-J.; Jung, J.; Cho, S.; Min, K.H.; Suh, Y.-G.; Kim, D.; et al. Direct activation of capsaicin receptors by products of lipoxygenases: endogenous capsaicin-like substances. *Proc. Natl. Acad. Sci. USA* **2000**, *97*, 6155–6160. [CrossRef] [PubMed]
109. Starowicz, K.; Niga, S.; Di Marzo, V. Biochemistry and pharmacology of endovanilloids. *Pharmacol. Ther.* **2007**, *114*, 13–33. [CrossRef] [PubMed]
110. Yue, H.-Y.; Fujita, T.; Kawasaki, Y.; Kumamoto, E. AM404 enhances the spontaneous release of L-glutamate in a manner sensitive to capsazepine in adult rat substantia gelatinosa neurones. *Brain Res.* **2004**, *1018*, 283–287. [CrossRef] [PubMed]
111. Niforatos, W.; Zhang, X.-F.; Lake, M.R.; Walter, K.A.; Neelands, T.; Holzman, T.F.; Scott, V.E.; Faltynek, C.R.; Moreland, R.B.; Chen, J. Activation of TRPA1 channels by the fatty acid amide hydrolase inhibitor 3′-carbamoylbiphenyl-3-yl cyclohexylcarbamate (URB597). *Mol. Pharmacol.* **2007**, *71*, 1209–1216. [CrossRef] [PubMed]
112. Cruz-Orengo, L.; Dhaka, A.; Heuermann, R.J.; Young, T.J.; Montana, M.C.; Cavanaugh, E.J.; Kim, D.; Story, G.M. Cutaneous nociception evoked by 15-delta PGJ2 via activation of ion channel TRPA1. *Mol. Pain* **2008**, *4*, 30. [CrossRef] [PubMed]
113. Wang, H.; Kohno, T.; Amaya, F.; Brenner, G.J.; Ito, N.; Allchorne, A.; Ji, R.-R.; Woolf, C.J. Bradykinin produces pain hypersensitivity by potentiating spinal cord glutamatergic synaptic transmission. *J. Neurosci.* **2005**, *25*, 7986–7992. [CrossRef] [PubMed]
114. Asuthkar, S.; Elustondo, P.A.; Demirkhanyan, L.; Sun, X.; Baskaran, P.; Velpula, K.K.; Thyagarajan, B.; Pavlov, E.V.; Zakharian, E. The TRPM8 protein is a testosterone receptor: I. Biochemical evidence for direct TRPM8-testosterone interactions. *J. Biol. Chem.* **2015**, *290*, 2659–2669. [CrossRef] [PubMed]
115. Asuthkar, S.; Demirkhanyan, L.; Sun, X.; Elustondo, P.A.; Krishnan, V.; Baskaran, P.; Velpula, K.K.; Thyagarajan, B.; Pavlov, E.V.; Zakharian, E. The TRPM8 protein is a testosterone receptor: II. Functional evidence for an ionotropic effect of testosterone on TRPM8. *J. Biol. Chem.* **2015**, *290*, 2670–2688. [CrossRef] [PubMed]
116. Leffler, A.; Fischer, M.J.; Rehner, D.; Kienel, S.; Kistner, K.; Sauer, S.K.; Gavva, N.R.; Reeh, P.W.; Nau, C. The vanilloid receptor TRPV1 is activated and sensitized by local anesthetics in rodent sensory neurons. *J. Clin. Investig.* **2008**, *118*, 763–776. [CrossRef] [PubMed]
117. Leffler, A.; Lattrell, A.; Kronewald, S.; Niedermirtl, F.; Nau, C. Activation of TRPA1 by membrane permeable local anesthetics. *Mol. Pain* **2011**, *7*, 62. [CrossRef] [PubMed]
118. Piao, L.-H.; Fujita, T.; Jiang, C.-Y.; Liu, T.; Yue, H.-Y.; Nakatsuka, T.; Kumamoto, E. TRPA1 activation by lidocaine in nerve terminals results in glutamate release increase. *Biochem. Biophys. Res. Commun.* **2009**, *379*, 980–984. [CrossRef] [PubMed]
119. Szallasi, A. Piperine: researchers discover new flavor in an ancient spice. *Trends Pharmacol. Sci.* **2005**, *26*, 437–439. [CrossRef] [PubMed]
120. Yang, L.; Fujita, T.; Jiang, C.-Y.; Piao, L.-H.; Yue, H.-Y.; Mizuta, K.; Kumamoto, E. TRPV1 agonist piperine but not olvanil enhances glutamatergic spontaneous excitatory transmission in rat spinal substantia gelatinosa neurons. *Biochem. Biophys. Res. Commun.* **2011**, *410*, 841–845. [CrossRef] [PubMed]
121. Liu, L.; Simon, S.A. Similarities and differences in the currents activated by capsaicin, piperine, and zingerone in rat trigeminal ganglion cells. *J. Neurophysiol.* **1996**, *76*, 1858–1869. [PubMed]
122. Liu, L.; Lo, Y.-C.; Chen, I.-J.; Simon, S.A. The responses of rat trigeminal ganglion neurons to capsaicin and two nonpungent vanilloid receptor agonists, olvanil and glyceryl nonamide. *J. Neurosci.* **1997**, *17*, 4101–4111. [PubMed]
123. Yang, B.H.; Piao, Z.G.; Kim, Y.-B.; Lee, C.-H.; Lee, J.K.; Park, K.; Kim, J.S.; Oh, S.B. Activation of vanilloid receptor 1 (VR1) by eugenol. *J. Dent. Res.* **2003**, *82*, 781–785. [CrossRef] [PubMed]
124. Inoue, M.; Fujita, T.; Goto, M.; Kumamoto, E. Presynaptic enhancement by eugenol of spontaneous excitatory transmission in rat spinal substantia gelatinosa neurons is mediated by transient receptor potential A1 channels. *Neuroscience* **2012**, *210*, 403–415. [CrossRef] [PubMed]
125. Yue, H.-Y.; Jiang, C.-Y.; Fujita, T.; Kumamoto, E. Zingerone enhances glutamatergic spontaneous excitatory transmission by activating TRPA1 but not TRPV1 channels in the adult rat substantia gelatinosa. *J. Neurophysiol.* **2013**, *110*, 658–671. [CrossRef] [PubMed]
126. Park, C.-K.; Xu, Z.-Z.; Berta, T.; Han, Q.; Chen, G.; Liu, X.-J.; Ji, R.-R. Extracellular microRNAs activate nociceptor neurons to elicit pain via TLR7 and TRPA1. *Neuron* **2014**, *82*, 47–54. [CrossRef] [PubMed]

127. Zhu, L.; Fujita, T.; Jiang, C.-Y.; Kumamoto, E. Enhancement by citral of glutamatergic spontaneous excitatory transmission in adult rat substantia gelatinosa neurons. *NeuroReport* **2016**, *27*, 166–171. [CrossRef] [PubMed]
128. Andersson, D.A.; Gentry, C.; Alenmyr, L.; Killander, D.; Lewis, S.E.; Andersson, A.; Bucher, B.; Galzi, J.-L.; Sterner, O.; Bevan, S.; et al. TRPA1 mediates spinal antinociception induced by acetaminophen and the cannabinoid Δ^9-tetrahydrocannabiorcol. *Nat. Commun.* **2011**, *2*, 551. [CrossRef] [PubMed]
129. Furue, H.; Narikawa, K.; Kumamoto, E.; Yoshimura, M. Responsiveness of rat substantia gelatinosa neurones to mechanical but not thermal stimuli revealed by *in vivo* patch-clamp recording. *J. Physiol.* **1999**, *521*, 529–535.
130. Yamanaka, M.; Taniguchi, W.; Nishio, N.; Hashizume, H.; Yamada, H.; Yoshida, M.; Nakatsuka, T. *In vivo* patch-clamp analysis of the antinociceptive actions of TRPA1 activation in the spinal dorsal horn. *Mol. Pain* **2015**, *11*, 20. [CrossRef] [PubMed]
131. Todd, A.J.; Watt, C.; Spike, R.C.; Sieghart, W. Colocalization of GABA, glycine and their receptors at synapses in the rat spinal cord. *J. Neurosci.* **1996**, *16*, 974–982. [PubMed]
132. Coggeshall, R.E.; Carlton, S.M. Receptor localization in the mammalian dorsal horn and primary afferent neurons. *Brain Res. Rev.* **1997**, *24*, 28–66. [CrossRef]
133. Moore, K.A.; Kohno, T.; Karchewski, L.A.; Scholz, J.; Baba, H.; Woolf, C.J. Partial peripheral nerve injury promotes a selective loss of GABAergic inhibition in the superficial dorsal horn of the spinal cord. *J. Neurosci.* **2002**, *22*, 6724–6731. [PubMed]
134. Kohno, T. A role of spinal inhibition in neuropathic pain. In *Cellular and Molecular Mechanisms for the Modulation of Nociceptive Transmission in the Peripheral and Central Nervous Systems*; Kumamoto, E., Ed.; Research Signpost: Kelara, India, 2007; pp. 131–145.
135. Coull, J.A.M.; Boudreau, D.; Bachand, K.; Prescott, S.A.; Nault, F.; Sik, A.; de Koninck, P.; de Koninck, Y. Trans-synaptic shift in anion gradient in spinal lamina I neurons as a mechanism of neuropathic pain. *Nature* **2003**, *424*, 938–942. [CrossRef] [PubMed]
136. Müller, F.; Heinke, B.; Sandkühler, J. Reduction of glycine receptor-mediated miniature inhibitory postsynaptic currents in rat spinal lamina I neurons after peripheral inflammation. *Neuroscience* **2003**, *122*, 799–805. [CrossRef] [PubMed]
137. Tanabe, M.; Takasu, K.; Yamaguchi, S.; Kodama, D.; Ono, H. Glycine transporter inhibitors as a potential therapeutic strategy for chronic pain with memory impairment. *Anesthesiology* **2008**, *108*, 929–937. [CrossRef] [PubMed]
138. Sandkühler, J. Models and mechanisms of hyperalgesia and allodynia. *Physiol. Rev.* **2009**, *89*, 707–758. [CrossRef] [PubMed]
139. Zeilhofer, H.U.; Wildner, H.; Yévenes, G.E. Fast synaptic inhibition in spinal sensory processing and pain control. *Physiol. Rev.* **2012**, *92*, 193–235. [CrossRef] [PubMed]
140. Baba, H.; Kohno, T.; Okamoto, M.; Goldstein, P.A.; Shimoji, K.; Yoshimura, M. Muscarinic facilitation of GABA release in substantia gelatinosa of the rat spinal dorsal horn. *J. Physiol.* **1998**, *508*, 83–93. [CrossRef] [PubMed]
141. Baba, H.; Goldstein, P.A.; Okamoto, M.; Kohno, T.; Ataka, T.; Yoshimura, M.; Shimoji, K. Norepinephrine facilitates inhibitory transmission in substantia gelatinosa of adult rat spinal cord (part 2): effects on somatodendritic sites of GABAergic neurons. *Anesthesiology* **2000**, *92*, 485–492. [CrossRef] [PubMed]
142. Baba, H.; Shimoji, K.; Yoshimura, M. Norepinephrine facilitates inhibitory transmission in substantia gelatinosa of adult rat spinal cord (part 1): effects on axon terminals of GABAergic and glycinergic neurons. *Anesthesiology* **2000**, *92*, 473–484. [CrossRef] [PubMed]
143. Takeda, D.; Nakatsuka, T.; Papke, R.; Gu, J.G. Modulation of inhibitory synaptic activity by a non-$\alpha4\beta2$, non-$\alpha7$ subtype of nicotinic receptors in the substantia gelatinosa of adult rat spinal cord. *Pain* **2003**, *101*, 13–23. [CrossRef]
144. Fukushima, T.; Ohtsubo, T.; Tsuda, M.; Yanagawa, Y.; Hori, Y. Facilitatory actions of serotonin type 3 receptors on GABAergic inhibitory synaptic transmission in the spinal superficial dorsal horn. *J. Neurophysiol.* **2009**, *102*, 1459–1471. [CrossRef] [PubMed]
145. Liu, T.; Fujita, T.; Kumamoto, E. Acetylcholine and norepinephrine mediate GABAergic but not glycinergic transmission enhancement by melittin in adult rat substantia gelatinosa neurons. *J. Neurophysiol.* **2011**, *106*, 233–246. [CrossRef] [PubMed]

146. Bíró, T.; Tóth, B.I.; Marincsák, R.; Dobrosi, N.; Géczy, T.; Paus, R. TRP channels as novel players in the pathogenesis and therapy of itch. *Biochim. Biophys. Acta* **2007**, *1772*, 1004–1021. [CrossRef] [PubMed]
147. Sikand, P.; Shimada, S.G.; Green, B.G.; LaMotte, R.H. Similar itch and nociceptive sensations evoked by punctate cutaneous application of capsaicin, histamine and cowhage. *Pain* **2009**, *144*, 66–75. [CrossRef] [PubMed]
148. Akiyama, T.; Carstens, E. Neural processing of itch. *Neuroscience* **2013**, *250*, 697–714. [CrossRef] [PubMed]
149. Liu, T.; Ji, R.-R. New insights into the mechanisms of itch: are pain and itch controlled by distinct mechanisms? *Pflügers Arch.* **2013**, *465*, 1671–1685. [CrossRef] [PubMed]
150. Fujita, T.; Liu, T.; Nakatsuka, T.; Kumamoto, E. Proteinase-activated receptor-1 activation presynaptically enhances spontaneous glutamatergic excitatory transmission in adult rat substantia gelatinosa neurons. *J. Neurophysiol.* **2009**, *102*, 312–319. [CrossRef] [PubMed]
151. Jordt, S.-E.; Julius, D. Molecular basis for species-specific sensitivity to "hot" chili peppers. *Cell* **2002**, *108*, 421–430. [CrossRef]
152. Gavva, N.R.; Klionsky, L.; Qu, Y.; Shi, L.; Tamir, R.; Edenson, S.; Zhang, T.J.; Viswanadhan, V.N.; Toth, A.; Pearce, L.V.; et al. Molecular determinants of vanilloid sensitivity in TRPV1. *J. Biol. Chem.* **2004**, *279*, 20283–20295. [CrossRef] [PubMed]
153. Chen, J.; Zhang, X.-F.; Kort, M.E.; Huth, J.R.; Sun, C.; Miesbauer, L.J.; Cassar, S.C.; Neelands, T.; Scott, V.E.; Moreland, R.B.; et al. Molecular determinants of species-specific activation or blockade of TRPA1 channels. *J. Neurosci.* **2008**, *28*, 5063–5071. [CrossRef] [PubMed]
154. Nagatomo, K.; Kubo, Y. Caffeine activates mouse TRPA1 channels but suppresses human TRPA1 channels. *Proc. Natl. Acad. Sci. USA* **2008**, *105*, 17373–17378. [CrossRef] [PubMed]
155. Chen, J.; Joshi, S.K.; DiDomenico, S.; Perner, R.J.; Mikusa, J.P.; Gauvin, D.M.; Segreti, J.A.; Han, P.; Zhang, X.-F.; Niforatos, W.; et al. Selective blockade of TRPA1 channel attenuates pathological pain without altering noxious cold sensation or body temperature regulation. *Pain* **2011**, *152*, 1165–1172. [CrossRef] [PubMed]
156. Banzawa, N.; Saito, S.; Imagawa, T.; Kashio, M.; Takahashi, K.; Tominaga, M.; Ohta, T. Molecular basis determining inhibition/activation of nociceptive receptor TRPA1 protein: a single amino acid dictates species-specific actions of the most potent mammalian TRPA1 antagonist. *J. Biol. Chem.* **2014**, *289*, 31927–31939. [CrossRef] [PubMed]

11

The Minimal Effect of Linker Length for Fatty Acid Conjugation to a Small Protein on the Serum Half-Life Extension

Jinhwan Cho [1,†], Junyong Park [2,†], Giyoong Tae [1], Mi Sun Jin [3] and Inchan Kwon [1,2,*]

1 School of Materials Science and Engineering, Gwangju Institute of Science and Technology (GIST), Gwangju 61005, Korea; kroea2002@gist.ac.kr (J.C.); gytae@gist.ac.kr (G.T.)
2 Department of Biomedical Science and Engineering, GIST, Gwangju 61005, Korea; happydragon@gist.ac.kr
3 School of Life Science, GIST, Gwangju 61005, Korea; misunjin@gist.ac.kr
* Correspondence: inchan@gist.ac.kr
† These authors contributed equally to this work.

Abstract: Conjugation of serum albumin or one of its ligands (such as fatty acid) has been an effective strategy to prolong the serum half-lives of drugs via neonatal Fc receptor (FcRn)–mediated recycling of albumin. So far, fatty acid (FA) has been effective in prolonging the serum half-lives for therapeutic peptides and small proteins, but not for large therapeutic proteins. Very recently, it was reported a large protein conjugated to FA competes with the binding of FcRn with serum albumin, leading to limited serum half-life extension, because primary FA binding sites in serum albumin partially overlap with FcRn binding sites. In order to prevent such competition, longer linkers between FA and the large proteins were required. Herein, we hypothesized that small proteins do not cause substantial competition for FcRn binding to albumin, resulting in the extended serum half-life. Using a small protein (28 kDa), we investigated whether the intramolecular distance in FA-protein conjugate affects the FcRn binding with albumin and serum half-life using linkers with varying lengths. Unlike with the FA-conjugated large protein, all FA-conjugated small proteins with different linkers exhibited comparable the FcRn binding to albumin and extended serum half-life.

Keywords: serum half-life extension; fatty acid conjugation; FcRn-mediated recycling; serum albumin

---

1. Introduction

Therapeutic proteins have been widely used for the treatment of human diseases [1]. However, therapeutic proteins are rapidly eliminated from the blood of patients due to several mechanisms, including renal filtration, proteolysis, intracellular degradation, and immune responses, which result in short serum half-lives [2,3]. Such short serum half-lives of therapeutic proteins result in the need for frequent administration [2–4]. Therefore, the extension of the serum half-life of therapeutic proteins is very important in developing new therapeutic proteins [2,4,5]. Conventionally, polyethylene glycol (PEG) chains have been conjugated to therapeutic proteins for serum half-life extension in order to reduce renal filtration and proteolysis [6]. However, recently several concerns have been raised about PEG conjugation, including PEG accumulation due to its poor degradability in the body and reduced efficacy resulting from immune responses to PEG [7].

As an alternative to PEG, human serum albumin (HSA) has been investigated as a half-life extender [8]. In contrast to PEG, HSA is biodegradable and minimally immunogenic [9,10]. Furthermore, HSA has an exceptionally long serum half-life (more than two weeks) partly due to evasion from intracellular degradation via neonatal Fc receptor (FcRn)–mediated recycling [2,3,10–13]. Direct coupling of therapeutic protein to HSA via either genetic fusion or chemical conjugation led to a significant extension of therapeutic protein serum half-life in vivo [11,12,14–17]. Recently, indirect coupling of therapeutics to HSA using albumin ligands such as fatty acids has received much attention, because fatty acids are cheaper than HSA and exhibit a much higher conjugation yield than HSA [9]. Furthermore, fatty acids are biocompatible and not immunogenic [18].

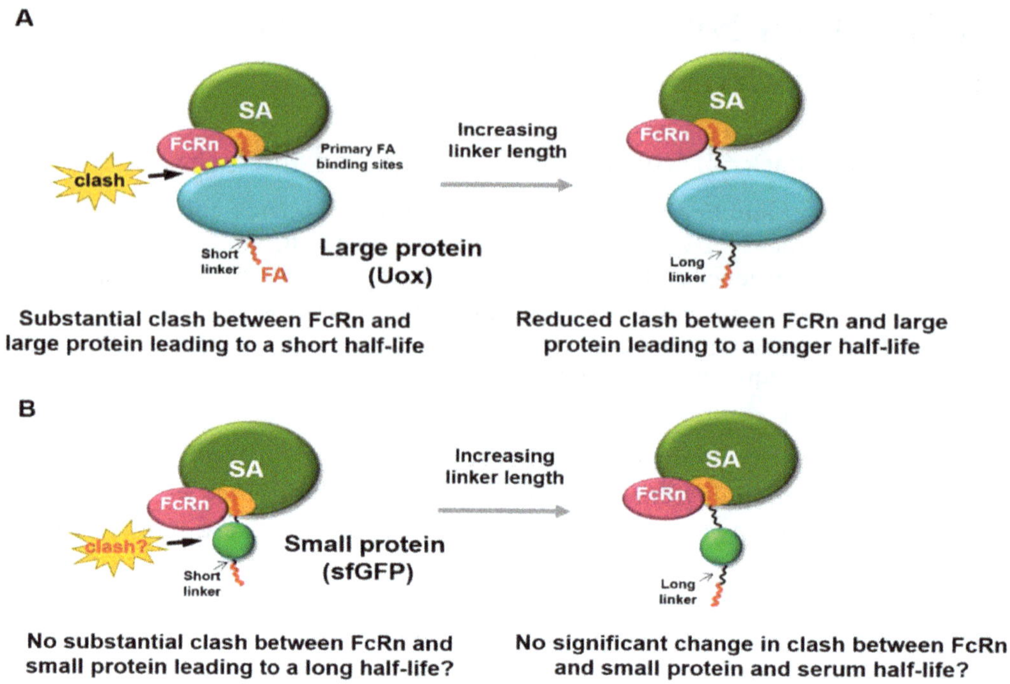

Figure 1. Effect of protein size of fatty acid-conjugated protein on the binding of FcRn with serum albumin. (**A**) For a large protein (Uox, 140 kDa), conjugation of fatty acid with a short linker leads to steric hindrance to binding of FcRn to serum albumin, due to its large size. Increasing the linker length reduces the steric hindrance to binding of FcRn to serum albumin, resulting in longer serum half-life. (**B**) For a small protein (superfolder green fluorescent protein [sfGFP], 28 kDa), conjugation of a fatty acid with a short linker may not exhibit substantial steric hindrance to binding of FcRn to serum albumin, due to its small size. Therefore, increasing linker length may not substantially alter the steric hindrance to the binding of FcRn to serum albumin.

Despite the numerous reports of serum half-life extension via fatty acid conjugation, its molecular mechanism was not yet fully revealed. It is noteworthy that fatty acid conjugation was effective for serum half-life extension of therapeutic peptides and small proteins (less than 28 kDa) [17,19–24]. Considering that a majority of therapeutic proteins and other candidates have molecular weights greater than 28 kDa [25], it is important to understand whether there is any protein size–dependent factor in serum half-life extension via fatty acid conjugation. Regarding this, a very recent report showed that fatty acid conjugation extends the serum half-life of urate oxidase (Uox) (140 kDa) [26], a large therapeutic protein used to treat hyperuricemia [27–31]. In this report, the conventional short linker between fatty acid (palmitic acid) and large protein (Uox) was shown not to be able to substantially extend the serum half-life of Uox, due to compromised FcRn binding to serum albumin. In order to avoid competition with FcRn binding and achieve the substantial serum half-life extension, longer linkers between fatty acid and Uox were required (Figure 1A) [26]. There are seven palmitic acid (PA) binding sites on serum albumin (FA1 to FA7) [32]. Two dominant PA binding sites at domain III of serum albumin (FA4 and FA5) [33–38] overlap with FcRn binding sites. With a short linker, PA-conjugated Uox (Uox-PA) was expected to be located near domain III of serum albumin. Therefore, the existence of bulky Uox near domain III was attributed to the significant reduction of FcRn binding to serum albumin in vitro, resulting in limited extension in serum half-life in vivo [26]. In contrast, longer linkers were expected to locate Uox-PA away from domain III, leading to the recovery of FcRn binding affinity to serum albumin in vitro and substantial extension of serum half-life in vivo [26].

Considering that fatty acid conjugation led to significant serum half-life extension of therapeutic peptides and small proteins [17,19–23], we hypothesized that small proteins exhibit minimal steric hindrance to binding of FcRn to serum albumin. Therefore, herein we investigated whether fatty acid conjugation to a small protein with linkers with various lengths affects binding of FcRn with serum albumin in vitro and serum half-life in vivo. For a small protein, if linkers with varying lengths do not substantially affect the binding affinity of FcRn to serum albumin in vitro and serum half-life in vivo (Figure 1B), that would demonstrate that protein size is an important factor in serum half-life extension via fatty acid conjugation. These results would facilitate our understanding of the molecular mechanism of fatty acid conjugation–mediated serum half-life extension of proteins.

2. Materials and Methods

2.1. Materials

Ampicillin; palmitic acid *N*-hydroxysuccinimide (NHS-PA); 3,3′,5,5′-tetramethylbenzidine (TMB); sinapinic acid; and deoxycholate (DCA) were obtained from Sigma-Aldrich (St. Louis, MO, USA). Mouse serum albumin (MSA) was obtained from Equitech-Bio Inc. (Kerrville, TX, USA). Isopropyl β-D-1-thiogalactopyranoside (IPTG), amine-binding plate, and phosphate-buffered saline (PBS) were obtained from Thermo Fisher Scientific (Waltham, MA, USA). Tween-20 was obtained from Bio-Rad (Hercules, CA, USA). Nickel-nitrilotriacetic acid (Ni-NTA) agarose beads and polypropylene columns were obtained from Qiagen Inc (Valencia, CA, USA). PD-10 column was obtained from GE Health care (Piscataway, NJ, USA). Vivaspin centrifugal concentrators with molecular weight cut-off (MWCO) of 10 kDa were purchased from Sartorius Corporation (Bohemia, NY, USA). Dibenzocyclooctyne (DBCO)-amine, DBCO-PEG4-amine, azidoacetic acid *N*-hydroxysuccinimide (NHS) ester, and azido-PEG4-NHS ester were obtained from Click Chemistry Tools LLC (Scottsdale, AZ, USA). 6×His tag antibody and horseradish peroxidase (HRP)–conjugated anti-rabbit Immunoglobulin G (IgG) were obtained from Cell Signaling Technology (Beverly, MA, USA). ZipTip with C18 resin was purchased from Millipore Corporation (Billerica, MA, USA). Protein Standard II was obtained from Bruker Daltonics (Bremen, Germany). Mouse FcRn was obtained from ACRO Biosystems (Newark, DE, USA).

2.2. Preparation of Purified Superfolder Green Fluorescent Protein (sfGFP) from E. coli

In order to obtain purified sfGFP using *E. coli*, cloning, expression, and purification of sfGFP were conducted as previously described [23]. Briefly, the pQE80-sfGFP plasmid was transformed into TOP10 *E. coli* competent cells. The transformed colony was precultured into 2×·YT medium containing 100 μg/mL ampicillin. After 8 h incubation at 37 °C, the precultured cells were inoculated into a 2×·YT medium containing 100 μg/mL ampicillin and incubated at 37 °C for the main culture. When the optical density at 600 nm reached 0.5, 1 mM IPTG was added to the main culture for sfGFP induction. After 5 h incubation at 37 °C, cells were collected by pellet down at 5000 g for 10 min. The cell pellets were stored at −80 °C until further use. In order to start the purification of sfGFP, the cell pellets were resuspended with lysis buffer (pH 7.4, 10 mM imidazole) by complete vortexing. The resuspended cell pellets were broken down by sonication for 1 h. Cell debris was removed by centrifugation at 12,000 rpm for 30 min. The supernatant was mixed with Ni-NTA agarose beads thoroughly and incubated at 15 °C and 220 rpm for 1 h, then was poured into a polypropylene column, followed by washing with washing buffer (pH 7.4, 20 mM imidazole) to remove impurities. The sfGFP was eluted with elution buffer (pH 7.4, 250 mM imidazole), and then was immediately subjected to buffer exchange into PBS buffer (pH 7.4) using a PD-10 column. Finally, the purified sfGFP was concentrated to a proper concentration with a Vivaspin column (MWCO: 10 kDa) according to the supplier's manual and stored at 4 °C before use. The molar extinction coefficient at 280 nm value of sfGFP was calculated to be 19,035 M^{-1} cm^{-1} by the following equation: ε_{280} = (5500 × number of tryptophan residues) + (1490 × number of tyrosine residues) + (125 × number of disulfide bonds) [39]. The concentration of sfGFP was then determined using the Beer-Lambert law.

2.3. Preparation of sfGFP-PA Conjugates with Various Linkers

The sfGFP-PA conjugates with various linker lengths were prepared as previously reported, except sfGFP was used instead of Uox [26]. The chemical structures of intermediates and linkers (LK01, 02, 03, and 04) are shown in Figure 2A and Figure S1 in Supplementary Materials. Briefly, each DBCO-amine or DBCO-PEG4-amine (180 μM) was reacted with NHS-PA (900 μM) at 37 °C for 20 h to make DBCO-PA or DBCO-PEG4-PA, respectively. The unreacted NHS-PA was quenched with excess Tris base (100 mM, pH 7.4). The sfGFP-PA conjugates with various linker lengths (SP01, SP02, SP03, and SP04) were generated using three different PA-containing reagents (NHS-PA, DBCO-PA, and DBCO-PEG4-PA). First, sfGFP (50 μM) and NHS-PA (500 μM) were reacted in PBS containing 0.40% (w/v) DCA at room temperature for 3 h, yielding SP01. Second, sfGFP (50 μM) and azidoacetic acid NHS ester (1500 μM) were reacted in PBS on ice for 2 h and quenched with excess Tris base (150 mM, pH 7.4) to make sfGFP-azides intermediate. After desalting and concentration by Vivaspin (MWCO: 10 kDa), the concentration of sfGFP-azides intermediate was measured using the Beer-Lambert law. sfGFP-azides intermediate (50 μM) was reacted with DBCO-PA (100 μM) in PBS with 0.80% (w/v) DCA at room temperature for 3 h, yielding SP02. Third, sfGFP (50 μM) and azido-PEG4-NHS ester (1500 μM) were reacted in PBS on ice for 2 h and quenched with excess Tris base (150 mM, pH 7.4) to make sfGFP-PEG4-azides intermediate. After desalting and concentration by Vivaspin (MWCO: 10 kDa), the concentration of sfGFP-PEG4-azides was measured using the Beer-Lambert law. sfGFP-PEG4-azides (50 μM) was reacted with DBCO-PA (100 μM) in PBS with 0.80% (w/v) DCA at room temperature for 3 h, yielding SP03. Fourth, sfGFP-PEG4-azides (50 μM) was reacted with DBCO-PEG4-PA (100 μM) in PBS with 0.80% (w/v) DCA at room temperature for 3 h, yielding SP04. Finally, all sfGFP-PA conjugates were desalted to PBS buffer (pH 7.4) using a PD-10 column and stored at 4 °C until required for use.

2.4. Matrix-Assisted Laser Desorption Ionization/Time-of-Flight (MALDI-TOF) Analysis of the sfGFP and sfGFP-PA Conjugates

In order to analyze the intact mass of the sfGFP or sfGFP-PA conjugate, the sample was desalted on a ZipTip C18 according to the manufacturer's (Millipore Corporation) protocol. The first layer applied to a polished steel plate using sinapinic acid in absolute ethanol. The desalted sfGFP or sfGFP-PA conjugate was mixed with 1:1 of sinapinic acid in TA30 solution (0.1% Trifluoroacetic acid:acetonitrile = 7:3) and then applied to the first layer prior to mass analysis via Microflex MALDI-TOF (Bruker Daltonics; Bremen, Germany). The MALDI-TOF was calibrated using a Protein Standard II (20–90 kDa) before measurement according to the manufacturer's instructions. The average masses of sfGFP, SP01, SP02, SP03, and SP04 were obtained by multiplying each area and its corresponding mass of all peaks and then dividing its average value by the average area of all peaks. The average numbers of conjugated PAs at SP01, SP02, SP03, and SP04 were obtained by using the molecular weight of the PA containing linker from the mass shift from sfGFP, sfGFP-azides, and sfGFP-PEG4-azides.

2.5. In Vitro Serum Albumin Binding Assay

MSA (10 μg/mL) in 100 μL of PBS (pH 7.4) was applied to amine-binding plates at 4 °C overnight. 5% skim milk in PBS containing 0.05% (v/v) of Tween-20 (PBS-T) (pH 7.4) was used for blocking nonspecific binding at room temperature for 2 h. sfGFP and sfGFP-PA conjugates (14 μM) in 50 μL of PBS were incubated on the plate at room temperature for 2 h. The amount of sfGFP bound was determined by enzyme-linked immunosorbent assay (ELISA) using the anti-6×His antibody. After that, the anti-6×His antibody (1:1000 diluted) was incubated at room temperature for 2 h and washed. Immediately after, HRP-conjugated anti-rabbit IgG (1:1000 diluted) was added and incubated for 1 h.

After washing, the TMB substrate was added, incubated for the appropriate time, and stopped with 1 M sulfuric acid. Absorbance at 450 nm was monitored using a Synergy H1 multimode microplate reader. (BioTek; Winooski, VT, USA).

2.6. *sfGFP Fluorescence Assay*

The fluorescence of sfGFP or sfGFP-PA conjugate was measured using a Synergy H1 multimode microplate reader. Each sfGFP or sfGFP-PA conjugate (1.7 μM) in 100 μL of PBS was added to a 96-well plate, and then the fluorescence was measured at an excitation wavelength of 480 nm and an emission wavelength of 510 nm. The relative fluorescence of sfGFP-PA conjugate was normalized by that of sfGFP.

2.7. *Serum Half-Life Determination in Mice*

The amounts of sfGFP and sfGFP-PA conjugate in vivo were investigated by injecting each protein (10 μM) in 200 μL of PBS into the tail veins of 9-week-old female BALB/c mice (n = 5). Experiments on mice were performed according to the guidelines of the Animal Care and Use Committee of the Gwangju Institute of Science and Technology (GIST) (GIST-2019-071). Blood samples (below 50 μL) were collected at 10, 20, 30, 40, and 50 min for sfGFP; 10 min and 1, 2, and 4 h for sfGFP-PA conjugates. Collected blood samples were allowed to clot at room temperature for 30 min, then centrifuged at 1500 rpm for 10 min at 4 °C to obtain the serum from the blood. The separated serum was stored at −20 °C until required for use. The concentrations of sfGFP and sfGFP-PA conjugates in the serum samples were measured by using a GFP ELISA kit according to the manufacturer's (Cell Biolabs Inc; San Diego, CA, USA) protocol.

2.8. *FcRn/Serum Albumin/sfGFP-PA Tertiary Complex Formation Assay*

Mouse FcRn (10 μg/mL) in 100 μL of PBS (pH 6.0) applied to an amine-binding plate at 4 °C overnight. In order to block nonspecific binding, 5% skim milk in PBS-T (pH 6.0) was added and incubated at room temperature for 2 h. MSA (1 mg/mL) in 100 μL of PBS (pH 6.0) was added at room temperature for 2 h. After washing, 14 μM of sfGFP or sfGFP-PA conjugates in 50 μL of PBS (pH 6.0) was added and incubated at room temperature for 2 h. After that, 100 μL of anti-6×His antibody (1:1000 diluted) was incubated at room temperature for 2 h. After washing, HRP-conjugated anti-rabbit IgG (1:1000 diluted) was added and incubated at room temperature for 1 h. Then, the TMB substrate was added, incubated for the appropriate time, and stopped with 1 M sulfuric acid. Absorbance at 450 nm was monitored with a Synergy H1 multimode microplate reader.

3. Results and Discussion

3.1. *PA-Conjugated sfGFP Conjugates with Various Linker Lengths*

We chose sfGFP as a small model protein to investigate the competition to binding of FcRn to serum albumin and the serum half-life extension upon fatty acid conjugation. Although green fluorescent protein is not a therapeutic protein, it has been widely used in biomedical applications [40–44]. In particular, its unique spectral properties including fluorescence and biocompatibility, make sfGFP a great surrogate for a therapeutic protein in drug delivery studies [41,42]. In order to investigate the protein-size dependency of serum half-life extension via fatty acid conjugation, a model protein should be much smaller than Uox (140 kDa). Considering that the molecular weight of sfGFP with an anti-hexahistidine (6×His) tag used in this study is about 28 kDa, sfGFP was suitable as a small model protein. Purified sfGFP was prepared as described previously [8,23,45]. Briefly, the gene of sfGFP was overexpressed in TOP 10 *E. coli* cells. Then, the recombinant sfGFP was purified via metal affinity chromatography using its 6×His tag. The band of purified sfGFP was observed in the Coomassie blue–stained protein gel (Figure 2B, lane 1), indicating that the purity of sfGFP was greater than 95%.

Next, four linkers with various lengths (LK01, 02, 03, and 04) were conjugated to sfGFP to generate sfGFP-PA conjugates (SP01, 02, 03, and 04) (Figure 2A). The same four linkers were previously used to prepare Uox-PA conjugates [26]. In general, properties of the fatty acid linker, such as solubility and length, may affect serum albumin binding affinity. However, for Uox-PA conjugates, the linkers did not exhibit substantial differences in serum albumin binding affinity [26]. Therefore, in order to minimize the effects of fatty acid linkers on serum albumin binding, we chose the same set of linkers for sfGFP-PA conjugates. The lengths of linkers were estimated as 0.25, 1.5, 2.8, and 4.8 nm, respectively [26]. Since these linker lengths were estimated at a maximal stretch, the actual linker lengths could be shorter than those theoretical values. The four sfGFP-PA conjugates (SP01, 02, 03, and 04) were prepared similarly to those of Uox-PA [26]. Briefly, for SP01, NHS-PA (Figure S1a in Supplementary Materials) was directly conjugated to lysine residues of sfGFP via NHS-amine reaction (Figure S1b in Supplementary Materials). In the case of SP02, azidoacetic acid NHS ester (Figure S1c in Supplementary Materials) was reacted with lysine residues of sfGFP to generate sfGFP-azides. DBCO-amine (Figure S1d in Supplementary Materials) was reacted with NHS-PA to generate an intermediate (DBCO-PA) (Figure S1e in Supplementary Materials). Then, DBCO-PA was reacted with sfGFP-azides via strain-promoted alkyne-azide cycloaddition (SPAAC) reactions (Figure S1f in Supplementary Materials) to obtain SP02. In the case of SP03, azido-PEG4-NHS (Figure S1g in Supplementary Materials) was reacted with lysine residues of sfGFP to generate sfGFP-PEG4-azides. Then, DBCO-PA was reacted with sfGFP-PEG4-azides to generate SP03. Finally, for SP04, NHS-PA was reacted with DBCO-PEG4-amine (Figure S1h in Supplementary Materials) to generate DBCO-PEG4-PA (Figure S1i in Supplementary Materials). Then, DBCO-PEG4-PA was reacted with sfGFP-PEG4-azides to generate SP04.

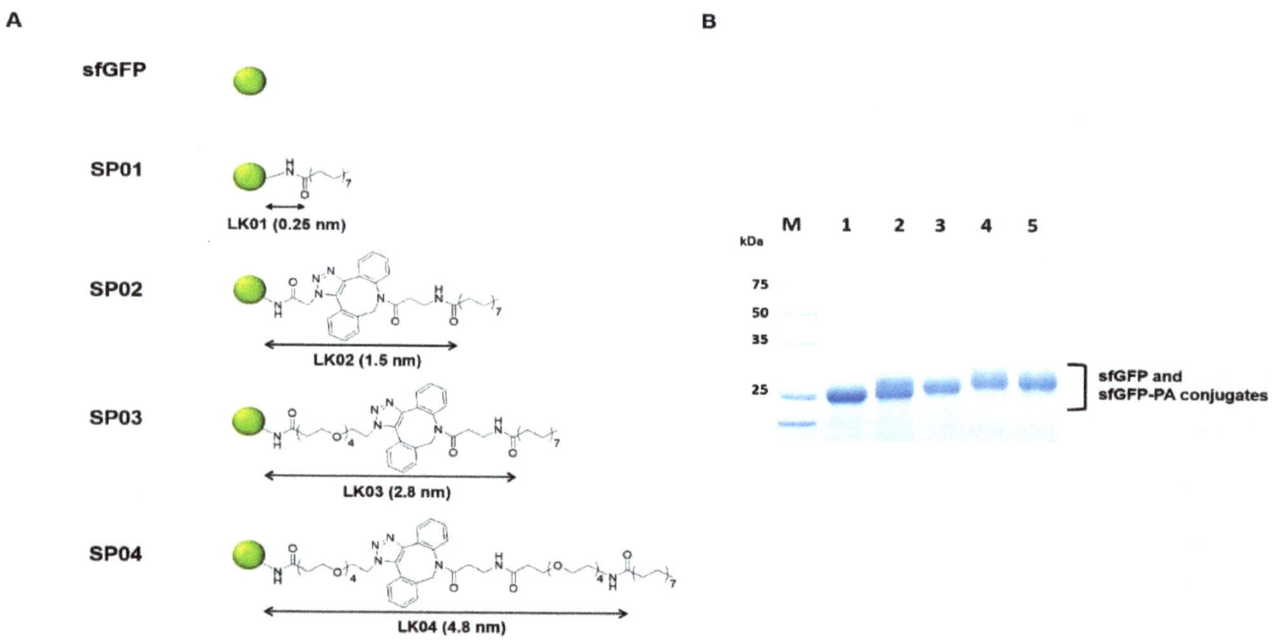

Figure 2. The structures and characterization of sfGFP-PA conjugates with various linker lengths. (**A**) sfGFP is represented as a green circle. The length of each linker was measured between the ε-carbon in a lysine residue of sfGFP and carbonyl carbon of PA when the linker was maximally stretched using Chem3D software and marked with black arrows. (**B**) Coomassie blue–stained protein gel image of purified sfGFP and sfGFP-PA conjugates was taken by Bio-Rad ChemiDoc XRS+. Lane M, molecular weight markers; Lane 1, sfGFP; Lane 2, SP01; Lane 3, SP02; Lane 4, SP03; Lane 5, SP04.

PA conjugation to the four sfGFP-PA conjugates was verified by protein band shifts in the protein gel and mass shifts in MALDI-TOF mass spectra (Figure 2B and Figure S2 in Supplementary Materials). In the protein gel, the bands of sfGFP-PA conjugates (SP01, 02, 03, and 04) were shifted up from the band of unmodified sfGFP, indicating the mass of sfGFP increased upon PA conjugation. Furthermore, we performed a MALDI-TOF spectrometric analysis of sfGFP and sfGFP-PA conjugates. The mass of unmodified sfGFP determined by MALDI-TOF analysis was 27,705 Da, which was consistent with its theoretical value (27,604 Da), with a 0.37% error. For sfGFP-PA conjugates, peaks were right-shifted, indicating that the mass of sfGFP increased upon PA conjugation. For all four sfGFP-PA conjugates, the mass differences between sfGFP-PA conjugate and unmodified sfGFP indicated that the average number of PA conjugated to single sfGFP was about one. Therefore, we speculated that the property differences among sfGFP-PA conjugates resulting from the different number of conjugated PAs were minimal.

3.2. *Serum Albumin Binding Affinity of sfGFP-PA Conjugates*

Using the sfGFP-PA conjugates, we first performed serum albumin binding assays at pH 7.4. 96-well plate was coated with MSA. Then, either the purified sfGFP-PA conjugate or unmodified sfGFP was incubated in a well. The amount of either sfGFP-PA conjugate or unmodified sfGFP bound MSA on the plate was analyzed by ELISA using anti-6×His antibody. The binding affinities sfGFP-PA conjugates (SP01, 02, 03, and 04) were comparable but significantly greater than that of unmodified sfGFP (Figure 3A). These results indicate that PA conjugation to sfGFP retained the albumin binding capacity. Furthermore, although linker properties may affect serum albumin binding affinity, the set of linkers used in this study did not substantially alter serum albumin binding affinity for all sfGFP-PA conjugates; this was consistent with the results for Uox-PA conjugates [26].

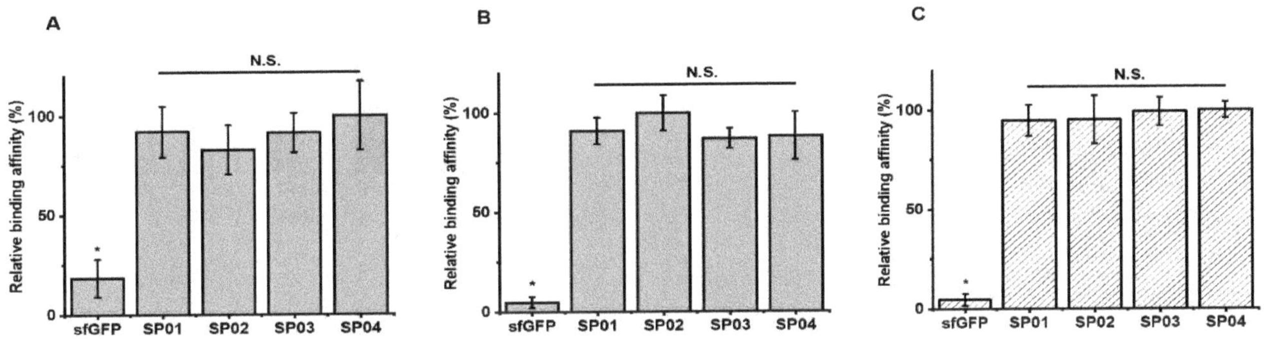

Figure 3. Relative albumin binding affinities of sfGFP-PA conjugate and tertiary complex formation of FcRn/MSA/sfGFP-PA conjugates. The amount of sfGFP or sfGFP-PA conjugate bound on MSA without mouse FcRn at pH 7.4 (**A**) or pH 6.0 (**B**). The amount of sfGFP or sfGFP-PA conjugate complexed with MSA and mouse FcRn at pH 6.0 (**C**). The amount of sfGFP or sfGFP-PA conjugate bound on the plate was normalized based on the highest signal to calculate relative binding affinity. The graph represents the mean ± standard deviations (SD) (n = 3). * $p < 0.01$; N.S.: not significant (two-tailed student *t*-test).

3.3. *Fluorescence of sfGFP-PA Conjugates*

Next, we investigated whether PA conjugation to sfGFP affected the fluorescence intensity of sfGFP. All sfGFP-PA conjugates (SP01, SP02, SP03, and SP04) exhibited about 20% reduction in fluorescence intensity compared to that of sfGFP (Figure S3 in Supplementary Materials). However, the fluorescence intensities of all sfGFP-PA conjugates were comparable. Such a reduction in fluorescence intensity is likely attributable to the use of DCA to increase the solubility of PAs during conjugation reaction [9,26]. Since DCA is a well-known detergent, it may perturb the folded structure of sfGFP, resulting in reduced fluorescence. Such a moderate reduction in fluorescence intensity of sfGFP-PA conjugate was not problematic in determining the serum half-life of sfGFP-PA because relative residual amounts of sfGFP-PA in serum were analyzed.

3.4. Serum Half-Lives of sfGFP-PA Conjugates

Then, the half-lives of sfGFP and sfGFP-PA conjugates were determined from the studies on mice. As reported previously [45], the percentages of residual sfGFP amounts were fitted to a two-phase model (Figure 4A). It was reported that FcRn-mediated recycling affects beta-phase in pharmacokinetics [46]. Therefore, beta-phase half-lives were plotted for sfGFP or sfGFP-PA conjugates in the order of increasing linker length. The half-life of sfGFP (single-phase) was 0.13 h. The beta-phase half-lives of sfGFP-PA conjugates were between 1.34 and 1.57 h, more than 10 times longer than that of sfGFP. This trend was notably different from that of Uox-PA conjugates [26]. In the case of Uox-PA conjugates up to a certain linker length, the half-life of Uox-PA conjugate increased as linker length increased (Figure 4B, light gray). However, the half-lives of sfGFP-PA conjugates were comparable, demonstrating that all linkers allow effective half-life extension of sfGFP in vivo (Figure 4B, dark gray). These results support our hypothesis that, for a small protein such as sfGFP, the distance between PA and small protein does not substantially alter serum half-life extension in vivo.

A

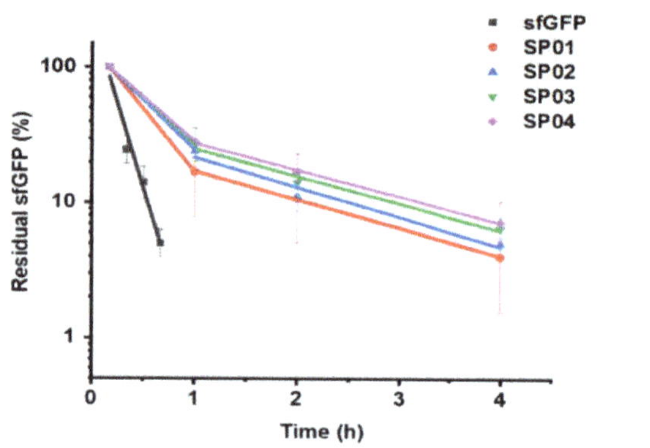

Samples	$t_{1/2}^{\alpha}$ (h)	$t_{1/2}^{\beta}$ (h)
sfGFP	0.13±0.02*	
SP01	0.37	1.57±0.01
SP02	0.41	1.34±0.12
SP03	0.45	1.51±0.20
SP04	0.46	1.50±0.10

* Single phase

B

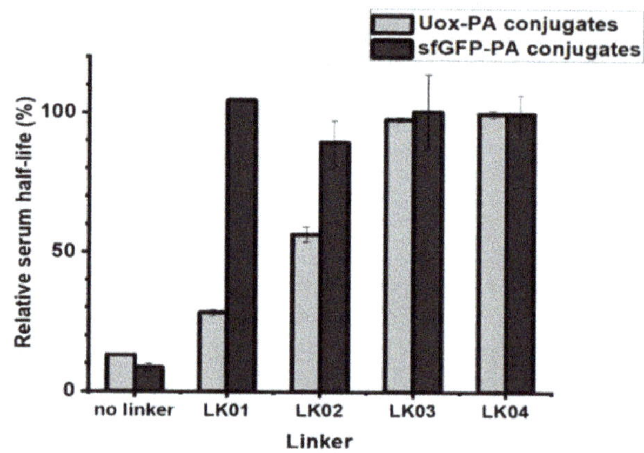

Figure 4. Pharmacokinetic studies of sfGFP and sfGFP-PA conjugates in mice. (**A**) Either purified sfGFP or sfGFP-PA conjugate was intravenously injected into the tail vein of a female Balb/c mouse (n = 4). The concentrations of sfGFP and sfGFP-PA conjugates were measured from blood samples taken at different time points: 10, 20, 30, 40, and 50 min for sfGFP; 10 min and, 1, 2, and 4 h for sfGFP-PA conjugates. The residual sfGFP amounts in serum were plotted on a logarithmic scale. Each data point represents the mean ± SD (n = 4). $t_{1/2}^{\alpha}$ and $t_{1/2}^{\beta}$ indicate the serum half-lives in the α- and β-phase, respectively. The serum half-lives of sfGFP and sfGFP-PA conjugates are summarized in the below table. (**B**) Comparison of relative serum half-lives of either Uox-PA (light gray) or sfGFP-PA conjugates (dark gray) versus corresponding linkers. The serum half-lives of unmodified protein and PA conjugates were normalized using those of PA conjugates with the LK04 linker. The serum half-life data of Uox and Uox-PA conjugates were obtained from the literature [26].

3.5. FcRn Binding Assays of sfGFP-PA Conjugates

In order to investigate whether sfGFP-PA conjugates compete with the binding of FcRn to serum albumin depending on linker length, we performed FcRn binding assays. The assays for sfGFP-PA conjugates were based on the formation of FcRn/serum albumin/sfGFP-PA tertiary structure, as reported previously for Uox-PA conjugates [26]. The dissociation constant between mouse FcRn and MSA was reported to be 546 nM [47]. Therefore, the tertiary structure formation should be dependent of binding of sfGFP-PA with MSA. The pH value of 6.0 was often used to confirm the interaction of albumin with FcRn [45,48]. Hu et al. reported that endo-lysosomal pH varies from 4.5 to 6.5 [49]. Therefore, we chose pH 6.0 for FcRn binding assays in our study. In order to evaluate albumin binding affinities of sfGFP-PA conjugates, the amount of sfGFP-PA bound on MSA was first determined. The albumin binding affinities of all four sfGFP-PA conjugates were comparable at pH 6.0 but significantly greater than that of unmodified sfGFP (Figure 3B). Then, we performed the FcRn binding assays. As expected for a small protein, all sfGFP-PA conjugates (SP01, 02, 03, and 04) showed the comparable formation of FcRn/MSA/sfGFP-PA tertiary complex (Figure 3C), indicating that none of the sfGFP-PA conjugates substantially interfere with FcRn binding to serum albumin in vitro. Combined with the FcRn/serum albumin/sfGFP-PA tertiary complex formation results, the sfGFP-PA conjugate, even with a short linker, does not hinder the FcRn binding to serum albumin; the result is effective half-life extension in vivo. Therefore, the results of sfGFP-PA conjugates support our previous results: Uox requires a long linker in the PA conjugate in order to achieve effective half-life extension in vivo for mitigating the steric hindrance between Uox and FcRn due to its large size. In view of the pharmacokinetics and FcRn binding assay results of large protein Uox-PA conjugates [26] and small protein sfGFP-PA conjugates, it can be concluded that the protein size is the dominating factor to consider for fatty acid conjugation.

4. Conclusions

In conclusion, our results showed that, for a small protein (sfGFP, 28 kDa), PA conjugation does not compromise the binding of FcRn to serum albumin in vitro or the serum half-life extension in vivo regardless of linker length. Combined with the previous results for a large protein (Uox, 140 kDa) [24], our results supported that the protein size in the fatty acid–protein conjugate is an important factor for effective binding of FcRn with serum albumin leading to prolonged serum half-life in vivo. We believe our findings can contribute to the successful design of other fatty acid–conjugated therapeutic proteins for serum half-life extension.

Author Contributions: Conceptualization, J.C. and I.K.; Formal analysis, J.C., J.P., G.T. and M.S.J.; Funding acquisition, I.K.; Investigation, J.C. and J.P.; Supervision, G.T. and I.K.; Visualization, M.S.J.; Writing—original draft, J.C., J.P., G.T. and I.K.; Writing—review & editing, M.S.J. and I.K. All authors have read and agreed to the published version of the manuscript.

References

1. Agyei, D.; Ahmed, I.; Akram, Z.; MN Iqbal, H.; K Danquah, M. Protein and peptide biopharmaceuticals: An overview. *Protein Pept. Lett.* **2017**, *24*, 94–101. [CrossRef] [PubMed]
2. Kontermann, R.E. Strategies for extended serum half-life of protein therapeutics. *Curr. Opin. Biotechnol.* **2011**, *22*, 868–876. [CrossRef] [PubMed]
3. Kontermann, R.E. Strategies to Extend Plasma Half-Lives of Recombinant Antibodies. *BioDrugs* **2009**, *23*, 93–109. [CrossRef] [PubMed]
4. Jevševa, S.; Kunstelj, M.; Porekar, V.G. PEGylation of therapeutic proteins. *Biotechnol. J.* **2010**, *5*, 113–128. [CrossRef] [PubMed]
5. Lim, H.-K.; Hong, S.H.; Bae, S.M.; Choi, I.Y.; Kim, H.H. A Liquid Formulation of a Long-acting Erythropoietin Conjugate. *Biotechnol. Bioprocess Eng.* **2020**, *25*, 117–125. [CrossRef]
6. Pelegri-O'Day, E.M.; Lin, E.-W.; Maynard, H.D. Therapeutic Protein–Polymer Conjugates: Advancing Beyond PEGylation. *J. Am. Chem. Soc.* **2014**, *136*, 14323–14332. [CrossRef]
7. Verhoef, J.J.F.; Anchordoquy, T.J. Questioning the use of PEGylation for drug delivery. *Drug Deliv. Transl. Res.* **2013**, *3*, 499–503. [CrossRef]
8. Yang, B.; Lim, S.I.; Kim, J.C.; Tae, G.; Kwon, I. Site-Specific Albumination as an Alternative to PEGylation for the Enhanced Serum Half-Life in Vivo. *Biomacromolecules* **2016**, *17*, 1811–1817. [CrossRef]
9. Cho, J.; Lim, S.I.; Yang, B.S.; Hahn, Y.S.; Kwon, I. Generation of therapeutic protein variants with the human serum albumin binding capacity via site-specific fatty acid conjugation. *Sci. Rep.* **2017**, *7*, 18041. [CrossRef]

10. Bern, M.; Sand, K.M.K.; Nilsen, J.; Sandlie, I.; Andersen, J.T. The role of albumin receptors in regulation of albumin homeostasis: Implications for drug delivery. *J. Control. Release* **2015**, *211*, 144–162. [CrossRef]
11. Sleep, D.; Cameron, J.; Evans, L.R. Albumin as a versatile platform for drug half-life extension. *Biochim. Biophys. Acta-Gen. Subj.* **2013**, *1830*, 5526–5534. [CrossRef] [PubMed]
12. Lim, S.I.; Hahn, Y.S.; Kwon, I. Site-specific albumination of a therapeutic protein with multi-subunit to prolong activity in vivo. *J. Control. Release* **2015**, *207*, 93–100. [CrossRef] [PubMed]
13. Zaman, R.; Islam, R.A.; Ibnat, N.; Othman, I.; Zaini, A.; Lee, C.Y.; Chowdhury, E.H. Current strategies in extending half-lives of therapeutic proteins. *J. Control. Release* **2019**, *301*, 176–189. [CrossRef]
14. Kratz, F. Albumin as a drug carrier: Design of prodrugs, drug conjugates and nanoparticles. *J. Control. Release* **2008**, *132*, 171–183. [CrossRef] [PubMed]
15. Madsbad, S.; Kielgast, U.; Asmar, M.; Deacon, C.F.; Torekov, S.S.; Holst, J.J. An overview of once-weekly glucagon-like peptide-1 receptor agonists-available efficacy and safety data and perspectives for the future. *Diabetes Obes. Metab.* **2011**, *13*, 394–407. [CrossRef] [PubMed]
16. Rosenstock, J.; Reusch, J.; Bush, M.; Yang, F.; Stewart, M.; Albiglutide Study Group, for the A.S. Potential of albiglutide, a long-acting GLP-1 receptor agonist, in type 2 diabetes: A randomized controlled trial exploring weekly, biweekly, and monthly dosing. *Diabetes Care* **2009**, *32*, 1880–1886. [CrossRef]
17. Elsadek, B.; Kratz, F. Impact of albumin on drug delivery—New applications on the horizon. *J. Control. Release* **2012**, *157*, 4–28. [CrossRef]
18. Carta, G.; Murru, E.; Banni, S.; Manca, C. Palmitic Acid: Physiological Role, Metabolism and Nutritional Implications. *Front. Physiol.* **2017**, *8*, 902. [CrossRef]
19. Knudsen, L.B.; Nielsen, P.F.; Huusfeldt, P.O.; Johansen, N.L.; Madsen, K.; Pedersen, F.Z.; Thøgersen, H.; Wilken, M.; Agersø, A. Potent Derivatives of Glucagon-like Peptide-1 with Pharmacokinetic Properties Suitable for Once Daily Administration. *J. Med. Chem.* **2000**, *43*, 1664–1669. [CrossRef]
20. Lee, J.; Lee, C.; Kim, I.; Moon, H.R.; Kim, T.H.; Oh, K.T.; Lee, E.S.; Lee, K.C.; Youn, Y.S. Preparation and evaluation of palmitic acid-conjugated exendin-4 with delayed absorption and prolonged circulation for longer hypoglycemia. *Int. J. Pharm.* **2012**, *424*, 50–57. [CrossRef]
21. Ramírez-Andersen, H.S.; Behrens, C.; Buchardt, J.; Fels, J.J.; Folkesson, C.G.; Jianhe, C.; Nørskov-Lauritsen, L.; Nielsen, P.F.; Reslow, M.; Rischel, C. Long-acting human growth hormone analogue by noncovalent albumin binding. *Bioconjug. Chem.* **2018**, *29*, 3129–3143. [CrossRef] [PubMed]
22. Shechter, Y.; Sasson, K.; Lev-Goldman, V.; Rubinraut, S.; Rubinstein, M.; Fridkin, M. Newly Designed Modifier Prolongs the Action of Short-Lived Peptides and Proteins by Allowing Their Binding to Serum Albumin. *Bioconjug. Chem.* **2012**, *23*, 1577–1586. [CrossRef] [PubMed]
23. Lim, S.I.; Mizuta, Y.; Takasu, A.; Hahn, Y.S.; Kim, Y.H.; Kwon, I. Site-specific fatty acid-conjugation to prolong protein half-life in vivo. *J. Control. Release* **2013**, *170*, 219–225. [CrossRef]
24. Gil, M.S.; Cho, J.; Thambi, T.; Giang Phan, V.H.; Kwon, I.; Lee, D.S. Bioengineered robust hybrid hydrogels enrich the stability and efficacy of biological drugs. *J. Control. Release* **2017**, *267*, 119–132. [CrossRef]
25. Milo, R.; Phillips, R. *Cell Biology by the Numbers*; Garland Science: New York, NY, USA, 2015. ISBN 1317230698.
26. Cho, J.; Park, J.; Kim, S.; Kim, J.C.; Tae, G.; Jin, M.S.; Kwon, I. Intramolecular distance in the conjugate of urate oxidase and fatty acid governs FcRn binding and serum half-life in vivo. *J. Control. Release* **2020**, *321*, 49–58. [CrossRef] [PubMed]
27. Vogt, B. Urate oxidase (rasburicase) for treatment of severe tophaceous gout. *Nephrol. Dial. Transplant.* **2005**, *20*, 431–433. [CrossRef]
28. Wang, L.-Y.; Shih, L.-Y.; Chang, H.; Jou, S.-T.; Lin, K.-H.; Yeh, T.-C.; Lin, S.-F.; Liang, D.-C. Recombinant Urate Oxidase (Rasburicase) for the Prevention and Treatment of Tumor Lysis Syndrome in Patients with Hematologic Malignancies. *Acta Haematol.* **2006**, *115*, 35–38. [CrossRef] [PubMed]
29. Richette, P.; Bardin, T. Successful treatment with rasburicase of a tophaceous gout in a patient allergic to allopurinol. *Nat. Clin. Pract. Rheumatol.* **2006**, *2*, 338–342. [CrossRef]
30. Edwards, N.L. Treatment-failure gout: A moving target. *Arthritis Rheum.* **2008**, *58*, 2587–2590. [CrossRef]
31. Fels, E.; Sundy, J.S. Refractory gout: What is it and what to do about it? *Curr. Opin. Rheumatol.* **2008**, *20*, 198–202. [CrossRef]
32. Bhattacharya, A.A.; Grüne, T.; Curry, S. Crystallographic analysis reveals common modes of binding of medium and long-chain fatty acids to human serum albumin. *J. Mol. Biol.* **2000**, *303*, 721–732. [CrossRef] [PubMed]

33. Curry, S.; Brick, P.; Franks, N.P. Fatty acid binding to human serum albumin: New insights from crystallographic studies. *Biochim. Biophys. Acta-Mol. Cell Biol. Lipids* **1999**, *1441*, 131–140. [CrossRef]
34. Simard, J.R.; Zunszain, P.A.; Hamilton, J.A.; Curry, S. Location of High and Low Affinity Fatty Acid Binding Sites on Human Serum Albumin Revealed by NMR Drug-competition Analysis. *J. Mol. Biol.* **2006**, *361*, 336–351. [CrossRef] [PubMed]
35. Fujiwara, S.; Amisaki, T. Identification of High Affinity Fatty Acid Binding Sites on Human Serum Albumin by MM-PBSA Method. *Biophys. J.* **2008**, *94*, 95–103. [CrossRef]
36. Fujiwara, S.; Amisaki, T. Fatty acid binding to serum albumin: Molecular simulation approaches. *Biochim. Biophys. Acta-Gen. Subj.* **2013**, *1830*, 5427–5434. [CrossRef]
37. Rizzuti, B.; Bartucci, R.; Sportelli, L.; Guzzi, R. Fatty acid binding into the highest affinity site of human serum albumin observed in molecular dynamics simulation. *Arch. Biochem. Biophys.* **2015**, *579*, 18–25. [CrossRef]
38. Hamilton, J.A. NMR reveals molecular interactions and dynamics of fatty acid binding to albumin. *Biochim. Biophys. Acta-Gen. Subj.* **2013**, *1830*, 5418–5426. [CrossRef]
39. Pace, C.N.; Vajdos, F.; Fee, L.; Grimsley, G.; Gray, T. How to measure and predict the molar absorption coefficient of a protein. *Protein Sci.* **1995**, *4*, 2411–2423. [CrossRef]
40. Pédelacq, J.-D.; Cabantous, S.; Tran, T.; Terwilliger, T.C.; Waldo, G.S. Engineering and characterization of a superfolder green fluorescent protein. *Nat. Biotechnol.* **2006**, *24*, 79–88. [CrossRef]
41. Feng, G.; Mellor, R.H.; Bernstein, M.; Keller-Peck, C.; Nguyen, Q.T.; Wallace, M.; Nerbonne, J.M.; Lichtman, J.W.; Sanes, J.R. Imaging Neuronal Subsets in Transgenic Mice Expressing Multiple Spectral Variants of GFP. *Neuron* **2000**, *28*, 41–51. [CrossRef]
42. Okabe, M.; Ikawa, M.; Kominami, K.; Nakanishi, T.; Nishimune, Y. 'Green mice' as a source of ubiquitous green cells. *FEBS Lett.* **1997**, *407*, 313–319. [CrossRef]
43. Jung, S.-K. A Review of Image Analysis in Biochemical Engineering. *Biotechnol. Bioprocess Eng.* **2019**, *24*, 65–75. [CrossRef]
44. Ahn, G.; Yu, G.; Abdullah, A.; Kim, Y.; Lee, D. Controlling the Release Profile Through Phase Control of Calcium Phosphate-Alginate Core-shell Nanoparticles in Gene Delivery. *Macromol. Res.* **2019**, *27*, 579–585. [CrossRef]
45. Yang, B.; Kim, J.C.; Seong, J.; Tae, G.; Kwon, I. Comparative studies of the serum half-life extension of a protein via site-specific conjugation to a species-matched or-mismatched albumin. *Biomater. Sci.* **2018**, *6*, 2092–2100. [CrossRef] [PubMed]
46. Datta-Mannan, A. Mechanisms Influencing the Pharmacokinetics and Disposition of Monoclonal Antibodies and Peptides. *Drug Metab. Dispos.* **2019**, *47*, 1100–1110. [CrossRef] [PubMed]
47. Nilsen, J.; Bern, M.; Sand, K.M.K.; Grevys, A.; Dalhus, B.; Sandlie, I.; Andersen, J.T. Human and mouse albumin bind their respective neonatal Fc receptors differently. *Sci. Rep.* **2018**, *8*, 14648. [CrossRef]
48. Seijsing, J.; Lindborg, M.; Höidén-Guthenberg, I.; Bönisch, H.; Guneriusson, E.; Frejd, F.Y.; Abrahmsén, L.; Ekblad, C.; Löfblom, J.; Uhlén, M.; et al. An engineered affibody molecule with pH-dependent binding to FcRn mediates extended circulatory half-life of a fusion protein. *Proc. Natl. Acad. Sci. USA* **2014**, *111*, 17110–17115. [CrossRef]
49. Hu, Y.-B.; Dammer, E.B.; Ren, R.-J.; Wang, G. The endosomal-lysosomal system: From acidification and cargo sorting to neurodegeneration. *Transl. Neurodegener.* **2015**, *4*, 18. [CrossRef]

12

Targeting TRPM2 in ROS-Coupled Diseases

Shinichiro Yamamoto and Shunichi Shimizu *

Division of Pharmacology, Faculty of Pharmaceutical Sciences, Teikyo Heisei University, Tokyo 164-8530, Japan; s.yamamoto@thu.ac.jp
* Correspondence: s.shimizu@thu.ac.jp

Academic Editors: Arpad Szallasi and Susan M. Huang

Abstract: Under pathological conditions such as inflammation and ischemia-reperfusion injury large amounts of reactive oxygen species (ROS) are generated which, in return, contribute to the development and exacerbation of disease. The second member of the transient receptor potential (TRP) melastatin subfamily, TRPM2, is a Ca^{2+}-permeable non-selective cation channel, activated by ROS in an ADP-ribose mediated fashion. In other words, TRPM2 functions as a transducer that converts oxidative stress into Ca^{2+} signaling. There is good evidence that TRPM2 plays an important role in ROS-coupled diseases. For example, in monocytes the influx of Ca^{2+} through TRPM2 activated by ROS contributes to the aggravation of inflammation via chemokine production. In this review, the focus is on TRPM2 as a molecular linker between ROS and Ca^{2+} signaling in ROS-coupled diseases.

Keywords: TRPM2; Ca^{2+} signaling; reactive oxygen species; ROS-coupled diseases

---

1. Introduction

The physiological concentration of Ca^{2+} in the intracellular compartment ($[Ca^{2+}]_i$) is on the order of 10^{-7} M; this is markedly lower than its extracellular concentration which is in the order of 10^{-3} M [1]. Due to this difference between intracellular and extracellular Ca^{2+} concentrations, Ca^{2+} can function as a second messenger. Recently, a subset of TRP channels has attracted attention because of their permeablity to Ca^{2+}. Indeed, the first *trp* gene was originally discovered in mutant fruit flies with impaired vision due to the lack of a specific Ca^{2+} influx pathway in photoreceptor cells [2]. Subsequently, a large number of TRP channel homologues were identified in vertebrates. As of today, the human TRP channel superfamily has 28 members that are divided into six subfamilies: canonical (C), vanilloid (V), melastatin (M), polycystic kidney disease (P), mucolipin (ML), and ankyrin (A), based on the homology of their protein sequences [3].

Generally speaking, the TRP protein has six putative transmembrane domains and a pore region between the fifth and sixth transmembrane domains. TRP proteins assemble into homo- or heterotetramers in order to form functional channels [4,5]. The TRPC subfamily shows the greatest homology to the *Drosophila* TRP protein. TRPC channels are downstream targets to phospholipase C activation following receptor stimulation [6–9].

The TRPV subfamily (TRPV1 to V6) was named after its founding member, the vanilloid (capsaicin) receptor TRPV1. TRPV channels are polymodal and their activators range from physical and chemical stimuli including heat (TRPV1, TRPV2, TRPV3, and TRPV4) [10–16], through protons (TRPV1) [17] and osmotic stress (TRPV4) [18,19], to capsaicin, the pungent principle in hot peppers (TRPV1) [10]. The TRPM subfamily has eight members. Its best known member is the cold-responsive menthol receptor, TRPM8 [20,21]. The TRPP subfamily includes TRPP1 and TRPP2, which are encoded by the *PKD1* and *PKD2* genes, respectively. *PKD1* and *PKD2* are the genes responsible for autosomal dominant polycystic kidney disease. TRPP1 is thought to interact with TRPP2, which functions as a receptor for mechanical stimuli such as shear stress [22,23].

The TRPML subfamily is composed of TRPML1 and its homologues. A mutation in the *MCOLN1* gene encoding TRPML1 causes mucolipidosis type IV. TRPML1 localizes in lysosomes and late endosomes and is activated by phosphoinositol (3,5)-bisphosphate [24,25].

TRPA1 (named after the large N-terminal domain with 17 predicted ankyrin repeats) is the sole member of the TRPA subfamily [26]. It is activated by irritant compounds such as exhaust fumes and allyl isothiocyanate in mustard oil. The cold activation of TRPA1 remains controversial [27,28]. Interestingly, TRPA1 is activated by both hyper- and hypoxia via oxidative modification of its cysteine residues and the dehydroxylation of the proline residues [29].

Traditionally, reactive oxygen species (ROS) are regarded as non-specific toxins that cause cell and tissue damage [30]. However, recently ROS have been identified as signal-transduction molecules [31]. For example, the oxidative stress-sensitive transcriptional factor Keap1, and the signal-transduction molecule ASK1, are activated by ROS to mediate a number of cellular responses [32,33]. The second member of the TRP melastatin subfamily, TRPM2, is a Ca^{2+}-permeable non-selective cation channel. TRPM2 is expressed broadly in neuronal cells, myocytes, pancreatic β cells, and immune cells such as T lymphocytes, monocytes/macrophages, and neutrophils [34–42]. TRPM2 is activated by oxidative stress including H_2O_2. In other words, TRPM2 functions as a sensor for oxidative stress. Indeed, TRPM2 is more sensitive to ROS than other TRPs including TRPC5, TRPV1 and TRPA1 (which is activated by ROS via oxidative modifications to its cysteine residues).

Large amounts of ROS are generated under pathological conditions that, in turn, contribute to the development and maintenance of various disease states [43]. TRPM2 converts ROS-induced oxidative stress into Ca^{2+} signaling; this Ca^{2+} signaling has been implicated in the aggravation of a number of diseases. In this review, the focus is on TRPM2 as a molecular linker between ROS and Ca^{2+} signaling.

2. TRPM2 Activators and Inhibitors

Among TRP channels TRPM2 is unique in that it contains a NudT9-Homology (NUDT9-H) domain at its cytosolic C-terminal region. Although NUDT9-H shares some homology with NUDT9 ADP-ribose hydrolase, its ADP-ribose hydrolase activity is low. In addition to the full-length TRPM2, several truncated splice variants have been described, including: (1) TRPM2-ΔN (containing a deletion of amino acids 538–557 in the N-terminus); (2) TRPM2-ΔC (deletion of amino acids 1292–1325 in the C-terminus), and (3) TRPM2-S (S for short) that lacks the four C-terminal transmembrane domains, putative Ca^{2+}-permeable pore region, and the entire C terminus [39,41,44].

The activation of TRPM2 is triggered by the binding of ADP-ribose to the NUDT9-H domain [45]. Since the NUDT9-H domain of TRPM2-ΔC is partially missing, TRPM2-ΔC is not activated by ADP-ribose. Nicotinic acid adenine dinucleotide phosphate (NAADP), cADP-ribose, and Ca^{2+} exert synergistic effects on ADP-ribose-induced TRPM2 activation. Moreover, these agents are also capable of activating TRPM2 by themselves [36,46–50].

In neutrophils, resting ADP-ribose levels approach 5 μM [50] which is sufficient to induce the activation of TRPM2 by increasing $[Ca^{2+}]_i$. The IQ-like motif in the calmodulin-binding domain at the N-terminal region, rather than the NUDT9-H domain, is thought to play a pivotal role in the Ca^{2+}-induced activation of TRPM2 [49]. Using inside-out patch recordings, Csanády and colleagues have investigated the direct activation of TRPM2; they found that neither cADP-ribose nor NAADP is able to directly activate TRPM2 [51]. On the other hand, they identified ADP-ribose-2′-phosphate as a direct TRPM2 agonist [52].

Silent information regulator-2 (SIR2), a member of the sirtuin family, is a nicotinamide adenine dinucleotide (NAD^+)-dependent protein deacetylase. SIR2 removes acetyl groups from acetylated substrates, and transfers them to NAD^+. Nicotinamide and O-acetylated-ADP-ribose (OAADPr) are produced as a result of this reaction. OAADPr was reported to activate TRPM2 by binding to the NUDT9-H domain. This implicates SIR2 in TRPM2 regulation [53].

NAD^+ was also reported to directly gate TRPM2, although a high concentration (in the mM range) of NAD^+ is required for this response [54]. However, purified NAD^+ fails to activate TRPM2 [52]. This apparent contradiction was explained by the presence of the NAD^+-degradation product ADP-ribose, a known TRPM2 agonist, in the non-purified NAD^+ [46,55]. CD38 is an ectoenzyme that catalyzes the production of cADP-ribose and ADP-ribose from its substrate, NAD^+ [56]. CD38 is implicated in the activation of TRPM2 via production of cADP-ribose and/or ADP-ribose [38,40,57].

Arguably the most important activator of TRPM2 is oxidative stress induced by ROS, including H_2O_2 [54]. It has been postulated that the activation of TRPM2 by oxidative stress is triggered via ADP-ribose production. Mitochondria are a major source of ADP-ribose. In mitochondria, ADP-ribose is generated by the oxidative stress-induced hydrolysis of NAD^+ [55]. In the nucleus, poly(ADP-ribose) polymerase-1 (PARP-1) plays an important role in repairing DNA damage in response to oxidative stress. The binding of PARP-1 to impaired DNA hydrolyzes NAD^+, leading to the production of nicotinamide and ADP-ribose. In turn, ADP-ribose is built into various nuclear proteins, resulting in the activation of DNA repair and stimulation of nuclear factor-mediated transcription [58–61]. Free ADP-ribose is generated following the degradation of poly(ADP-ribose) by poly(ADP-ribose) glycohydrolase (PARG) [61].

Pharmacological [62] or genetic manipulation of PARP-1 [63] blocks H_2O_2-induced TRPM2 activation. Conversely, H_2O_2-induced TRPM2 activation is enhanced at body temperature by hydroxyl radical production [64,65]. The hydroxyl radical produced by the reaction of H_2O_2 with intracellular Fe^{2+} (Fenton reaction) stimulates the PARP-1/PARG pathway, which leads to the activation of TRPM2. The phosphorylation of tyrosine residues in TRPM2 is thought to represent an important mechanism underlying the activation of TRPM2 by H_2O_2. The phosphorylation/dephosphorylation state is regulated by protein tyrosine phosphatase-L1 [66].

The short splice variant of TRPM2, TRPM2-S, was shown to interact with the full-length TRPM2. The TRPM2-S/full-length TRPM2 complex is not activated by H_2O_2 [39]. Therefore, TRPM2-S may function as a dominant negative modulator of TRPM2.

A large number of TRPM2 blockers have been reported. Adenosine monophosphate [46] and 8-bromo-ADP-ribose [38] inhibit ADP-ribose-induced TRPM2 activation by preventing the binding of ADP-ribose to the NUDT9-H domain. The antifungal agents clotrimazole and econazole [67], the antipyretic agent flufenamic acid [68], 2-aminoethoxydiphenyl borate (2-APB) [69], *N*-(p-amylcinnamoyl) anthranilic acid (ACA) [70], and curcumin, the active principle in turmeric [71], are TRPM2 channel blockers. PARP inhibitors (e.g., SB750139-B, PJ34, and DPQ) were also reported to prevent the activation of TRPM2 in response to oxidative stress. However, these inhibitors have no effect on ADP-ribose-induced TRPM2 activation.

Iron chelators were shown to attenuate H_2O_2-induced TRPM2 activation [64]. Surprisingly, the JAK2 inhibitor AG490 was also found to prevent TRPM2 activation by H_2O_2 [72]. It was, however, suggested that AG490 ameliorates H_2O_2-induced TRPM2 activation by scavenging hydroxyl radicals rather than inhibiting of JAK2. The AG490-related compounds, AG555 and AG556, exert an even stronger inhibitory effect on H_2O_2-induced TRPM2 activation than AG490 [73].

3. ROS Production under Pathological Conditions

3.1. *Inflammation*

Inflammation is a complex biological reaction to injury and/or infection. During inflammation, immune cells are transported from the blood stream into the damaged tissue in an attempt to eliminate the harmful agents and to initiate the process of healing and repair. However, when inflammation becomes chronic, it may exacerbate tissue damage and pose severe health risks.

At the inflamed sites, phagocytes (e.g., macrophages and neutrophils) digest the harmful agents which play an important role in their removal. During phagocytosis, oxygen consumption in the phagocytes is increased. This phenomenon is known as the "respiratory burst": oxygen is utilized for superoxide anion ($^{\cdot}O_2^{-}$) production by NADPH oxidase [74]. During bacterial phagocytosis, bacteria are engulfed by the plasma membrane, leading to the formation of phagosomes. Then NADPH oxidase activated and the resultant $^{\cdot}O_2^{-}$ contributes to bacterial killing. NADPH oxidase (NOX) is composed of several isoforms. Seven isoforms, termed as NOX1–5 and DUOX1–2, have been identified as catalytic subunits. These isoforms are localized in the plasma membrane and catalyze electron transport from the electron donor NADPH to oxygen, leading to the production of $^{\cdot}O_2^{-}$. In phagocytes, NOX2 is strongly expressed and interacts with the membrane protein $p22^{phox}$ [75]. The small G-protein RAC, and the cytosolic proteins $p40^{phox}$, $p47^{phox}$, and $p67^{phox}$ are also known to activate NOX2.

The production of $^{\cdot}O_2^{-}$ by NOX2 does not occur in a resting state. During phagocytosis, these activators translocate to the plasma membrane and interact with the NOX2/$p22^{phox}$ complex; this, in turn, triggers $^{\cdot}O_2^{-}$ production following the activation of NOX2 (Figure 1A). In addition, $^{\cdot}O_2^{-}$ is converted to H_2O_2 by the superoxide dismutase. These ROS contribute to killing bacteria.

Lipopolysaccharide (LPS), found in the outer membrane of Gram-negative bacteria, is a prototypical trigger of sepsis that elicits a strong immune response in animals. The LPS receptor is toll-like receptor-4 (TLR4) which associates with several adaptor molecules such as MyD88 [76]. The activation of TLR4 in response to LPS triggers immune responses including the production of cytokines and ROS accompanied by the activation of NADPH oxidase [77]. Cytokines (e.g., tumor necrosis factor, TNF) are released from immune cells and accumulate at the sites of inflammation. These molecules act in concert to organize the inflammatory network and produce large amount of ROS. The source of ROS appears to be the mitochondria rather than the NADPH oxidase [77–79].

3.2. *Ischemia-Reperfusion*

Ischemia-reperfusion injury is caused by re-oxygenation during reperfusion following the lack of oxygen during ischemia. Ischemia-reperfusion generates harmful substances that aggravate the tissue injury. This is a major mechanism of tissue damage during stroke and myocardial infarction. The hydroxyl radical scavenger, edaravone, is used as a neuroprotective agent in the management of patients with ischemic brain injury and amyotrophic lateral sclerosis (Lou Gehrig's Disease). During ischemia-reperfusion injury, mitochondria are the major source of ROS. Electrons leaked from the mitochondrial electron transport chain are transferred to molecular oxygen, resulting in the production of $^{\cdot}O_2^{-}$. The activity of the electron transport chain generates a relatively small amount of $^{\cdot}O_2^{-}$ under normal conditions, but its production may be greatly magnified by events occurring during ischemia-reperfusion (Figure 1B) [80].

NADPH oxidase also contributes to ROS production during ischemia-reperfusion. NOXs are present in blood vessels [81] where their expression is regulated by the hypoxia-sensitive transcriptional factor, hypoxia-inducible factor-1α (HIF1α) [81]. The expression of NOX isoforms is thus up-regulated by the lack of oxygen during ischemia. Then NOX generates large amounts of ROS during reperfusion (Figure 1B).

During ischemia, a failure in the generation of ATP also occurs concurrently with ATP consumption, leading to the depletion of ATP. ATP is eventually catabolized into hypoxanthine. Xanthine oxidase catalyzes two steps including the formation of xanthine from hypoxanthine, and the formation of uric acid from xanthine. Electrons are also generated in this process and transferred to molecular oxygen, leading to the formation of $^{\cdot}O_2^{-}$ [82] (Figure 1B). In summary, several factors contribute to ROS production during ischemia-reperfusion.

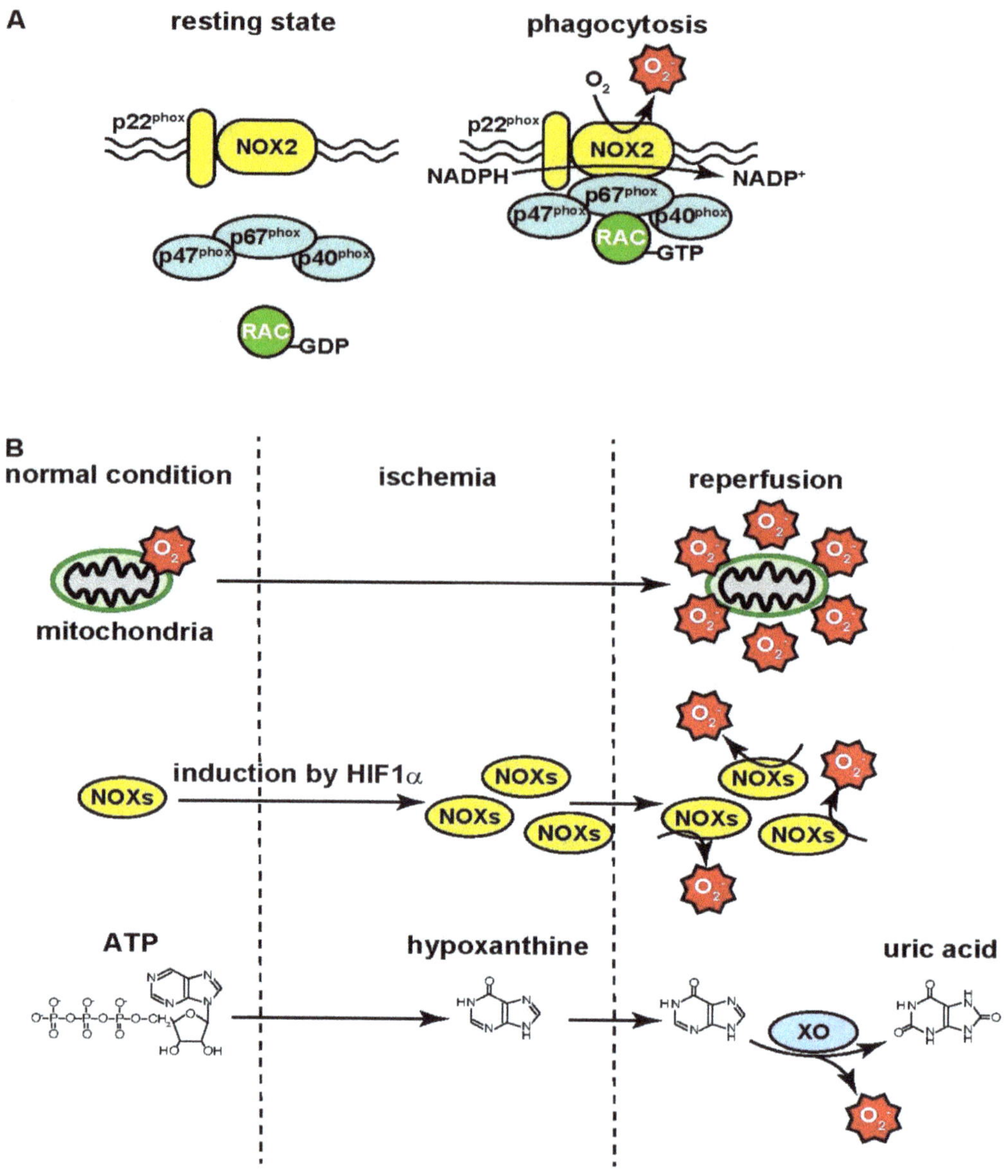

Figure 1. ROS production during inflammation and ischemia-reperfusion. (**A**) In resting state, cytosolic activators such as $p40^{phox}$, $p47^{phox}$, $p67^{phox}$ and small G protein RAC do not interact with NOX2-$p22^{phox}$ complex. These activators translocate to the plasma membrane during phagocytosis and interact with the NOX2-$p22^{phox}$ complex. Electrons derived from NADPH are transferred through the complex to molecular oxygen, leading to $^{\cdot}O_2^-$ production; (**B**) Oxidative phosphorylation is initiated by electron transport from NADH and/or $FADH_2$ to the electron transport chain in the mitochondrial inner membrane. The electron transport chain is composed of complexes I–IV. Electrons derived from NADH and $FADH_2$ are fed to complex I and complex II, respectively. They are then transferred to complexes in ascending order of the redox potential, which release free energy. Molecular oxygen accepts electrons for the formation of H_2O. On the other hand, the electron transport chain uses free energy derived from electron transport to pump H^+ out of the matrix, thereby creating proton gradient across the mitochondrial inner membrane. By utilizing energy released by the influx of H^+ into the matrix, ADP is phosphorylated, resulting in the generation of ATP. $^{\cdot}O_2^-$ is generated by the leakage of electrons from complexes I and III in the electron transport chain. The activity of the electron transport chain generates a relatively small amount of $^{\cdot}O_2^-$ under normal conditions, but its production may be greatly magnified by events occurring during ischemia-reperfusion. The expression of NOX isoforms is up-regulated by HIF1α during ischemia, and then NADPH oxidase then generates large amounts of ROS by reoxygenation during reperfusion. During ischemia, ATP is catabolized into hypoxanthine.

4. ROS-Coupled Diseases and TRPM2

4.1. *Inflammatory Diseases*

4.1.1. TRPM2-Mediated Chemokine Production

TRPM2 contributes to the aggravation of inflammation [40]. In monocytes/macrophages, Ca^{2+} influx through TRPM2 activated by ROS stimulates the production of the chemokine, CXCL2. CXC chemokines, such as macrophage inflammatory protein-2 (CXCL2), exhibit potent neutrophil chemotactic activity [83].

Dextran sulfate sodium (DSS)-induced colitis is a mouse model of human ulcerative colitis. In the colon of DSS-treated wild-type (WT) mice, the expression of CXCL2 was markedly increased in monocytes/macrophages. By contrast, CXCL2 expression was strongly suppressed in the colon of *Trpm2* KO mice following DSS challenge. The number of recruited neutrophils was also significantly reduced in the colon of DSS-treated *Trpm2* KO mice, presumably as a consequence of reduced CXCL2 levels, but their function was intact. No difference was noted in the number of macrophages in the inflamed colon of WT and *Trpm2* KO mice. The bone marrow output of neutrophils was normal, as was their accumulation into the abdominal cavity after intraperitoneal injection of chemokines. Last, DSS-treated *Trpm2* KO mice did not exhibit weight loss and/or ulceration of the colon, suggesting that *Trpm2* KO mice were largely protected from DSS-mediated colitis. Combined, these findings imply that TRPM2-mediated chemokine production in monocytes/macrophages is an important mechanism underlying the progression of DSS-induced ulcerative colitis.

TRPM2-dependent CXCL2 production was also implicated in the carrageenan-induced inflammatory pain and sciatic nerve ligation models [84]. The carrageenan-induced pain model is a widely used and reliable model for inflammatory pain. Sciatic nerve ligation causes neuropathic pain. Both CXCL2 production and neutrophil infiltration were attenuated in *Trpm2* KO mice. By contrast, the recruitment of F4/80-positive macrophages was not altered in the inflamed paw or around the injured sciatic nerve. Importantly, both mechanical allodynia and thermal hyperalgesia were attenuated in *Trpm2* KO mice. Based on these observations one may argue that TRPM2 expressed in macrophages aggravates pronociceptive inflammatory responses to induce inflammatory and neuropathic pain through neuroinflammation-mediated sensitization of the pain-signaling pathway.

TRPM2 in alveolar epithelial cells plays an important role in bleomycin-induced lung injury [85]. Bleomycin is a glycopeptide antibiotic with potent antitumor activity. It is used in the management of squamous cell carcinoma, testicular cancers, and lymphomas. The antitumor activity of bleomycin was attributed to its ability to cause DNA damage in the cancer cells through the production of oxygen radicals. A major dose-limiting side-effect of bleomycin is lung injury. In mice treated with bleomycin, the secretion of CXCL2 from alveolar epithelial cells was attenuated in *Trpm2* KO compared to WT. It was unexpected because alveolar macrophages (which have higher expression of TRPM2 than alveolar epithelial cells) were believed to be the main source of CXCL2 in response to bleomycin. The secretion of CXCL2 from alveolar epithelial cells was essential for neutrophil recruitment and the secretion of inflammatory cytokines including tumor necrosis factor α and interleukin-1β. Taken together, these findings imply that TRPM2-mediated CXCL2 production in alveolar epithelial cells is responsible for the aggravation of bleomycin-induced lung damage.

4.1.2. LPS-Induced Inflammatory Responses and TRPM2

The contribution of TRPM2 to LPS-induced lung inflammation is poorly understood. In vitro, activation by LPS of TRPM2 in monocytes and cultured microglia is involved in the generation of inflammatory cytokines [40,84,86]. By contrast, in vivo studies found no difference between WT and *Trpm2* KO mice in the secretion of inflammatory cytokines and the infiltration of inflammatory cells into the lungs following LPS administration [85,87]. Therefore, other signaling pathways (e.g., TLR4-mediated signaling) rather than Ca^{2+} signaling via TRPM2 may play a pivotal role in LPS-induced lung inflammation in vivo.

Adding to the confusion, recently Di et al suggested a protective anti-inflammatory role for TRPM2 during LPS-induced lung inflammation [88]. In LPS-treated *Trpm2* KO mice lung injury (including cytokine production and the infiltration of inflammatory cells into the lungs) was exacerbated compared to WT animals. In their experimental model, following LPS administration Ca^{2+} influx via TRPM2 was triggered in phagocytes such as neutrophils. The influx of Ca^{2+} depolarized the plasma membrane, contributing to the inhibition of NADPH oxidase. This protective mechanism was absent in the *Trpm2* KO animals. Therefore, *Trpm2* KO phagocytes overproduced ROS, resulting in the exacerbation of LPS-induced lung injury.

4.1.3. Functional Roles of TRPM2 during Infection

TRPM2 may play an important protective role during bacterial infections. For example, the Gram-negative bacterium *Francisella tularensis* (the agent responsible for tularemia) is equipped with an antioxidant system to escape the host immune response. Although *Francisella* is phagocytized by macrophages, it protects itself from ROS-mediated killing by inhibiting the formation of the NADPH oxidase complex [89]. Catalase (that converts H_2O_2 into H_2O and oxygen) also belongs to the antioxidant systems in *Francisella*.

By using a catalase-deficient *F. tularensis* strain, Shakerley et al. suggested that TRPM2 may play a central role in macrophages during bacterial infection [90]. Although macrophages infected with *F. tularensis* showed marginal TRPM2 activation, the influx of Ca^{2+} through TRPM2 was sufficient to induce immune responses such as interleukin-6 (IL-6) production in macrophages infected with catalase-deficient *F. tularensis*. During *Listeria monocytogenes* infection, TRPM2 was found to contribute to innate immunity [91]. In *Trpm2* KO mice infected by *L. monocytogenes*, the production of IL-12 and interferon-γ was diminished. Consequently, *Trpm2* KO mice were more susceptible to *L. monocytogenes* infection.

Formyl-methionyl-leucyl-phenylalanine (fMLP) is a secreted bacterial product that serves as a neutrophil chemotactic factor. fMLP activates CD38 by binding to its receptor. *Cd38*-deficient mice display disturbed Ca^{2+} signaling and neutrophil chemotaxis in response to fMLP [92]. As described above, CD38 is an ectoenzyme that catalyzes the production of cADP-ribose and ADP-ribose from its substrate, NAD^+. fMLP-induced Ca^{2+} influx and neutrophil chemotaxis were significantly suppressed in the *Trpm2*-deficient neutrophils, suggesting that TRPM2 is a molecular entity that links ADP-ribose produced by CD38 to Ca^{2+} signaling [38,40].

4.1.4. NLRP3 Inflammasome and TRPM2

The NOD-like receptor family pyrin domain containing-3 (NLRP3) "inflammasome" is composed of NLRP3, apoptosis-associated speck-like protein (ASC), and caspase-1. NLRP3 associates with the adaptor protein ASC in response to danger-associated stimuli. In order to form an active inflammasome complex, the NLRP3-ASC complex needs to bind caspase-1. This interaction results in the caspase-1-dependent processing of cytoplasmic targets, including the pro-inflammatory cytokines IL-1β and IL-18. Mature cytokines are then released from the cells [93]. The influx of Ca^{2+} via TRPM2 activated by ROS was suggested to participate in the activation of the NLRP3 inflammasome [94].

Particulate substances (e.g., liposomes and urate crystals) induce the production of ROS, partially mediated by the leakage of electrons from the mitochondrial electron transport chain [94,95]. These particulates also initiate a ROS-dependent Ca^{2+} influx via TRPM2; this, in turn, contributes to the secretion of IL-1β, accompanied by NLRP3 inflammasome activation. In *Trpm2*-disrupted macrophages, impaired NLRP3 inflammasome activation and interleukin-1β secretion was observed. Furthermore, *Trpm2* KO mice are resistant to particulate-induced and IL-1β-mediated peritonitis [94].

4.2. *Ischemia-Reperfusion Injury*

4.2.1. Brain

Ca^{2+} signaling influences a wide array of biological responses, including gene expression, neuronal growth, neurotransmitter release, and, ultimately, cell death. In other words, Ca^{2+} can exert both protective and deleterious effects on neuronal cells [96,97]. TRPM2 is believed to be responsible for the H_2O_2-induced Ca^{2+} influx that mediates cell death in various tissues [54] including rat cortical neurons [34]. There is good evidence that the influx of Ca^{2+} via TRPM2 contributes to neuronal cell death during ischemia-reperfusion injury both in vitro (oxygen and glucose deprivation, OGD, followed by re-oxygenation) and in vivo (brain ischemia-reperfusion induced by transient middle cerebral artery occlusion, tMCAO). Interestingly, there appears to be a sex-related difference in cell death [98–100]. When both male and female WT and *Trpm2* KO mice were subjected to tMCAO, male *Trpm2* KO mice had smaller infarct volumes than matched WT mice. By contrast, *Trpm2* KO had no protective effect on infarct volumes in female mice. In a second set of experiments, clotrimazole was used as a TRPM2 inhibitor. Clotrimazole reduced infarct volumes in male WT mice subjected to tMCAO. This beneficial effect was absent in *Trpm2* KO mice. Clotrimazole had no effects either on infarct volumes in castrated male mice. However, androgen replacement restored clotrimazole protection in castrated mice. Taken together, these findings suggest that androgen signaling contributes to TRPM2-dependent brain injury during ischemia-reperfusion. One may argue that androgen signaling stimulates PARP-1 which is necessary for the engagement of TRPM2 in ischemic injury in the male brain. However, other mechanisms may also exist because cell death was induced by OGD in neurons isolated from male embryos and cultured in sex steroid-free medium.

There is preliminary evidence that the *N*-methyl-D-aspartate glutamate receptor (NMDA-R) subunit expression pattern is altered in *Trpm2* KO mice [101]. NMDA-R is a heteromer composed of the obligatory GluN1 subunit along with other GluN subunits including GluN2A and GluN2B. An increase in the activity of GluN2A-containing NMDA-R is known to increase the phosphorylation of Extracellular Signal Regulated Kinase-1 (ERK) and AKT, thereby promoting pro-survival mechanisms in the cell. In contrast, an increase in the activity of GluN2B-containing NMDA-R inhibits pro-survival mechanisms [101]. *Trpm2* KO mice subjected to tMCAO showed smaller infarcts than WT mice, and OGD-induced cell death was reduced in hippocampal neurons prepared from *Trpm2* KO embryos. The expression of GluN2B and GluN2A was reduced and increased, respectively, in the hippocampus by the disruption of *Trpm2*. The ERK/AKT pathway was activated in the hippocampus of *Trpm2* KO mice.

As described above, stimulation of the NMDA-R (that contains GluN2A) activates the ERK/AKT pathway that, in turn, promotes pro-survival mechanisms. In the OGD model, the application of known GluN2A antagonists eliminated the neuroprotection in the hippocampal neurons isolated from *Trpm2* KO mouse embryos. This implies that increases in GluN2A by the disruption of *Trpm2* protect neurons from ischemia-reperfusion-induced cell death.

Migration of immune cells including neutrophils from the blood stream into the brain also plays an important role in ischemia-reperfusion brain injury [102]. As mentioned above, the size of the infarct induced by tMCAO was significantly smaller in *Trpm2* KO mice than in WT mice. WT mice transplanted with bone marrow obtained from *Trpm2* KO animals showed significantly smaller brain infract in the tMCAO model than *Trpm2* KO animals reconstituted with bone marrow from WT mice. This experiment supports the pivotal role of TRPM2 expressed in bone marrow-derived immune cells in the pathomechanism of ischemia-reperfusion brain injury.

4.2.2. Heart

Conflicting results have been reported regarding the function of TRPM2 in heart injury during ischemia-reperfusion. Cheung and colleagues reported that TRPM2 protected the heart against ischemia-reperfusion injury [35,103,104]. TRPM2 was expressed in the sarcolemma and transverse tubules of adult cardiomyocytes. After reperfusion following coronary artery occlusion, no significant differences were observed in infarct sizes between WT and *Trpm2* KO mice. The heart function was, however, compromised in *Trpm2* KO mice. ROS levels in left ventricular myocytes were significantly higher in *Trpm2* KO mice than in WT mice after ischemia-reperfusion. The levels of superoxide dismutase and its transcriptional factors, forkhead box transcription factor and HIF, were lower, whereas that of the NADPH oxidase catalytic subunit, NOX4, was higher in *Trpm2* KO mouse hearts subjected to ischemia-reperfusion [35]. In addition, mitochondrial proteins and complex I subunits were down-regulated in *Trpm2* KO mouse heart [103]. These alterations in protein expression triggered by ROS overproduction and mitochondrial dysfunction in *Trpm2* KO mouse heart may be responsible for the heart dysfunction.

Another study, by contrast, found that heart functions were improved in *Trpm2* KO mice, suggesting that a deficiency in TRPM2 protects heart against ischemia-reperfusion injury [105]. Albeit TRPM2 mRNA expression was observed in the heart, its level was markedly lower than that in neutrophils or neurons. Neutrophilic infiltration of the heart after ischemia-reperfusion was reduced in *Trpm2* KO mice. It was speculated that TRPM2 expressed in neutrophils, rather than the heart, is important for ischemia-reperfusion heart injury. Indeed, in isolated hearts infarct sizes were significantly smaller in the heart obtained from *Trpm2* KO mice and perfused with *Trpm2* KO neutrophils compared to *Trpm2* KO hearts perfused with WT neutrophils. Likewise, infarct sizes were significantly larger in the heart of *Trpm2* KO mice carrying WT neutrophils compared to the heart of *Trpm2* KO mice with TRPM2-deficient neutrophils, suggesting that the activation of neutrophil TRPM2 during reperfusion has an important role in the development of myocardial infarction.

By using a cardiac-specific *Trpm2* KO mice, Cheung and colleagues recently reported a functional role for TRPM2 in the heart [104]. Similar to their studies using conventional *Trpm2* KO mice, heart functions after ischemia-reperfusion were aggravated in the cardiac-specific *Trpm2* KO mice. On the other hand, significant differences in infarct sizes were not observed between the WT and cardiac-specific *Trpm2* KO animals. In summary, the role of TRPM2 in cardiac ischemia-reperfusion injury remains controversial.

4.2.3. Kidneys

In the kidneys, TRPM2 is thought to contribute to the aggravation of renal injury and ROS production after ischemia-reperfusion [106]. TRPM2 is expressed in the proximal tubules. The disruption of *Trpm2* protects kidneys against ischemia-reperfusion injury. This involvement of TRPM2 was shown to be linked to the presence of TRPM2 in parenchymal cells rather than hematopoietic cells. Oxidative stress accompanied by the activation of NADPH oxidase was triggered in WT, but in *Trpm2* KO, mouse kidneys subjected to ischemia-reperfusion. Ca^{2+} influx via TRPM2 participated in the activation of RAS-related C3 botulinum toxin substrate-1 (RAC1), an essential factor for the activation of NADPH oxidase.

4.3. Other Diseases and Injuries

4.3.1. Acetaminophen-Induced Liver Injury

Acetaminophen is an antipyretic analgesic drug. Acetaminophen overdose (accidental or intentional) is a well-known cause of potentially fatal liver injury [107,108]. Acetaminophen is mainly metabolized into a non-toxic compound via glucuronidation and a sulfation reaction. On the other hand, a small amount of acetaminophen is converted to the toxic compound, *N*-acetyl-parabenzo-quinoneimine (NAPQI). NAPQI is then metabolized into a non-toxic compound via glutathione conjugation. NAPQI is responsible for acetaminophen-induced liver injury. NAPQI was shown to deplete intracellular glutathione levels, leading to the production of ROS [109]. TRPM2 has been implicated in acetaminophen-induced liver injury [109]. H_2O_2 and acetaminophen induce

Ca^{2+} influx into hepatocytes in a TRPM2-dependent manner. Acetaminophen-induced liver injury is attenuated in *Trpm2* KO mice compared to WT animals.

4.3.2. Radiation-Induced Tissue Damage

Radiation is a mainstay of treatment for head and neck cancer. Unfortunately, it has significant adverse effects on healthy tissues that are in the field of the treatment. For example, xerostomia (dry mouth) is a result of salivary gland damage by radiation. The molecular mechanism of radiation injury is complex including generation of ROS and DNA damage [110]. TRPM2 was reported to exacerbate radiation-induced salivary gland dysfunction [110]. H_2O_2 and radiation induced the influx of Ca^{2+} in salivary gland acinar cells. This influx was reduced by the disruption of *Trpm2*. The irreversible loss of salivary gland fluid secretion in WT mice subjected to radiation was improved by using free radical scavengers and/or PARP inhibitors.

4.3.3. Alzheimer's Disease

Alzheimer's disease (AD) is a devastating form of progressive dementia of unknown cause and no effective treatment. Therefore, it is an attractive hypothesis that TRPM2 may be involved in neuronal cell death in AD patients [111]. The suggested pathology of AD includes an alteration in the proteolytic processing of the amyloid precursor protein, APP. In addition, amyloid β-peptide (Aβ) is accumulated in the AD brain. Although the molecular defect responsible for AD remain unknown, dysregulation of Ca^{2+} homeostasis is widely believed to be intimately associated with Aβ toxicity [112]. Proposed mechanisms of Aβ neurotoxicity include the production of ROS, as well as excitotoxicity with the intracellular accumulation of Ca^{2+} [113].

Previously, Lustbader *et al* reported that Aβ-binding alcohol dehydrogenase directly interacted with Aβ in the mitochondria of both AD patients and transgenic mice. This interaction promotes the leakage of ROS [114]. A recent study suggested that TRPM2 is involved in Aβ-induced neurotoxicity [112]. APP/PS1 animals are double transgenic mice that express a chimeric mouse/human APP and overproduce Aβ. They are widely used as model of AD. APP/PS1 mice were crossed with *Trpm2* KO animals. Synapse loss and decreased levels of synaptic proteins are early correlates of the severity of AD [112]. The level of the synaptic marker, synaptophysin, in the hippocampus was found to be lower in APP/PS1 mice than in WT mice. Synaptophysin levels in the hippocampus of *Trpm2*-disrupted APP/PS1 mice were similar to those in WT mice. In addition, age-dependent spatial memory deficits in APP/PS1 mice were reversed in *Trpm2*-disrupted APP/PS1 mice. These observations imply an important role for TRPM2 in Aβ-induced neuronal toxicity.

In addition, AD is associated with reductions in cerebral blood flow early in the course of the disease [115]. This Aβ-induced cerebrovascular dysfunction may be mediated by TRPM2 [115]. Indeed, TRPM2 is expressed in brain endothelial cells; in these cells, Aβ stimulated the influx of Ca^{2+} via TRPM2. The Aβ-induced activation of TRPM2 in brain endothelial cells was mediated by ROS derived from the activation of NADPH oxidase. Reduction in cerebral blood flow was induced by the neocortical superfusion of Aβ, and was attenuated by PARP and PARG inhibitors, as well as the disruption of *Trpm2*. Combined, these findings indicate that Aβ-induced TRPM2 activation contributes to endothelial dysfunction.

5. Conclusions

There is increasing evidence that TRPM2 plays an important role in the pathomechanism of ROS-coupled diseases. For example, TRPM2 contributes to aggravation of disease states in which monocytes/macrophages play a pivotal role via cytokine production. In the brain and kidney, TRPM2 is involved in ischemia-reperfusion injury. Moreover, TRPM2 is implicated in innate immunity and the pathobiology of Alzheimer disease.

On the other hand, there are conflicting findings with regard to the function of TRPM2 in myocardial infarction and in LPS-induced lung injury. Non-specific TRPM2 inhibitors (e.g., PARP inhibitors, clotrimazole, and 2-APB) have been shown to attenuate the exacerbation of ROS-coupled diseases. For instance, PARP inhibitors were found to attenuate radiation-induced tissue damage [110], and bleomycin-induced lung injury [85]. Furthermore, clotrimazole attenuated heart [105] and brain damage [98,100] induced by ischemia-reperfusion. 2-APB also exerted protective effects against ischemia-reperfusion-induced brain [102] and kidney [106] damage (Figure 2). These promising results, however, must be confirmed by yet-to-be-synthesized selective TRPM2 antagonists.

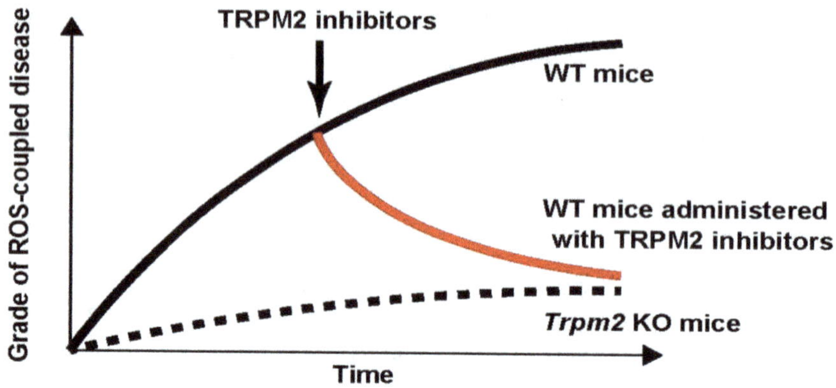

Figure 2. Does administration with TRPM2 inhibitors during ROS-coupled disease development improve the grade of these diseases? Pathological mouse model studies have been performed under *Trpm2*-disrupted conditions, and suggested that *Trpm2* KO mice are protected from ROS-coupled diseases. However, in terms of cure, it is important that the grade of these diseases is improved by the inhibition of TRPM2 during disease development. Therefore, the studies whether the inhibition of TRPM2 during ROS-coupled disease development has curative effects on the diseases should be done in the future.

Acknowledgments: The authors would like to thank Professor Arpad Szallasi in Drexel University College of Medicine for the English language review.

References

1. Clapham, D.E. Calcium signaling. *Cell* **1995**, *80*, 259–268. [CrossRef]
2. Montell, C.; Rubin, G.M. Molecular characterization of the Drosophila trp locus: A putative integral membrane protein required for phototransduction. *Neuron* **1989**, *2*, 1313–1323. [CrossRef]
3. Clapham, D.E. TRP channels as cellular sensors. *Nature* **2003**, *426*, 517–524. [CrossRef] [PubMed]
4. Goel, M.; Sinkins, W.G.; Schilling, W.P. Selective Association of TRPC Channel Subunits in Rat Brain Synaptosomes. *J. Biol. Chem.* **2002**, *277*, 48303–48310. [CrossRef] [PubMed]
5. Hofmann, T.; Schaefer, M.; Schultz, G.; Sudermann, T. Subunit composition of mammalian transient receptor potential channels in living cells. *Proc. Natl. Acad. Sci. USA* **2002**, *99*, 7461–7466. [CrossRef] [PubMed]
6. Zhu, X.; Jiang, M.; Peyton, M.; Boulay, G.; Hurst, R.; Stefani, E.; Birnbaumer, L. *trp*, a novel mammalian gene family essential for agonist-activated capacitative Ca^{2+} entry. *Cell* **1996**, *85*, 661–671. [CrossRef]
7. Hofmann, T.; Obukhov, A.G.; Schaefer, M.; Harteneck, C.; Gudermann, T.; Schultz, G. Direct activation of human TRPC6 and TRPC3 channels by diacylglycerol. *Nature* **1999**, *397*, 259–263. [PubMed]
8. Okada, T.; Inoue, R.; Yamazaki, K.; Maeda, A.; Kurosaki, T.; Yamakuni, T.; Tanaka, I.; Shimizu, S.; Ikenaka, K.; Imoto, K.; et al. Molecular and functional characterization of a novel mouse transient receptor potential protein homologue TRP7. *J. Biol. Chem.* **1999**, *274*, 27359–27370. [CrossRef] [PubMed]
9. Inoue, R.; Okada, T.; Onoue, H.; Hara, Y.; Shimizu, S.; Naitoh, S.; Ito, Y.; Mori, Y. The transient receptor potential protein homologue TRP6 is the essential component of vascular α_1-adrenoceptor-activated Ca^{2+}-permeable cation channel. *Circ. Res.* **2001**, *88*, 325–332. [CrossRef] [PubMed]
10. Caterina, M.J.; Schumacher, M.A.; Tominaga, M.; Rosen, T.A.; Levine, J.D.; Julius, D. The capsaicin receptor: A heat-activated ion channel in the pain pathway. *Nature* **1997**, *389*, 816–824. [PubMed]

11. Caterina, M.J.; Rosen, T.A.; Tominaga, M.; Brake, A.J.; Julius, D. A capsaicin-receptor homologue with a high threshold for noxious heat. *Nature* **1999**, *398*, 436–441. [PubMed]
12. Güler, A.D.; Lee, H.; Iida, T.; Shimizu, I.; Tominaga, M.; Caterina, M. Heat-evoked activation of the ion channel, TRPV4. *J. Neurosci.* **2002**, *22*, 6408–6414. [PubMed]
13. Peier, A.M.; Reeve, A.J.; Andersson, D.A.; Moqrich, A.; Earley, T.J.; Hergarden, A.C.; Story, G.M.; Colley, S.; Hogenesch, J.B.; McIntyre, P.; et al. A heat-sensitive TRP channel expressed in keratinocytes. *Science* **2002**, *296*, 2046–2049. [CrossRef] [PubMed]
14. Smith, G.D.; Gunthorpe, M.J.; Kelsell, R.E.; Hayes, P.D.; Reilly, P.; Facer, P.; Wright, J.E.; Jerman, J.C.; Walhin, J.P.; Ooi, L.; et al. TRPV3 is a temperature-sensitive vanilloid receptor-like protein. *Nature* **2002**, *418*, 186–190. [CrossRef] [PubMed]
15. Watanabe, H.; Vriens, J.; Suh, S.H.; Benham, C.D.; Droogmans, G.; Nilius, B. Heat-evoked activation of TRPV4 channels in a HEK293 cell expression system and in native mouse aorta endothelial cells. *J. Biol. Chem.* **2002**, *277*, 47044–47051. [CrossRef] [PubMed]
16. Xu, H.; Ramsey, I.S.; Kotecha, S.A.; Moran, M.M.; Chong, J.A.; Lawson, D.; Ge, P.; Lilly, J.; Silos-Santiago, I.; Xie, Y.; et al. TRPV3 is a calcium-permeable temperature-sensitive cation channel. *Nature* **2002**, *418*, 181–186. [CrossRef] [PubMed]
17. Tominaga, M.; Caterina, M.J.; Malmberg, A.B.; Rosen, T.A.; Gilbert, H.; Skinner, K.; Raumann, B.E.; Basbaum, A.I.; Julius, D. The cloned capsaicin receptor integrates multiple pain-producing stimuli. *Neuron* **1998**, *21*, 531–543. [CrossRef]
18. Liedtke, W.; Choe, Y.; Marti-Renom, M.A.; Bell, A.M.; Denis, C.S.; Sali, A.; Hudspeth, A.J.; Friedman, J.M.; Heller, S. Vanilloid receptor-related osmotically activated channel (VR-OAC), a candidate vertebrate osmoreceptor. *Cell* **2000**, *103*, 525–535. [CrossRef]
19. Strotmann, R.; Harteneck, C.; Nunnenmacher, K.; Schultz, G.; Plant, T.D. OTRPC4, a nonselective cation channel that confers sensitivity to extracellular osmolarity. *Nat. Cell Biol.* **2000**, *2*, 695–702. [PubMed]
20. McKemy, D.D.; Neuhausser, W.M.; Julius, D. Identification of a cold receptor reveals a general role for TRP channels in thermosensation. *Nature* **2002**, *416*, 52–58. [CrossRef] [PubMed]
21. Peier, A.M.; Moqrich, A.; Hergarden, A.C.; Reeve, A.J.; Andersson, D.A.; Story, G.M.; Earley, T.J.; Dragoni, I.; McIntyre, P.; Bevan, S.; et al. A TRP channel that senses cold stimuli and menthol. *Cell* **2002**, *108*, 705–715. [CrossRef]
22. Nauli, S.M.; Alenghat, F.J.; Luo, Y.; Williams, E.; Vassilev, P.; Li, X.; Elia, A.E.; Lu, W.; Brown, E.M.; Quinn, S.J.; et al. Polycystins 1 and 2 mediate mechanosensation in the primary cilium of kidney cells. *Nat. Genet.* **2003**, *33*, 129–137. [CrossRef] [PubMed]
23. Mochizuki, T.; Tsuchiya, K.; Nitta, K. Autosomal dominant polycystic kidney disease: Recent advances in pathogenesis and potential therapies. *Clin. Exp. Nephrol.* **2013**, *17*, 317–326. [CrossRef] [PubMed]
24. Jefferies, H.B.; Cooke, F.T.; Jat, P.; Boucheron, C.; Koizumi, T.; Hayakawa, M.; Kaizawa, H.; Ohishi, T.; Workman, P.; Waterfield, M.D.; et al. A selective PIKfyve inhibitor blocks PtdIns(3,5)P_2 production and disrupts endomembrane transport and retroviral budding. *EMBO Rep.* **2008**, *9*, 164–170. [CrossRef] [PubMed]
25. Dong, X.P.; Shen, D.; Wang, X.; Dawson, T.; Li, X.; Zhang, Q.; Cheng, X.; Zhang, Y.; Weisman, L.S.; Delling, M.; et al. PI(3,5)P_2 controls membrane trafficking by direct activation of mucolipin Ca^{2+} release channels in the endolysosome. *Nat. Commun.* **2010**, *1*, 38. [CrossRef] [PubMed]
26. Takahashi, N.; Mizuno, Y.; Kozai, D.; Yamamoto, S.; Kiyonaka, S.; Shibata, T.; Uchida, K.; Mori, Y. Molecular characterization of TRPA1 channel activation by cysteine-reactive inflammatory mediators. *Channels* **2008**, *2*, 287–298. [CrossRef] [PubMed]
27. Macpherson, L.J.; Geierstanger, B.H.; Viswanath, V.; Bandell, M.; Eid, S.R.; Hwang, S.; Patapoutian, A. The pungency of garlic: Activation of TRPA1 and TRPV1 in response to allicin. *Curr. Biol.* **2005**, *15*, 929–934. [CrossRef] [PubMed]
28. Jordt, S.E.; Bautista, D.M.; Chuang, H.H.; McKemy, D.D.; Zygmunt, P.M.; Hogestatt, E.D.; Meng, I.D.; Julius, D. Mustard oils and cannabinoids excite sensory nerve fibres through the TRP channel ANKTM1. *Nature* **2004**, *427*, 260–265. [CrossRef] [PubMed]
29. Takahashi, N.; Kuwaki, T.; Kiyonaka, S.; Numata, T.; Kozai, D.; Mizuno, Y.; Yamamoto, S.; Naito, S.; Knevels, E.; Carmeliet, P.; et al. TRPA1 underlies a sensing mechanism for O_2. *Nat. Chem. Biol.* **2011**, *10*, 701–711. [CrossRef] [PubMed]

30. Henricks, P.A.; Nijkamp, F.P. Reactive oxygen species as mediators in asthma. *Pulm. Pharmacol. Ther.* **2001**, *14*, 409–420. [CrossRef] [PubMed]
31. Dröge, W. Free radicals in the physiological control of cell function. *Physiol. Rev.* **2002**, *82*, 47–95. [CrossRef] [PubMed]
32. Taguchi, K.; Motohashi, H.; Yamamoto, M. Molecular mechanisms of Keap1-Nrf2 pathway in stress response and cancer evolution. *Genes Cells* **2011**, *16*, 123–140. [CrossRef] [PubMed]
33. Soga, M.; Matsuzawa, A.; Ichijo, H. Oxidative stress-induced diseases via the ASK1 signaling pathway. *Int. J. Cell Biol.* **2012**, *2012*. article ID 439587. [CrossRef] [PubMed]
34. Kaneko, S.; Kawakami, S.; Hara, Y.; Wakamori, M.; Itoh, E.; Minami, T.; Takada, Y.; Kume, T.; Katsuki, H.; Mori, Y.; et al. A critical role of TRPM2 in neuronal cell death by hydrogen peroxide. *J. Pharmacol. Sci.* **2006**, *101*, 66–76. [CrossRef] [PubMed]
35. Miller, B.A.; Wang, J.; Hirschler-Laszkiewicz, I.; Gao, E.; Song, J.; Zhang, X.; Koch, W.J.; Madesh, M.; Mallilankaraman, K.; Gu, T.; et al. The second member of transient receptor potential-melastatin channel family protects hearts from ischemia-reperfusion injury. *Am. J. Physiol. Heart Circ. Physiol.* **2013**, *304*, H1010–H1022. [CrossRef] [PubMed]
36. Togashi, K.; Hara, Y.; Tominaga, T.; Higashi, T.; Konishi, Y.; Mori, Y.; Tominaga, M. TRPM2 activation by cyclic ADP-ribose at body temperature is involved in insulin secretion. *EMBO J.* **2006**, *25*, 1804–1815. [CrossRef] [PubMed]
37. Lange, I.; Yamamoto, S.; Partida-Sánchez, S.; Mori, Y.; Fleig, A.; Penner, R. TRPM2 functions as lysosomal Ca^{2+} release channel in β-cells. *Sci. Signal.* **2009**, *71*, ra23. [CrossRef] [PubMed]
38. Partida-Sánchez, S.; Gasser, A.; Fliegert, R.; Siebrands, C.C.; Dammermann, W.; Shi, G.; Mousseau, B.J.; Sumazo-Toledo, A.; Bhagat, H.; Walseth, T.F.; et al. Chemotaxis of mouse bone marrow neutrophils and dendritic cell is controlled by ADP-ribose, the major product generated by the CD38 enzyme reaction. *J. Immunol.* **2007**, *179*, 7827–7839. [CrossRef] [PubMed]
39. Zhang, W.; Chu, X.; Tong, Q.; Cheung, J.Y.; Conrad, K.; Masker, K.; Miller, B.A. A novel TRPM2 isoform inhibits calcium influx and susceptibility to cell death. *J. Biol. Chem.* **2003**, *278*, 16222–16229. [CrossRef] [PubMed]
40. Yamamoto, S.; Shimizu, S.; Kiyonaka, S.; Takahashi, N.; Wajima, T.; Hara, Y.; Negoro, T.; Hiroi, T.; Kiuchi, Y.; Okada, T.; et al. TRPM2-mediated Ca^{2+} influx induces chemokine production in monocytes that aggravates inflammatory neutrophil infiltration. *Nat. Med.* **2008**, *14*, 738–747. [CrossRef] [PubMed]
41. Wehage, E.; Eisfeld, J.; Heiner, I.; Jungling, E.; Zitt, C.; Luckhoff, A. Activation of the cation channel long transient receptor potential channel 2 (LTRPC2) by hydrogen peroxide. A splice variant reveals a mode of activation independent of ADP-ribose. *J. Biol. Chem.* **2002**, *277*, 23150–23156. [CrossRef] [PubMed]
42. Sumoza-Toledo, A.; Lange, I.; Cortado, H.; Bhagat, H.; Mori, Y.; Fleig, A.; Penner, R.; Partida-Sánchez, S. Dendritic cell maturation and chemotaxis is regulated by TRPM2-mediated lysosomal Ca^{2+} release. *FASEB J.* **2011**, *25*, 3529–3542. [CrossRef] [PubMed]
43. Brieger, K.; Schiavone, S.; Miller, F.J.; Krause, K. Reactive oxygen species: From health to disease. *Swiss Med. Wkly.* **2012**, *142*, w13659. [CrossRef] [PubMed]
44. Kühn, F.J.; Lückhoff, A. Sites of the NUDT9-H domain critical for ADP-ribose activation of the cation channel TRPM2. *J. Biol. Chem.* **2004**, *279*, 46431–46437. [CrossRef] [PubMed]
45. Perraud, A.L.; Fleig, A.; Dunn, C.A.; Bagley, L.A.; Launay, P.; Schmitz, C.; Stokes, A.J.; Zhu, Q.; Bessman, M.J.; Penner, R.; et al. ADP-ribose gating of the calcium-permeable LTRPC2 channel revealed by Nudix motif homology. *Nature* **2001**, *411*, 595–599. [CrossRef] [PubMed]
46. Kolisek, M.; Beck, A.; Fleig, A.; Penner, R. Cyclic ADP-ribose and hydrogen peroxide synergize with ADP-ribose in the activation of TRPM2 channels. *Mol. Cell* **2005**, *18*, 61–69. [CrossRef] [PubMed]
47. Starkus, J.; Beck, A.; Fleig, A.; Penner, R. Regulation of TRPM2 by extra- and intracellular calcium. *J. Gen. Physiol.* **2007**, *130*, 427–440. [CrossRef] [PubMed]
48. Lange, I.; Penner, R.; Fleig, A.; Beck, A. Synergistic regulation of endogenous TRPM2 channels by adenine dinucleotides in primary human neutrophils. *Cell Calcium* **2008**, *44*, 604–615. [CrossRef] [PubMed]
49. Du, J.; Xie, J.; Yue, L. Intracellular calcium activates TRPM2 and tis alternative spliced isoforms. *Proc. Natl. Acad. Sci. USA* **2009**, *106*, 7239–7244. [CrossRef] [PubMed]

50. Heiner, I.; Eisfeld, J.; Warnstedt, M.; Radukina, N.; Jüngling, E.; Lückhoff, A. Endogenous ADP-ribose enables calcium-regulated cation currents through TRPM2 channels in neutrophil granulocytes. *Biochem. J.* **2006**, *398*, 225–232. [CrossRef] [PubMed]
51. Tóth, B.; Csanády, L. Identification of direct and indirect effectors of the transient receptor potential melastatin 2 (TRPM2) cation channel. *J. Biol. Chem.* **2010**, *285*, 30091–30102. [CrossRef] [PubMed]
52. Tóth, B.; Iordanov, I.; Csanády, L. Ruling out pyridine dinucleotides as true TRPM2 channel activators reveals novel direct agonist ADP-ribose-2′-phosphate. *J. Gen. Physiol.* **2015**, *145*, 419–430. [CrossRef] [PubMed]
53. Grubisha, O.; Rafty, L.A.; Takanishi, C.L.; Xu, X.; Tong, L.; Perraud, A.L.; Scharenberg, A.M.; Denu, J.M. Metabolite of SIR2 reaction modulates TRPM2 ion channel. *J. Biol. Chem.* **2006**, *281*, 14057–14065. [CrossRef] [PubMed]
54. Hara, Y.; Wakamori, M.; Ishii, M.; Maeno, E.; Nishida, M.; Yoshida, T.; Yamada, H.; Shimizu, S.; Mori, E.; Kudoh, J.; et al. LTRPC2 Ca^{2+}-permeable channel activated by changes in redox status confers susceptibility to cell death. *Mol. Cell* **2002**, *9*, 163–173. [CrossRef]
55. Perraud, A.L.; Takanishi, C.L.; Shen, B.; Kang, S.; Smith, M.K.; Schmitz, C.; Knowles, H.M.; Ferraris, D.; Li, W.; Zhang, J.; et al. Accumulation of free ADP-ribose from mitochondria mediates oxidative stress-induced gating of TRPM2 cation channels. *J. Biol. Chem.* **2005**, *280*, 6138–6148. [CrossRef] [PubMed]
56. Malavasi, F.; Deaglio, S.; Funaro, A.; Ferrero, E.; Horenstein, A.L.; Ortolan, E.; Vaisitti, T.; Aydin, S. Evolution and function of the ADP ribosyl cyclase/CD38 gene family in physiology and pathology. *Physiol. Rev.* **2008**, *88*, 841–886. [CrossRef] [PubMed]
57. Magnone, M.; Bauer, I.; Poggi, A.; Mannino, E.; Sturla, L.; Brini, M.; Zocchi, E.; De Flora, A.; Nencioni, A.; Bruzzone, S. NAD^+ levels control Ca^{2+} sore replenishment and mitogen-induced increase of cytosolic Ca^{2+} by cyclic ADP-ribose-dependent TRPM2 channel gating in human T lymphocytes. *J. Biol. Chem.* **2012**, *287*, 21067–21081. [CrossRef] [PubMed]
58. Tanuma, S.; Yagi, T.; Johnson, G.S. Endogenous ADP ribosylation of high mobility group proteins 1 and 2 and histone H1 following DNA damage in intact cells. *Arch. Biochem. Biophys.* **1985**, *237*, 38–42. [CrossRef]
59. De Murcia, G.; de Murcia, J.M. Poly(ADP-ribose) polymerase: A molecular nick-sensor. *Trends Biochem. Sci.* **1994**, *19*, 172–176. [CrossRef]
60. Oliver, F.J.; Menissier-de Murcia, J.; Nacci, C.; Decker, P.; Andriantsitohaina, R.; Muller, S.; de la Rubia, G.; Stoclet, J.C.; de Murcia, G. Resistance to endotoxic shock as a consequence of defective NF-κB activation in poly (ADP-ribose) polymerase-1 deficient mice. *EMBO J.* **1999**, *18*, 4446–4454. [CrossRef] [PubMed]
61. Virág, L.; Szabo, C. The therapeutic potential of poly(ADP-ribose) polymerase inhibitors. *Pharmacol. Rev.* **2002**, *54*, 375–429. [CrossRef] [PubMed]
62. Fonfria, E.; Marshall, I.C.; Benham, C.D.; Boyfield, I.; Brown, J.D.; Hill, K.; Hughes, J.P.; Skaper, S.D.; McNulty, S. TRPM2 channel opening in response to oxidative stress is dependent on activation of poly(ADP-ribose) polymerase. *Br. J. Pharmacol.* **2004**, *143*, 186–192. [CrossRef] [PubMed]
63. Buelow, B.; Song, Y.; Andrew, M.; Scharenberg, A.M. The poly(ADP-ribose) polymerase PARP-1 is required for oxidative stress-induced TRPM2 activation in lymphocytes. *J. Biol. Chem.* **2008**, *283*, 24571–24583. [CrossRef] [PubMed]
64. Ishii, M.; Shimizu, S.; Hara, Y.; Hagiwara, T.; Miyazaki, A.; Mori, Y.; Kiuchi, Y. Intracellular-produced hydroxyl radical mediates H_2O_2-induced Ca^{2+} influx and cell death in rat beta-cell line RIN-5F. *Cell Calcium* **2006**, *39*, 487–494. [CrossRef] [PubMed]
65. Shimizu, S.; Yonezawa, R.; Negoro, T.; Yamamoto, S.; Numata, T.; Ishii, M.; Mori, Y.; Toda, T. Sensitization of H_2O_2-induced TRPM2 activation and subsequent interleukin-8 (CXCL8) production by intracellular Fe^{2+} in human monocytic U937 cells. *Int. J. Biochem. Cell Biol.* **2015**, *68*, 119–127. [CrossRef] [PubMed]
66. Zhang, W.; Tong, Q.; Conrad, K.; Wozney, J.; Cheung, J.Y.; Miller, B.A. Regulation of TRP channel TRPM2 by the tyrosine phosphatase PTPL1. *Am. J. Physiol. Cell Physiol.* **2007**, *292*, C1746–C1758. [CrossRef] [PubMed]
67. Hill, K.; McNulty, S.; Randall, A.D. Inhibition of TRPM2 channels by the antifungal agents clotrimazole and econazole. *Naunyn-Schmiedeberg's Arch. Pharmacol.* **2004**, *370*, 227–237. [CrossRef] [PubMed]
68. Hill, K.; Benham, C. D.; McNulty, S.; Randall, A.D. Flufenamic acid is a pH-dependent antagonist of TRPM2 channels. *Neuropharmacology* **2004**, *47*, 450–460. [CrossRef] [PubMed]
69. Togashi, K.; Inada1, H.; Tominaga, M. Inhibition of the transient receptor potential cation channel TRPM2 by 2-aminoethoxydiphenyl borate (2-APB). *Br. J. Pharmacol.* **2008**, *153*, 1324–1330. [CrossRef] [PubMed]

70. Bari, M.R.; Akbar, S.; Eweida, M.; Kühn, F.J.; Gustafsson, A.J.; Lückhoff, A.; Islam, M.S. H_2O_2-induced Ca^{2+} influx and its inhibition by *N*-(p-amylcinnamoyl) anthranilic acid in the beta-cells: Involvement of TRPM2 channels. *J. Cell. Mol. Med.* **2009**, *13*, 3260–3267. [CrossRef] [PubMed]
71. Kheradpezhouh, E.; Barritt, G.J.; Rychkov, G.Y. Curcumin inhibits activation of TRPM2 channels in rat hepatocytes. *Redox Biol.* **2016**, *7*, 1–7. [CrossRef] [PubMed]
72. Shimizu, S.; Yonezawa, R.; Hagiwara, T.; Yoshida, T.; Takahashi, N.; Hamano, S.; Negoro, T.; Toda, T.; Wakamori, M.; Mori, Y.; et al. Inhibitory effects of AG490 on H_2O_2-induced TRPM2-mediated Ca^{2+} entry. *Eur. J. Pharmacol.* **2014**, *742*, 22–30. [CrossRef] [PubMed]
73. Toda, T.; Yamamoto, S.; Yonezawa, R.; Mori, Y.; Shimizu, S. Inhibitory effects of Tyrphostin AG-related compounds on oxidative stress-sensitive transient receptor potential channel activation. *Eur. J. Pharmacol.* **2016**, *786*, 19–28. [CrossRef] [PubMed]
74. Berton, G.; Castaldi, M.A.; Cassatella, M.A.; Nauseef, W.M. Celebrating the 50th anniversary of the seminal discovery that the phagocyte respiratory burst enzyme is an NADPH oxidase. *J. Leukoc. Biol.* **2015**, *97*, 1–2. [CrossRef] [PubMed]
75. Lambeth, J.D. NOX enzymes and the biology of reactive oxygen. *Nat. Rev. Immunol.* **2004**, *4*, 181–189. [CrossRef] [PubMed]
76. Akira, S.; Takeda, K. Toll-like receproe signaling. *Nat. Rev. Immunol.* **2004**, *4*, 499–511. [CrossRef] [PubMed]
77. Kohchi, C.; Inagawa, H.; Nishizawa, T.; Soma, G. ROS and innate immunity. *Anticancer Res.* **2009**, *29*, 817–822. [PubMed]
78. Schwabe, R.F.; Brenner, D.A. Mechanisms of liver injury. I. TNF-α-induced liver injury: Role of IKK, JNK, and ROS pathways. *Am. J. Physiol. Gastrointest. Liver Physiol.* **2006**, *290*, 583–589. [CrossRef] [PubMed]
79. Simon, H.U.; Haj-Yehia, A.; Levi-Schaffer, F. Role of reactive oxygen species (ROS) in apoptosis induction. *Apoptosis* **2000**, *5*, 415–418. [CrossRef] [PubMed]
80. Kalogeris, T.; Bao, Y.; Korthuis, R.J. Mitochondrial reactive oxygen species: A double edged sword in ischemia/reperfusion vs preconditioning. *Redox Biol.* **2014**, *2*, 702–714. [CrossRef] [PubMed]
81. Kleikers, P.W.; Wingler, K.; Hermans, J.J.; Diebold, I.; Altenhöfer, S.; Radermacher, K.A.; Janssen, B.; Görlach, A.; Schmidt, H.H. NADPH oxidases as a source of oxidative stress and molecular target in ischemia/reperfusion injury. *J. Mol. Med.* **2012**, *90*, 1391–1406. [CrossRef] [PubMed]
82. Pacher, P.; Nivorozhkin, A.; Szabó, C. Therapeutic effects of xanthine oxidase inhibitors: Renaissance half a century after the discovery of allopurinol. *Pharmacol. Rev.* **2006**, *58*, 87–114. [CrossRef] [PubMed]
83. Luster, A.D. Chemokines—Chemotactic cytokines that mediate inflammation. *N. Engl. J. Med.* **1998**, *338*, 436–445. [PubMed]
84. Haraguchi, K.; Kawamoto, A.; Isami, K.; Maeda, S.; Kusano, A.; Asakura, K.; Shirakawa, H.; Mori, Y.; Nakagawa, T.; Kaneko, S. TRPM2 contributes to inflammatory and neuropathic pain through the aggravation of pronociceptive inflammatory responses in mice. *J. Neurosci.* **2012**, *32*, 3931–3941. [CrossRef] [PubMed]
85. Yonezawa, R.; Yamamoto, S.; Takenaka, M.; Kage, Y.; Negoro, T.; Toda, T.; Ohbayashi, M.; Numata, T.; Nakano, Y.; Yamamoto, T.; et al. TRPM2 channels in alveolar epithelial cells mediate bleomycin-induced lung inflammation. *Free Radic. Biol.* **2016**, *90*, 101–113. [CrossRef] [PubMed]
86. Wehrhahn, J.; Kraft, R.; Harteneck, C.; Hauschildt, S. Transient receptor potential melastatin 2 is required for lipopolysaccharide-induced cytokine production in human monocytes. *J. Immunol.* **2010**, *184*, 2386–2393. [CrossRef] [PubMed]
87. Hardaker, L.; Bahra, P.; de Billy, B.C.; Freeman, M.; Kupfer, N.; Wyss, D.; Trifilieff, A. The ion channel transient receptor potential melastatin-2 does not play a role in inflammatory mouse models of chronic obstructive pulmonary diseases. *Respir. Res.* **2012**, *13*, 30. [CrossRef] [PubMed]
88. Di, A.; Gao, X.; Qian, F.; Kawamura, T.; Han, J.; Hecquet, C.; Ye, R.D.; Vogel, S.M.; Malik, A.B. The redox-sensitive cation channel TRPM2 modulates phagocyte ROS production and inflammation. *Nat. Immunol.* **2012**, *13*, 29–34. [CrossRef] [PubMed]
89. Mohapatra, N.P.; Soni, S.; Rajaram, M.V.; Dang, P.M.; Reilly, T.J.; El-Benna, J.; Clay, C.D.; Schlesinger, L.S.; Gunn, J.S. *Francisella* acid phosphatases inactivate the NADPH oxidase in human phagocytes. *J. Imunnol.* **2010**, *184*, 5141–5150. [CrossRef] [PubMed]
90. Shakerley, N.L.; Chandrasekaran, A.; Trebak, M.; Miller, B.A.; Melendez, J.A. *Francisella tularensis* catalase restricts immune function by impairing TRPM2 channel activity. *J. Imunnol.* **2016**, *291*, 3871–3881.

91. Knowles, H.; Heizer, J.W.; Li, Y.; Chapman, K.; Ogden, C.A.; Andreasen, K.; Shapland, E.; Kucera, G.; Mogan, J.; Humann, J.; et al. Transient receptor potential melastatin 2 (TRPM2) ion channel is required for innate immunity against *Listeria monocytogenes*. *Proc. Natl. Acad. Sci. USA* **2011**, *108*, 11578–11583. [CrossRef] [PubMed]
92. Partida-Sánchez, S.; Cockayne, D.A.; Monard, S.; Jacobson, E.L.; Oppenheimer, N.; Garvy, B.; Kusser, K.; Goodrich, S.; Howard, M.; Harmsen, A.; et al. Cyclic ADP-ribose production by CD38 regulates intracellular calcium release, extracellular calcium influx and chemotaxis in neutrophils and is required for bacterial clearance in vivo. *Nat. Med.* **2001**, *7*, 1209–1216. [CrossRef] [PubMed]
93. Tschopp, J.; Schroder, K. NLRP3 inflammasome activation: The convergence of multiple signaling pathways on ROS production? *Nat. Rev. Immunol.* **2010**, *10*, 210–215. [CrossRef] [PubMed]
94. Zhong, Z.; Zhai, Y.; Liang, S.; Mori, Y.; Han, R.; Sutterwala, F.S.; Qiao, L. TRPM2 links oxidative stress to NLRP3 inflammasome activation. *Nat. Commun.* **2013**, *4*, 1611. [CrossRef] [PubMed]
95. West, A.P.; Shadel, G.S.; Ghosh, S. Mitochondria in innate immune responses. *Nat. Rev. Immunol.* **2011**, *11*, 389–402. [CrossRef] [PubMed]
96. Chen, Q.; Surmeier, D.J.; Reiner, A. NMDA and non-NMDA receptor-mediated excitotoxicity are potentiated in cultured striatal neurons by prior chronic depolarization. *Exp. Neurol.* **1999**, *159*, 283–296. [CrossRef] [PubMed]
97. Burgoyne, R.D. Neuronal calcium sensor proteins: Generating diversity in neuronal Ca^{2+} signaling. *Nat. Rev. Neurosci.* **2007**, *8*, 182–193. [CrossRef] [PubMed]
98. Jia, J.; Verma, S.; Nakayama, S.; Quillinan, N.; Grafe, M.R.; Hurn, P.D.; Herson, P.S. Sex differences in neuroprotection provided by inhibition of TRPM2 channels following experimental stroke. *J. Cereb. Blood Flow Metab.* **2011**, *31*, 2160–2168. [CrossRef] [PubMed]
99. Verma, S.; Quillinan, N.; Yang, Y.; Nakayama, S.; Cheng, J.; Kelley, M.H.; Herson, P.S. TRPM2 channel activation following in vitro ischemia contributes to male hippocampal cell death. *Neurosci. Lett.* **2012**, *530*, 41–46. [CrossRef] [PubMed]
100. Shimizu, T.; Macey, T.A.; Quillinan, N.; Klawitter, J.; Perraud, A.L.; Traystman, R.J.; Herson, P.S. Androgen and PARP-1 regulation of TRPM2 channels after ischemic injury. *J. Cereb. Blood Flow Metab.* **2013**, *33*, 1549–1555. [CrossRef] [PubMed]
101. Alim, I.; Teves, L.; Li, R.; Mori, Y.; Tymianski, M. Modulation of NMDAR subunit expression by TRPM2 channels regulates neuronal vulnerability of ischemic cell death. *J. Neurosci.* **2013**, *33*, 17264–17277. [CrossRef] [PubMed]
102. Gelderblom, M.; Melzer, N.; Schattling, B.; Gob, E.; Hicking, G.; Arunachalam, P.; Bittner, S.; Ufer, F.; Herrmann, A.M.; Bernreuther, C.; et al. Transient receptor potential melastatin subfamily member 2 cation channel regulates detrimental immune cell invasion in ischemic stroke. *Stroke* **2014**, *45*, 3395–3402. [CrossRef] [PubMed]
103. Miller, B.A.; Hoffman, N.E.; Merali, S.; Zhang, X.Q.; Wang, J.; Rajan, S.; Shanmughapriya, S.; Gao, E.; Barrero, C.A.; Mallilankaraman, K.; et al. TRPM2 cahnnels protect against cardiac ischemia-reperfusion injury. *J. Biol. Chem.* **2014**, *289*, 7615–7629. [CrossRef] [PubMed]
104. Hoffman, N.E.; Miller, B.A.; Wang, J.; Elrod, J.W.; Rajan, S.; Gao, E.; Song, J.; Zhang, X.; Hirschler-Laszkiewicz, I.; Shanmughapriya, S.; et al. Ca^{2+} entry via Trpm2 is essential for cardiac myocyte bioenergetics maintenance. *Am. J. Physiol. Heart Circ. Physiol.* **2015**, *308*, H637–H650. [CrossRef] [PubMed]
105. Hiroi, T.; Wajima, T.; Nrgoro, T.; Ishii, M.; Nakano, Y.; Kiuchi, Y.; Mori, Y.; Shimizu, S. Neutrophil TRPM2 channels are implicated in the exacerbation of myocardial ishchemia/reperfusion injury. *Cardiovasc. Res.* **2013**, *97*, 271–281. [CrossRef] [PubMed]
106. Gao, G.; Wang, W.; Tadagavadi, R.K.; Briley, N.E.; Love, M.I.; Miller, B.A.; Reeves, W.B. TRPM2 mediates ischemic kidney injury and oxidant stress through RAC1. *J. Clin. Investig.* **2014**, *124*, 4989–5001. [CrossRef] [PubMed]
107. Davidson, D.G.; Eastham, W.N. Acute liver necrosis following overdose of paracetamol. *BMJ* **1966**, *2*, 497–499. [CrossRef] [PubMed]
108. Mitchell, J.R.; Jollow, D.J.; Potter, W.Z.; Davis, D.C.; Gillette, J.R.; Brodie, B.B. Acetaminophen-induced hepatic necrosis. I. role of drug metabolism. *J. Pharmacol. Exp. Ther.* **1971**, *187*, 185–194.

109. Kheradpezhouh, E.; Ma, L.; Morphett, A.; Barritt, G.J.; Rychkov, G.Y. TRPM2 channels mediate acetaminophen-induced liver damage. *Proc. Natl. Acad. Sci. USA* **2014**, *111*, 3176–3181. [CrossRef] [PubMed]
110. Liu, X.; Cotrim, A.; Teos, L.; Zheng, C.; Swaim, W.; Mitchell, J.; Mori, Y.; Ambudkar, I. Loss of TRPM2 function protects against irradiation-induced salivary gland dysfunction. *Nat. Commun.* **2013**, *4*, 1515. [CrossRef] [PubMed]
111. Yamamoto, S.; Wajima, T.; Hara, Y.; Nishida, M.; Mori, Y. Transient receptor potential channels in Alzheimer's disease. *Biochim. Biophys. Acta* **2007**, *1772*, 958–967. [CrossRef] [PubMed]
112. Ostapchenko, V.G.; Chen, M.; Guzman, M.S.; Xie, Y.F.; Lavine, N.; Fan, J.; Beraldo, F.H.; Martyn, A.C.; Belrose, J.C.; Mori, Y.; et al. The transient receptor potential melastatin 2 (TRPM2) channel contributes to β-amyloid oligomer-related neurotoxicity and memory impairment. *J. Neurosci.* **2015**, *35*, 15157–15169. [CrossRef] [PubMed]
113. Zuo, L.; Hemmelgarn, B.T.; Chuang, C.; Besr, T.M. The role of oxidative stress-induced epigenetic alterations in amyloid-β production in Alzheimer's disease. *Oxid. Med. Cell. Longev.* **2015**, *2015*, Article ID 604658. [CrossRef] [PubMed]
114. Lustbader, J.W.; Cirilli, M.; Lin, C.; Xu, H.W.; Takuma, K.; Wang, N.; Caspersen, C.; Chen, X.; Pollak, S.; Chaney, M.; et al. ABAD directly links Aβ to mitochondrial toxicity in Alzheimer's disease. *Science* **2004**, *304*, 448–452. [CrossRef] [PubMed]
115. Park, L.; Wang, G.; Moore, J.; Girouard, H.; Zhou, P.; Anrather, J.; Iadecola, C. The key role of transient receptor potential melastatin-2 channels in amyloid-β-induced neurovascular dysfunction. *Nat. Commun.* **2014**, *5*, 5318. [CrossRef] [PubMed]

13

Development of TRPM8 Antagonists to Treat Chronic Pain and Migraine

Andy D. Weyer [1] and Sonya G. Lehto [2,*]

1 Pacific University School of Physical Therapy, Hillsboro, OR 97123, USA; andy.weyer@pacificu.edu
2 One Amgen Center Dr, Thousand Oaks, CA 91320, USA
* Correspondence: slehto@amgen.com

Academic Editors: Susan M. Huang, Arpad Szallasi and Jean Jacques Vanden Eynde

Abstract: A review. Development of pharmaceutical antagonists of transient receptor potential melastatin 8 (TRPM8) have been pursued for the treatment of chronic pain and migraine. This review focuses on the current state of this progress.

Keywords: transient receptor potential melastatin 8 (TRPM*); pain; menthol; cold hyperalgesia; cold analgesia; mechanical hyperalgesia; migraine

---

1. Introduction

Transient receptor potential melastatin 8 (TRPM8) is a non-selective cation channel encoded by the *TRPM8* gene, first characterized as a detector of cold [1,2]. TRPM8 is found on both Aδ and C fiber afferents, and in addition to activation by cold temperatures, TRPM8 is activated by a number of chemical agonists that are known to produce cool sensations such as menthol, icilin, and eucalyptol [3,4]. As a natural extension of these findings, much research over the past decade has been devoted to the role of TRPM8-expressing afferents in the complex interpretation of hot and cold temperatures. Furthermore, the role of TRPM8 in pain sensation has been debated; indeed, while a large body of research has supported a role for TRPM8 in reducing or limiting pain sensation under injury conditions, an equally large number of publications propose that TRPM8 actually exaggerates pain after injury. From a pharmaceutical perspective, this complicates whether specific agonists or antagonists of TRPM8 should be developed to treat different pain conditions. In this review, we summarize the literature concerning the contribution of TRPM8 to both analgesia and nociception, and provide an update on the current state of drug development involving this versatile protein.

2. The Role for TRPM8 in Mechanical and Heat Analgesia

Intimately tied to our understanding of a potential role for TRPM8 in promoting analgesia is the effect of one of its prime agonists, menthol. Menthol is a common component of topical creams that have long been used to reduce pain and provide a cooling sensation [5]. Although some data has indicated that menthol may activate a variety of other channels, including transient receptor potential Ankyrin 1 (TRPA1), gamma-aminobutyric acid (GABA), and voltage-gated calcium and sodium channels [6,7], more recent studies have demonstrated that the prime target of menthol is indeed TRPM8, as genetic deletion of this receptor in mice prevents responsiveness to menthol at both the behavioral and cellular levels [8].

In animal studies, menthol has been shown to block the mechanical and heat hyperalgesia caused by injection of inflammatory compounds such as Complete Freund's Adjuvant (CFA) or the transient receptor potential vanilloid 1 (TRPV1) agonist capsaicin [7,9,10]. Furthermore, injection of the TRPM8 agonist icilin significantly reduced the colonic damage observed in two different mouse models of inflammatory bowel disease [11]. In support of these inflammatory studies, it has been shown that components of the "inflammatory soup" that develops after an injury can inhibit TRPM8. Andersson and colleagues reported that low pH inactivates TRPM8, making it less responsive to the TRPM8 agonist icilin and cold temperatures (but interestingly not menthol) [12]. Similarly, another study found that bradykinin, a key potentiator of pain and component of the inflammatory soup, reduces TRPM8 activity through the action of protein kinase C in both the periphery and at the central synapse in the dorsal horn [10].

Adding to the view that TRPM8 promotes analgesia following injury are data from studies in which TRPM8 is either genetically deleted or experimentally knocked down. Proudfoot and colleagues first demonstrated this concept in a chronic constriction injury (CCI) model. Experimental rats in this study exhibited significantly reduced heat and mechanical pain behaviors when topical icilin was applied to the paw, but this effect was completely reversed when TRPM8 expression was knocked down via intrathecal injection of antisense oligonucleotides [13]. In similar experiments utilizing the CCI model, cooling or applying menthol to the affected paw resulted in reduced hypersensitivity in response to mechanical stimuli [14,15], but this effect was not seen when TRPM8 was knocked out or when TRPM8-expressing afferents were ablated [14]. Likewise, one of the first studies to utilize TRPM8 knockout mice demonstrated that TRPM8 was responsible for the analgesia provided by a cold plate during the first phase of the formalin test [16], and later studies using mice deficient in TRPM8 showed that menthol was unable to exert its analgesic effects in models of inflammatory pain using capsaicin or CFA [7].

A number of studies in humans also point toward a role for TRPM8 in mediating analgesia. In a recent study, injections of the TRPA1 agonist cinnamaldehyde into the forearm resulted in significant pain and neurogenic flare; however, simultaneous injection of menthol resulted in lower pain ratings, elevated mechanical pain thresholds, and reduced neurogenic flare as compared to cinnamaldehyde alone [17]. Two case studies also demonstrate the analgesic role of TRPM8 in patients suffering from chronic neuropathic pain. One individual developed neuropathic pain after long-term dosing with the chemotherapeutic Bortezomib, which causes neuropathy in up to 35% of patients. This individual suffered from a severe burning sensation in his lower limbs and "lightning-like" sensations in his hands. However, topical application of a 0.5% menthol cream to his lower extremities in a stocking distribution and the lumbosacral region overlying the affected nerve roots resulted in a significant improvement in response to suprathreshold mechanical stimuli and overall pain ratings [18]. Similarly, in another case where a patient suffered from severe allodynia following a case of post-herpetic neuralgia, application of menthol oil in concentrations of 2 or 10% resulted in a significant abatement of symptoms [19]. Further proof of the analgesic effects through TRPM8 can be observed in the ability of menthol or eucalyptol (another TRPM8 agonist) to prevent the irritant effects of acrolein and other cigarette smoke components [20].

3. The Role of TRPM8 in Cold Hyperalgesia

Much data also suggests that TRPM8 plays a role in amplifying pain sensation after injury, especially in models of neuropathic pain. Hypersensitivity to cold is a common complaint of individuals with neuropathies, with 20–30% of individuals diagnosed with different types of neuropathies complaining of cold hyperalgesia and elevated cold pain thresholds [21–23]. Likewise, other studies report significant elevations in cold pain thresholds in patients treated with the chemotherapeutic oxaliplatin, indicating that innocuous temperatures had become painful for these individuals [23,24]. In addition to alterations in cold thresholds, these individuals also rated specific cold temperatures as 3–4 times more painful than at baseline.

The cold hypersensitivity following neuropathic injury observed in human subjects has been consistently paralleled in animal models of nerve injury, and has been further extended to identify a definitive role for TRPM8 in mediating this pain. For instance, oxaliplatin-induced neuropathies in mice cause cold hypersensitivity on the behavioral level and also result in an increased percentage of isolated sensory neurons that respond to cold temperatures [25,26]. When TRPM8 knockout mice are utilized for these same experiments, this cold hyperalgesia is absent, implicating TRPM8 as a critical player in this phenomenon [25]. At this time it is unclear whether TRPM8 expression increases after installation of oxaliplatin-induced neuropathy, with one study reporting increased mRNA expression [27] and another reporting no change in mRNA expression levels [25].

Another popular neuropathic model is the CCI, in which ligatures are tied around the sciatic nerve. This model has consistently been shown to cause cold hypersensitivity, and multiple studies have reported that the increased responsiveness to the acetone evaporative cooling test following CCI was significantly reduced when TRPM8 was genetically deleted or when TRPM8-expressing afferents were chemically ablated [15,26]. Similarly, another study has reported that knockdown of TRPM8 with antisense oligonucleotides results in reduced responsiveness to cold as compared to animals injected with the missense oligonucleotide [14]. Additionally, this study and others have reported an increase in the number of neurons expressing TRPM8 [14,28,29] and an increase in total amount of TRPM8 protein in the DRG following CCI surgery [14]. Functionally, an increased number of isolated sensory neurons are responsive to cold and menthol after CCI, and these responses are potentiated as compared to controls [28].

4. The Role of TRPM8 in Bladder Pain

Interstitial cystitis/bladder pain syndrome is a condition characterized by pain in the bladder region and by urinary urgency and increased urination frequency [30]. Current therapeutics are often insufficient for treating this condition, so the identification of new drug targets is of particular interest. Much like in animal models of neuropathic pain, animal models of bladder pain reveal TRPM8 to be pro-nociceptive. For instance, the use of a novel TRPM8 antagonist, AMTB, increased intercontraction intervals in a rodent model of overactive bladder syndrome, and also decreased the visceromotor reflex [31]. A similar phenomenon was observed in guinea pigs, as a novel TRPM8 antagonist reversed the reduction in bladder voiding volume induced by cold saline and menthol infusion in to the bladder [32]. Whether these effects are mediated via inhibition of TRPM8 channels on bladder-projecting afferents or on TRPM8 located in the bladder itself is unclear, as TRPM8 expression at the mRNA and protein levels has been observed in both afferents innervating the bladder [31,33,34] and in the bladder itself [34,35]. A recent study may shed some light on this, as recordings from C-fiber afferents demonstrated reduced firing in response to bladder distention in the presence of menthol when a novel TRPM8 antagonist was infused into the bladder [36]. Interestingly, increased TRPM8 immunostaining was observed in bladder samples from individuals with bladder pain syndrome, and this was moderately correlated with increased pain scores in those patients [34].

5. The Role of TRPM8 in Migraine

In addition to its role in somatic pain sensation, recent genome-wide association studies have found a significant correlation between migraine incidence and single nucleotide polymorphisms (SNPs) located near the TRPM8 coding region (for a review see [37]). Interestingly, this connection seems to be present only for individuals of Northern European ancestry [38–42], as studies involving populations from Spain, India, and China found either no association or weak associations between migraine incidence and SNPs near the *TRPM8* locus [43–47].

These human studies have naturally sparked interest in exploring the contribution of TRPM8 to migraine through the use of rodent models. Unfortunately, these studies have found opposing results concerning TRPM8's involvement. Burgos-Vega and colleagues observed that application of icilin to the dura mater resulted in reduced paw and facial withdrawal thresholds in response to a mechanical stimulus, indicating that activation of TRPM8 caused migraine-like behaviors [48]. These behaviors were then subsequently blocked by dosing animals with a novel TRPM8 antagonist. Perhaps most interesting, however, was that sumatriptan, a drug commonly used to treat migraines, also prevented the migraine-like behaviors, which strongly implicates a role for TRPM8 in migraine generation. Conversely, a recent study by Ren and colleagues found opposing results, with application of menthol to the dura mater relieving migraine-like symptoms brought on by the application of inflammatory mediators to the dura. Symptom relief could then be subsequently blocked by injection of a TRPM8 antagonist. Finally, adding even more confusion to the matter is a study from Huang et al. that reported that TRPM8-expressing afferents were virtually absent from the dura [49]. However, further interest in strategies targeting TRP channels as migraine therapeutics is supported by clinical success of CGRP receptor antagonism since activation of TRP channels can elicit CGRP release [50].

6. Why is TRPM8 Analgesic in Some Cases and Nociceptive in Others?

An important point about TRPM8's roles in nociception and analgesia is that activation of TRPM8 seems to consistently cause cold pain following injury, while simultaneously reducing mechanical and heat pain. Therefore, whether to target TRPM8 with either an agonist or antagonist may depend on which symptom is most troublesome to the patient; individuals with a primary complaint of mechanical hyperalgesia may respond best to TRPM8 agonists, while those with cold hyperalgesia may respond best to TRPM8 antagonists. Importantly, this is not to suggest that TRPM8 itself is sensitive to both mechanical and cold stimuli; indeed, afferent recordings indicate that pharmacological blockade of TRPM8 has no effect on baseline mechanical responsiveness [51] and genetic deletion of TRPM8 or pharmacological ablation of TRPM8-expressing afferents does not impact behavioral responses to mechanical stimuli [15]. Rather, it seems that the effects of TRPM8 agonism/antagonism are due to effects at the spinal level, with TRPM8-expressing afferents either directly or indirectly inhibiting mechanonociceptive afferents. Indeed, Proudfoot et al. reported that the analgesic effects of TRPM8 activation may be due to axoaxonic synapses on mechanonociceptive and heat-nociceptive afferent terminals, which contain inhibitory mGluRII and mGluRIII receptors [13]. Thus, release of glutamate from TRPM8-expressing afferents may decrease the amount of excitatory neurotransmitters released onto nociceptive projection neurons in lamina I and II of the dorsal horn. There is also a suggestion that topical menthol-induced pain relief may occur through blockade of voltage gated sodium channels [52].

At the same time, cold hyperalgesia following injury may be due to activation of a separate population of TRPM8-expressing nociceptors that relay painful information to the central nervous system. These nociceptors may have reduced thresholds for activation under injury conditions, leading to the observed strong hyperalgesic responses to cold. Additionally, they may be triggered by especially strong stimuli that facilitate TRPM8 activation; indeed, studies in humans consistently report that application of high concentrations of menthol (30%–40%) induces pain, cold allodynia, and cold hyperalgesia [53–55], whereas the lower concentrations used in topical agents induce analgesia.

7. Development of TRPM8 Antagonists for Chronic Pain

Antagonists of TRPM8 as therapeutics for chronic pain, migraine or inflammation have been pursued over the recent decade by many pharmaceutical companies such as Hydra Biosciences, Glenmark, Janssen, Pfizer, Bayer, Grunenthal, Mitsubishi Tanabe, RaQualia, Dompe/Axxam, BASF, Dendreon and Amgen. These efforts have led to the publication of many patents (for a review see [56–58]).

Janssen has published several potent and selective small molecule antagonists that suppresses icilin-induced wet-dog shakes, cold pressor response, as well as cold-induced allodynia in a neuropathic pain model in rats with a similar resulting dose-response range of effect in either of the cold-induced endpoints [59–63]. Glenmark also similarly reported efficacy with their antagonist in both wet-dog shakes and oxaliplatin-induced cold allodynia at the same 30 mg/kg dose [64]. RaQualia published RQ-00203078 which is a single digit nM antagonist at human or rat TRPM8 that also potently blocks icilin-induced wet-dog shakes in rats and is now commercially available, though evaluation in analgesic models has not been published [65].

AMG2850 is a ~200 nM potent and selective antagonist from Amgen that blocks both TRPM8 agonist-induced behavioral responses (wet-dog shakes) and cold-induced increases in blood pressure (cold pressor test)—both considered pharmacodynamic models of TRPM8 antagonism in vivo. Although the effect in cold allodynia was not evaluated, the effective dose would presumably be similar to that in the reported cold endpoint, the cold pressor test. There was, however, no evidence of meaningful reversal of inflammatory nor neuropathic-induced mechanical hypersensitivities in rats. This lack of efficacy occurred even at unbound plasma concentrations in excess of 21-fold the IC_{90} pharmacodynamic model suggesting that TRPM8 does not play a role in these mechanical pain behaviors at what would be reasonably considered more than enough target coverage [51,66,67], thus casting doubt on the therapeutic potential of TRPM8 as an analgesic in non-cold related conditions.

Pfizer did advance to clinical trials with a ~100 nM molecule, PF-05105679, which successfully inhibited the cold pressor response in humans, but also produced hot sensations that were both unexpected and considered adverse. The lack of therapeutic index to this event coupled with the short half-life in humans limited further clinical progression as well as the ability to evaluate the analgesic effect [32,68]. It has been demonstrated that cutaneous TRPM8 controls autonomic and behavioral thermoeffectors involved in body temperature maintenance with antagonists decreasing body temperature in rodents [26,69–71]. While the Pfizer antagonist did not produce a significant alteration of body temperature in healthy volunteers, further understanding is needed to elucidate whether and how these hot sensations may be on-target side effects in humans.

Chemotherapeutic drug-induced cold allodynia can be dose limiting, resulting in the cessation of treatment, enduring years beyond treatment, and for which there are currently no proven therapies [72–74]. Since chemotherapy is associated with changes in TRPM8 expression [25,75], perhaps TRPM8 antagonists could be beneficial in the prevention and/or reversal of this chemotherapy-induced cold allodynia. Or, perhaps TRPM8 antagonists could still be useful therapeutics for any other cold-related painful allodynia or hyperalgesia associated with other neuropathic or inflammatory conditions or even migraine or bladder pain. Currently, there are no ongoing trials with TRPM8 antagonists [76].

Acknowledgments: Funding to publish this review was paid by Amgen Inc.

References

1. Peier, A.M.; Moqrich, A.; Hergarden, A.C.; Reeve, A.J.; Andersson, D.A.; Story, G.M.; Earley, T.J.; Dragoni, I.; McIntyre, P.; Bevan, S.; et al. A TRP channel that senses cold stimuli and menthol. *Cell* **2002**, *108*, 705–715. [CrossRef]
2. McKemy, D.D.; Neuhausser, W.M.; Julius, D. Identification of a cold receptor reveals a general role for TRP channels in thermosensation. *Nature* **2002**, *416*, 52–58. [CrossRef] [PubMed]
3. Behrendt, H.J.; Germann, T.; Gillen, C.; Hatt, H.; Jostock, R. Characterization of the mouse cold-menthol receptor TRPM8 and vanilloid receptor type-1 VR1 using a fluorometric imaging plate reader (FLIPR) assay. *Br. J. Pharmacol.* **2004**, *141*, 737–745. [CrossRef] [PubMed]
4. Dai, Y. TRPs and pain. *Semin. Immunopathol.* **2016**, *38*, 277–291. [CrossRef] [PubMed]
5. Eccles, R. Menthol and related cooling compounds. *J. Pharm. Pharmacol.* **1994**, *46*, 618–630. [CrossRef] [PubMed]
6. Karashima, Y.; Damann, N.; Prenen, J.; Talavera, K.; Segal, A.; Voets, T.; Nilius, B. Bimodal action of menthol on the transient receptor potential channel TRPA1. *J. Neurosci.* **2007**, *27*, 9874–9884. [CrossRef] [PubMed]
7. Pan, R.; Tian, Y.; Gao, R.; Li, H.; Zhao, X.; Barrett, J.E.; Hu, H. Central mechanisms of menthol-induced analgesia. *J. Pharm. Exp. Ther.* **2012**, *343*, 661–672. [CrossRef] [PubMed]
8. Liu, B.; Fan, L.; Balakrishna, S.; Sui, A.; Morris, J.B.; Jordt, S.E. TRPM8 is the principal mediator of menthol-induced analgesia of acute and inflammatory pain. *Pain* **2013**, *154*, 2169–2177. [CrossRef] [PubMed]
9. Alpizar, Y.A.; Boonen, B.; Gees, M.; Sanchez, A.; Nilius, B.; Voets, T.; Talavera, K. Allyl isothiocyanate sensitizes TRPV1 to heat stimulation. *Pflugers Arch. EJP* **2014**, *466*, 507–515. [CrossRef] [PubMed]

10. Premkumar, L.S.; Raisinghani, M.; Pingle, S.C.; Long, C.; Pimentel, F. Downregulation of transient receptor potential melastatin 8 by protein kinase C-mediated dephosphorylation. *J. Neurosci.* **2005**, *25*, 11322–11329. [CrossRef] [PubMed]
11. Ramachandran, R.; Hyun, E.; Zhao, L.; Lapointe, T.K.; Chapman, K.; Hirota, C.L.; Ghosh, S.; McKemy, D.D.; Vergnolle, N.; Beck, P.L.; et al. TRPM8 activation attenuates inflammatory responses in mouse models of colitis. *Proc. Natl. Acad. Sci. USA* **2013**, *110*, 7476–7481. [CrossRef] [PubMed]
12. Andersson, D.A.; Chase, H.W.; Bevan, S. TRPM8 activation by menthol, icilin, and cold is differentially modulated by intracellular pH. *J. Neurosci.* **2004**, *24*, 5364–5369. [CrossRef] [PubMed]
13. Proudfoot, C.J.; Garry, E.M.; Cottrell, D.F.; Rosie, R.; Anderson, H.; Robertson, D.C.; Fleetwood-Walker, S.M.; Mitchell, R. Analgesia mediated by the TRPM8 cold receptor in chronic neuropathic pain. *Curr. Boil.* **2006**, *16*, 1591–1605. [CrossRef] [PubMed]
14. Su, L.; Wang, C.; Yu, Y.-H.; Ren, Y.-Y.; Xie, K.-L.; Wang, G.-L. Role of TRPM8 in dorsal root ganglion in nerve injury-induced chronic pain. *BMC Neurosci.* **2011**, *12*, 120. [CrossRef] [PubMed]
15. Knowlton, W.M.; Palkar, R.; Lippoldt, E.K.; McCoy, D.D.; Baluch, F.; Chen, J.; McKemy, D.D. A sensory-labeled line for cold: TRPM8-expressing sensory neurons define the cellular basis for cold, cold pain, and cooling-mediated analgesia. *J. Neurosci.* **2013**, *33*, 2837–2848. [CrossRef] [PubMed]
16. Dhaka, A.; Murray, A.N.; Mathur, J.; Earley, T.J.; Petrus, M.J.; Patapoutian, A. TRPM8 is required for cold sensation in mice. *Neuron* **2007**, *54*, 371–378. [CrossRef] [PubMed]
17. Andersen, H.H.; Gazerani, P.; Arendt-Nielsen, L. High-Concentration L-Menthol Exhibits Counter-Irritancy to Neurogenic Inflammation, Thermal and Mechanical Hyperalgesia Caused by Trans-cinnamaldehyde. *J. Pain* **2016**, *17*, 919–929. [CrossRef] [PubMed]
18. Colvin, L.A.; Johnson, P.R.; Mitchell, R.; Fleetwood-Walker, S.M.; Fallon, M. From bench to bedside: A case of rapid reversal of bortezomib-induced neuropathic pain by the TRPM8 activator, menthol. *J. Clin. Oncol.* **2008**, *26*, 4519–4520. [CrossRef] [PubMed]
19. Davies, S.J.; Harding, L.M.; Baranowski, A.P. A novel treatment of postherpetic neuralgia using peppermint oil. *Clin. J. Pain* **2002**, *18*, 200–202. [CrossRef] [PubMed]
20. Willis, D.N.; Liu, B.; Ha, M.A.; Jordt, S.E.; Morris, J.B. Menthol attenuates respiratory irritation responses to multiple cigarette smoke irritants. *FASEB J.* **2011**, *25*, 4434–4444. [CrossRef] [PubMed]
21. Eberle, T.; Doganci, B.; Kramer, H.H.; Geber, C.; Fechir, M.; Magerl, W.; Birklein, F. Warm and cold complex regional pain syndromes: Differences beyond skin temperature? *Neurology* **2009**, *72*, 505–512. [CrossRef] [PubMed]
22. Maier, C.; Baron, R.; Tolle, T.R.; Binder, A.; Birbaumer, N.; Birklein, F.; Gierthmuhlen, J.; Flor, H.; Geber, C.; Huge, V.; et al. Quantitative sensory testing in the German Research Network on Neuropathic Pain (DFNS): Somatosensory abnormalities in 1236 patients with different neuropathic pain syndromes. *Pain* **2010**, *150*, 439–450. [CrossRef] [PubMed]
23. Attal, N.; Bouhassira, D.; Gautron, M.; Vaillant, J.N.; Mitry, E.; Lepere, C.; Rougier, P.; Guirimand, F. Thermal hyperalgesia as a marker of oxaliplatin neurotoxicity: A prospective quantified sensory assessment study. *Pain* **2009**, *144*, 245–252. [CrossRef] [PubMed]
24. Binder, A.; Stengel, M.; Maag, R.; Wasner, G.; Schoch, R.; Moosig, F.; Schommer, B.; Baron, R. Pain in oxaliplatin-induced neuropathy—sensitisation in the peripheral and central nociceptive system. *Eur. J. Cancer* **2007**, *43*, 2658–2663. [CrossRef] [PubMed]
25. Descoeur, J.; Pereira, V.; Pizzoccaro, A.; Francois, A.; Ling, B.; Maffre, V.; Couette, B.; Busserolles, J.; Courteix, C.; Noel, J.; et al. Oxaliplatin-induced cold hypersensitivity is due to remodelling of ion channel expression in nociceptors. *EMBO Mol. Med.* **2011**, *3*, 266–278. [CrossRef] [PubMed]
26. Knowlton, W.M.; Daniels, R.L.; Palkar, R.; McCoy, D.D.; McKemy, D.D. Pharmacological blockade of TRPM8 ion channels alters cold and cold pain responses in mice. *PLoS ONE* **2011**, *6*, e25894. [CrossRef] [PubMed]
27. Gauchan, P.; Andoh, T.; Kato, A.; Kuraishi, Y. Involvement of increased expression of transient receptor potential melastatin 8 in oxaliplatin-induced cold allodynia in mice. *Neurosci. Lett.* **2009**, *458*, 93–95. [CrossRef] [PubMed]
28. Xing, H.; Chen, M.; Ling, J.; Tan, W.; Gu, J.G. TRPM8 mechanism of cold allodynia after chronic nerve injury. *J. Neurosci.* **2007**, *27*, 13680–13690. [CrossRef] [PubMed]

29. Frederick, J.; Buck, M.E.; Matson, D.J.; Cortright, D.N. Increased TRPA1, TRPM8, and TRPV2 expression in dorsal root ganglia by nerve injury. *Biochem. Biophys. Res. Commun.* **2007**, *358*, 1058–1064. [CrossRef] [PubMed]
30. Berry, S.H.; Elliott, M.N.; Suttorp, M.; Bogart, L.M.; Stoto, M.A.; Eggers, P.; Nyberg, L.; Clemens, J.Q. Prevalence of symptoms of bladder pain syndrome/interstitial cystitis among adult females in the United States. *J. Urol.* **2011**, *186*, 540–544. [CrossRef] [PubMed]
31. Lashinger, E.S.; Steiginga, M.S.; Hieble, J.P.; Leon, L.A.; Gardner, S.D.; Nagilla, R.; Davenport, E.A.; Hoffman, B.E.; Laping, N.J.; Su, X. AMTB, a TRPM8 channel blocker: Evidence in rats for activity in overactive bladder and painful bladder syndrome. *Am. J. Physiol. Renal Physiol.* **2008**, *295*, F803–F810. [CrossRef] [PubMed]
32. Winchester, W.J.; Gore, K.; Glatt, S.; Petit, W.; Gardiner, J.C.; Conlon, K.; Postlethwaite, M.; Saintot, P.P.; Roberts, S.; Gosset, J.R.; et al. Inhibition of TRPM8 channels reduces pain in the cold pressor test in humans. *J. Pharm. Exp. Ther.* **2014**, *351*, 259–269. [CrossRef] [PubMed]
33. Hayashi, T.; Kondo, T.; Ishimatsu, M.; Yamada, S.; Nakamura, K.; Matsuoka, K.; Akasu, T. Expression of the TRPM8-immunoreactivity in dorsal root ganglion neurons innervating the rat urinary bladder. *J. Neurosci. Res.* **2009**, *65*, 245–251. [CrossRef] [PubMed]
34. Mukerji, G.; Yiangou, Y.; Corcoran, S.L.; Selmer, I.S.; Smith, G.D.; Benham, C.D.; Bountra, C.; Agarwal, S.K.; Anand, P. Cool and menthol receptor TRPM8 in human urinary bladder disorders and clinical correlations. *BMC Urol.* **2006**, *6*, 6. [CrossRef] [PubMed]
35. Kobayashi, H.; Yoshiyama, M.; Zakoji, H.; Takeda, M.; Araki, I. Sex differences in the expression profile of acid-sensing ion channels in the mouse urinary bladder: A possible involvement in irritative bladder symptoms. *BJU Int.* **2009**, *104*, 1746–1751. [CrossRef] [PubMed]
36. Ito, H.; Aizawa, N.; Sugiyama, R.; Watanabe, S.; Takahashi, N.; Tajimi, M.; Fukuhara, H.; Homma, Y.; Kubota, Y.; Andersson, K.E.; et al. Functional role of the transient receptor potential melastatin 8 (TRPM8) ion channel in the urinary bladder assessed by conscious cystometry and ex vivo measurements of single-unit mechanosensitive bladder afferent activities in the rat. *BJU Int.* **2016**, *117*, 484–494. [CrossRef] [PubMed]
37. Dussor, G.; Cao, Y.Q. TRPM8 and Migraine. *Headache* **2016**, *56*, 1406–1417. [CrossRef] [PubMed]
38. Chasman, D.I.; Anttila, V.; Buring, J.E.; Ridker, P.M.; Schurks, M.; Kurth, T. Selectivity in genetic association with sub-classified migraine in women. *PLoS Genet.* **2014**, *10*, e1004366. [CrossRef] [PubMed]
39. Chasman, D.I.; Schurks, M.; Anttila, V.; de Vries, B.; Schminke, U.; Launer, L.J.; Terwindt, G.M.; van den Maagdenberg, A.M.; Fendrich, K.; Volzke, H.; et al. Genome-wide association study reveals three susceptibility loci for common migraine in the general population. *Nat. Genet.* **2011**, *43*, 695–698. [CrossRef] [PubMed]
40. Freilinger, T.; Anttila, V.; de Vries, B.; Malik, R.; Kallela, M.; Terwindt, G.M.; Pozo-Rosich, P.; Winsvold, B.; Nyholt, D.R.; van Oosterhout, W.P.; et al. Genome-wide association analysis identifies susceptibility loci for migraine without aura. *Nat. Genet.* **2012**, *44*, 777–782. [CrossRef] [PubMed]
41. Esserlind, A.L.; Christensen, A.F.; Le, H.; Kirchmann, M.; Hauge, A.W.; Toyserkani, N.M.; Hansen, T.; Grarup, N.; Werge, T.; Steinberg, S.; et al. Replication and meta-analysis of common variants identifies a genome-wide significant locus in migraine. *Eur. J. Neurol.* **2013**, *20*, 765–772. [CrossRef] [PubMed]
42. Zhao, H.; Eising, E.; de Vries, B.; Vijfhuizen, L.S.; International Headache Genetics Consortium; Anttila, V.; Winsvold, B.S.; Kurth, T.; Stefansson, H.; Kallela, M.; et al. Gene-based pleiotropy across migraine with aura and migraine without aura patient groups. *Cephalalgia* **2016**, *36*, 648–657. [CrossRef] [PubMed]
43. Carreno, O.; Corominas, R.; Fernandez-Morales, J.; Camina, M.; Sobrido, M.J.; Fernandez-Fernandez, J.M.; Pozo-Rosich, P.; Cormand, B.; Macaya, A. SNP variants within the vanilloid TRPV1 and TRPV3 receptor genes are associated with migraine in the Spanish population. *Am. J. Med. Genet. B Neuropsychiatr. Genet.* **2012**, *159B*, 94–103. [CrossRef] [PubMed]
44. An, X.K.; Ma, Q.L.; Lin, Q.; Zhang, X.R.; Lu, C.X.; Qu, H.L. PRDM16 rs2651899 variant is a risk factor for Chinese common migraine patients. *Headache* **2013**, *53*, 1595–1601. [CrossRef] [PubMed]
45. Ghosh, J.; Pradhan, S.; Mittal, B. Genome-wide-associated variants in migraine susceptibility: A replication study from North India. *Headache* **2013**, *53*, 1583–1594. [CrossRef] [PubMed]
46. Sintas, C.; Fernandez-Morales, J.; Vila-Pueyo, M.; Narberhaus, B.; Arenas, C.; Pozo-Rosich, P.; Macaya, A.; Cormand, B. Replication study of previous migraine genome-wide association study findings in a Spanish sample of migraine with aura. *Cephalalgia* **2015**, *35*, 776–782. [CrossRef] [PubMed]

47. Fan, X.; Wang, J.; Fan, W.; Chen, L.; Gui, B.; Tan, G.; Zhou, J. Replication of migraine GWAS susceptibility loci in Chinese Han population. *Headache* **2014**, *54*, 709–715. [CrossRef] [PubMed]
48. Burgos-Vega, C.C.; Ahn, D.D.; Bischoff, C.; Wang, W.; Horne, D.; Wang, J.; Gavva, N.; Dussor, G. Meningeal transient receptor potential channel M8 activation causes cutaneous facial and hindpaw allodynia in a preclinical rodent model of headache. *Cephalalgia* **2016**, *36*, 185–193. [CrossRef] [PubMed]
49. Huang, D.; Li, S.; Dhaka, A.; Story, G.M.; Cao, Y.Q. Expression of the transient receptor potential channels TRPV1, TRPA1 and TRPM8 in mouse trigeminal primary afferent neurons innervating the dura. *Mol. Pain* **2012**, *8*, 66. [CrossRef] [PubMed]
50. Dussor, G.; Yan, J.; Xie, J.Y.; Ossipov, M.H.; Dodick, D.W.; Porreca, F. Targeting TRP channels for novel migraine therapeutics. *ACS Chem. Neurosci.* **2014**, *5*, 1085–1096. [CrossRef] [PubMed]
51. Lehto, S.G.; Weyer, A.D.; Zhang, M.; Youngblood, B.D.; Wang, J.; Wang, W.; Kerstein, P.C.; Davis, C.; Wild, K.D.; Stucky, C.L.; et al. AMG2850, a potent and selective TRPM8 antagonist, is not effective in rat models of inflammatory mechanical hypersensitivity and neuropathic tactile allodynia. *Naunyn Schmiedebergs Arch. Pharmacol.* **2015**, *388*, 465–476. [CrossRef] [PubMed]
52. Gaudioso, C.; Hao, J.; Martin-Eauclaire, M.F.; Gabriac, M.; Delmas, P. Menthol pain relief through cumulative inactivation of voltage-gated sodium channels. *Pain* **2012**, *153*, 473–484. [CrossRef] [PubMed]
53. Namer, B.; Seifert, F.; Handwerker, H.O.; Maihofner, C. TRPA1 and TRPM8 activation in humans: Effects of cinnamaldehyde and menthol. *Neuroreport* **2005**, *16*, 955–959. [CrossRef] [PubMed]
54. Wasner, G.; Schattschneider, J.; Binder, A.; Baron, R. Topical menthol–a human model for cold pain by activation and sensitization of C nociceptors. *Brain* **2004**, *127*, 1159–1171. [CrossRef] [PubMed]
55. Hatem, S.; Attal, N.; Willer, J.C.; Bouhassira, D. Psychophysical study of the effects of topical application of menthol in healthy volunteers. *Pain* **2006**, *122*, 190–196. [CrossRef] [PubMed]
56. DeFalco, J.; Duncton, M.A.; Emerling, D. TRPM8 biology and medicinal chemistry. *Curr. Top. Med. Chem.* **2011**, *11*, 2237–2252. [CrossRef] [PubMed]
57. Eid, S.R. Therapeutic targeting of TRP channels–the TR(i)P to pain relief. *Curr. Top. Med. Chem.* **2011**, *11*, 2118–2130. [CrossRef] [PubMed]
58. Premkumar, L.S.; Abooj, M. TRP channels and analgesia. *Life Sci.* **2013**, *92*, 415–424. [CrossRef] [PubMed]
59. Feketa, V.V.; Zhang, Y.; Cao, Z.; Balasubramanian, A.; Flores, C.M.; Player, M.R.; Marrelli, S.P. Transient receptor potential melastatin 8 channel inhibition potentiates the hypothermic response to transient receptor potential vanilloid 1 activation in the conscious mouse. *Crit. Care Med.* **2014**, *42*, e355–e363. [CrossRef] [PubMed]
60. Zhu, B.; Xia, M.; Xu, X.; Ludovici, D.W.; Tennakoon, M.; Youngman, M.A.; Matthews, J.M.; Dax, S.L.; Colburn, R.W.; Qin, N.; et al. Arylglycine derivatives as potent transient receptor potential melastatin 8 (TRPM8) antagonists. *Bioorg. Med. Chem. Lett.* **2013**, *23*, 2234–2237. [CrossRef] [PubMed]
61. Matthews, J.M.; Qin, N.; Colburn, R.W.; Dax, S.L.; Hawkins, M.; McNally, J.J.; Reany, L.; Youngman, M.A.; Baker, J.; Hutchinson, T.; et al. The design and synthesis of novel, phosphonate-containing transient receptor potential melastatin 8 (TRPM8) antagonists. *Bioorg. Med. Chem. Lett.* **2012**, *22*, 2922–2926. [CrossRef] [PubMed]
62. Calvo, R.R.; Meegalla, S.K.; Parks, D.J.; Parsons, W.H.; Ballentine, S.K.; Lubin, M.L.; Schneider, C.; Colburn, R.W.; Flores, C.M.; Player, M.R. Discovery of vinylcycloalkyl-substituted benzimidazole TRPM8 antagonists effective in the treatment of cold allodynia. *Bioorg. Med. Chem. Lett.* **2012**, *22*, 1903–1907. [CrossRef] [PubMed]
63. Parks, D.J.; Parsons, W.H.; Colburn, R.W.; Meegalla, S.K.; Ballentine, S.K.; Illig, C.R.; Qin, N.; Liu, Y.; Hutchinson, T.L.; Lubin, M.L.; et al. Design and optimization of benzimidazole-containing transient receptor potential melastatin 8 (TRPM8) antagonists. *J. Med. Chem.* **2011**, *54*, 233–247. [CrossRef] [PubMed]
64. Chaudhari, S.S.; Kadam, A.B.; Khairatkar-Joshi, N.; Mukhopadhyay, I.; Karnik, P.V.; Raghuram, A.; Rao, S.S.; Vaiyapuri, T.S.; Wale, D.P.; Bhosale, V.M.; et al. Synthesis and pharmacological evaluation of novel *N*-aryl-3,4-dihydro-1′H-spiro[chromene-2,4′-piperidine]-1′-carboxamides as TRPM8 antagonists. *Bioorg. Med. Chem. Lett.* **2013**, *21*, 6542–6553. [CrossRef] [PubMed]
65. Ohmi, M.; Shishido, Y.; Inoue, T.; Ando, K.; Fujiuchi, A.; Yamada, A.; Watanabe, S.; Kawamura, K. Identification of a novel 2-pyridyl-benzensulfonamide derivative, RQ-00203078, as a selective and orally active TRPM8 antagonist. *Bioorg. Med. Chem. Lett.* **2014**, *24*, 5364–5368. [CrossRef] [PubMed]

66. Tamayo, N.A.; Bo, Y.; Gore, V.; Ma, V.; Nishimura, N.; Tang, P.; Deng, H.; Klionsky, L.; Lehto, S.G.; Wang, W.; et al. Fused piperidines as a novel class of potent and orally available transient receptor potential melastatin type 8 (TRPM8) antagonists. *J. Med. Chem.* **2012**, *55*, 1593–1611. [CrossRef] [PubMed]
67. Horne, D.B.; Tamayo, N.A.; Bartberger, M.D.; Bo, Y.; Clarine, J.; Davis, C.D.; Gore, V.K.; Kaller, M.R.; Lehto, S.G.; Ma, V.V.; et al. Optimization of Potency and Pharmacokinetic Properties of Tetrahydroisoquinoline Transient Receptor Potential Melastatin 8 (TRPM8) Antagonists. *J. Med. Chem.* **2014**, *57*, 2989–3004. [CrossRef] [PubMed]
68. Andrews, M.D.; Af Forselles, K.; Beaumont, K.; Galan, S.R.; Glossop, P.A.; Grenie, M.; Jessiman, A.; Kenyon, A.S.; Lunn, G.; Maw, G.; et al. Discovery of a Selective TRPM8 Antagonist with Clinical Efficacy in Cold-Related Pain. *ACS Med. Chem. Lett.* **2015**, *6*, 419–424. [CrossRef] [PubMed]
69. Almeida, M.C.; Hew-Butler, T.; Soriano, R.N.; Rao, S.; Wang, W.; Wang, J.; Tamayo, N.; Oliveira, D.L.; Nucci, T.B.; Aryal, P.; et al. Pharmacological blockade of the cold receptor TRPM8 attenuates autonomic and behavioral cold defenses and decreases deep body temperature. *J. Neurosci.* **2012**, *32*, 2086–2099. [CrossRef] [PubMed]
70. Miller, S.; Rao, S.; Wang, W.; Liu, H.; Wang, J.; Gavva, N.R. Antibodies to the extracellular pore loop of TRPM8 act as antagonists of channel activation. *PLoS ONE* **2014**, *9*, e107151. [CrossRef] [PubMed]
71. Gavva, N.R.; Davis, C.; Lehto, S.G.; Rao, S.; Wang, W.; Zhu, D.X. Transient receptor potential melastatin 8 (TRPM8) channels are involved in body temperature regulation. *Mol. Pain* **2012**, *8*, 36. [CrossRef] [PubMed]
72. Grisold, W.; Cavaletti, G.; Windebank, A.J. Peripheral neuropathies from chemotherapeutics and targeted agents: Diagnosis, treatment, and prevention. *Neuro-Oncology* **2012**. [CrossRef] [PubMed]
73. Windebank, A.J.; Grisold, W. Chemotherapy-induced neuropathy. *J. Peripher. Nerv. Syst.* **2008**, *13*, 27–46. [CrossRef] [PubMed]
74. Pachman, D.R.; Barton, D.L.; Watson, J.C.; Loprinzi, C.L. Chemotherapy-induced peripheral neuropathy: Prevention and treatment. *Clin. Pharmacol. Ther.* **2011**, *90*, 377–387. [CrossRef] [PubMed]
75. Basso, L.; Altier, C. Transient Receptor Potential Channels in neuropathic pain. *Curr. Opin. Pharmacol.* **2016**, *32*, 9–15. [CrossRef] [PubMed]
76. Clinical Trials.gov. Available online: https://clinicaltrials.gov/ (accessed on 24 March 2017).

14

Blocking TRPA1 in Respiratory Disorders: Does it Hold a Promise?

Indranil Mukhopadhyay, Abhay Kulkarni and Neelima Khairatkar-Joshi *

Biological Research, Glenmark Research Centre, Glenmark Pharmaceuticals Ltd. Navi Mumbai, Maharashtra 400709, India; Indranil.Mukhopadhyay@glenmarkpharma.com (I.M.); Abhay.Kulkarni@glenmarkpharma.com (A.K.)

* Correspondence: Neelima.Joshi@glenmarkpharma.com

Academic Editors: Arpad Szallasi and Jean Jacques Vanden Eynde

Abstract: Transient Receptor Potential Ankyrin 1 (TRPA1) ion channel is expressed abundantly on the C fibers that innervate almost entire respiratory tract starting from oral cavity and oropharynx, conducting airways in the trachea, bronchi, terminal bronchioles, respiratory bronchioles and upto alveolar ducts and alveoli. Functional presence of TRPA1 on non-neuronal cells got recognized recently. TRPA1 plays a well-recognized role of "chemosensor", detecting presence of exogenous irritants and endogenous pro-inflammatory mediators that are implicated in airway inflammation and sensory symptoms like chronic cough, asthma, chronic obstructive pulmonary disease (COPD), allergic rhinitis and cystic fibrosis. TRPA1 can remain activated chronically due to elevated levels and continued presence of such endogenous ligands and pro-inflammatory mediators. Several selective TRPA1 antagonists have been tested in animal models of respiratory disease and their performance is very promising. Although there is no TRPA1 antagonist in advanced clinical trials or approved on market yet to treat respiratory diseases, however, limited but promising evidences available so far indicate likelihood that targeting TRPA1 may present a new therapy in treatment of respiratory diseases in near future. This review will focus on in vitro, animal and human evidences that strengthen the proposed role of TRPA1 in modulation of specific airway sensory responses and also on preclinical and clinical progress of selected TRPA1 antagonists.

Keywords: TRPA1; airway inflammation; airway sensory responses; asthma; COPD; cough

---

1. TRPA1 Receptor

TRPA1 ion channel and its biology is known for more than a decade now. It has attracted academic scientists due to its interesting tissue distribution and functions. TRPA1 is abundantly expressed in peripheral nervous system and has demonstrated a chemosensory function. Hence, it has been assigned a role of "warning system" against external as well as internal assaults. Industrial researchers are interested in TRPA1 as a target for therapeutic intervention due to its implicated role in miscellaneous diseases. Evidence for potential role of TRPA1 in pain signaling based on TRPA1 knockout (TRPA1 KO) mice and siRNA studies emerged much earlier compared to its involvement in airway diseases—which is relatively recent and still emerging. TRPA1 is highly expressed on pulmonary innervation—an anatomically relevant region for respiratory diseases, and could be one of the major players in orchestration of airway inflammatory response. A large number of recent studies have implicated TRPA1 in the pathogenesis of several respiratory diseases including chronic cough, asthma, COPD, allergic rhinitis and cystic fibrosis. Blockade of TRPA1 is perceived as a novel strategy for its therapeutic intervention.

2. TRPA1—Expression and Activation in Airways

TRPA1 was first identified in cultured human lung fibroblasts [1]. Later on, TRPA1 expression on mouse lung was reported, albeit to a lesser extent compared to other tissues [2]. TRPA1 is abundantly expressed on the innervations of almost entire respiratory tract including the C-fibers of the trigeminal and vagal ganglia, which innervate upper regions of oral cavity and oropharynx and on conducting airways in the trachea, bronchi, terminal bronchioles, respiratory bronchioles, alveolar ducts and alveoli. C-fibers largely "sense" the presence of potentially toxic inhaled irritants and toxicants. TRPA1 was initially recognized as an irritant sensing ion channel on majority of vagal nociceptive C-fibers in the bronchopulmonary region [3]. It is well known now that unlike traditional chemoreceptors, TRPA1 is activated by a wide variety of structurally different molecules with high chemical reactivity spanning from exogenous irritants to endogenously produced reactive reagents [4–11]. Functional presence of TRPA1 on non-neuronal cells got recognized recently. TRPA1 is shown to be expressed on lung fibroblasts, epithelial and smooth muscle cells [12–15].

The role of TRPA1 in airway pathologies has been corroborated by studies using the TRPA1 KO mice and TRPA1 antagonists. In wild-type mice, airway exposure to hypochlorite or Hydrogen peroxide (H_2O_2) evoke respiratory depression as manifested by a reduction in breathing frequency and increase in end expiratory pause, both of which were attenuated in TRPA1 KO mice [6]. A host of chemicals are known to be specifically associated with respiratory diseases and airway reflex responses such as coughing, sneezing and bronchoconstriction. Acrolein and crotonaldehyde induce strong tussive response in animals as well as in man. H_2O_2, 4-Hydroxynonenal (4-HNE), photochemical smog, zinc, toluene diisocyanate are associated with allergic asthma in humans. All the above listed chemicals are direct and potent activators of TRPA1. α,β-unsaturated aldehydes are earliest recognized TRPA1 activators, and are detected in air spaces, breath, sputum, lungs, and blood from patients with asthma as well as COPD. Fragrance chemicals like menthol, 1,8-Cineole, borneol, fenchyl alcohol etc. are associated with TRPA1 activation and play a key role in allergic reactions [16]. Cigarette smoke, wood smoke, diesel exhaust, and other combustion-derived particles activate TRPA1, causing irritation and inflammation in the respiratory tract [17,18]. TRPA1 is a molecular sensor for wood smoke particulate and several chemical constituents such as 3,5-ditert-butylphenol, coniferaldehyde, formaldehyde, perinaphthenone, agathic acid, and isocupressic acid are TRPA1 agonists [18]. Nassini R et al. [14] demonstrated that TRPA1 is expressed in non-neuronal cells in human and murine airways, and promote a non-neurogenic inflammatory response. This raises an alternate possibility that airway inflammation may also be promoted by non-neuronal mediators. Thus, TRPA1 ion channel with its wide range of expression in neuronal and non-neuronal cells and its activation by several exogenous and endogenous stimuli relevant to airway sensory responses may be a major regulator in driving several respiratory diseases.

3. TRPA1 in Chronic Cough

Cough is a vagally mediated defensive mechanism to protect the airway to clear respiratory tract from continuously exposed airborne environmental irritants. Despite wide prevalence of chronic cough, therapy options are very inadequate and often symptomatic. Currently available treatments such as dextromethorphan, hydrocodone and codeine are inadequate due to limited efficacy, central nervous system (CNS) side effects or abuse liability, respiratory depression and gastrointestinal disturbances. The paucity, if not absence of effective medicine to treat cough is mainly because the molecular mechanisms that orchestrate chronic cough are not clearly understood in experimental animal models as well as in man. Scientists are attempting to shed some light on the possible mechanism behind the occurrence of chronic cough. A number of TRP channels (TRPA1, TRPV1 and TRPV4) have been linked to sensory perception relevant to cough response [19]. A large number of in vitro and in vivo studies have recently indicated important role of TRPA1 activation in driving cough reflex. Acrolein and crotonaldehyde are contained in cigarette smoke and polluted air which are well recognized cough inducers. TRPA1 agonists are shown to induce activation of recombinant human TRPA1 channels in vitro in human embryonic kidney cells (HEK293), depolarization of murine, guinea pig and human vagal sensory nerves and produce cough in healthy human volunteers [20]. Allyl isothiocyanate (AITC), acrolein, crotonaldehyde and cinnamaldehyde—all are potent TRPA1 agonists and shown to induce dose dependent and robust tussive response in guinea pigs which was attenuated by non-selective TRP channel blockers (camphor, gentamicin) as well as by selective TRPA1 antagonist from Hydra Biosciences—HC-030031 (Figure 1) [9]. The cough response however remained unchanged upon administration of capsazepine which is a TRPV1 antagonist as well as desensitizing TRPA1 agonist [21]. We demonstrated direct in vitro activation of TRPA1 receptor by citric acid which is routinely used to evoke cough in preclinical and clinical studies [22]. Citric acid induced tussive response in guinea pigs was inhibited by a potent and selective TRPA1 antagonist from our laboratory, GRC 17536 (structure not disclosed). Anti-tussive effect of other TRPA1 antagonists is also demonstrated in animal cough model. Recently, a poster from Almirall at European Respiratory Society Conference (2015) reported a potent oral TRPA1 antagonist-Compound A, that showed inhibition of isolated guinea pig vagus nerve depolarization with EC_{50} of 80 nM. Furthermore, in the in vivo model of AITC induced cough, Compound-A showed dose dependent inhibition of cough response with ED_{50} of 0.17 mg/kg dose [23].

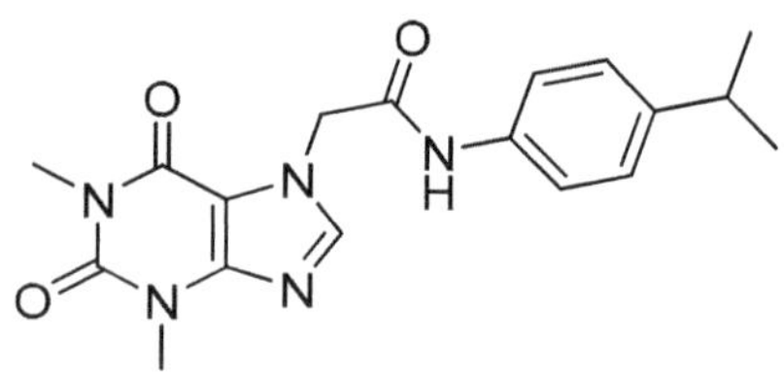

HC-030031

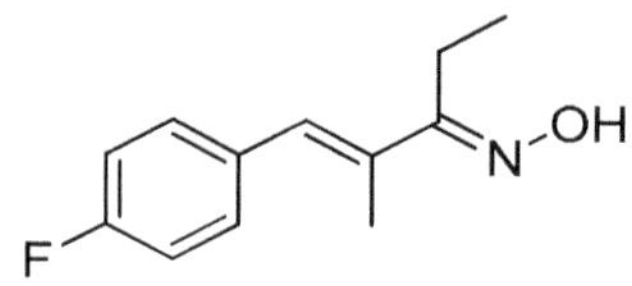

A-967079

Figure 1. Chemical structure of Hydra Biosciences (HC-030031) and Abbott (A-967079).

Importantly, TRPA1 mediated tussive response is associated with both exogenous TRPA1 agonists as well as endogenous biochemicals that are produced during diseases associated with cough. For example, prostaglandin E2 (PGE_2) and bradykinin are produced during tissue inflammation. Mucoid secretions containing similar pro-tussive inflammatory mediators are produced in patients with post nasal drip syndrome (PNDS). 4-HNE, reactive oxygen species (ROS), reactive nitrogen species (RNS), 15-deoxy-delta-12,14-prostaglandin J2 (15d-PGJ_2) are produced in the airways during asthma, COPD and in the esophagus during gastroesophageal reflux disease (GERD) [24] and lastly, toll like receptors (TLRs) that are produced during post viral cough condition. [25–27]. Thus, TRPA1 could have a central role in producing chronic cough associated with diverse pathologies but via a common mechanism of vagal nerve activation due to its activators prevailing during specific diseases as described above [9,20,28,29]. Hence TRPA1 has emerged as one of the most promising targets for the development of medicines to treat chronic cough.

4. TRPA1 and Asthma

Asthma is an inflammatory disease of the lungs characterized by bronchoconstriction and airway hyperreactivity, leading to shortness of breath, wheezing, and coughing. It is triggered by exposure to allergen or irritant and manifested as episodes or attacks of airway narrowing that are mediated by airway nerves and muscles. Studies focusing on airway smooth muscle and epithelial function strongly indicate involvement of immunogenic and neurogenic mechanisms in airway inflammation. TRPA1 could be a key integrator of immune and neuronal signaling in the airways [30].

Various noxious chemicals and environmental/industrial irritants that activate TRPA1 happen to be triggers for asthma or reactive airways dysfunction syndrome (RADS) and are known to worsen asthma attacks [31]. Toluene diisocyanate is a potent TRPA1 activator and exposure to this chemical is the leading cause of occupational asthma. Exposure to cigarette smoke strongly correlates with asthma severity. Cigarette smoke ingredients-acrolein and crotonaldehyde activate native and recombinant TRPA1 and produce tracheal extravasation in wild type animals in TRPA1 dependent manner. Asthmatics are sensitive to photochemical smog that contains acrolein and other oxidant species which are also known to activate TRPA1. Several TRPA1 activators or sensitizers are endogenously produced in lungs of patients which are also efficient triggers of asthma e.g., H_2O_2, 4-HNE, cyclic prostaglandin PGJ_2 and bradykinin. Elevated levels of bradykinin and nerve growth factor (NGF) are found in bronchoalveolar lavage of asthma and rhinitis patients while elevated 4-HNE and acrolein are detected in lungs, air spaces, breath, sputum and blood of asthma and COPD patients. Experiments with TRPA1 KO mice revealed reduced airway infiltration by inflammatory leukocytes accompanied by decreased production of pro-inflammatory cytokines and neuropeptide release in the airways in the ovalbumin (OVA) asthma model [30]. In the wild type mice that developed asthma upon OVA challenge, pharmacological blockade of TRPA1 receptor with HC-030031 reiterated the above observation. HC-030031 also inhibited OVA-induced late asthmatic response in dose dependent manner in B/N rats [32]. During late asthmatic response, allergen challenge is implicated to trigger airway sensory nerves via TRPA1 activation to further initiate a central reflex event. A couple of recent posters presented in conferences have reported similar findings as above using TRPA1 selective antagonists [33,34]. GRC 17536 showed significant inhibition of lung eosinophilia, mucus production and airway hyperresponsiveness in mouse asthma model, and, inhibition of eosinophils and early airway reactivity in guinea pig allergic asthma model [33]. Another TRPA1 antagonist from Cubist Pharmaceuticals, CB-625 (structure not disclosed), was effective in reducing the late asthmatic response and antigen induced airway hyperresponsiveness upon oral dosing in sheep model of asthma [34]. Epidemiological evidence has linked therapeutic acetaminophen doses with risk of COPD and asthma [35]. Recent studies by Nassini et al. [36] demonstrated that *N*-acetyl-p-benzoquinoneimine (NAPQ1), a metabolite of acetaminophen, evoked pro-inflammatory responses in the lung. They further demonstrated that NAPQ1 selectively activates TRPA1, and selective inhibition of TRPA1 abated the pro-inflammatory effect of acetaminophen. It remains to be seen if TRPA1 antagonists attenuate asthma in clinics.

5. Role of TRPA1 in COPD

COPD is a disease characterized by increased infiltration of inflammatory cells in the lung, increased oxidative and nitrosative burden in the lung and parenchymal destruction, associated with progressive decline in lung function. COPD is strongly associated with smoking status of an individual but other environmental factors such as bio mass fuel exposure are also implicated in the etiology of COPD [37].

TRPA1 is shown to be a major neuronal sensor for oxidants in the airways [6]. Various pollutants, oxidants, cigarette smoke extract (CSE) and cigarette smoke (CS) ingredients such as acrolein, crotonaldehyde, 4-HNE that are associated with the pathobiology of COPD, are potent agonists of TRPA1. Some of these are associated with interleukin 8 (IL8) release in the human macrophagic cell lines [7,38]. Our TRPA1 antagonist GRC 17536 was effective in inhibiting CSE, crotonaldehyde and acrolein induced Ca^{2+} influx in vitro and AITC induced Ca^{2+} influx and IL8 production in human lung fibroblast cells (CCD19-Lu) and human pulmonary alveolar epithelial cell line (A549) [22]. CSE induced increase in TRPA1 expression and IL8 release in human bronchial epithelial cells (HBEC) was attenuated by HC-030031 [39].

Further corroborating evidence to support the role of TRPA1 in COPD came from the studies in animal models of COPD. CS and acrolein induced release of keratinocyte chemoattractant (KC) (CXCL1/GRO alpha; mouse homolog of human IL-8) in bronchoalveolar lavage fluid (BALf) of mice was significantly reduced in TRPA1 KO mice [14]. Pretreatment of animals with HC-030031 showed protection from CS induced plasma protein extravasation whereas capsazepine was not effective suggesting selective involvement of TRPA1 in inducing CS associated inflammation. When C57BL/6 mice was exposed to CS for 4 weeks, significant increase in TRPA1 mRNA was observed in trigeminal and nodose/jugular ganglia of CS-exposed mice with a positive correlation to cellular infiltration. An increase in leukocytes, macrophages and neutrophils was observed in BALf of mice [40]. Increased immunostaining for TRPA1 was observed in wild type mice chronically exposed to CS whereas TRPA1 KO mice revealed reduced inflammation and structural changes [39]. All these observations suggest strong involvement of TRPA1 in mediating CS induced inflammation in the animal models.

Although COPD is directly linked to the smoking history, recently it was shown that other factors like biomass fuels and biomass smoke exposure is also a risk factor for COPD development [41]. Wood smoke and its chemical constituents are activators of TRPA1 and are known for their damaging effects on respiratory system. Wood smoke particulate matter (WSPM) at low concentration, which is relevant in terms of potential human exposure levels are known to activate TRPA1 [18]. There is ample evidence to show involvement of TRPA1 in COPD and TRPA1 antagonists seem promising treatment options in clinical management of COPD.

6. Role of TRPA1 in Allergic Rhinitis

Allergic rhinitis and asthma are chronic inflammatory atopic disorders characterized by overlapping symptoms and pathophysiology. Toluene diisocyanate (TDI) is a highly reactive chemical associated with respiratory symptoms resembling allergic rhinitis and a most prevalent cause of occupational asthma [42,43]. Exposure of mice to TDI showed decreased breathing rates, increased cytokines accompanied by increased eosinophils and allergic inflammation in nasal cavity [44]. It is an effective TRPA1 activator with in vitro EC_{50} of 10 μM which is a physiologically relevant concentration known to cause decreased breathing rate and sensory irritation in mice. Interestingly, these symptoms were absent in TRPA1 KO mice [45] suggesting an important role of TRPA1 in allergic or occupational asthma and rhinitis. A recent study showed increased level of TRPA1 mRNA in subjects with rhinitis compared to normal controls ($p = 0.03$) suggesting potential involvement of TRPA1 in allergic rhinitis [46].

7. Role of TRPA1 in Cystic Fibrosis

Cystic fibrosis (CF) is a disease associated with mutation in the gene for cystic fibrosis transmembrane conductance regulator (CFTR) and can affect many organs. When upper and lower airways are involved, it causes impaired mucociliary clearance leading to mucus plugging in the airways, failure in effective clearing of inhaled bacteria and lung neutrophilia. Respiratory failure is a major cause of mortality associated with CF. Recently TRPA1 expression was reported on different epithelial cells obtained from lung tissues of CF patients [47]. IL8 expression was observed in the bronchial epithelial cells co-expressing TRPA1. Furthermore TRPA1 specific inhibitors from Hydra Biosciences (HC-030031) and Abbott (A-967079) (Figure 1) [48] inhibited *P. aeruginosa* induced transcription of IL8, IL1b, IL6 and tumor necrosis factor α (TNFα) in A549 and human cystic fibrosis cell line (CuFi-1). *P. aeruginosa* is a gram negative bacteria and releases lipopolysaccharide (LPS) which is a direct TRPA1 agonist and sensitizer [49]. Silencing TRPA1 significantly reduced the release of IL-8, IL-1β and TNF-α from HBECs from CF patients. This is the first study which revealed the potential of TRPA1 antagonists in controlling inflammation associated with CF.

8. TRPA1 Antagonists: What's the Status?

Till date, there is limited published literature showing efficacy of TRPA1 antagonists in respiratory diseases. The accumulating evidence supporting TRPA1 as an attractive target in respiratory disease has resulted in large number of small molecules patents (Table 1). Some of the compounds have been evaluated in animal models of respiratory diseases as summarized in earlier sections and the data is very encouraging. However it remains to be seen if such promising results in animal will eventually translate to efficacy in humans. Until then, translational studies to assess their pharmacological effects on patient derived lung tissues ex vivo could strengthen the claim of their potential utility to treat human respiratory diseases. Such study tools are established for assessing translatability of TRPA1 antagonist pharmacology in pain where in calcitonin gene-related peptide (CGRP) release from human dental pulp is assayed as a biomarker. Recently, TRPA1 antagonist—GRC 17536 from our laboratory has shown positive proof of concept in reducing peripheral diabetic neuropathic pain in patients with intact nerves [50]. The clinical features of chronic pain and refractory chronic cough seem overlapping. Clinical presentation of chronic pain typically includes paraesthesia (abnormal sensation in the absence of a stimulus), hyperalgesia (pain triggered by a low exposure to a known painful stimulus), and allodynia (pain triggered by a non-painful stimulus) and shows similarities with the clinical features of refractory chronic cough, such as an abnormal throat sensation or tickle (laryngeal paraesthesia), increased cough sensitivity in response to known tussigens (hypertussia), and cough triggered in response to non-tussive stimuli such as talking or cold air (allotussia). Gabapentin, which is used to treat neuropathic pain, is also reported to show antitussive effect in human chronic cough patients recently [51]. Hence there is optimism to believe that TRPA1 antagonists could work in treatment of chronic cough.

Table 1. TRPA1 in Respiratory Diseases: A Patent Update.

Patent Number	Owner Companies	Indications
WO2013084153; WO2013014597; WO2012176143; WO2012172475; WO2012176105; WO2011132017; WO2014203210; WO2010125469; WO2010004390; WO2010109287; WO2013183035; WO2009118596; WO2012085662; WO2009144548; WO2011114184	Glenmark Pharmaceuticals SA	Asthma; COPD; Bronchitis, COPD, Cough, Respiratory disorder
WO2009140517; WO2010132838; WO2007073505; WO2010039289; WO2015164643; WO2016044792; WO2010036821	Hydra Biosciences Inc.	Asthma, Cough; Respiratory disease; Asthma; COPD; Lung injury
WO2009071631; WO2010141805	Janssen Pharmaceutica NV	COPD; Lung disease; Cough
WO2015052264; WO2014060341; WO2014056958; WO2014049047; WO2014072325	F Hoffmann-La Roche AG; Hoffmann-La Roche Inc.; Roche Holding AG Genentech Inc.	Asthma; COPD; Cough; Allergic rhinitis; Respiratory disease; Bronchospasm
WO2015144976; WO2012152983; WO2014053694; WO2015144977	Orion Corp	Asthma; COPD; Cough
WO2013023102; WO2014113671	Cubist Pharmaceuticals Inc.; Hydra Biosciences Inc.	Asthma; COPD; Respiratory disease
WO2015115507; WO2014098098; WO2013108857	Ajinomoto Co Inc.	Asthma; COPD; Cough; Lung disease
JP2014024810	Kao Corp	Respiratory failure
WO2009089082	AbbVie Deutschland GmbH & Co KG; Abbott Laboratories	Lung disease
WO2016028325	Duke University; University of California	Fibrosis
WO2015155306	Almirall Prodesfarma SA	Respiratory disease
WO2014135617	Ario Pharma Ltd; PharmEste SRL	Asthma; COPD; Cough

As far as COPD is concerned, cigarette smoke and wood smoke have a close and proven involvement in COPD pathobiology. Constituents of cigarette smoke and wood smoke are potent activators of TRPA1. Hence, TRPA1 antagonists such as GRC 17536, which have started to show promising clinical benefits in human pain proof of concept trials, could also be effective in treating respiratory diseases. Several pharmaceutical companies have active drug discovery programs targeting TRPA1 receptor for potential treatment of miscellaneous respiratory disorders (Table 1).

9. TRPA1 Antagonists: Any Safety Concerns?

TRPA1 KO mice are viable, normal in appearance and fertile with no auditory dysfunction [4,52]. Unlike TRPV1 or TRPM8, TRPA1 is not involved in body temperature regulation at basal level or under cold challenge [53,54]. Hence TRPA1 antagonists are expected to be devoid of adverse effects on body temperature unlike the TRPV1 antagonists (hyperthermia) or TRPM8 antagonists (hypothermia). Human healthy volunteers administered with CB-625 show normal body temperature and also unimpaired thermosensation in heat and cold tests [55]. This is in line with TRPA1 KO mice data that exhibits unimpaired heat and cold sensitivity [4]. Also, wild type (WT) animals in spinal nerve ligation (SNL) nerve injury model when treated with antisense TRPA1 were protected against cold hyperalgesia while showing no effect on normal cold sensitivity [56]. Animals treated with TRPA1 antagonist have normal performance in hot and cold plate tests and no paradoxical sensation [53].

Although TRPA1 is predominantly expressed in sensory neurons, it is also expressed in other non-neuronal tissues, albeit at a much lower level. This raises a question if targeting TRPA1 could have unintended/unrecognized adverse effects on physiological functions or on known protective functions such as sensing environmental irritants. TRPA1 KO mice are recently reported to show physical hyperactivity [57]. Since several TRPA1 antagonists are at different stages of evaluation including chemical synthesis, preclinical studies and clinical trials, their long term safety in patients is likely to be addressed soon.

10. Summary

The role of TRPA1 in the respiratory system has been summarized in Figure 2. TRPA1 is expressed on pulmonary innervation - an anatomically relevant region for respiratory diseases and implicated in the orchestration of inflammatory response in animal models of airway diseases, including chronic cough, asthma, COPD, allergic rhinitis and cystic fibrosis. TRPA1 can remain activated chronically due to elevated levels and continued presence of endogenous ligands and pro-inflammatory mediators. Phenotype of TRPA1 KO mice in allergen-induced asthma model and CS model is in line with this since these animals show reduced leukocyte infiltration in the airways, reduction of cytokine and mucus production.

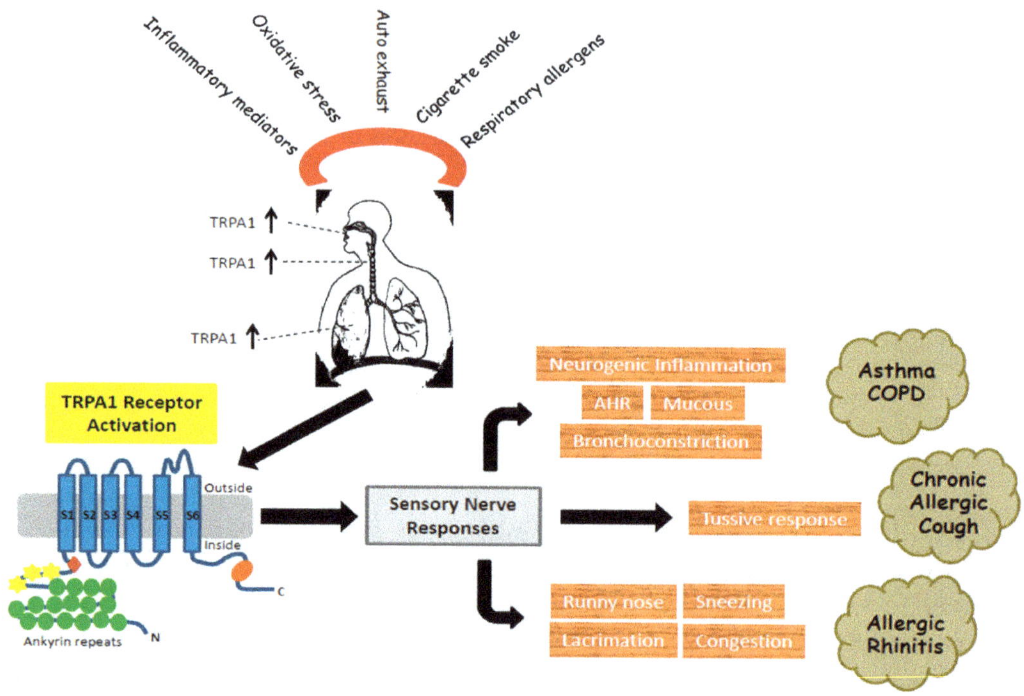

Figure 2. TRPA1 in respiratory diseases.

Preclinical performance of TRPA1 antagonists in respiratory disease models is promising. There is no TRPA1 antagonist in advanced clinical trials or approved on market yet to treat respiratory diseases. We are in the wait to see if they can attenuate undesirable airway sensory responses in man and additionally if they are capable of reversing disease progression and outperform current standard of care such as anti-inflammatory drugs. Available evidences and underlying science indicate likelihood that they may live up to the expectations and help clinicians in treatment of chronic airway diseases with unmet medical need in near future.

Abbreviations

TRPA1	Transient Receptor Potential Ankyrin 1
COPD	Chronic obstructive pulmonary disease
TRPA1 KO	TRPA1 knockout
H_2O_2	Hydrogen peroxide
4-HNE	4-Hydroxynonenal
CNS	Central nervous system
HEK293	Human embryonic kidney cells
AITC	Allyl isothiocyanate
PGE_2	Prostaglandin E2
PNDS	Post nasal drip syndrome
ROS	Reactive oxygen species
RNS	Reactive nitrogen species
15d-PGJ_2	15-deoxy-delta-12,14-prostaglandin J2
GERD	Gastroesophageal reflux disease
TLRs	Toll like receptors
RADS	Reactive airways dysfunction syndrome
NGF	Nerve growth factor
OVA	Ovalbumin
NAPQ1	*N*-acetyl-p-benzoquinoneimine
CSE	Cigarette smoke extract
CS	Cigarette smoke
IL8	Interleukin 8
CCD19-Lu	Human lung fibroblast cells
A549	Human pulmonary alveolar epithelial cell line
HBEC	Human bronchial epithelial cells
KC	Keratinocyte chemoattractant
BALf	Bronchoalveolar lavage fluid
WSPM	Wood smoke particulate matter
TDI	Toluene diisocyanate
CF	Cystic fibrosis
CFTR	Cystic fibrosis transmembrane conductance regulator
TNFα	Tumor necrosis factor α
CuFi-1	Human cystic fibrosis cell line
LPS	Lipopolysaccharide
CGRP	Calcitonin gene-related peptide
WT	Wild type
SNL	Spinal nerve ligation

References

1. Jaquemar, D.; Schenker, T.; Trueb, B. An ankyrin-like protein with transmembrane domains is specifically lost after oncogenic transformation of human fibroblasts. *J. Biol. Chem.* **1999**, *274*, 7325–7333. [CrossRef]
2. Kunert-Keil, C.; Bisping, F.; Krüger, J.; Brinkmeier, H. Tissue-specific expression of TRP channel genes in the mouse and its variation in three different mouse strains. *BMC Genom.* **2006**, *7*, 159. [CrossRef]
3. Nassenstein, C.; Kwong, K.; Taylor-Clark, T.; Kollarik, M.; Macglashan, D.M.; Braun, A.; Undem, B.J. Expression and function of the ion channel TRPA1 in vagal afferent nerves innervating mouse lungs. *J. Physiol.* **2008**, *586*, 1595–1604. [CrossRef]
4. Bautista, D.M.; Jordt, S.E.; Nikai, T.; Tsuruda, P.R.; Read, A.J.; Poblete, J.; Yamoah, E.N.; Basbaum, A.I.; Julius, D. TRPA1 mediates the inflammatory actions of environmental irritants and proalgesic agents. *Cell* **2006**, *124*, 1269–1282. [CrossRef]
5. Trevisani, M.; Siemens, J.; Materazzi, S.; Bautista, D.M.; Nassini, R.; Campi, B.; Imamachi, N.; Andrè, E.; Patacchini, R.; Cottrell, G.S.; et al. 4-Hydroxynonenal, an endogenous aldehyde, causes pain and neurogenic inflammation through activation of the irritant receptor TRPA1. *Proc. Natl. Acad. Sci. USA* **2007**, *104*, 13519–13524. [CrossRef]
6. Bessac, B.F.; Sivula, M.; von Hehn, C.A.; Escalera, J.; Cohn, L.; Jordt, S.E. TRPA1 is a major oxidant sensor in murine airway sensory neurons. *J. Clin. Invest.* **2008**, *118*, 1899–1910. [CrossRef]
7. Andrè, E.; Campi, B.; Materazzi, S.; Trevisani, M.; Amadesi, S.; Massi, D.; Creminon, C.; Vaksman, N.; Nassini, R.; Civelli, M.; et al. Cigarette smoke-induced neurogenic inflammation is mediated by α,β-unsaturated aldehydes and the TRPA1 receptor in rodents. *J. Clin. Invest.* **2008**, *118*, 2574–2582. [CrossRef]
8. Matta, J.A.; Cornett, P.M.; Miyares, R.L.; Abe, K.; Sahibzada, N.; Ahern, G.P. General anesthetics activate a nociceptive ion channel to enhance pain and inflammation. *Proc. Natl. Acad. Sci. USA* **2008**, *105*, 8784–8789. [CrossRef]
9. Andrè, E.; Gatti, R.; Trevisani, M.; Preti, D.; Baraldi, P.G.; Patacchini, R.; Geppetti, P. Transient receptor potential ankyrin receptor 1 is a novel target for pro-tussive agents. *Br. J. Pharmacol.* **2009**, *158*, 1621–1628. [CrossRef]
10. Hu, H.; Bandell, M.; Petrus, M.J.; Zhu, M.X.; Patapoutian, A. Zinc activates damage-sensing TRPA1 ion channels. *Nat. Chem. Biol.* **2009**, *5*, 183–190. [CrossRef]
11. Taylor-Clark, T.E.; Ghatta, S.; Bettner, W.; Undem, B.J. Nitrooleic acid, an endogenous product of nitrative stress, activates nociceptive sensory nerves via the direct activation of TRPA1. *Mol. Pharmacol.* **2009**, *75*, 820–829. [CrossRef]
12. Nagata, K.; Duggan, A.; Kumar, G.; García-Añoveros, J. Nociceptor and hair cell transducer properties of TRPA1, a channel for pain and hearing. *J. Neurosci.* **2005**, *25*, 4052–4061. [CrossRef]
13. Mukhopadhyay, I.; Gomes, P.; Aranake, S.; Shetty, M.; Karnik, P.; Damle, M.; Kuruganti, S.; Thorat, S.; Khairatkar-Joshi, N. Expression of functional TRPA1 receptor on human lung fibroblast and epithelial cells. *J. Recept. Signal Transduct.* **2011**, *31*, 350–358. [CrossRef]
14. Nassini, R.; Pedretti, P.; Moretto, N.; Fusi, C.; Carnini, C.; Facchinetti, F.; Viscomi, A.R.; Pisano, A.R.; Stokesberry, S.; Brunmark, C.; et al. Transient receptor potential ankyrin 1 channel localized to non-neuronal airway cells promotes non-neurogenic inflammation. *PLoS ONE* **2012**, *7*, e42454. [CrossRef]
15. Büch, T.R.; Schäfer, E.A.; Demmel, M.T.; Boekhoff, I.; Thiermann, H.; Gudermann, T.; Steinritz, D.; Schmidt, A. Functional expression of the transient receptor potential channel TRPA1, a sensor for toxic lung inhalants, in pulmonary epithelial cells. *Chem. Biol. Interact.* **2013**, *206*, 462–471. [CrossRef]
16. Mihara, S.; Shibamoto, T. The role of flavor and fragrance chemicals in TRPA1 (transient receptor potential cation channel, member A1) activity associated with allergies. *Allergy Asthma Clin. Immunol.* **2015**, *11*. [CrossRef]
17. Kichko, T.I.; Kobal, G.; Reeh, P.W. Cigarette smoke has sensory effects through nicotinic and TRPA1 but not TRPV1 receptors on the isolated mouse trachea and larynx. *Am. J. Physiol. Lung Cell. Mol. Physiol.* **2015**, *309*, L812–L820. [CrossRef]

18. Shapiro, D.; Deering-Rice, C.E.; Romero, E.G.; Hughen, R.W.; Light, A.R.; Veranth, J.M.; Reilly, C.A. Activation of transient receptor potential ankyrin-1 (TRPA1) in lung cells by wood smoke particulate material. *Chem. Res. Toxicol.* **2013**, *26*, 750–758. [CrossRef]
19. Grace, M.S.; Dubuis, E.; Birrell, M.A.; Belvisi, M.G. Pre-clinical studies in cough research: Role of Transient Receptor Potential (TRP) channels. *Pulm. Pharmacol. Ther.* **2013**, *26*, 498–507. [CrossRef]
20. Birrell, M.A.; Belvisi, M.G.; Grace, M.; Sadofsky, L.; Faruqi, S.; Hele, D.J.; Maher, S.A.; Freund-Michel, V.; Morice, A.H. TRPA1 agonists evoke coughing in guinea pig and human volunteers. *Am. J. Respir. Crit. Care Med.* **2009**, *180*, 1042–1047. [CrossRef]
21. Kistner, K.; Siklosi, N.; Babes, A.; Khalil, M.; Selescu, T.; Zimmermann, K.; Wirtz, S.; Becker, C.; Neurath, M.F.; Reeh, P.W.; et al. Systemic desensitization through TRPA1 channels by capsazepine and mustard oil—A novel strategy against inflammation and pain. *Sci. Rep.* **2016**, *6*, 28621. [CrossRef]
22. Mukhopadhyay, I.; Kulkarni, A.; Aranake, S.; Karnik, P.; Shetty, M.; Thorat, S.; Ghosh, I.; Wale, D.; Bhosale, V.; Khairatkar-Joshi, N. Transient receptor potential ankyrin 1 receptor activation in vitro and in vivo by pro-tussive agents: GRC 17536 as a promising anti-tussive therapeutic. *PLoS ONE* **2014**, *9*, e97005. [CrossRef]
23. Aparici, M.; Tarrasón, G.; Jover, I.; Carcasona, C.; Fernández-Blanco, J.; Eichhorn, P.; Gavaldà, A.; De Alba, J.; Roberts, R.; Miralpeix, M. Pharmacological profile of a novel, potent and oral TRPA1 antagonist. Characterization in a preclinical model of induced cough. *Eur. Respir. J.* **2015**, *46*, PA3948. [CrossRef]
24. Canning, B.J. Afferent nerves regulating the cough reflex: Mechanisms and mediators of cough in disease. *Otolaryngol. Clin. North Am.* **2010**, *43*, 15–25. [CrossRef]
25. Bezemer, G.F.G.; Sagar, S.; van Bergenhenegouwen, J.; Georgiou, N.A.; Garssen, J.; Kraneveld, A.D.; Folkerts, G. Dual Role of Toll-Like Receptors in Asthma and Chronic Obstructive Pulmonary Disease. *Pharmacol. Rev.* **2012**, *64*, 337–358. [CrossRef]
26. Zhang, L.; Liu, J.; Bai, J.; Wang, X.; Li, Y.; Jiang, P. Comparative expression of Toll-like receptors and inflammatory cytokines in pigs infected with different virulent porcine reproductive and respiratory syndrome virus isolates. *J. Virol.* **2013**, *10*, 135. [CrossRef]
27. Qi, J.; Buzas, K.; Fan, H.; Cohen, J.I.; Wang, K.; Mont, E.; Klinman, D.; Oppenheim, J.J.; Howard, O.M. Painful pathways induced by TLR stimulation of dorsal root ganglion neurons. *J. Immunol.* **2011**, *186*, 6417–6426. [CrossRef]
28. Belvisi, M.G.; Dubuis, E.; Birrell, M.A. Transient receptor potential A1 channels: Insights into cough and airway inflammatory disease. *Chest* **2011**, *140*, 1040–1047. [CrossRef]
29. Lavinka, P.C.; Dong, X. Molecular signaling and targets from itch: Lessons for cough. *Cough* **2013**, *9*, 8. [CrossRef]
30. Caceres, A.I.; Brackmann, M.; Elia, M.D.; Bessac, B.F.; del Camino, D.; D'Amours, M.; Witek, J.S.; Fanger, C.M.; Chong, J.A.; Hayward, N.J.; et al. A sensory neuronal ion channel essential for airway inflammation and hyperreactivity in asthma. *Proc Natl Acad Sci USA* **2009**, *106*, 9099–9104. [CrossRef]
31. Facchinetti, F.; Patacchini, R. The rising role of TRPA1 in asthma. *Open Drug Discov. J.* **2010**, *2*, 71–80. [CrossRef]
32. Raemdonck, K.; de Alba, J.; Birrell, M.A.; Grace, M.; Maher, S.A.; Irvin, C.G.; Fozard, J.R.; O'Byrne, P.M.; Belvisi, M.G. A role for sensory nerves in the late asthmatic response. *Thorax* **2012**, *67*, 19–25. [CrossRef]
33. Anupindi, R.; Mukhopadhyay, I.; Thomas, A.; Kumar, S.; Chaudhari, S.S.; Kulkarni, A.; Gudi, G.; Khairatkar-Joshi, N. GRC 17536, a novel, selective TRPA1 antagonist for potential treatment of respiratory disorders. *Eur. Respir. J.* **2010**, *36*, E5645.
34. Camino, D.; Chong, J.A.; Hayward, N.J.; Monsen, J.; Moran, M.M.; Curtis, R.; Murphy, C.; Mortin, L.I.; Abraham, W.M. Effects of blocking TRPA1 in a sheep model of asthma. In Proceedings of the International Workshop on Transient Receptor Potential Channels, a TRiP to Spain, Valencia, Spain, 12–14 September 2012; p. 68.
35. Beasley, R.; Clayton, T.; Crane, J.; von Mutius, E.; Lai, C.K.; Montefort, S.; Stewart, A. Association between paracetamol use in infancy and childhood, and risk of asthma, rhinoconjunctivitis, and eczema in children aged 6–7 years: Analysis from phase three of the ISAAC programme. *Lancet* **2008**, *372*, 1039–1048. [CrossRef]
36. Nassini, R.; Materazzi, S.; Andre', E.; Sartiani, L.; Aldini, G.; Trevisani, M.; Carnini, C.; Massi, D.; Pedretti, P.; Carini, M.; et al. Acetaminophen, *via* its reactive metabolite *N*-acetyl-*p*benzo-quinoneimine and transient receptor potential ankyrin-1 stimulation, causes neurogenic inflammation in the airways and other tissues in rodents. *FASEB J.* **2010**, *24*, 4904–4916. [CrossRef]

37. Liu, S.; Zhou, Y.; Wang, X.; Wang, D.; Lu, J.; Zheng, J.; Zhong, N.; Ran, P. Biomass fuels are the probable risk factor for chronic obstructive pulmonary disease in rural South China. *Thorax* **2007**, *62*, 889–897. [CrossRef]
38. Facchinetti, F.; Amadei, F.; Geppetti, P.; Tarantini, F.; Serio, C.; Dragotto, A.; Gigli, P.M.; Catinella, S.; Civelli, M.; Patacchini, R. α,β-Unsaturated aldehydes in cigarette smoke release inflammatory mediators from human macrophages. *Am. J. Respir. Cell Mol. Biol.* **2007**, *37*, 617–623. [CrossRef]
39. Lin, A.H.; Liu, M.H.; Ko, H.K.; Perng, D.W.; Lee, T.S.; Kou, Y.R. Lung epithelial TRPA1 transduces the extracellular ROS into transcriptional regulation of lung inflammation induced by cigarette smoke: The role of influxed Ca^{2+}. *Mediat. Inflamm.* **2015**, *2015*, 148367. [CrossRef]
40. Dupont, L.L.; Alpizar, Y.A.; Brusselle, G.G.; Bracke, K.R.; Talavera, K.; Joos, G.F.; Maes, T. Expression of transient receptor potential (TRP) channels in a murine model of cigarette smoke exposure. In Proceedings of the C34. Insights into COPD Pathogenesis from Pre-Clinical Studies, San Diego, CA, USA, 16–21 May 2014; Volume 189, p. A4286.
41. Hu, G.; Zhou, Y.; Tian, J.; Yao, W.; Li, J.; Li, B.; Ran, P. Risk of COPD from exposure to biomass smoke: A metaanalysis. *Chest* **2010**, *1381*, 20–31. [CrossRef]
42. Hur, G.Y.; Kohw, D.H.; Choi, G.S.; Park, H.J.; Choi, S.J.; Ye, Y.M.; Kimw, K.S.; Park, H.S. Clinical and immunologic findings of methylene Diphenyl diisocyanate-induced occupational asthma in a car upholstery factory. *Clin. Exp. Allergy* **2008**, *38*, 586–593. [CrossRef]
43. Fisseler-Eckhoff, A.; Bartsch, H.; Zinsky, R.; Schirren, J. Environmental isocyanate-induced asthma: Morphologic and pathogenetic aspects of an increasing occupational disease. *Int. J. Environ. Res. Public Health* **2011**, *8*, 3672–3687. [CrossRef]
44. Johnson, V.J.; Yucesoy, B.; Reynolds, J.S.; Fluharty, K.; Wang, W.; Richardson, D.; Luster, M.I. Inhalation of toluene diisocyanate vapor induces allergic rhinitis in mice. *J. Immunol.* **2007**, *179*, 1864–1871. [CrossRef]
45. Taylor-Clark, T.E.; Kiros, F.; Carr, M.J.; McAlexander, M.A. Transient receptor potential ankyrin 1 mediates toluene diisocyanate–evoked respiratory irritation. *Am. J. Respir. Cell Mol. Biol.* **2009**, *40*, 756–762. [CrossRef]
46. Tourangeau, L.M.; Christiansen, S.C.; Herschbach, J.; Brooks, S.M.; Eddleston, J.; Zuraw, B. Nasal mucosal TRPA1 and TRPV1 levels in human rhinitis. *J. Allergy Clin. Immunol.* **2011**, *127*, AB52. [CrossRef]
47. Prandini, P.; De Logu, F.; Fusi, C.; Provezza, L.; Nassini, R.; Montagner, G.; Materazzi, S.; Munari, S.; Gilioli, E.; Bezzerri, V.; et al. TRPA1 channels modulate inflammatory response in respiratory cells from cystic fibrosis patients. *Am. J. Respir. Cell. Mol. Biol.* **2016**, *55*. [CrossRef]
48. Chen, J.; Hackos, D.H. TRPA1 as drug target-Promise and challenges. *Naunyn-Schmiedeberg's Arch. Pharmacol.* **2015**, *388*, 451–463. [CrossRef]
49. Meseguer, V.; Alpizar, Y.A.; Luis, E.; Tajada, S.; Denlinger, B.; Fajardo, O.; Manenschijn, J.A.; Fernández-Peña, C.; Talavera, A.; Kichko, T.; et al. TRPA1 channels mediate acute neurogenic inflammation and pain produced by bacterial endotoxins. *Nat. Commun.* **2014**, *5*, 3125. [CrossRef]
50. Tandon, M.; Jain, S.M.; Balamurugan, R.; Koslowski, M.; Keohane, P. Treatment of pain associated with diabetic peripheral neuropathy with the novel TRPA1 antagonist GRC 17536 in patients with intact peripheral nerve function. In Proceedings of the Fifth International Meeting of The Special Interest Group on Neuropathic Pain (NeuPSIG), Nice, France, 14–17 May 2015.
51. Ryan, N.M.; Birring, S.S.; Gibson, P.G. Gabapentin for refractory chronic cough: A randomised, double-blind, placebo-controlled trial. *Lancet* **2012**, *380*, 1583–1589. [CrossRef]
52. Kwan, K.Y.; Allchorne, A.J.; Vollrath, M.A.; Christensen, A.P.; Zhang, D.S.; Woolf, C.J.; Corey, D.P. TRPA1 contributes to cold, mechanical, and chemical nociception but is not essential for hair-cell transduction. *Neuron* **2006**, *50*, 277–289. [CrossRef]
53. Chen, J.; Joshi, S.K.; DiDomenico, S.; Perner, R.J.; Mikusa, J.P.; Gauvin, D.M.; Segreti, J.A.; Han, P.; Zhang, X.F.; Niforatos, W.; et al. Selective blockade of TRPA1 channel attenuates pathological pain without altering noxious cold sensation or body temperature regulation. *Pain* **2011**, *152*, 1165–1172. [CrossRef]
54. de Oliveira, C.; Garami, A.; Lehto, S.G.; Pakai, E.; Tekus, V.; Pohoczky, K.; Youngblood, B.D.; Wang, W.; Kort, M.E.; Kym, P.R.; et al. Transient receptor potential channel ankyrin-1 is not a cold sensor for autonomic thermoregulation in rodents. *J. Neurosci.* **2014**, *34*, 4445–4452. [CrossRef]
55. Curtis, R.; Coleman, S.; Camino, D.D.; Hayward, N.J.; Moran, M.M.; Bokesch, P. Transient Receptor Potential A1 (TRPA1) is not involved in thermoregulation in dogs and humans. In Proceedings of the A Trip to Spain: International workshop on transient receptor potential channels, Valencia, Spain, 12–14 September 2012; p. 65.

56. Obata, K.; Katsura, H.; Mizushima, T.; Yamanaka, H.; Kobayashi, K.; Dai, Y.; Fukuoka, T.; Tokunaga, A.; Tominaga, M.; Noguchi, K. TRPA1 induced in sensory neurons contributes to cold hyperalgesia after inflammation and nerve injury. *J. Clin. Invest.* **2005**, *115*, 2393–2401. [CrossRef]
57. Bodkin, J.V.; Thakore, P.; Aubdool, A.A.; Liang, L.; Fernandes, E.S.; Nandi, M.; Spina, D.; Clark, J.E.; Aaronson, P.I.; Shattock, M.J.; et al. Investigating the potential role of TRPA1 in locomotion and cardiovascular control during hypertension. *Pharmacol. Res. Perspect.* **2014**, *2*, e00052. [CrossRef]

15

TRPV3 in Drug Development

Lisa M. Broad [1,*], Adrian J. Mogg [1], Elizabeth Eberle [2], Marcia Tolley [2], Dominic L. Li [3] and Kelly L. Knopp [3]

1. Lilly Research Centre, Eli Lilly and Company Ltd., Erl Wood Manor, Windlesham, Surrey GU20 6PH, UK; mogg_adrian@lilly.com
2. Covance Greenfield Laboratories, Greenfield, Indianapolis, IN 46140, USA; eberle_elizabeth_lutz@network.lilly.com (E.E.); tolley_marcia_k@network.lilly.com (M.T.)
3. Lilly Research Laboratories, Eli Lilly and Company Inc., Indianapolis, IN 46285, USA; dominic.li5702@gmail.com (D.L.L.); knopp_kelly_l@lilly.com (K.L.K.)

* Correspondance: broad_lisa@lilly.com

Academic Editors: Arpad Szallasi and Susan M. Huang

Abstract: Transient receptor potential vanilloid 3 (TRPV3) is a member of the TRP (Transient Receptor Potential) super-family. It is a relatively underexplored member of the thermo-TRP sub-family (Figure 1), however, genetic mutations and use of gene knock-outs and selective pharmacological tools are helping to provide insights into its role and therapeutic potential. TRPV3 is highly expressed in skin, where it is implicated in skin physiology and pathophysiology, thermo-sensing and nociception. Gain of function TRPV3 mutations in rodent and man have enabled the role of TRPV3 in skin health and disease to be particularly well defined. Pre-clinical studies provide some rationale to support development of TRPV3 antagonists for therapeutic application for the treatment of inflammatory skin conditions, itch and pain. However, to date, only one compound directed towards block of the TRPV3 receptor (GRC15300) has progressed into clinical trials. Currently, there are no known clinical trials in progress employing a TRPV3 antagonist.

Keywords: TRPV3; keratinocytes; itch; pain; Olmsted syndrome

1. Introduction

TRPV3 is a non-selective cation channel, displaying relatively high permeability to calcium. It was first cloned in 2002 and displays ~30%–40% sequence homology with other TRPV channels.

Other features in common include the predicted protein structure encompassing six transmembrane spanning domains (1–6), a pore-forming loop between domains 5–6, cytoplasmic amino and carboxyl termini, ankyrin repeats and coiled-coil domains at the amino terminus and several putative phosphorylation sites [1–3] (see Figure 2). The channel is formed from four subunits, with homo-tetrameric TRPV3 receptors being commonly studied. Hetero-tetrameric channels containing TRPV3 and TRPV1, for example, are reported to be able to form by some [3–5], but not all researchers [6]; however, the nature, role and expression of native TRPV3 containing heteromers is far from clear.

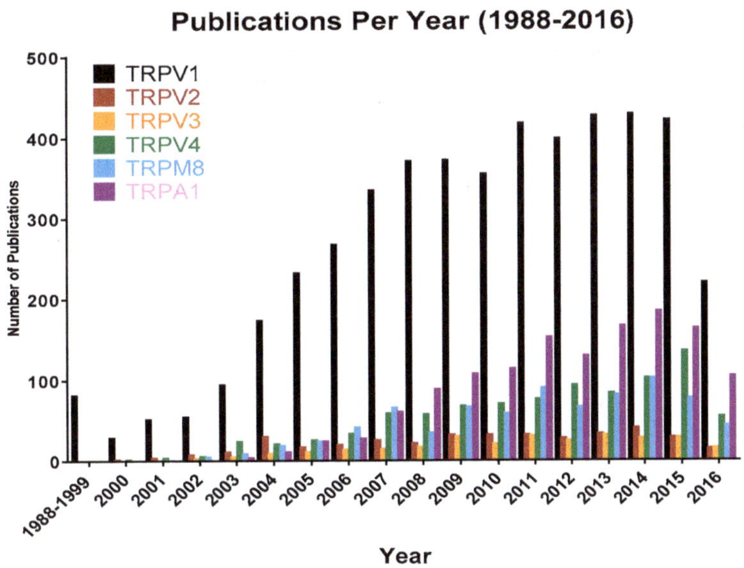

Figure 1. Total publications per year around TRPV3 (orange bars) relative to other thermo-TRPs (TRPV1, TRPV2, TRPV4, TRPM8 and TRPA1). Data as of 25/05/2016. Searches were conducted using PubMed and, where applicable, included alternative nomenclature (e.g., TRPV1 and VR1).

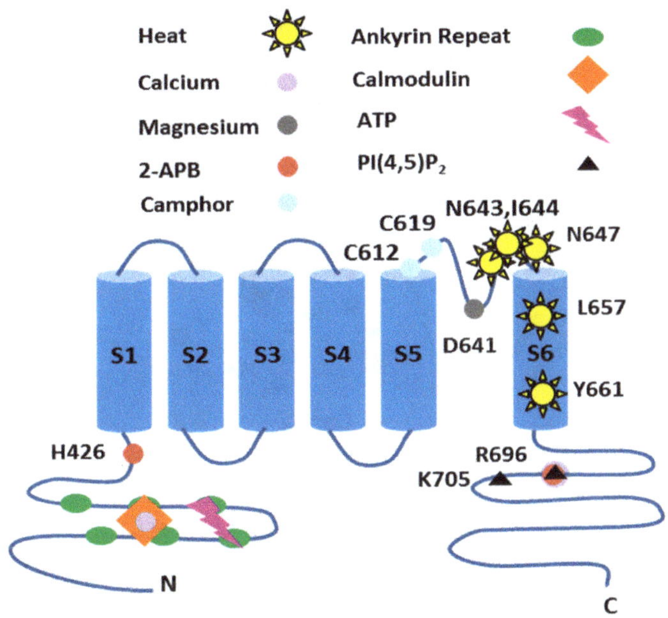

Figure 2. Membrane topology of TRPV3. Residues involved in heat activation (N643, I644, N647, L658 and Y661), activation by 2-APB (H426 and R696), Camphor (C612 and C619) and modulation by phosphatidylinositol 4,5-bisphosphate (PI(4,5)P_2; R696 and K705), ATP (K169 and K174), Mg^{2+} (D641) and Ca^{2+} (R696) are highlighted, in addition to the location of ankyrin repeats [7–13].

In common with other TRP channels, TRPV3 acts as a polymodal signal integrator. It is activated by numerous physical and chemical modulators and by posttranslational modifications, and the impact of individual stimuli is influenced by the presence of other stimuli (see Figure 3 for summary). TRPV3 is activated by innocuous temperature, with the threshold for channel opening at 31–39 °C, and activity is retained over temperatures extending into the noxious range [14]. Chemical agonists include spice extracts (such as camphor and carvacrol), synthetic agents (including 2-aminoethoxy diphenylborate, 2-APB) and endogenous ligand farnesyl pyrophosphate (FPP), [1–3,15,16]. Repeated exposure to heat or chemical agonists leads to sensitization of the receptor [8,17], through hysteresis of gating [14], while co-application of diverse stimuli, such as heat and chemical agonists, is synergistic [17,18]. Activation of G_q coupled GPCRs also sensitizes TRPV3 [19], with key components in the downstream signalling cascade including protein kinase C [20], Ca^{2+}-calmodulin [8,10], phosphatidylinositol 4,5-bisphosphate ($PI(4,5)P_2$) [11] and unsaturated fatty acids [18,20]. Other modulators include voltage [11], ATP [10], Mg^{2+} [12], and intracellular acidification [21,22].

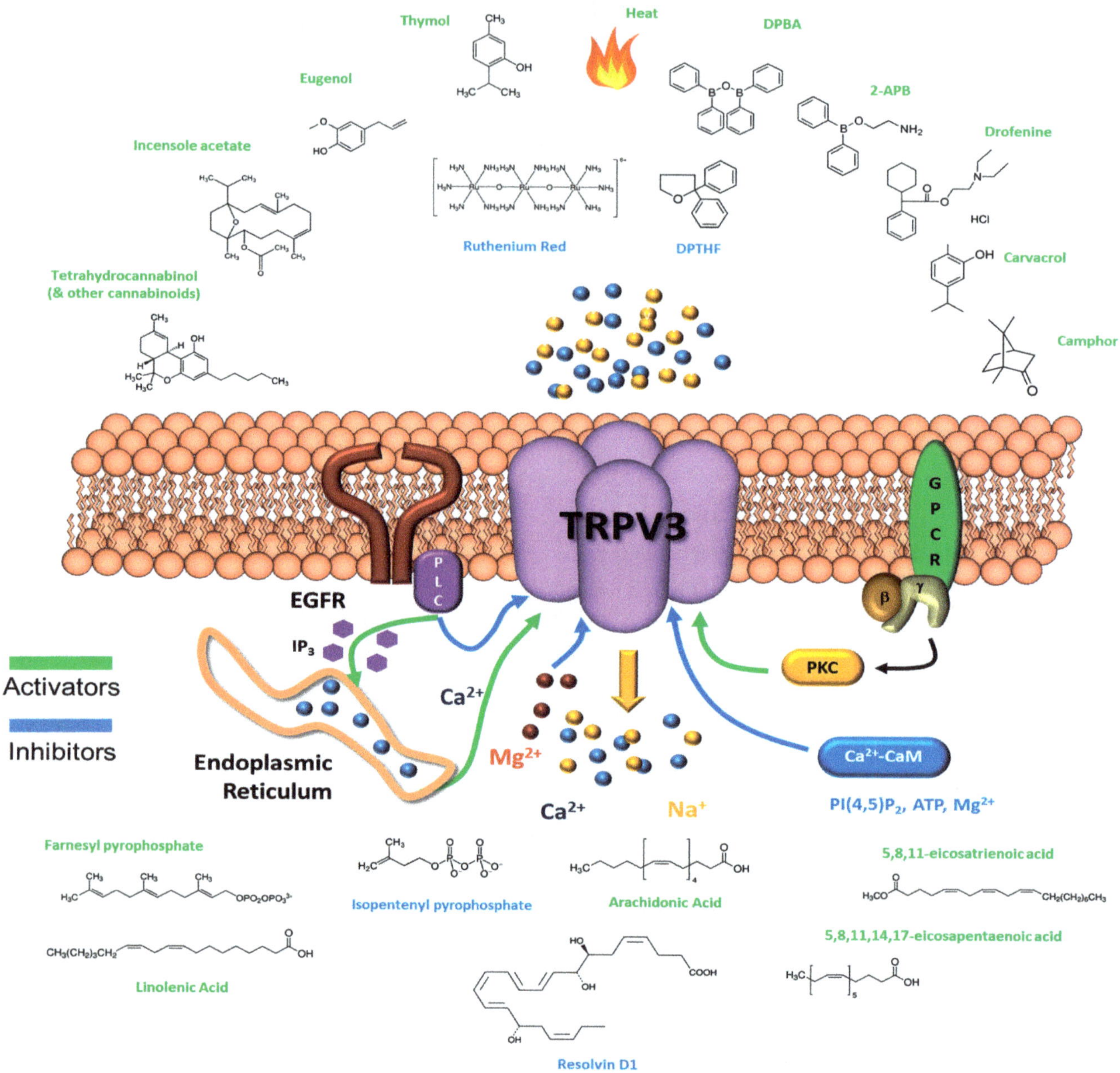

Figure 3. Activators, inhibitors and modulators of TRPV3. Quaternary structure of TRPV3 with compounds and signalling pathways known to activate, inhibit or modulate the receptor. See Introduction for references–additional references [23–26].

The amino acid residues and regions underlying activation of TRPV3 by a number of stimuli have been mapped. Information relating to the mechanism of activation by heat [14,27,28], 2-APB [9] and camphor [13] is available. Likewise, residues involved in mediating modulation by Ca^{2+}/Ca^{2+}-calmodulin; [8,10]; Mg^{2+} [12]; pH [21] and voltage [11] have been defined (Figure 2, see Yang and Zhu for recent detailed review [29]).

2. Expression and Function of TRPV3

In contrast to TRPV1, TRPA1 and TRPM8, a direct role for TRPV3 in the peripheral nervous system is controversial, as expression in sensory neurons is not conserved across species, with minimal detection in rodents [1–3,30]. TRPV3 is however expressed in skin keratinocytes (Figure 4) across species [1,2,31] and in humans, TRPV3 gene expression in skin is the highest of the >50 tissues profiled in the GTEx project [32] (Supplementary Figure S1). TRPV3 expression is also reported in other epithelial cells including oral and nasal epithelium [19,33], distal colon [34] and cornea [35]. In oral epithelia, use of TRPV3 knock mice implicate this channel in wound healing [33]. Likewise, although TRPV3 gene expression in brain overall appears to be very low (Supplementary Figure S1), studies utilising TRPV3 knock-out mice are suggestive of a role for TRPV3 in regulating hippocampal synaptic plasticity [36] and incensole acetate, a reported TRPV3 agonist, broadly modulated brain activity in wild-type, but not TRPV3 knock-out mice [37]. Interestingly, there are several reports detailing TRPV1 channel expression on the endoplasmic reticulum of dorsal root ganglia and sarcoplasmic reticulum of skeletal muscle cells [38,39]. Indeed, it has recently been reported that there is functional expression of TRPV3 on the ER of mouse embryonic stem cells, with the channel having a putative role in controlling cell cycle and cellular proliferation [40]. These novel findings, if confirmed in native adult tissues, may need to be taken into account when developing compounds for TRPV3.

Until recently, reliance on non-selective agonist and antagonist tools, such as Ruthenium Red, has hampered progress in clearly defining a functional role for native TRPV3. For example, evidence for a role of TRPV3 in modulating the CNS dopaminergic system [41,42] and colonic [34] and corneal epithelia responses [35] is largely circumstantial for this very reason. Perhaps unsurprisingly, keratinocytes have been the most commonly utilized preparation for the study of native TRPV3 function by far, and provide the most compelling data package. Early studies in m308 keratinocytes identified whole cell currents, increases in intracellular calcium and release of IL-1α in response to application or co-application of known TRPV3 agonists and modulators, including eugenol, DPBA, camphor, 2-APB and arachidonic acid [19,20]. This work was later extended by Grubisha et al. (2014) [18], who confirmed that these responses could be blocked by a selective TRPV3 antagonist and by shRNA knock-down of TRPV3. In primary cultures of keratinocytes from wild-type mice, whole cell currents, increases in intracellular calcium or production of nitric-oxide were observed in response to TRPV3 agonists, or agonist combinations, including heat, 2-APB, carvacrol and camphor, these responses were sensitized on repeat application [12,17,43–46] and were absent in TRPV3 knock-out mice [17,45,46]. In transgenic mice over-expressing TRPV3 in skin keratinocytes, co-application of heat and 2-APB led to augmented TRPV3 mediated PGE_2 release from keratinocytes [30]. In addition, application of 2-APB and carvacrol has been shown to promote TGF-α release from primary cultures of human keratinocytes [45], and in human keratinocyte HaCaT cells, 2-APB and acidic pH promoted whole cell currents blocked by Ruthenium Red [21].

Studies using keratinocytes have provided several insights for how TRPV3 regulates skin function and the function of neighbouring cells (Figure 4). A key protein interaction partner appears to be the epidermal growth factor receptor (EGFR). This receptor is proposed to form a signalling complex with TRPV3, whereby activation of the EGFR results in increased TRPV3 channel activity, stimulation of TGF-α release and epidermal homeostasis [45]. TRPV3 plays a role in maintenance of the skin barrier, as deletion of TRPV3 evokes deleterious changes in epidermal barrier structure. Hair morphogenesis is also disrupted in TRPV3 null mice [17,45]. In cultures of human outer root sheath keratinocytes, activation of TRPV3 induced membrane currents, elevated intracellular calcium, inhibited proliferation, induced apoptosis, inhibited hair shaft elongation and promoted premature hair follicle regression. These cellular effects, including inhibition of hair growth, were blocked by siRNA mediated TRPV3 knock-down [47]. α-Hydroxyl acids, commonly used in the cosmetic industry in chemical peels to promote exfoliation, have also been proposed to exert their effects through activation of keratinocyte TRPV3 [21]. Once again, the suggested mechanism is calcium influx through keratinocyte TRPV3 channels, leading to overload in intracellular calcium and cell death [21]. Of relevance to pain, TRPV3 mediated ATP release from keratinocytes has been shown to activate purinoceptors in dorsal root ganglion neurons [48], thereby influencing nociceptive function. Consistent with this, in transgenic mice over-expressing TRPV3 in skin keratinocytes, increased pain sensitivity was observed [30]. A number of related findings demonstrate that indirect modulation by keratinocytes can strongly influence pain signalling, for example in a recent study in TRPV1-knockout mice selectively expressing TRPV1 in keratinocytes, keratinocyte stimulation was sufficient to evoke acute nociception-related responses [49] and keratinocytes are also reported to induce neuronal excitability after nerve injury [50]. Of note, however, although TRPV3 null mice show disrupted responses to acute noxious heat and innocuous thermal sensation in thermotaxis endpoints [17], responses in other types of pain models are largely unaltered. In addition, the role of TRPV3 in innocuous temperature perception and acute thermal nociception appears to be somewhat dependent on gender and genetic background [46,51], for recent review, see Reference [52].

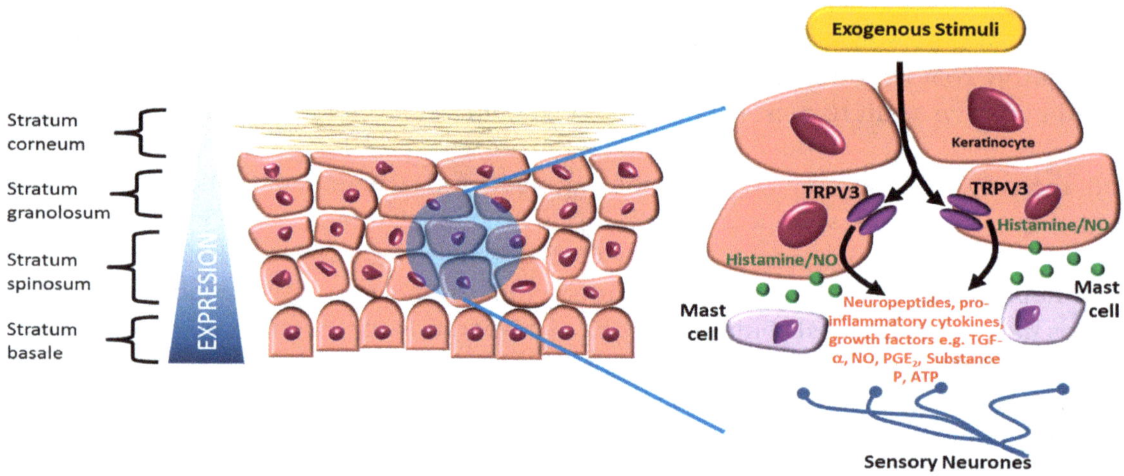

Figure 4. Summary of TRPV3 expression and function in epidermal keratinocytes. TRPV3 protein has been found throughout the epidermis and around hair follicles, with protein elevated under certain inflammatory skin conditions.

Several studies have reported alterations in TRPV3 mRNA and/or protein expression in pathological states, including in the skin of burns victims [53]; in rosacea, a chronic inflammatory skin condition [54]; in psoriasis [55] and in breast tissue biopsies from patients with breast pain [56]. Of note, aberrant TRPV3 function might be anticipated in some pathological states. For example, arachidonic acid, which is a strong potentiator of keratinocyte TRPV3, is present at high concentrations in psoriatic dermatitis (>100 μM; [57]) indicating that TRPV3 activity may be potentiated in psoriatic epidermis. Interestingly, a recent preliminary report describes a mechanistic link between TRPV3 activity in psoriasis through IL-1α and EGFR signalling [55].

3. Insights from Genetic Mutations

Adding further support to the role of TRPV3 in skin physiology and pathology, a TRPV3 gain-of-function G573S/C mutation was identified to underlie the spontaneously hairless, dermatitis phenotype of two rodent strains, DS-Nh mice and WBN/kob-HT rats, used as animal models of atopy [31,58,59]. Development of a TRPV3Gly573Ser transgenic mouse, recapitulated this phenotype, with significantly increased scratching behavior [58]. These transgenic mice also displayed augmented release of NGF in response to heat and significantly increased levels of serum chemokines and interleukins [58]. The increased release of pro-inflammatory and pro-nociceptive factors might be hypothesized to alter nociception, however data from exploration of the pain phenotype of TRPV3 gain-of-function rodents is only just emerging [60].

More recently, similar gain-of-function mutations in TRPV3, including but not limited to the Gly573 mutation, have been identified as the cause of Olmsted syndrome (OS) in humans (for review see [61]). OS is a rare keratinizing disorder characterized by marked thickening of the skin on the soles of the feet and palms of the hands, periorificial keratotic plaques, diffuse alopecia, and pruritus. In a few cases, atypical OS is reported with erythromelalgia. Pain and itching are variable in OS but are reported to be particularly severe in atypical OS patients with erythromelalgia, which leads to acute flares of hyperalgesia and some features of neuropathic pain.

4. TRPV3 Indications

Whilst activation of keratinocyte TRPV3 has been shown to mediate the release of pro-inflammatory and pro-nociceptive mediators and pruritogens, and the gain-of-function mutations implicate TRPV3 in skin conditions where a predominant feature is itch [62], there is a surprising lack of preclinical in vivo data exploring this aspect.

Selective TRPV3 antagonists have recently been introduced by Hydra Biosciences, Glenmark Pharmaceuticals and AbbVie (Section 5), and afford the opportunity to investigate the therapeutic potential of blockade of the TRPV3 channel.

We previously reported that Hydra's FTP-THQ (Figure 5) was a potent and selective in vitro antagonist of recombinant and native TRPV3 receptors, having virtually no activity at TRPV1, TRPV4, TRPM8 and TRPA1 [18]. We have now assessed FTP-THQ in vitro in m308 keratinocytes and confirmed that it can prevent release of ATP and GM-CSF by concentrations of DPBA and 2-APB that are known to selectively activate TRPV3 in these cells ([18]; Figure 6).

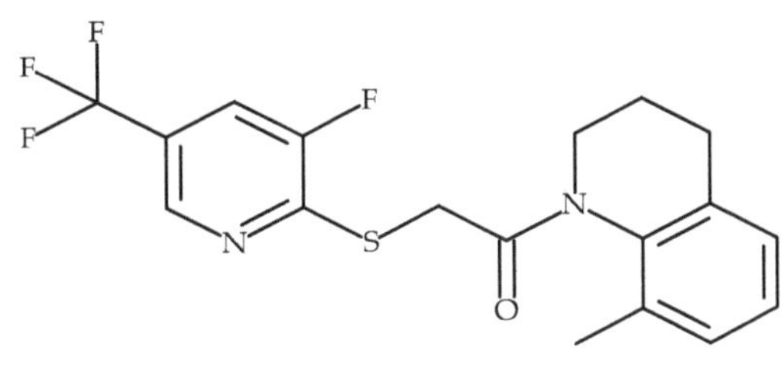

Figure 5. Structure of TRPV3 selective antagonist FTP-THQ [63].

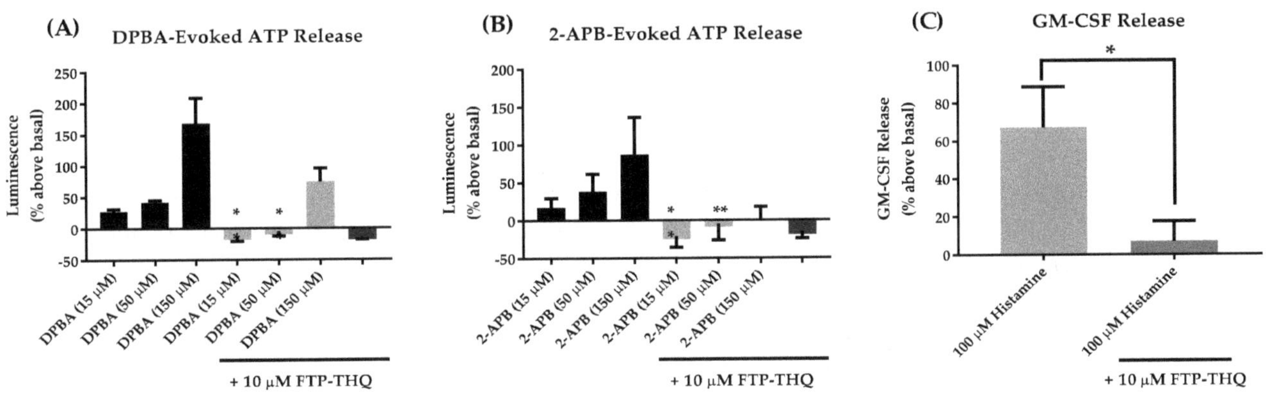

Figure 6. FTP-THQ [1-([3-fluoro-5-(trifluoromethyl)pyridine-2-yl]sulfanylacetyl)-8-methyl-1,2,3,4-tetrahydroquinoline], a potent and selective TRPV3 receptor antagonist blocked TRPV3 mediated release of ATP (**A** & **B**) and GM-CSF (**C**) from mouse keratinocytes in vitro. Results are mean ± SEM of 3 independent experiments. Statistical significance was assessed using the paired Student's *t*-test, * $p < 0.05$, ** $p < 0.001$.

FTP-THQ also has appropriate pharmacokinetic properties to assess its profile in vivo with an in vitro IC_{50} of 117 nM at the rat recombinant receptor and 186 nM at the mouse native receptor [18], and a Brain/Plasma ratio of approximately 7. In mice, after intraperitoneal administration, it dose-dependently blocked histamine-induced itch (Figure 7) with unbound exposure in brain (152 nM) consistent with the in vitro potency value, while the plasma levels where significantly less (37 nM). These data suggest TRPV3 can be pharmacologically modulated in a manner that is consistent with the gain-of-function mutations described in Table 1.

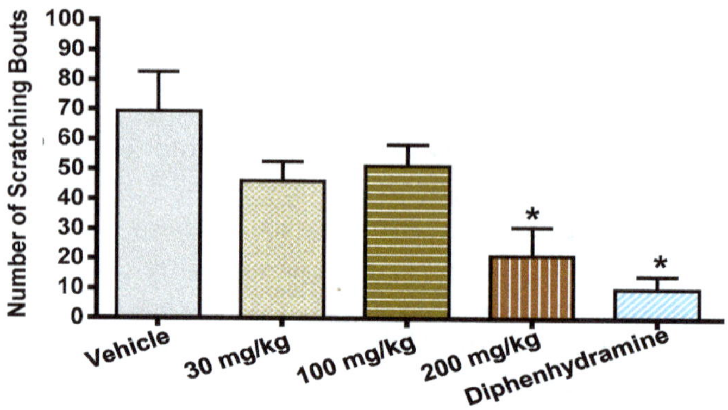

Figure 7. Effects of FTP-THQ on histamine-induced scratching behavior. Harlan CD-1 mice ($n = 7$–8/treatment group), 4–5 weeks old were acclimated to testing room for 1 h. FTP-THQ was administered at 30, 100, or 200 mg/kg i.p., 1 h prior to histamine, while diphenhyramine was administered at 20 mg/kg, 30 min prior to histamine. Animals were then placed inside a clear plexiglass chamber and the number of scratching bouts was scored for 20 min. Data were collected via Abacus software; one-way ANOVA with post-hoc Dunnett's was used for analysis. * $p < 0.05$ vs. vehicle control.

From the pain perspective, the genetic data are less compelling, but small molecule manipulation of the receptor with multiple compounds is suggestive of a role in nociceptive processing. For recent reviews, see References [64–66]. The TRPV3 agonist FPP is reported to elicit pain behaviors after intraplantar injection into inflamed animals [16]. The same group has also reported that 17(R)-resolvin D, an endogenous TRPV3 antagonist, is anti-nociceptive in acute and inflammatory pain states [24]. Complementarily, tool antagonist molecules from Hydra, Glenmark and AbbVie described below have attenuated pain behaviors in a number of pre-clinical pain models, including primarily carrageenan and Complete Freund's Adjuvant-induced thermal and/or tactile hypersensitivity, but also in nerve ligation models [63,67,68].

We also evaluated FTP-THQ in a number of pre-clinical pain behavior models and replicated the previous findings in CFA-induced thermal hypersensitivity at the 200 mg/kg dose, and as exemplified in Figure 8, observed effects in the formalin-induced nocifensive responding assay. Interestingly, effects in this assay were observed at lower plasma/brain exposures. Confounding side effects, such as alterations in locomotor activity, were not observed, however, unlike previous reports (see [65]) we did observe a dose-dependent hypothermia with the antagonist. The thermo-sensing TRP channels have collectively been implicated as having the potential to alter normal thermal sensation and temperature regulation, due to findings with TRPV1 antagonists. Our data would suggest, at least in rodents, an alteration in body temperature should be closely monitored. It is unknown if these effects would translate into higher species. Taken together, the collective data indicate that potent and selective TRPV3 antagonists effectively attenuate scratching and pain behavior in pre-clinical animal models, and pharmacological blockade of this target may afford some therapeutic benefit.

By way of summary, Table 1 provides the potential therapeutic utility of TRPV3 modulators. However, as mentioned previously, no current clinical trials are ongoing.

Table 1. Summary of Physiological and Pathophysiological roles of TRPV3.

Potential Roles	Summary of Evidence	Reference(s)
Olmsted Syndrome	Several independent clinical reports identify mutations in the TRPV3 gene as a cause of gain-of-function mutations and recessive Olmsted's Syndrome. Characteristic features include palmoplantar keratoderma, periorificial hyperkeratotic lesions and alopecia. Less common presentations include digit constriction, onychodystrophy and pruritus	[66,69–73]
Olmsted Syndrome with Erythromelalgia	Clinical data of three patients whose disease presentation included intense flares of inflammation, itching, burning pain, vasodilatation, and redness of the extremities consistent with erythromelalgia. Whole exome sequencing identified a de novo heterozygous missense mutation within TRPV3, p.Leu673Phe.	[74,75]
Pruitic and Atopic Dermatitis	Clinical data suggest TRPV3 expression is increased in lesional skin in patients with atopic dermatitis. Preclinical data suggest DS-Nh mice develop allergic and pruritic dermatitis	[58,76]
Psoriasis	Clinical data suggest TRPV3 expression is significantly increased in psoriatic lesions, and that these channels are functional in keratinocytes isolated from lesioned skin. A novel antagonist of TRPV3 dose-dependently inhibited 2APB/carvacrol induced IL-1α release keratinocytes. Similarly, inhibition of EGFR signaling was observed with the antagonist. Inhibitors of both IL-1α release and EGFR signaling have previously attenuated psoriatic symptoms and thus a linkage with TRPV3 is suggested	[55]
Wound Healing	Pre-clinical data suggest higher expression of TRPV3 in mouse oral epithelia versus skin, and expression was upregulated in wounded oral epithelial tissue. TRPV3 activation promoted oral epithelial cell proliferation, which was diminished in TRPV3 knockout mice. Subsequent knock out profiling in a molar tooth extraction model suggest oral wound closure was delayed	[33]
Burn/Post-burn pruritus	Clinical data suggest increased TRPV3 expression in the epidermis of burn scars with pruritus	[29,53]
Hair growth	Pre-clinical data suggest TRPV3 agonists eugenol and 2-aminoethoxydiphenyl borate inhibited hair shaft elongation, suppressed proliferation, and induced apoptosis in human organ-cultured hair follicles. Similarly, functional effects of TRPV3 activation in human ORS keratinocytes were demonstrated as on-target via siRNA	[47]
Skin Barrier Formation	Pre-clinical data suggest TRPV3 forms a direct complex with transglutaminases, thereby regulating growth factor signaling for the formation of the skin barrier	[45]
Rosacea	Clinical data suggest increased TRPV3 expression in epidermal keratinocytes, and dermal labeling was observed in a subset of immune cells and fibroblasts in erythematotelangiectatic rosacea and phymatous rosacea-affected skin. Increased gene expression was also observed in patients with phymatous rosacea	[54]
Cerebral Ischemia	Pre-clinical data suggest the TRPV3 agonist incensole acetate protects against ischemic neuronal damage and reperfusion injury in mice. Reduced infarct volumes, inhibition of TNF-α, IL-1β and TGF-β expression, and NF-κB activation were demonstrated as on-target using TRPV3 knock-out mice	[77,78]
Mastalgia	Clinical data suggest increased expression of TRPV3 in basal keratinocytes that correlated with disease score	[56]
Traumatic Peripheral Nerve Injury	Clinical data suggest increased TRPV3 expression in the DRG neurons of patients with DRG avulsion injury, in the peripheral nerve proximal to the site of brachial plexus injury. However, a decrease in TRPV3 expression was observed in the skin of patients with diabetic neuropathy	[3,79]
Cold- and Heat-evoked Pain	Pre-clinical data showed TRPV3 knockout mice have impaired responses to noxious heat. WBN/Kob-Ht rats, which have a TRPV3 gain-of-function mutation, showed an increased sensitivity to noxious heat and cold stimuli. Multiple antagonists have shown efficacy in inflammatory insult-induced hypersensitivity and nerve ligation-induced hypersensitivity	[45,60,64,65]

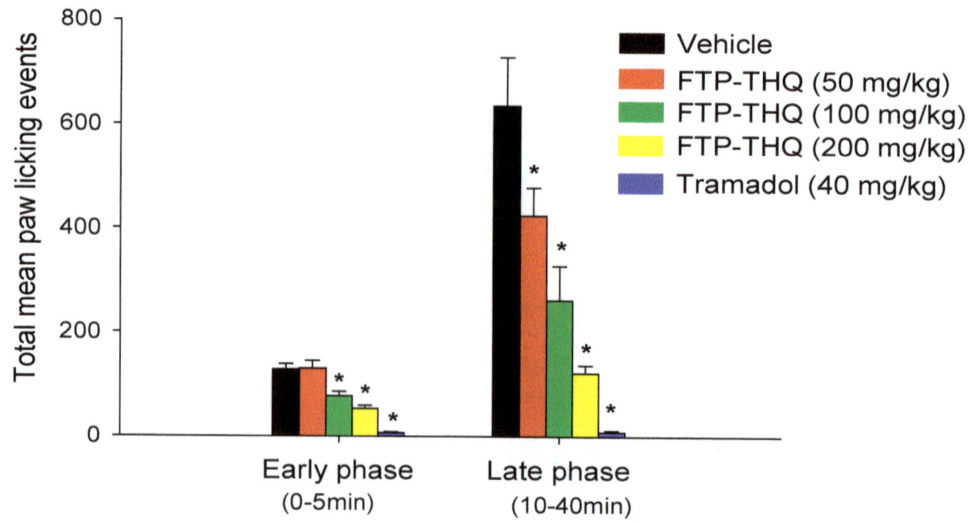

Figure 8. Effects of FTP-THQ on formalin-induced nocifensive behavior. Harlan Sprague Dawley Rats ($n = 7–8$/treatment group), were acclimated to the testing room for 1 h. FTP-THQ was administered at 50, 100, or 200 mg/kg i.p. 15 min prior to formalin, while the positive control tramadol was administered at 40 mg/kg i.p. 30 min prior to formalin. The animals were placed in Startle Behavior Chambers and behavior events (licking, guarding, flinching) binned in 5-min intervals and plotted as Early and Late Phase. Data were analyzed using 1-way ANOVA, and comparisons of drug treatment groups were compared with control groups using a post-hoc Dunnett's comparison. * $p < 0.05$ vs. vehicle control.

5. TRPV3 Drug Development Overview

Major milestones in the area of TRPV3 drug development are highlighted in Figure 9 and in comparison to TRPV1, the number of patents describing TRPV3 modulators has been modest (Figure 10) with Hydra Biosciences and Glenmark Pharmaceuticals being the main players.

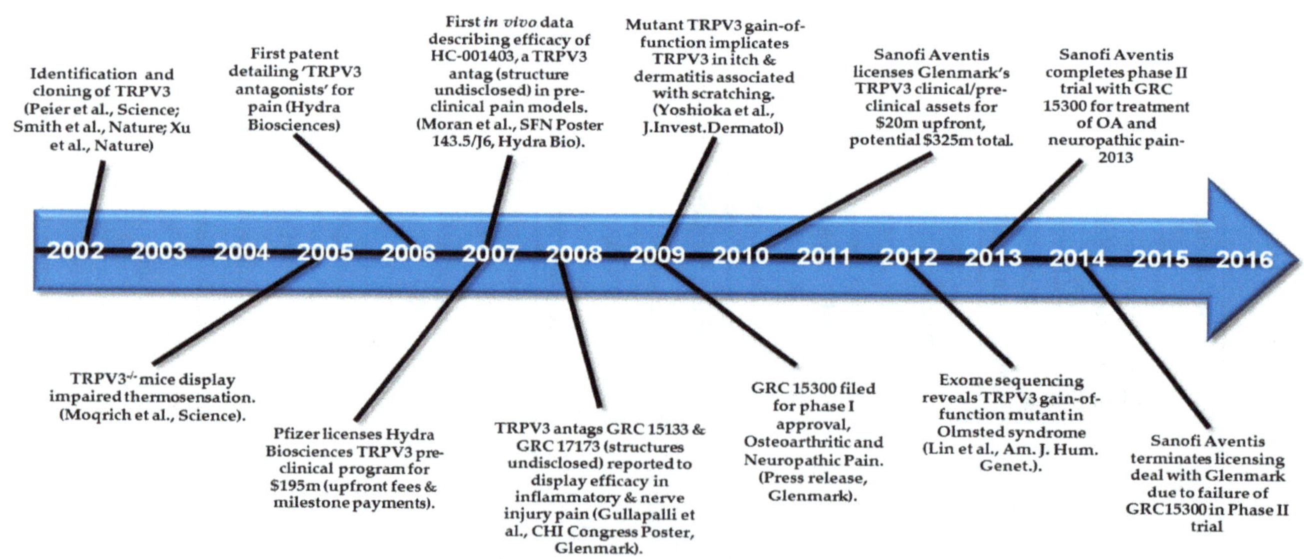

Figure 9. Timeline of major TRPV3 development activities.

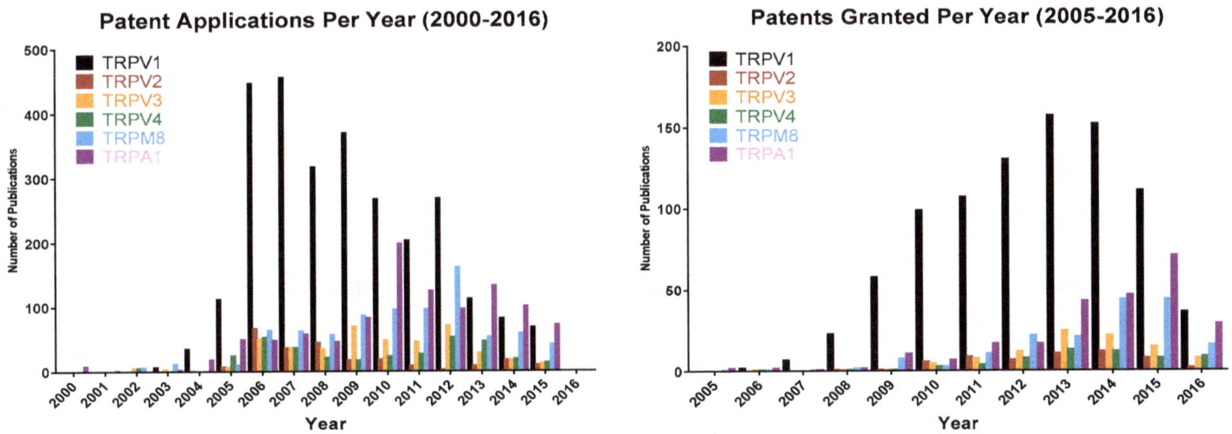

Figure 10. Number of patents applied for and granted per year for each of the thermo-TRPs compared to TRPV3 (orange bars).

5.1. *Glenmark Pharmaceuticals Ltd.*

Glenmark have patented a range of TRPV3 antagonists [80–84], Figure 11. In 2010, Glenmark entered into an out-licensing agreement with Sanofi Aventis and subsequently progressed their lead molecule (GRC15300, structure unknown) into the clinic for the treatment of osteoarthritic and neuropathic pain. In 2012, GRC15300 entered into Phase II trials for treatment of neuropathic pain; however, by the end of 2013, these trials had been discontinued. The Sanofi-Glenmark agreement was terminated in 2014 and since that date, no further development has been reported.

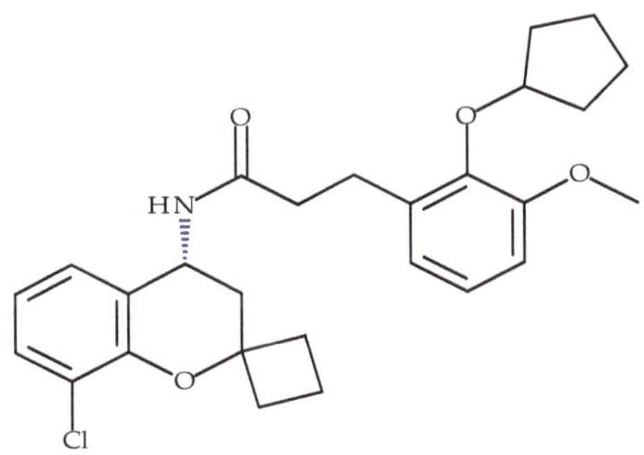

Glenmark - CPC-MPP

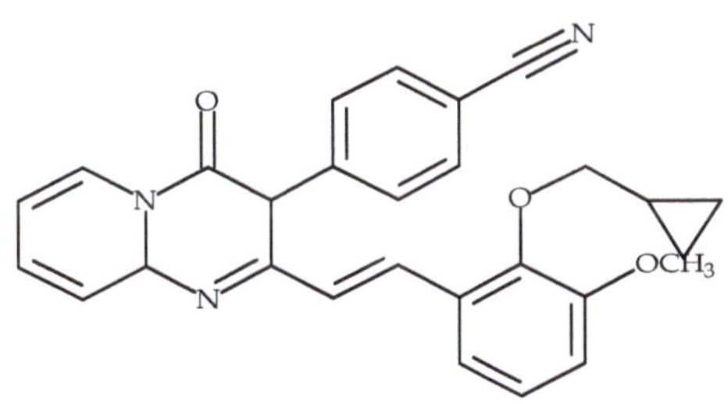

Glenmark - Example 19 - US2010/0292254A1

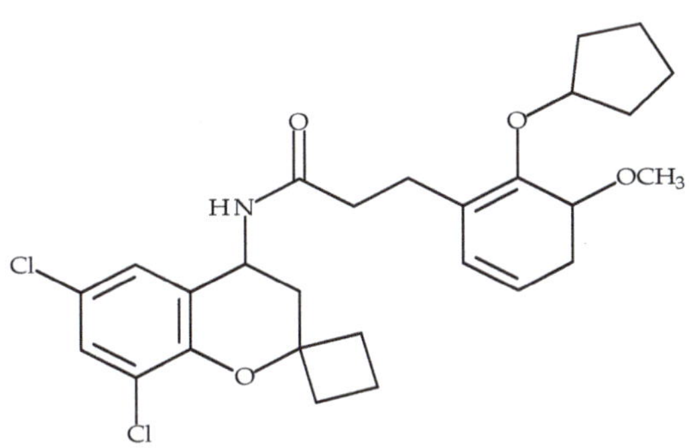

Glenmark - Example 59 - US2010/0311778A1

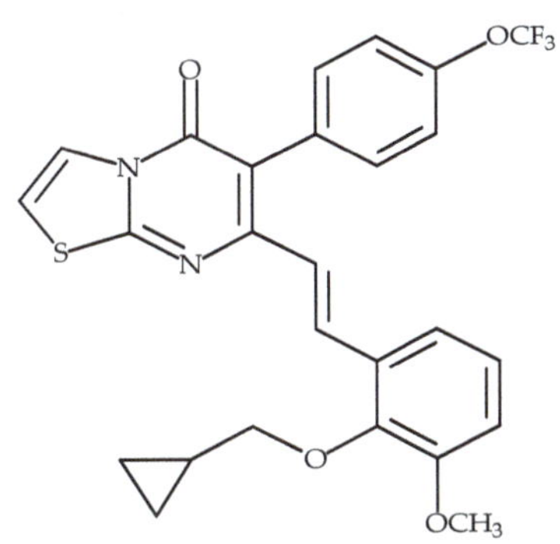

Glenmark - Example 58 - US2009/0286811A1

Figure 11. Examples of patented TRPV3 antagonists from Glenmark Pharmaceuticals.

5.2. Hydra Biosciences Inc.

Hydra Biosciences have also published several patents and publications on TRPV3 antagonists. In 2007, they entered into a collaboration with Pfizer to develop TRPV3 antagonists for pain. The company web page currently reports an active TRPV3 program directed toward dermatological disorders. In the published patents, there are descriptions of two compounds (Compound 15 and Compound 64 in Reference [68]; Figure 12). Compounds were described as having modest potency (<1 μM) in vitro and were shown to be effective in models of thermal injury, the formalin model, Carrageenan, and CFA. An additional patent [63] discloses FTP-THQ that we have assessed above in a number of in vitro and in vivo assays (Figures 6–8).

5.3. Abbvie Inc.

In recent years, AbbVie have been active in the TRPV3 arena, publishing several patents [85,86] and more recently a paper [67]. They describe a series of compounds, some displaying mid-nanomolar potency in blocking 2-APB-stimulated calcium influx in assays using recombinant human and mouse TRPV3 channels. Their recent publication describes synthesis and biological properties of a series of (Pyridin-2-yl)methanol derivatives, with the lead molecule (Figure 13) having modest in vitro potency (Kb = 0.56 μM) and efficacy in rat models of neuropathic pain (CCI and SNL).

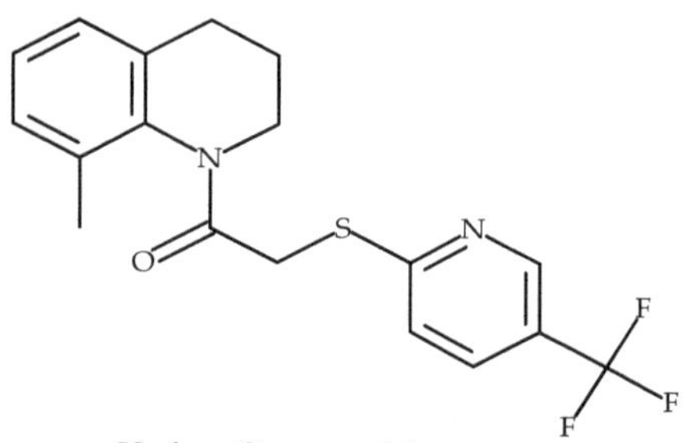

Hydra - Compound 8

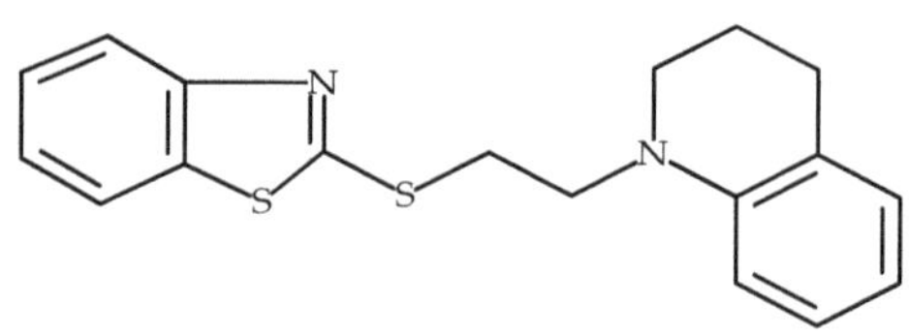

Hydra - Compound 64

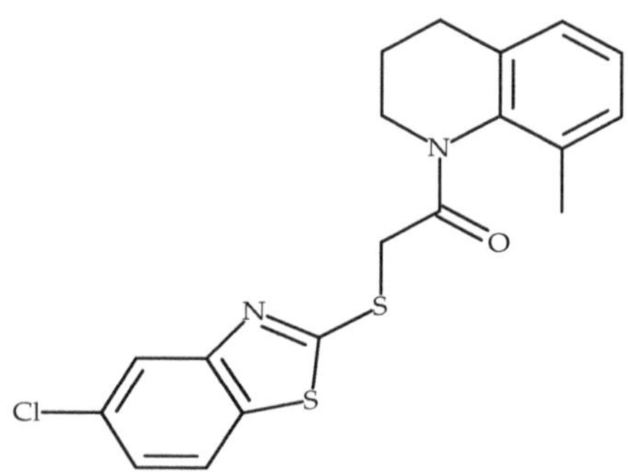

Hydra - Compound 15

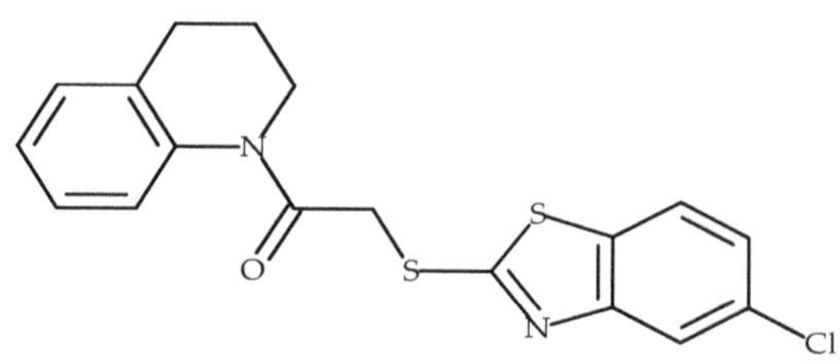

Hydra - Compound 101

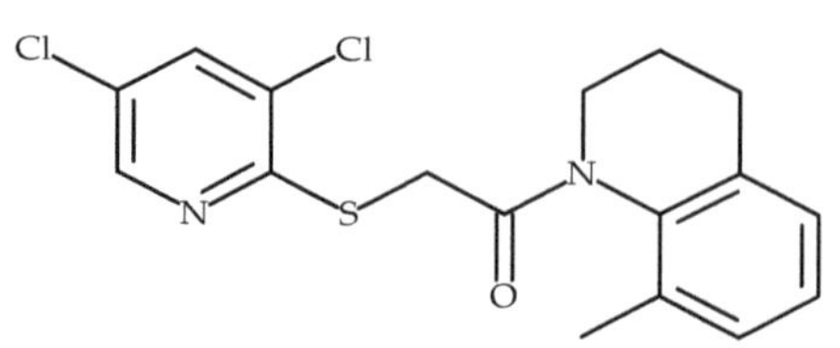

Hydra - DCP-THQ

Figure 12. Representatives from Hydra Biosciences patented TRPV3 antagonist series.

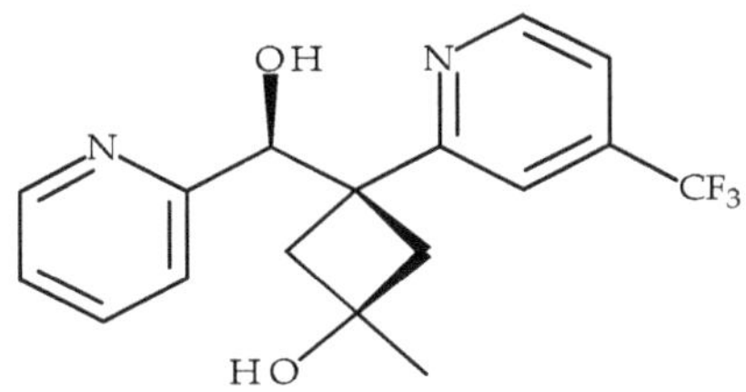

Abbvie - Compound 74a

Figure 13. A leading representative from Abbvie's TRPV3 antagonist series.

5.4. Miscellaneous

Interestingly, there are also several patents detailing the utility of TRPV3 agonists. One describes derivatives of incensole acetate for use as antidepressants [37,87]. Another details TRPV3 agonists for the treatment of TRPV3-associated skin conditions such as acne, psoriasis, dermatitis, and wound healing, and describes the TRPV3 activity of peptides derived from soricidin (a fifty-four amino acid paralytic peptide isolated from the submaxilary saliva gland of the Northern Short-tailed Shrew, *Blanina brevieauda* [88]).

6. Conclusions and Outlook

In summary, we are making headway in understanding the role of TRPV3 in health and disease and this appears to be a promising therapeutic target for itch and skin-related conditions and for the treatment of patients with TRPV3 causally related conditions, such as Olmsted syndrome. To date information from gain of function mutations in rodent and man, coupled with data from gene knock out studies do not provide an overwhelmingly compelling case for targeting TRPV3 as a pain therapeutic; however, pre-clinical data utilizing structurally diverse TRPV3 antagonists do provide some support that blockade of this channel may provide analgesia in chronic pain states. Questions remain however as to how much clinical efficacy for pain can be realized through selectively targeting this mechanism and how results from rodents will translate to humans given the differences in expression in the pain pathway. Given the issues with the side effects associated with targeting other TRP family members, such as TRPV1, including body temperature changes and altered thermal sensitivity, there may be an opportunity to develop topical treatments for TRPV3 given the compelling role in skin.

Acknowledgments: We thank Jeff Kennedy for scientific input and Jeff Kennedy and Denise Morrow for early studies evaluating the in vivo efficacy of FTP-THQ in preventing itch related behaviors. We thank Brian Spegal for the body temperature studies conducted with FTP-THQ, Jeff Cramer for pharmacokinetic studies on FTP-THQ and Rosa Simmons for technical assistance with the figures and legends. We thank David Collier and Cara Lee Ann Ruble for inputs relating to the expression profile of TRPV3.

References

1. Peier, A.M.; Reeve, A.J.; Andersson, D.A.; Moqrich, A.; Earley, T.J.; Hergarden, A.C.; Story, G.M.; Colley, S.; Hogenesch, J.B.; McIntyre, P.; et al. A heat-sensitive TRP channel expressed in keratinocytes. *Science* **2002**, *296*, 2046–2049. [CrossRef] [PubMed]
2. Xu, H.; Ramsey, I.S.; Kotecha, S.A.; Moran, M.M.; Chong, J.A.; Lawson, D.; Ge, P.; Lilly, J.; Silos-Santiago, I.; Xie, Y.; et al. TRPV3 is a calcium-permeable temperature-sensitive cation channel. *Nature* **2002**, *418*, 181–186. [CrossRef] [PubMed]

3. Smith, G.D.; Gunthorpe, M.J.; Kelsell, R.E.; Hayes, P.D.; Reilly, P.; Facer, P.; Wright, J.E.; Jerman, J.C.; Walhin, J.-P.; Ooi, L.; et al. TRPV3 is a temperature-sensitive vanilloid receptor-like protein. *Nature* **2002**, *418*, 186–190. [CrossRef] [PubMed]
4. Cheng, W.; Yang, F.; Takanishi, C.L.; Zheng, J. Thermosensitive TRPV channel subunits coassemble into heteromeric channels with intermediate conductance and gating properties. *J. Gen. Physiol.* **2007**, *129*, 16. [CrossRef] [PubMed]
5. Cheng, W.; Yang, F.; Liu, S.; Colton, C.K.; Wang, C.; Cui, Y.; Cao, X.; Zhu, M.X.; Sun, C.; Wang, K.; et al. Heteromeric heat-sensitive transient receptor potential channels exhibit distinct temperature and chemical response. *J. Biol. Chem.* **2012**, *287*, 7279–7288. [CrossRef] [PubMed]
6. Hellwig, N.; Albrecht, N.; Harteneck, C.; Gunter, S.; Schaefer, M. Homo- and heteromeric assembly of TRP channel subunits. *J. Cell. Sci.* **2005**, *118*, 917–928. [CrossRef] [PubMed]
7. Grandl, J.; Hu, H.; Bandell, M.; Bursulaya, B.; Schmidt, M.; Petrus, M.; Patapoutian, A. Pore region of TRPV3 ion channel is specifically required for heat activation. *Nat. Neurosci.* **2008**, *11*, 1007–1013. [CrossRef] [PubMed]
8. Xiao, R.; Tang, J.; Wang, C.; Colton, C.K.; Tian, J.; Zhu, M.X. Calcium plays a central role in the sensitization of TRPV3 channel to repetitive stimulations. *J. Biol. Chem.* **2008**, *283*, 6162–6174. [CrossRef] [PubMed]
9. Hu, H.; Grandl, J.; Bandell, M.; Petrus, M.; Patapoutian, A. Two amino acid residues determine 2-APB sensitivity of the ion channels TRPV3 and TRPV4. *Proc. Natl. Acad. Sci. USA* **2009**, *106*, 1626–1631. [CrossRef] [PubMed]
10. Phelps, C.B.; Wang, R.R.; Choo, S.S.; Gaudet, R. Differential regulation of TRPV1, TRPV3, and TRPV4 sensitivity through a conserved binding site on the ankyrin repeat domain. *J. Biol. Chem.* **2010**, *285*, 731–740. [CrossRef] [PubMed]
11. Doerner, J.F.; Hatt, H.; Ramsey, I.S. Voltage- and temperature-dependent activation of TRPV3 channels is potentiated by receptor-mediated PI(4,5)P2 hydrolysis. *J. Gen. Physiol.* **2011**, *137*, 271–288. [CrossRef] [PubMed]
12. Luo, J.; Stewart, R.; Berdeaux, R.; Hu, H. Tonic inhibition of TRPV3 by Mg^{2+} in mouse epidermal keratinocytes. *J. Investig. Dermatol.* **2012**, *132*, 2158–2165. [CrossRef] [PubMed]
13. Sherkheli, M.A.; Vogt-Eisele, A.K.; Weber, K.; Hatt, H. Camphor modulates TRPV3 cation channels activity by interacting with critical pore-region cysteine residues. *Pak. J. Pharm. Sci.* **2013**, *26*, 431–438. [PubMed]
14. Liu, B.; Yao, J.; Zhu, M.X.; Qin, F. Hysteresis of gating underlines sensitization of TRPV3 channels. *J. Gen. Physiol.* **2011**, *138*, 509–520. [CrossRef] [PubMed]
15. Vogt-Eisele, A.K.; Weber, K.; Sherkheli, M.A.; Vielhaber, G.; Panten, J.; Gisselmann, G.; Hatt, H. Monoterpenoid agonists of TRPV3. *Br. J. Pharmacol.* **2007**, *151*, 530–540. [CrossRef] [PubMed]
16. Bang, S.; Yoo, S.; Yang, T.-J.; Cho, H.; Hwang, S.W. Farnesyl pyrophosphate is a novel pain-producing molecule via specific activation of TRPV3. *J. Biol. Chem.* **2010**, *285*, 19362–19371. [CrossRef] [PubMed]
17. Moqrich, A.; Hwang, S.W.; Earley, T.J.; Petrus, M.J.; Murray, A.N.; Spencer, K.S.R.; Andahazy, M.; Story, G.M.; Patapoutian, A. Impaired thermosensation in mice lacking TRPV3, a heat and camphor sensor in the skin. *Science* **2005**, *307*, 1468–1472. [CrossRef] [PubMed]
18. Grubisha, O.; Mogg, A.J.; Sorge, J.L.; Ball, L.-J.; Sanger, H.; Ruble, C.L.A.; Folly, E.A.; Ursu, D.; Broad, L.M. Pharmacological profiling of the TRPV3 channel in recombinant and native assays. *Br. J. Pharmacol.* **2014**, *171*, 2631–2644. [CrossRef] [PubMed]
19. Xu, H.; Delling, M.; Jun, J.C.; Clapham, D.E. Oregano, thyme and clove-derived flavors and skin sensitizers activate specific TRP channels. *Nat. Neurosci.* **2006**, *9*, 628–635. [CrossRef] [PubMed]
20. Hu, H.-Z.; Xiao, R.; Wang, C.; Gao, N.; Colton, C.K.; Wood, J.D.; Zhu, M.X. Potentiation of TRPV3 channel function by unsaturated fatty acids. *J. Cell. Physiol.* **2006**, *208*, 201–212. [CrossRef] [PubMed]
21. Cao, X.; Yang, F.; Zheng, J.; Wang, K. Intracellular proton-mediated activation of TRPV3 channels accounts for the exfoliation effect of alpha-hydroxyl acids on keratinocytes. *J. Biol. Chem.* **2012**, *287*, 25905–25916. [CrossRef] [PubMed]
22. Gao, L.; Yang, P.; Qin, P.; Lu, Y.; Li, X.; Tian, Q.; Li, Y.; Xie, C.; Tian, J.-B.; Zhang, C.; et al. Selective potentiation of 2-APB-induced activation of TRPV1–3 channels by acid. *Sci. Rep.* **2016**, *6*, 20791. [CrossRef] [PubMed]

23. Bang, S.; Yoo, S.; Yang, T.-J.; Cho, H.; Hwang, S.W. Isopentenyl pyrophosphate is a novel antinociceptive substance that inhibits TRPV3 and TRPA1 ion channels. *Pain* **2011**, *152*, 1156–1164. [CrossRef] [PubMed]
24. Bang, S.; Yoo, S.; Yang, T.J.; Cho, H.; Hwang, S.W. 17(R)-resolvin D1 specifically inhibits transient receptor potential ion channel vanilloid 3 leading to peripheral antinociception. *Br. J. Pharmacol.* **2012**, *165*, 683–692. [CrossRef] [PubMed]
25. de Petrocellis, L.; Orlando, P.; Moriello, A.S.; Aviello, G.; Stott, C.; Izzo, A.A.; di Marzo, V. Cannabinoid actions at TRPV channels: Effects on TRPV3 and TRPV4 and their potential relevance to gastrointestinal inflammation. *Acta Physiol.* **2012**, *204*, 255–266. [CrossRef] [PubMed]
26. Chung, M.-K.; Guler, A.D.; Caterina, M.J. Biphasic currents evoked by chemical or thermal activation of the heat-gated ion channel, TRPV3. *J. Biol. Chem.* **2005**, *280*, 15928–15941. [CrossRef] [PubMed]
27. Grandl, J.; Kim, S.E.; Uzzell, V.; Bursulaya, B.; Petrus, M.; Bandell, M.; Patapoutian, A. Temperature-induced opening of TRPV1 ion channel is stabilized by the pore domain. *Nat. Neurosci.* **2010**, *13*, 708–714. [CrossRef] [PubMed]
28. Kim, S.E.; Patapoutian, A.; Grandl, J. Single residues in the outer pore of TRPV1 and TRPV3 have temperature-dependent conformations. *PLoS ONE* **2013**, *8*, e59593. [CrossRef] [PubMed]
29. Yang, P.; Zhu, M.X. TRPV3. *Handb. Exp. Pharmacol.* **2014**, *222*, 273–291. [PubMed]
30. Huang, S.M.; Lee, H.; Chung, M.-K.; Park, U.; Yu, Y.Y.; Bradshaw, H.B.; Coulombe, P.A.; Walker, J.M.; Caterina, M.J. Overexpressed transient receptor potential vanilloid 3 ion channels in skin keratinocytes modulate pain sensitivity via prostaglandin E2. *J. Neurosci.* **2008**, *28*, 13727–13737. [CrossRef] [PubMed]
31. Asakawa, M.; Yoshioka, T.; Matsutani, T.; Hikita, I.; Suzuki, M.; Oshima, I.; Tsukahara, K.; Arimura, A.; Horikawa, T.; Hirasawa, T.; et al. Association of a mutation in TRPV3 with defective hair growth in rodents. *J. Investig. Dermatol.* **2006**, *126*, 2664–2672. [CrossRef] [PubMed]
32. Lonsdale, J.; Thomas, J.; Salvatore, M.; Phillips, R.; Lo, E.; Shad, S.; Hasz, R.; Walters, G.; Garcia, F.; Young, N.; et al. The genotype-tissue expression (GTEx) project. *Nat. Genet.* **2013**, *45*, 580–585. [CrossRef] [PubMed]
33. Aijima, R.; Wang, B.; Takao, T.; Mihara, H.; Kashio, M.; Ohsaki, Y.; Zhang, J.-Q.; Mizuno, A.; Suzuki, M.; Yamashita, Y.; et al. The thermosensitive TRPV3 channel contributes to rapid wound healing in oral epithelia. *FASEB J.* **2015**, *29*, 182–192. [CrossRef] [PubMed]
34. Ueda, T.; Yamada, T.; Ugawa, S.; Ishida, Y.; Shimada, S. TRPV3, a thermosensitive channel is expressed in mouse distal colon epithelium. *Biochem. Biophys. Res. Commun.* **2009**, *383*, 130–134. [CrossRef] [PubMed]
35. Yamada, T.; Ueda, T.; Ugawa, S.; Ishida, Y.; Imayasu, M.; Koyama, S.; Shimada, S. Functional expression of transient receptor potential vanilloid 3 (TRPV3) in corneal epithelial cells: involvement in thermosensation and wound healing. *Exp. Eye Res.* **2010**, *90*, 121–129. [CrossRef] [PubMed]
36. Brown, T.E.; Chirila, A.M.; Schrank, B.R.; Kauer, J.A. Loss of interneuron LTD and attenuated pyramidal cell LTP in TRPV1 and TRPV3 KO mice. *Hippocampus* **2013**, *23*, 662–671. [CrossRef] [PubMed]
37. Moussaieff, A.; Rimmerman, N.; Bregman, T.; Straiker, A.; Felder, C.C.; Shoham, S.; Kashman, Y.; Huang, S.M.; Lee, H.; Shohami, E.; et al. Incensole acetate, an incense component, elicits psychoactivity by activating TRPV3 channels in the brain. *FASEB J.* **2008**, *22*, 3024–3034. [CrossRef] [PubMed]
38. Gallego-Sandín, S.; Rodríguez-García, A.; Alonso, M.T.; García-Sancho, J. The endoplasmic reticulum of dorsal root ganglion neurons contains functional TRPV1 channels. *J. Biol. Chem.* **2009**, *284*, 32591–32601. [CrossRef] [PubMed]
39. Lotteau, S.; Ducreux, S.; Romestaing, C.; Legrand, C.; Van Coppenolle, F. Characterization of Functional TRPV1 Channels in the Sarcoplasmic Reticulum of Mouse Skeletal Muscle. *PLoS ONE* **2013**, *8*, e58673. [CrossRef] [PubMed]
40. Lo, I.C.; Chan, H.C.; Qi, Z.; Ng, K.L.; So, C.; Tsang, S.Y. TRPV3 channel negatively regulates cell cycle progression and safeguards the pluripotency of embryonic stem cells. *J. Cell. Physiol.* **2016**, *231*, 403–413. [CrossRef] [PubMed]
41. Guatteo, E.; Chung, K.K.H.; Bowala, T.K.; Bernardi, G.; Mercuri, N.B.; Lipski, J. Temperature sensitivity of dopaminergic neurons of the substantia nigra pars compacta: involvement of transient receptor potential channels. *J. Neurophysiol.* **2005**, *94*, 3069–3080. [CrossRef] [PubMed]

42. Singh, U.; Kumar, S.; Shelkar, G.P.; Yadhav, M.; Kokare, D.M.; Goswami, C.; Lechan, R.M.; Singru, P.S. Transient receptor potential vanilloid (TRPV3) in the ventral tegmental area of rat: Role in modulation of the mesolimbic-dopamine reward pathway. *Neuropharmacology* **2016**, *110*, 198–210. [CrossRef] [PubMed]
43. Chung, M.-K.; Lee, H.; Mizuno, A.; Suzuki, M.; Caterina, M.J. 2-aminoethoxydiphenyl borate activates and sensitizes the heat-gated ion channel TRPV3. *J. Neurosci.* **2004**, *24*, 5177–5182. [CrossRef] [PubMed]
44. Chung, M.-K.; Lee, H.; Mizuno, A.; Suzuki, M.; Caterina, M.J. TRPV3 and TRPV4 mediate warmth-evoked currents in primary mouse keratinocytes. *J. Biol. Chem.* **2004**, *279*, 21569–21575. [CrossRef] [PubMed]
45. Cheng, X.; Jin, J.; Hu, L.; Shen, D.; Dong, X.-P.; Samie, M.A.; Knoff, J.; Eisinger, B.; Liu, M.-L.; Huang, S.M.; et al. TRP channel regulates EGFR signaling in hair morphogenesis and skin barrier formation. *Cell* **2010**, *141*, 331–343. [CrossRef] [PubMed]
46. Miyamoto, T.; Petrus, M.J.; Dubin, A.E.; Patapoutian, A. TRPV3 regulates nitric oxide synthase-independent nitric oxide synthesis in the skin. *Nat. Commun.* **2011**, *2*, 369. [CrossRef] [PubMed]
47. Borbíró, I.; Lisztes, E.; Tóth, B.I.; Czifra, G.; Oláh, A.; Szöllosi, A.G.; Szentandrássy, N.; Nánási, P.P.; Péter, Z.; Paus, R.; et al. Activation of transient receptor potential vanilloid-3 inhibits human hair growth. *J. Investig. Dermatol.* **2011**, *131*, 1605–1614. [CrossRef] [PubMed]
48. Mandadi, S.; Sokabe, T.; Shibasaki, K.; Katanosaka, K.; Mizuno, A.; Moqrich, A.; Patapoutian, A.; Fukumi-Tominaga, T.; Mizumura, K.; Tominaga, M. TRPV3 in keratinocytes transmits temperature information to sensory neurons via ATP. *Pflugers Arch. Eur. J. Physiol.* **2009**, *458*, 1093–1102. [CrossRef] [PubMed]
49. Pang, Z.; Sakamoto, T.; Tiwari, V.; Kim, Y.-S.; Yang, F.; Dong, X.; Güler, A.D.; Guan, Y.; Caterina, M.J. Selective keratinocyte stimulation is sufficient to evoke nociception in mice. *Pain* **2015**, *156*, 656–665. [CrossRef] [PubMed]
50. Radtke, C.; Vogt, P.M.; Devor, M.; Kocsis, J.D. Keratinocytes acting on injured afferents induce extreme neuronal hyperexcitability and chronic pain. *Pain* **2010**, *148*, 94–102. [CrossRef] [PubMed]
51. Huang, S.M.; Li, X.; Yu, Y.; Wang, J.; Caterina, M.J. TRPV3 and TRPV4 ion channels are not major contributors to mouse heat sensation. *Mol. Pain* **2011**, *7*, 37. [CrossRef] [PubMed]
52. Nilius, B.; Bíró, T.; Owsianik, G. TRPV3: Time to decipher a poorly understood family member! *J. Physiol.* **2014**, *592*, 295–304. [CrossRef] [PubMed]
53. Yang, Y.S.; Cho, S.I.; Choi, M.G.; Choi, Y.H.; Kwak, I.S.; Park, C.W.; Kim, H.O. Increased expression of three types of transient receptor potential channels (TRPA1, TRPV4 and TRPV3) in burn scars with post-burn pruritus. *Acta Derm. Venereol.* **2015**, *95*, 20–24. [CrossRef] [PubMed]
54. Sulk, M.; Seeliger, S.; Aubert, J.; Schwab, V.D.; Cevikbas, F.; Rivier, M.; Nowak, P.; Voegel, J.J.; Buddenkotte, J.; Steinhoff, M. Distribution and expression of non-neuronal transient receptor potential (TRPV) ion channels in rosacea. *J. Investig. Dermatol.* **2012**, *132*, 1253–1262. [CrossRef] [PubMed]
55. Scott, V.E.; Patel, H.; Wetter, J.; Edlmayer, R.; Neelands, T.; Miller, L.; Huang, S.; Gauld, S.; Todorovic, V.; Gomtsian, A.; et al. Defining a mechanistic link between TRPV3 activity and psoriasis through IL-1α and EGFR signaling pathways. *J. Investig. Dermatol.* **2016**, *136*, S94. [CrossRef]
56. Gopinath, P.; Wan, E.; Holdcroft, A.; Facer, P.; Davis, J.B.; Smith, G.D.; Bountra, C.; Anand, P. Increased capsaicin receptor TRPV1 in skin nerve fibres and related vanilloid receptors TRPV3 and TRPV4 in keratinocytes in human breast pain. *BMC Women's Health* **2005**, *5*, 2. [CrossRef] [PubMed]
57. Brash, A.R. Arachidonic acid as a bioactive molecule. *J. Clin. Investig.* **2001**, *107*, 1339–1345. [CrossRef] [PubMed]
58. Yoshioka, T.; Imura, K.; Asakawa, M.; Suzuki, M.; Oshima, I.; Hirasawa, T.; Sakata, T.; Horikawa, T.; Arimura, A. Impact of the Gly573Ser substitution in TRPV3 on the development of allergic and pruritic dermatitis in mice. *J. Investig. Dermatol.* **2009**, *129*, 714–722. [CrossRef] [PubMed]
59. Xiao, R.; Tian, J.; Tang, J.; Zhu, M.X. The TRPV3 mutation associated with the hairless phenotype in rodents is constitutively active. *Cell Calcium* **2008**, *43*, 334–343. [CrossRef] [PubMed]
60. Maruyama, M.; Sakai, A.; Suzuki, H.; Akimoto, T. Analysis of TRPV3 function in pain sensation using a gain-of-function mutant rat. *Exp. Anim.* **2015**, *64*, S69–S135.
61. Duchatelet, S.; Hovnanian, A. Olmsted syndrome: clinical, molecular and therapeutic aspects. *Orphanet. J. Rare Dis.* **2015**, *10*, 33. [CrossRef] [PubMed]
62. Nilius, B.; Biro, T. TRPV3: A "more than skinny" channel. *Exp. Dermatol.* **2013**, *22*, 447–452. [CrossRef] [PubMed]

63. Moran, M.M.; Chong, J.; Fanger, C.A.; Ripka, A.; Larsen, G.R.; Zhen, X.; Underwood, D.J.; Weigele, M. Compounds for Modulating TRPV3 Function. WO2008033564A1, 2008.
64. Reilly, R.M.; Kym, P.R. Analgesic potential of TRPV3 antagonists. *Curr. Top. Med. Chem.* **2011**, *11*, 2210–2215. [CrossRef] [PubMed]
65. Joshi, N. The TRPV3 Receptor as a Pain Target: A therapeutic promise or just some more new biology? *Open Drug Discov. J.* **2010**, *2*, 89–97. [CrossRef]
66. Huang, S.M.; Chung, M.-K. Targeting TRPV3 for the Development of Novel Analgesics. *Open Pain J.* **2013**, *6*, 119–126. [CrossRef] [PubMed]
67. Gomtsyan, A.R.; Schmidt, R.G.; Bayburt, E.K.; Gfesser, G.A.; Voight, E.A.; Daanen, J.F.; Schmidt, D.L.; Cowart, M.D.; Liu, H.; Altenbach, R.J.; et al. Synthesis and pharmacology of (pyridin-2-yl)methanol derivatives as novel and selective transient receptor potential vanilloid 3 antagonists. *J. Med. Chem.* **2016**, *59*, 4926–4947. [CrossRef] [PubMed]
68. Chong, J.A.; Fanger, C.M.; Larsen, G.R.; Lumma, W.C.; Moran, M.M.; Ripka, A.; Underwood, D.J.; Weigele, M.; Zhen, X. Compounds for Modulating TRPV3 Function. US20060270688A1, 2006.
69. Lin, Z.; Chen, Q.; Lee, M.; Cao, X.; Zhang, J.; Ma, D.; Chen, L.; Hu, X.; Wang, H.; Wang, X.; et al. Exome sequencing reveals mutations in TRPV3 as a cause of Olmsted syndrome. *Am. J. Hum. Genet.* **2012**, *90*, 558–564. [CrossRef] [PubMed]
70. Lai-Cheong, J.E.; Sethuraman, G.; Ramam, M.; Stone, K.; Simpson, M.A.; McGrath, J.A. Recurrent heterozygous missense mutation, p.Gly573Ser, in the TRPV3 gene in an Indian boy with sporadic Olmsted syndrome. *Br. J. Dermatol.* **2012**, *167*, 440–442. [CrossRef] [PubMed]
71. Eytan, O.; Fuchs-Telem, D.; Mevorach, B.; Indelman, M.; Bergman, R.; Sarig, O.; Goldberg, I.; Adir, N.; Sprecher, E. Olmsted syndrome caused by a homozygous recessive mutation in TRPV3. *J. Investig. Dermatol.* **2014**, *134*, 1752–1754. [CrossRef] [PubMed]
72. Ni, C.; Yan, M.; Zhang, J.; Cheng, R.; Liang, J.; Deng, D.; Wang, Z.; Li, M.; Yao, Z. A novel mutation in TRPV3 gene causes atypical familial Olmsted syndrome. *Sci. Rep.* **2016**, *6*, 21815. [CrossRef] [PubMed]
73. Kariminejad, A.; Barzegar, M.; Abdollahimajd, F.; Pramanik, R.; McGrath, J.A. Olmsted syndrome in an Iranian boy with a new de novo mutation in TRPV3. *Clin. Exp. Dermatol.* **2014**, *39*, 492–495. [CrossRef] [PubMed]
74. Duchatelet, S.; Guibbal, L.; de Veer, S.; Fraitag, S.; Nitschke, P.; Zarhrate, M.; Bodemer, C.; Hovnanian, A. Olmsted syndrome with erythromelalgia caused by recessive transient receptor potential vanilloid 3 mutations. *Br. J. Dermatol.* **2014**, *171*, 675–678. [CrossRef] [PubMed]
75. Duchatelet, S.; Pruvost, S.; de Veer, S.; Fraitag, S.; Nitschke, P.; Bole-Feysot, C.; Bodemer, C.; Hovnanian, A. A new TRPV3 missense mutation in a patient with Olmsted syndrome and erythromelalgia. *JAMA Dermatol.* **2014**, *150*, 303–306. [CrossRef] [PubMed]
76. Yamamoto-Kasai, E.; Yasui, K.; Shichijo, M.; Sakata, T.; Yoshioka, T. Impact of TRPV3 on the development of allergic dermatitis as a dendritic cell modulator. *Exp. Dermatol.* **2013**, *22*, 820–824. [CrossRef] [PubMed]
77. Lipski, J.; Park, T.I.H.; Li, D.; Lee, S.C.W.; Trevarton, A.J.; Chung, K.K.H.; Freestone, P.S.; Bai, J.-Z. Involvement of TRP-like channels in the acute ischemic response of hippocampal CA1 neurons in brain slices. *Brain Res.* **2006**, *1077*, 187–199. [CrossRef] [PubMed]
78. Moussaieff, A.; Yu, J.; Zhu, H.; Gattoni-Celli, S.; Shohami, E.; Kindy, M.S. Protective effects of incensole acetate on cerebral ischemic injury. *Brain Res.* **2012**, *1443*, 89–97. [CrossRef] [PubMed]
79. Facer, P.; Casula, M.A.; Smith, G.D.; Benham, C.D.; Chessell, I.P.; Bountra, C.; Sinisi, M.; Birch, R.; Anand, P. Differential expression of the capsaicin receptor TRPV1 and related novel receptors TRPV3, TRPV4 and TRPM8 in normal human tissues and changes in traumatic and diabetic neuropathy. *BMC Neurol.* **2007**, *7*, 11. [CrossRef] [PubMed]
80. Lingam, V.S.P.; Chaudhari, S.S.; Thomas, A.; Khairatkar-Joshi, N.; Kattige, V.G. Fused Pyrimidineone Compounds as TRPV3 Modulators. U.S. Patent 20090286811, 19 November 2009.
81. Lingam, V.S.P.; Thomas, A.; Phatangare, S.K.; Mindhe, A.S.; Khatik, J.Y.; Khairatkar-Joshi, N.; Kattige, V.G. Fused Imidazole Derivatives as TRPV3 Antagonist. U.S. Patent 20110257193, 20 October 2011.
82. Lingam, V.S.P.; Chaudhari, S.S.; Thomas, A.; Khairatkar-Joshi, N.; Kattige, V.G. Fused Pyrimidineone Compounds as TRPV3 Modulators. U.S. Patent 20120115886, 10 May 2012.

83. Lingam, V.S.P.; Thomas, A.; Dattaguru, A.M.; Khatik, J.Y.; Khairatkar-Joshi, N.; Kattige, V.G. Fused Pyramine Derivatives As TRPV3 Modulators. U.S. Patent 20100292254, 18 November 2010.
84. Lingam, V.S.P.; Thomas, A.; Gharat, L.A.; Ukirde, D.V.; Phatangare, S.K.; Mindhe, A.S.; Khairatkar-Joshi, N.; Kattige, V.G. Chromane Derivatives As TRPV3 Modulators. U.S. Patent 20100311778, 9 December 2010.
85. Bayburt, E.K.; Clapham, B.; Cox, P.B.; Daanen, J.F.; Gomtsyan, A.R.; Kort, M.E.; Kym, P.R.; Voight, E.A. Novel TRPV3 Modulators. U.S. Patent 20130150409, 13 June 2013.
86. Bayburt, E.K.; Clapham, B.; Cox, P.B.; Daanen, J.F.; Dart, M.J.; Gfesser, G.A.; Gomtsyan, A.R.; Kort, M.E.; Kym, P.R.; Schmidt, R.G.; et al. Novel TRPV3 Modulators. U.S. Patent 20130131036, 23 May 2009.
87. Moussaieff, A.; Shohami, E.; Kashman, Y.; Fride, E.; Schmitz, M.L.; Renner, F.; Fiebich, B.L.; Munoz, E.; Ben-Neriah, Y.; Mechoulam, R. Incensole acetate, a novel anti-inflammatory compound isolated from Boswellia resin, inhibits nuclear factor-kappa B activation. *Mol. Pharmacol.* **2007**, *72*, 1657–1664. [CrossRef] [PubMed]
88. Stewart, J.M. TRPV3 Agonists for the Treatment of Skin Conditions. U.S. Patent 20150250699, 10 September 2015.

Permissions

All chapters in this book were first published by MDPI; hereby published with permission under the Creative Commons Attribution License or equivalent. Every chapter published in this book has been scrutinized by our experts. Their significance has been extensively debated. The topics covered herein carry significant findings which will fuel the growth of the discipline. They may even be implemented as practical applications or may be referred to as a beginning point for another development.

The contributors of this book come from diverse backgrounds, making this book a truly international effort. This book will bring forth new frontiers with its revolutionizing research information and detailed analysis of the nascent developments around the world.

We would like to thank all the contributing authors for lending their expertise to make the book truly unique. They have played a crucial role in the development of this book. Without their invaluable contributions this book wouldn't have been possible. They have made vital efforts to compile up to date information on the varied aspects of this subject to make this book a valuable addition to the collection of many professionals and students.

This book was conceptualized with the vision of imparting up-to-date information and advanced data in this field. To ensure the same, a matchless editorial board was set up. Every individual on the board went through rigorous rounds of assessment to prove their worth. After which they invested a large part of their time researching and compiling the most relevant data for our readers.

The editorial board has been involved in producing this book since its inception. They have spent rigorous hours researching and exploring the diverse topics which have resulted in the successful publishing of this book. They have passed on their knowledge of decades through this book. To expedite this challenging task, the publisher supported the team at every step. A small team of assistant editors was also appointed to further simplify the editing procedure and attain best results for the readers.

Apart from the editorial board, the designing team has also invested a significant amount of their time in understanding the subject and creating the most relevant covers. They scrutinized every image to scout for the most suitable representation of the subject and create an appropriate cover for the book.

The publishing team has been an ardent support to the editorial, designing and production team. Their endless efforts to recruit the best for this project, has resulted in the accomplishment of this book. They are a veteran in the field of academics and their pool of knowledge is as vast as their experience in printing. Their expertise and guidance has proved useful at every step. Their uncompromising quality standards have made this book an exceptional effort. Their encouragement from time to time has been an inspiration for everyone.

The publisher and the editorial board hope that this book will prove to be a valuable piece of knowledge for researchers, students, practitioners and scholars across the globe.

List of Contributors

Magda Kondej and Piotr Stępnicki
Department of Synthesis and Chemical Technology of Pharmaceutical Substances, Faculty of Pharmacy with Division of Medical Analytics, Medical University of Lublin, 4A Chodźki St., Lublin PL-20093, Poland

Agnieszka A. Kaczor
Department of Synthesis and Chemical Technology of Pharmaceutical Substances, Faculty of Pharmacy with Division of Medical Analytics, Medical University of Lublin, 4A Chodźki St., Lublin PL-20093, Poland
School of Pharmacy, University of Eastern Finland, Yliopistonranta 1, Kuopio FI-70211, Finland

Xiguang Qi, Mingzhe Shen, Peihao Fan, Xiaojiang Guo, Levent Kirisci and Lirong Wang
Department of Pharmaceutical Sciences, Computational Chemical Genomics Screening Center, University of Pittsburgh School of Pharmacy, 3501 Terrace St Pittsburgh, PA 15261, USA

Tianqi Wang
Department of Biological Sciences, University of Pittsburgh School of Arts & Sciences, Pittsburgh, PA 15260, USA

Ning Feng and Manling Zhang
Division of Cardiology, Vascular Medicine Institute, University of Pittsburgh School of Medicine, Pittsburgh, PA 15213, USA

Robert A. Sweet
Department of Neurology, University of Pittsburgh School of Medicine, Pittsburgh, PA 15213, USA
Department of Psychiatry, University of Pittsburgh School of Medicine, Pittsburgh, PA 15213, USA

Nidal Zeineh and Moshe Gavish
The Ruth and Bruce Rappaport Faculty of Medicine, Technion Institute of Technology, Haifa 31096, Israel

Nunzio Denora
Department of Pharmacy–Pharmaceutical Sciences, University of Bari "Aldo Moro", 70125 Bari, Italy
Institute for Chemical and Physical Processes (IPCF)-CNR SS Bari, Via Orabona 4, 70126 Bari, Italy

Valentino Laquintana and Massimo Franco
Department of Pharmacy–Pharmaceutical Sciences, University of Bari "Aldo Moro", 70125 Bari, Italy

AbrahamWeizman
Research Unit at Geha Mental Health Center and Laboratory of Biological Psychiatry at Felsenstein Medical Research Center, Petah Tikva 4910002, Israel
Sackler Faculty of Medicine, Tel Aviv University, Tel Aviv 6997801, Israel

Andrei V. Derbenev
Department of Physiology, School of Medicine, Tulane University, New Orleans, LA 70112, USA

Andrea Zsombok
Department of Physiology, School of Medicine, Tulane University, New Orleans, LA 70112, USA
Department of Medicine, Endocrinology Section, School of Medicine, Tulane University, New Orleans, LA 70112, USA

Hajar Sirous
Bioinformatics Research Center, School of Pharmacy and Pharmaceutical Sciences, Isfahan University of Medical Sciences, Isfahan 81746-73461, Iran

Giuseppe Campiani and Giulia Chemi
Department of Biotechnology, Chemistry and Pharmacy, DoE Department of Excellence 2018–2022, University of Siena, via Aldo Moro 2, 53100 Siena, Italy

Simone Brogi and Vincenzo Calderone
Department of Pharmacy, University of Pisa, via Bonanno 6, 56126 Pisa, Italy

Sherif T. S. Hassan
Department of Applied Ecology, Faculty of Environmental Sciences, Czech University of Life Sciences Prague, Kamýcká 129, 6-Suchdol, 16521 Prague, Czech Republic

Yagnesh Nagarajan and Daniel J. Peet
School of Biological Sciences, University of Adelaide, Adelaide 5005, SA, Australia

Grigori Y. Rychkov
School of Medicine, University of Adelaide, Adelaide 5005, SA, Australia
South Australian Health and Medical Research Institute (SAHMRI), Adelaide 5005, SA, Australia

Michael J. Caterina and Zixuan Pang
Departments of Neurosurgery, Biological Chemistry and Neuroscience, Neurosurgery Pain Research Institute, Johns Hopkins School of Medicine, 725 N. Wolfe St., Baltimore, MD 21205, USA

Gabriel Zazeri, Ana Paula Ribeiro Povinelli and Marinônio Lopes Cornélio
Departamento de Física, Instituto de Biociências, Letras e Ciências Exatas (IBILCE), UNESP, Rua Cristovão Colombo 2265, CEP 15054-000 São José do Rio Preto, SP, Brazil

Marcelo de Freitas Lima
Departamento de Química, Instituto de Biociências, Letras e Ciências Exatas (IBILCE), UNESP, Rua Cristovão Colombo 2265, CEP 15054-000 São José do Rio Preto, SP, Brazil

Eiichi Kumamoto and Tsugumi Fujita
Department of Physiology, Saga Medical School, 5-1-1 Nabeshima, Saga 849-8501, Japan

Jinhwan Cho and Giyoong Tae
School of Materials Science and Engineering, Gwangju Institute of Science and Technology (GIST), Gwangju 61005, Korea

Junyong Park
Department of Biomedical Science and Engineering, GIST, Gwangju 61005, Korea

Inchan Kwon
School of Materials Science and Engineering, Gwangju Institute of Science and Technology (GIST), Gwangju 61005, Korea
Department of Biomedical Science and Engineering, GIST, Gwangju 61005, Korea

Mi Sun Jin
School of Life Science, GIST, Gwangju 61005, Korea

Shinichiro Yamamoto and Shunichi Shimizu
Division of Pharmacology, Faculty of Pharmaceutical Sciences, Teikyo Heisei University, Tokyo 164-8530, Japan

Andy D. Weyer
Pacific University School of Physical Therapy, Hillsboro, OR 97123, USA

Sonya G. Lehto
One Amgen Center Dr, Thousand Oaks, CA 91320, USA

Indranil Mukhopadhyay, Abhay Kulkarni and Neelima Khairatkar-Joshi
Biological Research, Glenmark Research Centre, Glenmark Pharmaceuticals Ltd. Navi Mumbai, Maharashtra 400709, India

Lisa M. Broad and Adrian J. Mogg
Lilly Research Centre, Eli Lilly and Company Ltd., Erl Wood Manor, Windlesham, Surrey GU20 6PH, UK

Elizabeth Eberle and Marcia Tolley
Covance Greenfield Laboratories, Greenfield, Indianapolis, IN 46140, USA

Dominic L. Li and Kelly L. Knopp
Lilly Research Laboratories, Eli Lilly and Company Inc., Indianapolis, IN 46285, USA

Index

Printed in the USA
CPSIA information can be obtained
at www.ICGtesting.com
LVHW080036211023
761596LV00010BA/1788